NEUROMUSCULAR MANIFESTATIONS OF SYSTEMIC DISEASE

CONTEMPORARY NEUROLOGY SERIES AVAILABLE:

Fred Plum, M.D., ***Editor-in-Chief***
J. Richard Baringer, M.D., ***Associate Editor***
Sid Gilman, M.D., ***Associate Editor***

12 TOPICS ON TROPICAL NEUROLOGY
R. W. Hornabrook, M.D., F.R.A.C.P., *Editor*

13 LEGAL ASPECTS OF NEUROLOGIC PRACTICE
H. Richard Beresford, M.D., J.D.

14 CLINICAL NEUROENDOCRINOLOGY
Joseph B. Martin, M.D.,
Seymour Reichlin, M.D., Ph.D., and
Gregory M. Brown, M.D., Ph.D., F.R.C.P.(C.)

17 MENTAL RETARDATION AND RELATED DISORDERS
Charles F. Barlow, M.D.

18 CLINICAL NEUROPHYSIOLOGY OF THE VESTIBULAR SYSTEM
Robert W. Baloh, M.D., and
Vincent Honrubia, M.D.

19 THE DIAGNOSIS OF STUPOR AND COMA, EDITION 3
Fred Plum, M.D., and
Jerome B. Posner, M.D.

20 MANAGEMENT OF HEAD INJURIES
Bryan Jennett, M.D., F.R.C.S., and
Graham Teasdale, M.R.C.P., F.R.C.S.

21 DISORDERS OF THE CEREBELLUM
Sid Gilman, M.D.
James R. Bloedel, M.D., Ph.D., and
Richard Lechtenberg, M.D.

22 THE NEUROLOGY OF AGING
Robert Katzman, M.D., and
Robert D. Terry, M.D.

23 THE NEUROLOGY OF EYE MOVEMENT
R. John Leigh, M.D., and
David S. Zee, M.D.

24 DISORDERS OF PERIPHERAL NERVES
Herbert H. Schaumburg, M.D.,
Peter S. Spencer, Ph.D., MRC Path., and
P. K. Thomas, M.D., D.Sc., F.R.C.P.

NEUROMUSCULAR MANIFESTATIONS OF SYSTEMIC DISEASE

ROBERT B. LAYZER, M.D.

Professor of Neurology
University of California, San Francisco
School of Medicine
San Francisco, California

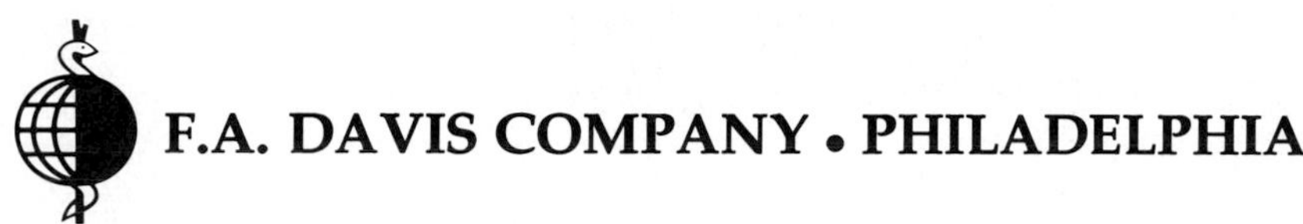

Printed in the United States of America

NOTE: As new scientific information becomes available through basic and clinical research, recommended treatments and drug therapies undergo changes. The author(s) and publisher have done everything possible to make this book accurate, up-to-date, and in accord with accepted standards at the time of publication. However, the reader is advised always to check product information (package inserts) for changes and new information regarding dose and contraindications before administering any drug. Caution is especially urged when using new or infrequently ordered drugs.

Library of Congress Cataloging in Publication Data
Layzer, Robert B., 1931–
Neuromuscular manifestations of systemic disease.

Includes bibliographies and index.
1. Neuromuscular manifestations of general diseases.
I. Title. [DNLM: 1. Neurologic Manifestations.
2. Neuromuscular Diseases. WE550 L431n]
RC925.55.L39 1985 616′.047 84-10096
ISBN 0-8036-5521-5

PREFACE

This book is about the peripheral motor disorders that accompany diseases of other organ systems, including the complications of medical and surgical treatment.

The medical literature on this subject is already voluminous and is growing rapidly, but the information is widely dispersed among a great many articles, chapters, and monographs. Existing textbooks devote much less space to these common, remediable disorders than to the primary and hereditary neuromuscular diseases, most of which are untreatable.

Over the years I have often wished for a comprehensive guide to the diagnosis and management of the acquired or "secondary" neuromuscular diseases. At last, no such book having appeared, I decided to write it myself. In doing so I tried to provide useful information for practicing physicians in all fields of medicine. In addition to the detailed descriptions of individual neuromuscular complications that occupy most of the volume, the opening chapter offers a problem oriented approach to the diagnosis of neuromuscular syndromes, as well as a guide to the use and interpretation of laboratory tests. Despite this practical orientation, I have also indulged my abiding fascination with disease mechanisms by including many critical discussions of pathophysiology and pathogenesis, which for some readers may be the most interesting sections.

Many colleagues and friends have sharpened my thinking about neuromuscular problems in the past 20 years, but a good part of this book grew out of my work with the superb neurology residents at the University of California, San Francisco. My constant struggle to stay a few references ahead of them may account for the rather extensive bibliography. I am grateful to Gareth J. Parry, M.D., David Norman, M.D., and Meredith Halks-Miller, M.D. for supplying some of the illustrations, and to Susan Quan for making the drawings in Figures 7, 11, 15, 16, 22, 27 to 32, 43 to 45, and 47.

Robert B. Layzer, M.D.

CONTENTS

Chapter 1

DIAGNOSIS OF NEUROMUSCULAR DISORDERS

GENERAL APPROACH TO NEUROMUSCULAR DISEASE

Achieving success in the diagnosis of neuromuscular disorders depends on adopting the same type of *anatomic approach* that is used for other neurologic disorders. First, conjectures about anatomic localization are formulated from the medical history and physical examination; next, preliminary laboratory tests are used to evaluate these conjectures and to obtain additional localizing data. A sound pathologic differential diagnosis can then be constructed, and additional laboratory investigations can be selected to reach a specific diagnosis. This approach is a neurologic commonplace, if not actually a shibboleth; but it is true that most diagnostic errors occur when clinicians neglect anatomic analysis and depend on laboratory tests or a "gestalt" approach based on clusters of familiar symptoms and signs.

In dealing with neuromuscular problems, the anatomic focus is the *motor unit*, that is, the motor nerve cell, its single axon and terminal axonal branches, and the many muscle fibers that they supply (Fig. 1). Neuromuscular diseases tend to be confined to one segment of the motor unit: anterior horn cells, nerve roots, peripheral nerves, nerve terminals, neuromuscular junctions, or muscle fibers. Finer anatomic distinctions can be made as our understanding of neuromuscular diseases expands; we now recognize disorders of the muscle membrane (myotonia, periodic paralysis), and we distinguish demyelinative from axonal peripheral neuropathies.

Admittedly, clinical localization may be difficult, since disorders located in different portions of the motor unit have similar signs and symptoms. Only a few of the clinical manifestations listed in Table 1 are anatomically specific: muscle swelling and induration nearly always designate a myopathy; fasciculations are closely linked to motor nerve disorders; and sensory findings always imply a neural disease. The task of clinical localization becomes easier, however, if we adopt the strategy of classifying the large array of neuromuscular disorders into a small number of clinical syn-

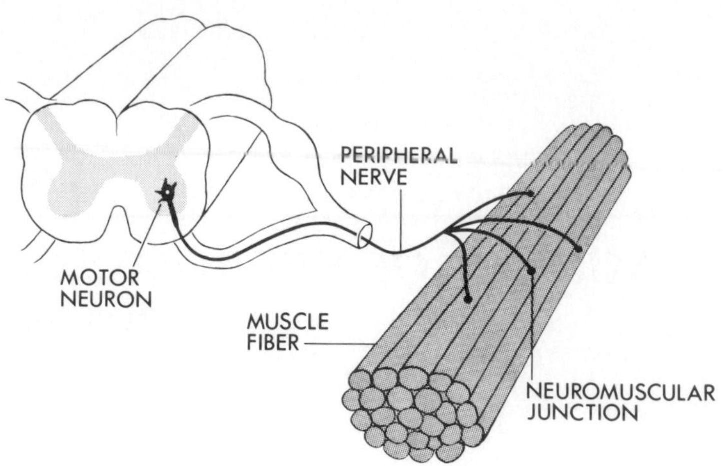

FIGURE 1. The motor unit. (From Layzer, R.: Primary Care 2:235, 1975, with permission.)

dromes, based on their presenting problems (Table 2). These syndromes can be subdivided according to their salient features, thus reducing the number of disorders in each category to a manageable size. The next section of this chapter deals with the differential diagnosis of these clinical syndromes, which include most of the neuromuscular manifestations of systemic disease.

The last section of this chapter is concerned with the interpretation of laboratory investigations that are especially useful in the diagnosis of neuromuscular disorders: serum enzyme measurements, electrodiagnostic tests, muscle imaging procedures, and muscle and nerve biopsy. Laboratory studies can serve several purposes: they can supplement clinical information about localization or pathophysiology, reveal tissue pathology, or identify specific diseases. Serum enzyme determinations and electrodiagnostic tests are used for the first purpose; they are indispensable at an early stage of the diagnostic workup. Muscle and nerve biopsy are occasionally needed for localization, and in a few diseases they provide a specific diagnosis. Tests for specific diseases should not be done until the differential diagnosis has been reduced to a manageable size. There is a logical weakness in attributing a patient's neuromuscular disorder to a systemic illness merely because the two conditions are present in the same patient. For example, a polyneuropathy occurring in a patient with diabetes mellitus could be diabetic neuropathy, but not when it has the clinical, electrophysiologic, and pathologic features of an inflammatory neuropathy.

Figure 2 provides an idealized scheme for integrating laboratory investigations into a diagnostic workup. Of course, most clinicians do not

TABLE 1. Muscle Symptoms and Signs in Motor Unit Disorders

Symptoms	Signs
Weakness	Flaccid weakness and hyporeflexia
Wasting	Atrophy
Twitching	Fasciculations
Pain	Tenderness
Swelling	Mass, enlargement, induration
Spasms	Spasms, delayed relaxation
Stiffness	Persistent contraction at rest; fibrous contracture

TABLE 2. Neuromuscular Problem List

1. Acute generalized weakness
2. Myoglobinuria
3. Subacute and chronic generalized weakness
4. Peripheral neuropathy
5. Muscle pain and swelling
6. Muscle spasms and stiffness
7. Asthenia and fatigue

follow this sequence strictly; the diagnostic process is too complex and circuitous to be captured in a simple diagram. Nevertheless, this scheme serves as a reminder of the hierarchical logic that underlies the diagnostic process; errors will occur if one strays too far from these guidelines.

NEUROMUSCULAR SYNDROMES

Acute Generalized Weakness

Management of Acute Respiratory Insufficiency

Rapidly progressive weakness becomes a medical emergency when airway obstruction and ventilatory weakness threaten to produce respiratory fail-

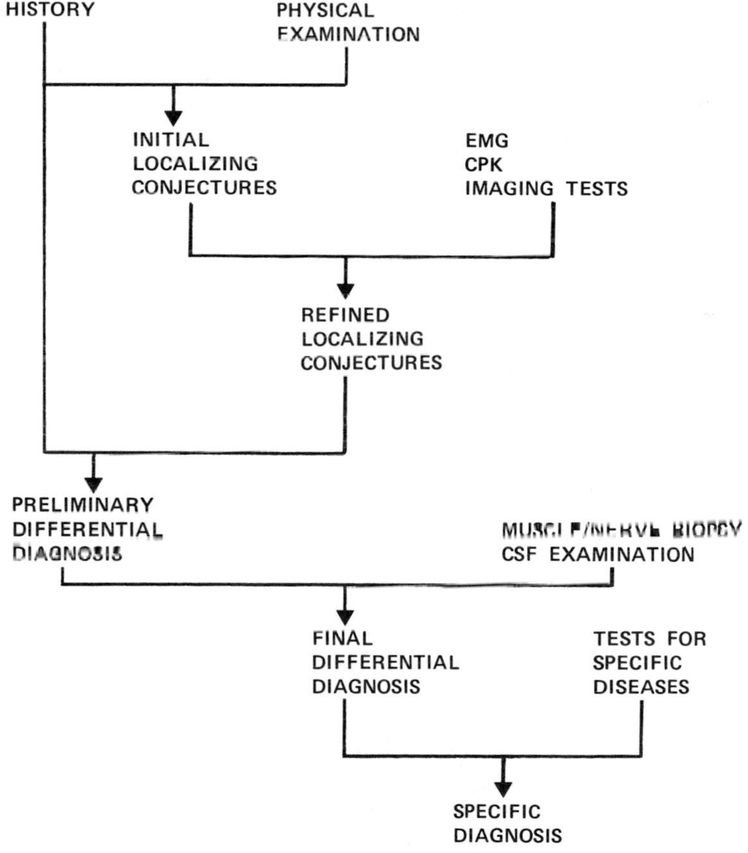

FIGURE 2. A general approach to the diagnosis of neuromuscular disorders.

ure. This complication carries a high mortality rate, primarily because many physicians do not recognize the signs of impending respiratory failure, or do not realize how rapidly respiratory function can deteriorate in a patient with progressive weakness. The combination of oropharyngeal and respiratory weakness is especially hazardous, because it leads to pooling of secretions in the hypopharynx, allows aspiration of secretions or food into the trachea, and produces a weak cough that does not clear the airway effectively.

The key to good management is careful and continuous observation of the patient—preferably in an intensive care unit staffed by physicians skilled at tracheal intubation. The vital capacity should be determined on admission and followed closely afterwards; when it approaches 25 percent of normal the patient will soon need intubation. A patient who is short of breath at rest or who is choking on his secretions should be intubated at once. It is dangerous to wait until hypoxia occurs: normal blood gases are *not* reassuring in this setting, since "respiratory arrest" can occur moments later.

When specific treatment is available (in patients with myasthenia gravis, for instance), the physician may be tempted to defer tracheal intubation while endeavoring to improve the patient's muscle strength with medication. This approach is dangerous; it is safer to intubate the patient first and treat him afterward. Similarly, when the cause of the weakness is not known, diagnostic investigations should be deferred until the airway is secure and respiration is assured.

Differential Diagnosis

Some of the many causes of acute generalized weakness are listed in Table 3. Most of these disorders are rare; the ones most likely to be encountered in industrialized countries are the Guillain-Barré syndrome, myasthenia gravis, botulism, the various types of periodic paralysis, and the acute necrotic myopathies.

When weakness is widespread and severe it may be difficult to localize the pathologic process within the motor unit from the clinical findings alone. Much can be learned, however, by considering the *early* pattern of weakness; the presence or absence of muscle pain, tenderness, and swelling; the state of the reflexes; and whether there are sensory symptoms or signs.

In *acute anterior horn cell disease,* typified by poliomyelitis, weakness is patchy and asymmetrical; the bulbar muscles may be weak but the facial and ocular muscles are usually spared. Myalgia and muscle tenderness are commonly present, but the muscles are not swollen, and other sensory manifestations rarely occur.

Acute polyneuropathies may cause distal, proximal, or diffuse weakness. The weakness may start in the upper or lower extremities or may involve all four limbs simultaneously. Facial weakness is common and often affects one side of the face more than the other; weakness of the throat and tongue also occurs, but ocular weakness is unusual. The muscle stretch reflexes tend to be lost even in muscles that are not very weak, owing to involvement of the sensory limb of the reflex arc. Pain in the back and limbs may be prominent, and distal sensory symptoms and signs are usually present.

Acute disorders of neuromuscular transmission involve the cranial muscles early, causing ptosis, ocular weakness, symmetric facial weakness, and oropharyngeal weakness. In the limbs, weakness tends to be greater in the proximal muscles. There is no pain or sensory involvement.

TABLE 3. Causes of Acute Generalized Weakness

A. Motor neuron disorders
   1. Poliomyelitis
   2. Other enterovirus infections
   3. Paralytic (dumb) rabies
B. Polyneuropathy
   1. Guillain-Barré syndrome
   2. Hepatic porphyrias*
   3. Diphtheria
   4. Arsenic poisoning
   5. Tick paralysis
   6. Podophyllum poisoning
   7. Acute hypophosphatemia†
   8. Acute exacerbation of chronic hyperkalemia†
   9. Shellfish and food fish poisoning
C. Disorders of neuromuscular transmission
   1. Myasthenia gravis
   2. Botulism
   3. Magnesium excess
   4. Drugs: neuromuscular blocking agents, trimethaphan, antibiotics
   5. Neurotoxic snake bite
D. Myopathy
   1. Acute hypokalemic paralysis
      a. Chronic potassium depletion
      b. Thyrotoxic periodic paralysis
      c. Familial hypokalemic periodic paralysis*
   2. Familial hyperkalemic periodic paralysis*
   3. Necrotic myopathies‡

*Hereditary disease.
†Anatomic localization uncertain.
‡See Table 6.

In *acute hypokalemic paralysis,* symmetric weakness often begins in the proximal leg muscles and ascends to the trunk, proximal arms, and anterior neck. The bulbar muscles and face are affected in severe cases, but the ocular muscles are spared. The muscles may feel tight or full but they are not tender or swollen and there are no sensory symptoms or signs. A similar picture occurs in familial hyperkalemic periodic paralysis.

The *acute necrotic myopathies* produce a myopathic distribution of weakness similar to the pattern of hypokalemic paralysis, except that the cranial muscles are usually spared. The affected muscles are painful and tender and may be swollen. Myoglobinuria may be evident as a red or brown discoloration of the urine.

Laboratory Studies

The serum creatine kinase (CPK) activity is markedly elevated in the necrotic myopathies. It may also be elevated in potassium-deficient hypokalemic paralysis and in acute hypophosphatemic polyneuropathy, conditions in which a necrotic myopathy may accompany the primary cause of weakness. CPK activity is normal in the other syndromes.

Electrodiagnosis is an invaluable localizing tool in acute weakness (Table 4), though unfortunately the tests must often be carried out in an intensive care unit, where electrical interference can cause problems. The examination should be thorough and flexible, because many of the familiar findings associated with chronic motor unit disorders are not seen in acute weakness.

TABLE 4. Electrodiagnostic Findings in Acute Generalized Weakness

		Motor Nerve Conduction		Sensory Nerve Conduction		
Syndrome	**EMG**	**Amplitude**	**Velocity**	**Amplitude**	**Latency**	**Repetitive Stimulation**
Motor neuron disorders	Sparse recruitment pattern; rapid firing	Normal	Normal	Normal	Normal	Normal
Polyneuropathy	Sparse recruitment pattern; rapid firing	May be reduced	May be reduced	May be reduced	May be prolonged	Normal
Disorders of neuromuscular transmission	Recruitment full for effort; MUPs* small, brief in weak muscles	Reduced in weak muscles	Normal	Normal	Normal	Abnormal decrement or increment (may be normal)
Myopathy	Recruitment full for effort; MUPs* small, brief in weak muscles	Reduced in weak muscles	Normal	Normal	Normal	Normal

*MUPs: Motor unit potentials.

In acute lower motor neuron disease, fibrillations do not appear within the first week, and any motor unit potentials that can be activated have a normal configuration. Thus, the only EMG finding in acute anterior horn cell or peripheral nerve disease is reduced voluntary recruitment of the motor unit potentials.

Nerve conduction may not be slow in acute neuropathies, even in the Guillain-Barré syndrome: the disease process may be proximal to the nerve segment being tested, or the diseased nerves may not conduct at all. If the distal portions of the nerves are involved, the amplitude of motor and sensory nerve responses will be reduced; if they are not involved, the amplitude of these responses will be normal. However, normal findings have localizing significance in the presence of severe weakness; they indicate that the lesions are proximal to the stimulating and recording electrodes.

Repetitive motor nerve stimulation often gives abnormal results in disorders of neuromuscular transmission. A decrementing response at slow rates of stimulation is observed in both postsynaptic and presynaptic disorders, while an incrementing response at fast rates of stimulation is found only in presynaptic disorders. In some cases, no abnormality can be demonstrated by repetitive stimulation, but the amplitude of the muscle response to nerve stimulation is low in extremely weak muscles, and motor unit potentials are small and brief, indicating that the disease process is at or distal to the motor nerve terminals. If the electromyographer stimulates the muscle *directly* (employing a higher voltage than is used for nerve stimulation), the visible muscle twitch will be much larger than that obtained by indirect stimulation. A normal direct muscle response, with a poor indirect response, locates the disorder in the nerve terminals or neuromuscular junctions. In myopathies, the EMG findings are similar, but direct and indirect muscle stimulation both give a weak muscle twitch.

Muscle and nerve biopsies are of little value in the diagnosis of acute, generalized weakness. Microscopic examination of a muscle biopsy sample from a patient with myoglobinuria may show muscle necrosis, but this can be deduced from the clinical picture and the serum enzyme levels, and biopsy rarely reveals the specific cause of the necrosis. Sural nerve biopsy might disclose inflammatory changes in the Guillain-Barré syndrome, but this diagnosis is readily made from clinical, electrodiagnostic, and spinal fluid findings.

Myoglobinuria

Clinical Features

Myoglobinuria is an external manifestation of focal or diffuse muscle necrosis (rhabdomyolysis) that is severe enough for pigment escaping from muscle to be visible in the urine. The affected muscles are weak, painful, tender, and sometimes swollen, and there may be blue discoloration of the overlying skin. The urine has a pink or red color when fresh and turns brown or brownish-black on standing.

For myoglobinuria to be visible, the urine myoglobin concentration must be at least 1 mg per ml (Knochel 1982). Skeletal muscle contains about 2 mg of myoglobin per gram, so it would take at least 15 g of skeletal muscle to supply the myoglobin for 300 ml of pigmented urine. Light microscopic examination of muscle samples from patients with generalized rhabdomyolysis often shows remarkably extensive necrosis of muscle fibers. In a few days the necrotic fibers are invaded by mononuclear cells and undergo phagocytosis, and during the next few weeks muscle fiber regeneration rapidly restores the muscle architecture. Despite the extensive muscle necrosis, recovery of muscle bulk and strength after a bout of myoglobinuria is usually surprisingly good, except in cases of ischemic necrosis or where muscle circulation is hampered by swelling within a closed compartment (see Chapter 8).

Complications

Aside from causing muscle weakness, which may be severe enough to cause respiratory failure, myoglobinuria has important indirect consequences.

Acute tubular necrosis tends to occur when a substantial amount of myoglobin passes through the kidneys, and transient oliguria can occur even in mild cases (Cadnapaphornchai et al. 1980). It is not known whether myoglobin damages the kidney directly, but even subclinical myoglobinuria may be harmful. In a recent study of military recruits, creatinine clearance fell significantly following several episodes of asymptomatic myoglobinemia induced by long marches (Melamed et al. 1982). Acute tubular necrosis can usually be prevented by administering large volumes of intravenous fluid with 25 g mannitol and 200 mg furosemide to induce diuresis (Knochel 1982).

Hyperkalemia is a life-threatening complication of rhabdomyolysis. It is caused by diminished renal clearance of potassium in the face of massive release of potassium from muscle into the bloodstream. The plasma potassium level must be monitored closely so that measures may be taken to prevent ventricular arrhythmia (Chapter 2). Release of muscle contents also causes *hyperphosphatemia* and *hyperuricemia,* and the latter may contribute to the kidney damage. *Hypocalcemia* occurs as a consequence of the deposition of calcium salts in the injured muscle, especially in oliguric patients (Meroney et al. 1957). The hypocalcemia does not usually require treatment, although tetany may occur. When renal function recovers, the blood calcium levels return to normal and may even become elevated as calcium moves from the muscle into the blood (Peiffer and Bundschu 1978).

Massive muscle swelling sometimes produces a *compartment syndrome,* which can permanently damage major nerve trunks and muscle tissue; this complication can be forestalled by fasciotomy (Chapter 8). Severe rhabdomyolysis may also lead to *shock,* in part because fluid accumulates in damaged muscle, and to *disseminated intravascular coagulation.*

Differential Diagnosis

A systematic classification of myoglobinuria is difficult to devise because the various categories overlap each other. For practical convenience, the disorders listed in Table 5 are arranged according to the *clinical setting* in which they occur, rather than the supposed physiologic mechanism. Using this classification, it should be possible in most cases to deduce the etiology of myoglobinuria from the medical history alone.

Laboratory Diagnosis

Too much emphasis has been placed on expensive laboratory tests for detecting myoglobinuria or myoglobinemia. In patients with acute weakness, myoglobinuria has no more diagnostic significance than a high serum

TABLE 5. Causes of Myoglobinuria

A. Heavy muscle exertion
   1. Military recruits, marathon runners, etc.
   2. Involuntary muscle contraction (seizures, tetanus, dystonia, catatonic rigidity, delirium tremors, neuroleptic malignant syndrome)
   3. Metabolic myopathies

B. Ischemia
   1. Acute occlusion of major limb artery
   2. Compression of artery (knee-chest position)
   3. Air embolism
   4. Azotemic hyperparathyroidism

C. Toxic infections
   1. Influenza, other viruses
   2. Gram-negative bacteria
   3. Leptospirosis
   4. Toxic shock
   5. Kawasaki syndrome

D. Hyperthermia

E. Hypothermia

F. Coma owing to drug or chemical poisoning (barbiturates, heroin, carbon monoxide)

G. Muscle injury
   1. Burns
   2. Mechanical injury
   3. Electrical injury

H. Mineral and electrolyte disorders
   1. Potassium deficiency
   2. Phosphorus deficiency

I. Drugs and toxins
   1. Drug abuse (alcohol, i.v. heroin, i.v. amphetamines)
   2. Neuroleptics; phencyclidine
   3. Malignant hyperthermia during anesthesia
   4. Epsilon-aminocaproic acid
   5. Myotoxic snake bite, brown recluse spider bite
   6. Food poisoning (Mediterranean quail, Haff disease)

J. Recurrent spontaneous myoglobinuria
   1. Carnitine palmityltransferase deficiency
   2. Idiopathic

CPK level. Myoglobinuria never occurs without a marked elevation of serum CPK activity, and the CPK elevation persists longer than the myoglobinuria. When a patient is admitted to the hospital with acute renal failure, a high serum CPK may be the first indication that recent rhabdomyolysis was the underlying cause.

In patients with acute weakness and pigmented urine, a positive dipstick test for heme pigment is sufficient evidence of myoglobinuria, provided that the urine is free of red blood cells. The dipstick test can detect myoglobin in a concentration as low as .01 mg per ml, which is too dilute to be visible to the naked eye.

Radionuclide scanning with technetium diphosphonate can demonstrate focal areas of muscle necrosis (Chaikin 1980). Muscle deposits of calcium are sometimes demonstrable in plain radiographs taken during the oliguric period (Clark et al. 1966). When fasciotomy is under consideration, computed tomography can delineate necrosis and swelling in deep muscle masses (Vukanovic et al. 1980); the necrotic areas are hypodense and fail to enhance after intravenous contrast administration. (However, intravenous injection of contrast material is contraindicated in such patients because of their precarious renal function.) Nuclear magnetic resonance (NMR) scanning will probably be very useful for this purpose.

Subacute and Chronic Generalized Weakness

This category contains most of the common neuromuscular manifestations of systemic disease (Table 6). The traditional clinical and electrodiagnostic guides to anatomic localization can usually be relied upon in these conditions.

Clinical and Laboratory Features

MOTOR NEURON DISORDERS. The typical picture consists of muscle weakness, atrophy, and fasciculations in a patchy, asymmetric distribution that conforms neither to a nerve root nor a peripheral nerve pattern. The cranial muscles are often spared except for the muscles supplied by the tenth and twelfth nerves. Muscle cramps may be prominent, but there are no sensory symptoms or signs. The reflexes are diminished in proportion

TABLE 6. Causes of Subacute and Chronic Generalized Weakness

A. Motor neuron disorders
  1. Amyotrophic lateral sclerosis
  2. Carcinomatous polioencephalomyelitis
  3. Subacute motor neuronopathy in lymphoma
  4. Carcinomatous proximal neuromyopathy
B. Polyneuropathy (see Table 10)
C. Disorders of neuromuscular transmission
  1. Myasthenia gravis
  2. Lambert-Eaton syndrome
  3. Drugs (beta-blockers, lithium)
D. Myopathy
  1. Mineral and electrolyte disorders
    a. Chronic potassium deficiency*
    b. Chronic phosphorus deficiency†
  2. Endocrine disorders
    a. Hyperthyroidism†
    b. Hypothyroidism†‡
    c. Hyperadrenalism†
    d. Nelson syndrome‡
    e. Acromegaly†
    f. Vitamin-D deficiency or resistance†
    g. Hyperparathyroidism†
  3. Infections
    a. Toxoplasmosis*
    b. Trichinosis*
    c. Cysticercosis§
  4. Immune disorders
    a. Polymyositis, dermatomyositis*
    b. Sarcoidosis*§
    c. Amyloidosis of muscle§
  5. Neoplastic and paraneoplastic disorders
    a. Dermatomyositis*
    b. Noninflammatory necrotic myopathy*
    c. Metastatic carcinomatous myopathy§
  6. Drugs and toxins
    a. Subacute and chronic alcoholic myopathy*†
    b. Corticosteroids, rifampicin, colchicine†
    c. Clofibrate, drugs causing potassium deficiency, beta blockers, emetine*
    d. Chloroquine‡

*Necrotic myopathy.
†Atrophic myopathy.
‡Degenerative myopathy.
§Infiltrative myopathy.

to the amount of weakness, unless upper motor neuron involvement is also present. There may be other central nervous system findings, such as upper motor neuron signs in amyotrophic lateral sclerosis, or cerebellar signs in carcinomatous polioencephalomyelitis. The serum CPK activity is normal except in amyotrophic lateral sclerosis, in which mild or moderate elevations are often found (Welch and Goldberg 1972). Electromyography shows typical changes of acute and chronic denervation and reinnervation, and fasciculations are often present. Motor and sensory nerve conduction tests give normal results except for low amplitudes of motor responses in weak muscles.

PERIPHERAL NEUROPATHIES. Motor or sensorimotor polyneuropathies tend to occur in two clinical patterns. The most familiar picture consists of distal, symmetric weakness and atrophy, affecting the lower extremities more than the upper extremities. Alcoholic neuropathy is a typical example. In the second pattern, the limb weakness has a diffuse distribution, with proximal accentuation in some cases. Chronic inflammatory polyneuropathies often give this clinical picture. In most neuropathies the reflexes are reduced or absent even in relatively strong muscles, and there are sensory symptoms or signs that have a distal distribution. Weakness occasionally involves the neck, trunk, and lower cranial nerves. The serum CPK activity is normal. The EMG and nerve conduction findings depend on the pathologic character of the neuropathy, as described in the next section of this chapter.

DISORDERS OF NEUROMUSCULAR TRANSMISSION. The two diseases in this category are clinically rather dissimilar. Myasthenia gravis causes fluctuating muscle weakness that has a predilection for the cranial muscles, neck, breathing muscles, and proximal limb muscles. Muscle bulk and reflexes are normal. The Lambert-Eaton syndrome resembles a myopathy, with weakness of the proximal limbs, neck, and trunk. The weak muscles are flabby and mildly wasted but there are no fasciculations. Weakness of the respiratory and cranial muscles is not prominent, although there may be mild ptosis. The tendon reflexes are diminished or absent, but reflex activity improves after a few seconds of strong muscle contraction. There are no sensory symptoms or signs in either condition.

In both of these disorders serum CPK levels, EMG, and nerve conduction tests generally give normal results. Repetitive nerve stimulation tends to show abnormal decrement in both disorders and regularly shows an abnormal increment in the Lambert-Eaton syndrome.

MYOPATHIES. The well-known clinical picture of myopathy consists of symmetric limb weakness that is more pronounced in the proximal muscles and worse in the lower extremities than in the upper. The anterior neck and trunk are also weak. There are no fasciculations; the reflexes are either normal or are reduced in proportion to the degree of weakness, and sensation is normal. This pattern is discernible in most of the myopathies listed in Table 6.

Based on muscle pathology and laboratory data, the acquired myopathies can be classified into four types, which may also have distinctive clinical features (Table 7).

The *atrophic myopathies* are characterized pathologically by scattered muscle fiber atrophy, often involving type 2 fibers predominantly. There is little or no degeneration of muscle fibers, and the muscle architecture is

TABLE 7. Laboratory Findings in Subacute and Chronic Myopathies

Test	Type of Myopathy			
	Atrophic	Necrotic	Degenerative	Infiltrative
CPK	Normal	Moderately or markedly elevated	Normal or mildly elevated	Normal
EMG	Myopathic or normal	Myopathic with fibrillations and irritability	Myopathic with fibrillations and irritability	Normal or myopathic with fibrillations and irritability
Muscle biopsy	Selective or unselective muscle fiber atrophy (ungrouped)	Segmental necrosis; phagocytosis; regeneration	Vacuolar degeneration	Interstitial deposition or infiltration

undisturbed by fibrosis or fatty infiltration. The serum CPK levels are normal. The EMG shows simple myopathic changes but it may be normal in mild cases, since the motor units activated by weak effort tend to consist of type 1 muscle fibers. The clinical picture consists of painless muscle weakness and flabby muscle atrophy in a standard myopathic distribution.

In the *necrotic myopathies* there is scattered, segmental necrosis of muscle fibers, some of which are seen to be undergoing phagocytosis. Regenerating muscle fibers may also be present. The serum CPK activity is moderately or markedly elevated. EMG often shows fibrillations in addition to the usual myopathic abnormalities. Muscle weakness in a myopathic distribution is sometimes accompanied by muscle pain, tenderness, or swelling. In inflammatory myopathies muscle induration and fibrotic contracture also occur, and there may be unusual patterns of muscle involvement, such as prominent distal weakness.

The term *degenerative myopathy* refers to a more gradual type of muscle fiber degeneration, sometimes associated with vacuolar changes reflecting storage of some substance within muscle fibers. There is little histologic evidence of active muscle fiber necrosis, phagocytosis, or regeneration. The serum CPK activity is normal or slightly elevated. EMG tends to show marked irritability of the muscle fibers in addition to the usual myopathic changes.

The *infiltrative myopathies* result from interstitial infiltration or accumulation of some extraneous material like amyloid or parasitic cysts. The muscle fibers themselves show little or no abnormality, the CPK is normal, and the EMG may be normal or myopathic, sometimes with muscle fiber irritability. There is usually diffuse muscle enlargement; there may be weakness, myalgia, and muscle tenderness in a proximal distribution, or the muscles may be strong and not tender.

Peripheral Neuropathy

Until recently, diagnostic workups failed to yield a specific diagnosis in 50 percent of patients with peripheral neuropathy (Prineas 1970). This discouraging picture has improved considerably thanks to many advances in our clinical and laboratory knowledge during the past 10 or 15 years. It is now possible to make an etiologic diagnosis in a large majority of the cases, usually without the assistance of sophisticated laboratory investigations.

The neuropathies fall into two main groups: focal or multifocal neuropathies, and diffuse or generalized neuropathies. These categories can be subdivided according to the temporal course of the illness; the anatomic distribution of the muscle weakness; and the results of nerve conduction tests and spinal fluid analysis.

Focal Neuropathies

A focal deficit implies a localized cause. The first step in diagnosis, therefore, is to determine where the lesion is located: in a spinal nerve root, in a nerve plexus, or in the proximal or distal part of a limb. For example, a median neuropathy causing weakness or EMG signs of denervation in the forearm muscles is not due to the carpal tunnel syndrome.

The next step is to decide whether the problem involves a single nerve, multiple nerves in one limb or region, or multiple nerves in widely separate locations.

Finally, the temporal course should be analyzed. An abrupt or apoplectic onset, in which the deficit is maximal at once, is due to either trauma or a vascular cause, such as diabetic angiopathy or vasculitis. A series of step-like, sudden worsenings also suggests an angiopathic neuropathy. A rapid onset over several hours or a few days occurs in postinfectious neuritis, mechanical entrapment, and global limb ischemia. A slower onset and progression over a period of weeks or months suggests nerve entrapment, infiltration by neoplasm, radiation injury, or a focal inflammatory process.

Table 8 summarizes the differential diagnosis of the focal neuropathies. Each subcategory contains only a few diseases, which are easy to distinguish from each other with the aid of a few laboratory tests.

Diffuse or Generalized Neuropathies

These types of neuropathies— also called polyneuropathies—present much more diagnostic difficulty than the focal neuropathies. A classification based

TABLE 8. Focal Neuropathies

Mode of Onset	Single Nerve or Root	Multiple Nerves in One Region	Multiple, Widely Separated Nerves
Abrupt	Trauma Diabetes mellitus Vasculitis	Trauma Diabetes mellitus	Trauma Diabetes mellitus Vasculitis
Rapid	Entrapment Postinfectious H. zoster	Postinfectious H. zoster Arterial embolism or thrombosis Arteriovenous fistula	
Gradual	Entrapment Intrinsic or extrinsic tumor	Radiation Malignant tumor invading soft tissue Meningeal cancer Diabetic amyotrophy, thoracoabdominal neuropathy	Entrapment Sarcoidosis Leprosy Meningeal cancer Multiple conduction block neuropathy

on the temporal course of the disease simplifies the task somewhat (Table 9). However, most of the polyneuropathies pursue a subacute or chronic course, and even when we omit the pure sensory polyneuropathies, which are outside the scope of this book, this category is unmanageably large. Some of these neuropathies eventually exhibit a relapsing course, a helpful diagnostic feature, but this may not be evident for many months. At this point, we can get additional help from two types of laboratory data: nerve conduction measurements and spinal fluid analysis. Electrodiagnostic tests help to determine whether the neuropathic process involves demyelination, axonal degeneration, or a mixture of both. A high spinal fluid protein concentration suggests that the neuropathy involves the spinal nerve roots, while a lymphocytic pleocytosis, a raised IgG index, or the presence of oligoclonal bands suggests nerve root inflammation.

Using clinical and laboratory information, we can recognize four main types of subacute or chronic polyneuropathy (Table 10):

1. A distal, symmetric pattern of weakness with "axonal" motor nerve conduction velocities and normal spinal fluid. This group includes nearly all of the nutritional, metabolic, and toxic neuropathies. A few cases of inflammatory and paraneoplastic neuropathy also present these features. The amyloid neuropathies can be distinguished by their predilection for the small-diameter pain, temperature, and autonomic nerve fibers.

2. A distal, symmetric pattern of weakness with "axonal" motor nerve conduction velocities and elevated spinal fluid protein concentration. This category includes most cases of diabetic polyneuropathy, the neuropathy of myxedema, and a few cases of inflammatory and paraproteinemic polyneuropathy.

TABLE 9. Polyneuropathies Classified According to Temporal Course

A. Fulminating (hours)
   1. Food poisoning (shellfish, food fish)
   2. Acute exacerbation of chronic hyperkalemia
   3. Acute hypophosphatemia
   4. Podophyllum poisoning
B. Acute (days)
   1. Guillain-Barré syndrome
   2. Porphyria
   3. Diphtheria
   4. Arsenic poisoning
   5. Tick paralysis
C. Subacute (weeks or months) (see Table 10)
   1. Inflammatory
   2. Nutritional
   3. Toxic
   4. Metabolic
   5. Paraneoplastic
D. Chronic (years)
   1. Chronic idiopathic polyneuritis
   2. Benign paraproteinemia
   3. Primary amyloidosis
   4. Diabetes mellitus
   5. Genetic diseases
E. Relapsing
   1. Idiopathic polyneuritis
   2. Benign paraproteinemia
   3. Collagen-vascular disease
   4. Paraneoplastic
   5. Repeated toxic exposure
   6. Refsum's disease

TABLE 10. Causes of Subacute Polyneuropathy

Disease	Clinical Syndrome*
A. Inflammatory	4 (1,2)
1. Idiopathic polyneuritis	
2. Benign paraproteinemia	
3. Collagen-vascular disease	
B. Nutritional	
1. Vitamin deficiency (B_1, B_6, B_{12})	1
2. Intestinal malabsorption	
a. Sprue	1
b. Postgastrectomy	3
C. Toxic	
1. Alcoholism	1
2. Heavy metals	1
3. Carbon disulfide, tri-orthocresyl phosphate, acrylamide	1
4. Hexacarbons	3
5. Disulfiram, ethambutol, gold, isoniazide, nitrofurantoin, vincristine	1
6. Amiodarone, gold, perhexiline	4
D. Metabolic	
1. Uremia	1
2. Diabetes mellitus	2 (1)
3. Hypoglycemia	1
4. Myxedema	2
E. Paraneoplastic	
1. Carcinoma, lymphoma	1,2,4
2. B-cell dyscrasias	
a. Amyloid neuropathy	1
b. Non-amyloid neuropathy	
1) Multiple myeloma, Waldenström's macroglobulinemia	1
2) Solitary myeloma	4

*Types of subacute neuropathy:
1: Distal, axonal polyneuropathy with normal CSF.
2: Distal, axonal polyneuropathy with high CSF protein.
3: Distal, demyelinative polyneuropathy with normal CSF.
4: Diffuse, demyelinative polyneuropathy with high CSF protein.

3. A distal, symmetric pattern with "demyelinative" motor nerve conduction velocities and normal spinal fluid. The main examples are the polyneuropathy occurring in patients with malabsorption following gastric resection, and the toxic neuropathies caused by hexacarbon solvents.

4. Diffuse muscle weakness with "demyelinative" motor nerve conduction velocities and a high spinal fluid protein concentration. In these cases the muscle weakness may have a proximal or distal accentuation, and cranial and respiratory muscles may be affected. There may be no sensory involvement, but when sensory loss is present it has a stocking-glove pattern in the limbs and sometimes involves the anterior face and trunk. The temporal course may be steadily progressive or relapsing. Electrodiagnostic tests indicate either pure demyelination or a mixture of demyelination and axonal degeneration. The spinal fluid protein is moderately or markedly elevated, and inflammatory changes may be present. This category contains most of the inflammatory and paraneoplastic neuropathies and some cases of gold neuropathy. The drug-induced lipid storage neuropathies caused by perhexilene and amiodarone have elevated spinal fluid protein levels without inflammatory features.

Group 1, the axonal polyneuropathies with normal spinal fluid, is still awkwardly large, but an adequate screening workup for these causes can be defined. It consists of a focused history and physical examination, a sedimentation rate, tests for occult blood in the feces, an SMA-12, chest radiographs, serum immunoglobulin studies, a serum vitamin B_{12} level, malabsorption screening tests, and analysis of the urine for arsenic, mercury, and coproporphyrins. If this workup is unrevealing, an occult carcinoma is still possible, but a laboratory search for cancer will very likely be fruitless. A sural nerve biopsy may be done to look for evidence of an inflammatory process.

In Groups 2 and 4, the differential diagnosis lies mainly between paraneoplastic, paraproteinemic, and idiopathic inflammatory polyneuropathy. If the screening workup fails to disclose a paraproteinemia or a malignancy, a sural nerve biopsy should be done prior to a trial of steroid or immunosuppressive therapy.

Muscle Pain and Swelling

Muscle pain is usually a temporary annoyance related to a minor injury, strenuous exercise, or some other easily identified cause. Yet muscle pain is one of the most frequent medical complaints, and it occurs in so many different diseases that diagnosis may be difficult. In analyzing this symptom it is helpful to consider the problem of *focal* muscle pain separately from the problem of *generalized* myalgia.

Focal Muscle Pain

The differential diagnosis of painful muscle masses is aided by paying close attention to the mode of onset and the clinical setting (Table 11). An *acute onset,* measured in hours or a few days, is associated with intramuscular hemorrhage, muscle infarction, toxic myopathies, the virulent types of bacterial myositis, exertional muscle damage, and nonmusucular conditions like thrombophlebitis, a ruptured tendon, or a ruptured synovial cyst. A *subacute onset* occurs in pyomyositis, tumors, inflammatory pseudotumors, and parasitic cysts. A *gradual onset* over several months is seen in nodular sarcoid myopathy.

A marked elevation of serum enzyme levels occurs in many of these disorders, but the CPK is usually normal in cases of tumor, inflammatory processes confined to the connective tissue, parasitic cysts, thrombophlebitis, ruptured tendon, or ruptured synovial cyst. Computed tomography and NMR imaging may provide useful diagnostic and localizing information.

In some conditions, focal muscle pain occurs without swelling or induration. Among these disorders are several types of chronic or episodic leg pain that characteristically occur at rest.

Growing pains are a complaint of early childhood characterized by episodes of nocturnal leg pain lasting up to an hour, without muscle spasms or other abnormal signs (Peterson 1977). The pains are more likely to occur after unaccustomed exercise. This syndrome tends to be familial and is often associated with episodic headaches and episodic abdominal pain (Oster 1972). The symptoms generally disappear during adolescence.

The restless legs syndrome occurs in adults and also has a familial tendency. When resting in a chair or in bed, the sufferer experiences an intolerable sensation in his legs that forces him to move his legs about or to get up and walk, whereupon the unpleasant sensation subsides, only to return when his legs become quiet. This leg discomfort has been variously described as aching, pulling, crawling, or burning, but the essence of the

TABLE 11. Causes of Focal Muscle Pain

A. With swelling or induration
  1. Neoplasm
  2. Trauma (hematoma)
  3. Ruptured tendon
  4. Ruptured Baker cyst
  5. Thrombophlebitis
  6. Infection
    a. Streptococcal myositis
    b. Gas gangrene
    c. Pyomyositis
    d. Trichinosis, hydatid cysts, sparganosis
    e. Painful leg weakness in children with influenza
  7. Inflammation
    a. Localized nodular myositis
    b. Proliferative myositis
    c. Pseudomalignant myositis ossificans
    d. Eosinophilic fasciitis
    e. Sarcoidosis (nodular form)
  8. Ischemia
    a. Muscle necrosis following relief of large artery occlusion
    b. Diabetes (infarction of thigh muscle)
    c. Embolism (marantic endocarditis)
    d. Azotemic hyperparathyroidism (muscle and skin necrosis)
  9. Toxic and metabolic disorders
    a. Acute alcoholic myopathy
    b. Myoglobinuria in drug-induced coma
    c. Exertional muscle damage
      (1) Normal persons (e.g., military recruits)
      (2) Metabolic myopathies

B. No swelling or induration
  1. Exertional myalgia
    a. Normal persons
    b. Vascular insufficiency (intermittent claudication)
    c. Metabolic myopathies
  2. Acute brachial neuritis
  3. Ischemic mononeuropathy
  4. Parkinsonism
  5. Resting leg pain of obscure cause
    a. Growing pains
    b. Restless legs
    c. Painful legs and moving toes
    d. Idiopathic leg pain

complaint lies in the irresistible urge to move the legs rather than in the quality of the uncomfortable sensation (Ekbom 1970). Some subjects even thrash their legs periodically while they are asleep; these movements must be distinguished from nocturnal leg myoclonus (night starts). There is a high incidence of the restless legs syndrome in uremia. The most effective medication for this complaint is 0.5 mg clonazepam taken at bedtime or twice a day (Matthews 1979).

Idiopathic leg pain is a constant aching pain of the lower extremities that is most noticeable at rest, especially after exercise. The intensity of the pain diminishes during light exercise such as walking, but the pain never disappears entirely, and these patients do not exhibit the peculiar motor behavior typical of the restless legs syndrome. The pain is usually felt deep in the muscles but it may not be of muscular origin, since it is also located in the knees, ankles, or feet. The complaint may persist for many years, and it is remarkably resistant to medical treatment.

Generalized Muscle Pain

Within this category it is useful to distinguish painful disorders associated with muscle weakness from those without weakness (Table 12). Most of the former conditions are myopathies characterized by inflammation or necrosis of muscle and are thus associated with elevated serum enzyme levels and myopathic EMG abnormalities, often with irritable features. Cysticercosis and amyloidosis, however, are infiltrative myopathies that cause generalized myalgia and muscle enlargement without muscle fiber necrosis or serum enzyme elevation. The atrophic myopathies associated with osteomalacia and hyperparathyroidism do not cause muscle pain, but the accompanying bone disease causes much pain during limb movement and weight-bearing. Poliomyelitis and some acute polyneuropathies, like the Guillain-Barré syndrome and porphyria, tend to be associated with severe myalgia, but the serum CPK level is usually normal.

Diffuse myalgia without muscle weakness is ordinarily not associated with serum enzyme elevation. An exception is hypothyroidism, which raises the serum enzyme levels even when no myopathy is present.

The most common cause of chronic, generalized muscle pain is a controversial syndrome known variously as *primary fibromyalgia,* fibrositis, or myofascial syndrome (Yunus et al. 1981). The controversy centers on whether this is a genuine physical disorder or a form of psychogenic pain caused by depression, hypochondriasis, or hysteria. The patients complain of multifocal, migratory muscle pain and tenderness, commonly located in the posterior neck, trapezius muscles, lower back, upper buttocks, and lateral thighs. There are no objective neuromuscular findings, although

TABLE 12. Causes of Generalized Muscle Pain

A. With muscle weakness
  1. Inflammation (polymyositis, dermatomyositis)
  2. Infection
     a. Toxoplasmosis
     b. Trichinosis
     c. Toxic myopathy (influenza or other viral infections, leptospirosis, gram-negative infections, toxic shock syndrome, Kawasaki syndrome)
     d. Poliomyelitis
  3. Toxic and metabolic disorders
     a. Acute alcoholic myopathy
     b. Hypophosphatemia
     c. Potassium deficiency
     d. Total parenteral nutrition (essential fatty acid deficiency)
     e. Necrotic myopathy caused by carcinoma
     f. Hypothyroid myopathy
     g. Drugs (epsilon-aminocaproic acid, clofibrate, emetine)
     h. Carnitine palmityltransferase deficiency
  4. Amyloidosis
  5. Bone pain and myopathy (osteomalacia, hyperparathyroidism)
  6. Acute polyneuropathy (Guillain-Barré syndrome, porphyria)

B. Without muscle weakness
  1. Polymyalgia rheumatica
  2. Muscle pain-fasciculation syndrome
  3. Myalgia in infection or fever
  4. Myalgia in collagen-vascular disease
  5. Steroid withdrawal
  6. Hypothyroidism
  7. Primary fibromyalgia (fibrositis)
  8. Fabry's disease
  9. Parkinsonism

patients often claim that they can feel lumps in the painful muscles. A characteristic finding on physical examination is the presence of exquisitely tender "trigger points" in the painful muscles, especially near tendinous insertions. Injection of these regions with a local anesthetic, a steroid drug, or isotonic saline (Frost et al. 1980) often provides temporary relief, but "dry needling" is also efficacious (Lewit 1979). Laboratory tests are unrevealing. Whether or not "primary fibromyalgia" is a genuine neuromuscular disorder, effective treatment relies mainly on reassurance, administration of tricyclic antidepressants, and a program of gradually increasing physical activity.

Painless Muscle Swelling

Not all muscle masses are painful. Rhabdomyosarcoma, a rare, highly malignant tumor of skeletal muscle, presents as a deep muscle mass that generally enlarges rapidly over a period of several weeks. At this stage pain is typically absent unless a nerve is being compressed. Focal parasitic cysts caused by echinococcosis or sparganosis are painless in the majority of cases. The gradual muscle enlargement that occurs in a few patients with cysticercosis whose muscles are heavily infiltrated with parasitic cysts is usually not painful. The diffuse muscle hypertrophy of hypothyroidism is usually asymptomatic in young children, though adults with muscle enlargement often complain of muscle pain and stiffness.

Muscle Spasms and Stiffness

It is not uncommon for patients and physicians to speak loosely of "cramps" when they mean muscle pain. A true cramp, however, is a type of painful muscle spasm, one of many "motor unit hyperactivity states" that have, as their chief manifestation, either continuous muscle stiffness; muscle twitching, jerking, or spasm; or delayed muscle relaxation after voluntary contraction (Layzer 1979). Table 13 summarizes the clinical features of several motor unit disorders marked by muscle spasms or stiffness. Ordinarily a diagnosis can be made from the clinical picture and electromyographic examination of the involuntary muscle activity. In difficult cases, however, it may be useful to locate the origin of the abnormal motor activity, by observing whether it persists during sleep, general anesthesia, spinal anesthesia, peripheral nerve block, or block of neuromuscular transmission (Layzer 1979).

Most of the motor unit hyperactivity states are primary neurologic or neuromuscular disorders that are outside the scope of this book. However, five syndromes do turn up as manifestations of systemic disease or treatment: slow muscle relaxation in hypothyroidism; muscle contracture induced by anesthesia (malignant hyperthermia); tetany induced by alkalosis or hypocalcemia; tetanus; and ordinary muscle cramps. All but the last of these will be described in later chapters.

Muscle Cramps

A muscle cramp is a sudden, forceful, painful, involuntary contraction of one muscle or part of a muscle, lasting anywhere from a few seconds to several minutes. The clinical features of ordinary cramps are listed in Table 14. The cramps experienced by normal persons are usually triggered by brief contraction of a muscle that is already shortened, though sometimes

TABLE 13. Motor Unit Hyperactivity States

		Manifestations								
Syndrome	Motor Unit Localization	Percussion Myotonia	Slow Relaxation	Continuous Stiffness	Myokymia	Spontaneous Spasms	Spasms Induced by Exercise	Reflex Spasms	Carpopedal Spasms	EMG of Involuntary Muscle Activity
Myotonia	Muscle membrane	+	+				+			Myotonia
Myxedema contracture*	Muscle SR		+				+			Silent
McArdle's syndrome	Muscle SR						+			Silent
Malignant hyperthermia	Muscle SR			+†						Silent
Ordinary cramps	Motor nerve terminals					+	+			High-frequency high-amplitude discharge
Neuromyotonia	Distal motor nerves		+	+	+		+		+	Continuous high-frequency discharge of MUPs & MUP fragments
Tetany	Motor & sensory nerves					+			+‡	Repetitive discharge of single or grouped MUPs at 5–15 Hz
Tetanus	Motor neurons of spinal cord and brain stem			+		+	+	+		Continuous discharge of MUPs resembling voluntary contraction
Stiff-man syndrome	Motor neurons of spinal cord			+		+	+	+		Continuous discharge of MUPs resembling voluntary contraction

Abbreviations: SR, sarcoplasmic reticulum; MUP, motor unit potential.
*Ordinary cramps also occur.
†Induced by anesthesia.
‡Provoked by ischemia and alkalosis.

TABLE 14. Clinical Features of Cramps

1. Explosive onset, variable rate of resolution. Visible, palpable contraction.
2. Painful. May leave soreness, swelling, and high CPK.
3. Tend to be confined to one muscle or part of a muscle.
4. Start and end with twitching. Wax and wane independently in different parts of muscle.
5. Occur after trivial movement but also after forceful contraction (especially when muscle shortens).
6. Can usually be terminated by passive stretching of muscle.

they seem to occur spontaneously. *Nocturnal leg cramps* generally involve the calf muscles or the plantar foot muscles, causing plantar flexion of the foot or toes. Nocturnal leg cramps are frequent in the elderly but they occur at any age. Some people are more troubled by frequent *daytime cramps* that occur during or after strenuous exercise; these cramps can involve nearly any muscle of the limbs, trunk, or neck, but in other respects they are identical to nocturnal leg cramps. Some people with frequent daytime cramps have rather large muscles, are subject to frequent benign fasciculations, and have myokymia of the calf muscles. Both nocturnal and diurnal cramps occur frequently in patients with diseases of the lower motor neuron and with certain metabolic disturbances (Table 15).

Cramps are painful in proportion to the size of the muscle involved and the duration of the muscle spasm. The initial pain is presumably caused by stimulation of pain nerves sensitive to stretch, but severe cramps leave behind a persistent soreness that tends to be maximal 24 or 48 hours later and to be accompanied by muscle tenderness and swelling and elevated serum enzyme levels. As a consequence, people with frequent muscle cramps may have high serum enzyme levels much of the time.

Electromyography performed during a muscle cramp (Denny-Brown 1953; Norris et al. 1957) shows a high-frequency, high-amplitude electrical discharge, the intensity of which fluctuates with the passage of time and varies in different parts of the same muscle (Fig. 3). The onset and subsidence of cramps are associated with fasciculations that are evident both clinically and electromyographically. These facts, and the strong clinical association of cramps with lower motor neuron diseases, leave little doubt that ordinary muscle cramps originate in spontaneous discharges of motor nerves. The precise anatomic and physiologic causes, however, are still unknown.

TABLE 15. Conditions Associated with Frequent Muscle Cramps

A. No apparent cause
   1. Nocturnal leg cramps in the elderly
   2. Large muscles and fasciculations
   3. Diurnal cramps related to exercise
B. Lower motor neuron disorders
   1. Amyotrophic lateral sclerosis, old polio, other motor neuron diseases
   2. Radiculopathy and neuropathy
C. Metabolic disorders
   1. Pregnancy
   2. Uremia
   3. Hypothyroidism
   4. Hypoadrenalism
D. Acute extracellular volume depletion
   1. Perspiration
   2. Diarrhea, vomiting
   3. Diuretic therapy
   4. Hemodialysis

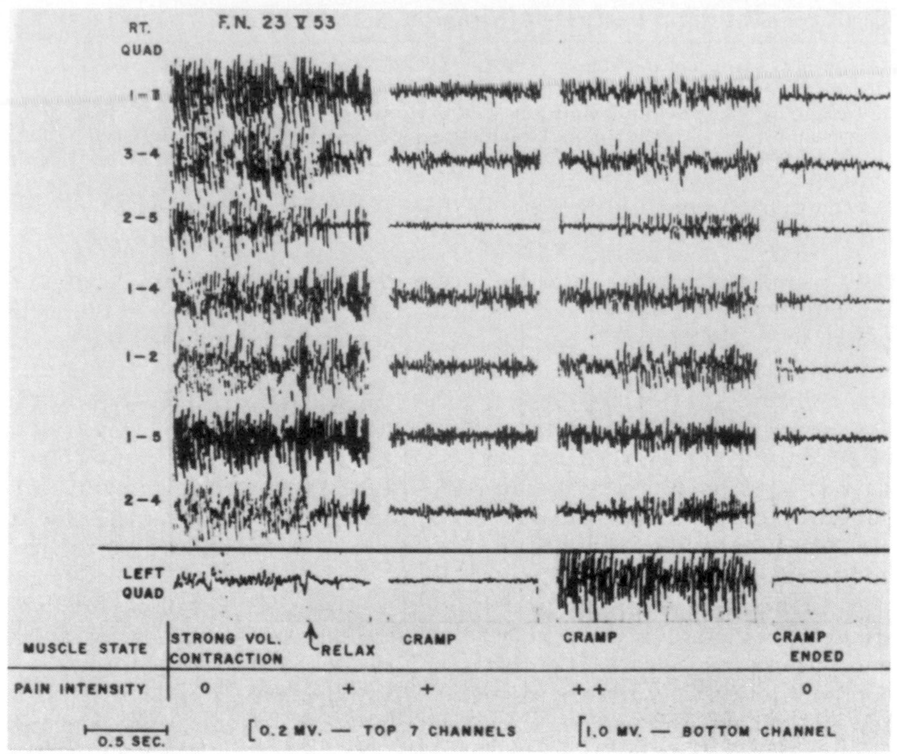

FIGURE 3. EMG recordings during a muscle cramp. Needle electrodes were inserted in five different locations in the right quadriceps muscle, and potential differences between various electrode pairs were recorded with an ink-writer. *(First column)* The right quadriceps muscle was contracted isometrically until a cramp developed. *(Second column)* Four seconds later, the cramp persists. Electrical activity varies in different parts of the muscle. *(Third column)* Five seconds later, the cramp increases during voluntary contraction of the *left* quadriceps muscle. *(Fourth column)* One second after cessation of cramp, some spontaneous activity continues. (From Norris et al. 1957, with permission.)

Pathophysiology. Denny-Brown (1953) suggested that cramps originate in the distal portions of the motor nerves, and I have speculated elsewhere (Layzer 1984) that most cramps, like fasciculations, arise in the intramuscular portion of the motor nerve terminals. In this location the axonal branches, being unmyelinated, have different physiologic properties from the extramuscular nerve fibers. Motor nerve terminals are prone to develop repetitive activity following tetanic stimulation (Standaert 1963) or on exposure to certain drugs (Noebels and Prince 1977); they are also subject to mechanical deformation when the muscle changes length, and to the chemical influences of the muscle extracellular space. These speculations remain to be investigated, for there has been very little research into the pathophysiology of cramps in the past 25 years.

An individual cramp can nearly always be terminated by stretching the affected muscle firmly for several seconds. Patients who complain of frequent muscle cramps should be evaluated for the presence of one of the predisposing neurologic or metabolic disorders. If there is no correctable metabolic disturbance, and the complaint is sufficiently distressing, prophylactic therapy may be appropriate. For nocturnal cramps, a bedtime dose of quinine or carbamazepine is usually effective. Diurnal cramps often respond to maintenance therapy with phenytoin or carbamazepine in standard anticonvulsant dosage.

TABLE 16. Medical Causes of Asthenia Without Muscle Weakness

1. Endocrine disorders: hypoadrenalism, hypothyroidism, apathetic hyperthyroidism
2. Metabolic disorders: uremia
3. Infection: hepatitis, mononucleosis, tuberculosis, chronic bacterial infections, postviral syndrome
4. Cancer: carcinoma of lung or gastrointestinal tract, leukemia
5. Anemia
6. Low cardiac output: heart failure, constrictive pericarditis, restrictive cardiomyopathy, heart block
7. Orthostatic hypotension: hypovolemia (diuretic therapy, vomiting, diarrhea), hypotensive drug therapy, autonomic insufficiency
8. Hypoxic pulmonary diseases
9. Collagen-vascular diseases
10. Drugs: beta blockers, bretylium, guanethidine

Asthenia

Patients who complain of "weakness" or "fatigue" often have no demonstrable neuromuscular disorder. The most accurate term for these symptoms is *asthenia,* which is a feeling of weariness and a disinclination to physical or mental effort. It is important to realize that asthenia has an entirely different diagnostic significance from objective weakness. All too often, in medical articles and textbooks, "weakness" is listed as a symptom of disease without any mention of objective muscle strength.

Complaints of chronic asthenia are common in psychiatric disorders, especially depression and anxiety neurosis. However, asthenia is also a prominent symptom in a wide variety of physical ailments, and persistent asthenia in the absence of specific psychiatric symptoms merits a thorough screening workup (Table 16). This is especially true if asthenia is accompanied by medical symptoms such as weight loss or fever. An important feature of psychiatric asthenia, usually not present in physical illness, is a disinclination to *mental* effort that is as debilitating as the sensation of physical fatigue and weakness.

INTERPRETATION OF LABORATORY TESTS

Serum Enzymes

Serum enzyme measurements are an important tool in neuromuscular diagnosis. While the activity of many serum enzymes is elevated in muscle disease, creatine kinase has proven to be the most sensitive and specific indicator of muscle abnormality.

Source of Serum Enzymes

The cellular enzymes that appear in the serum are nearly all cytoplasmic proteins that are not tightly bound to subcellular structures. This suggests that the escape of cellular enzymes into the blood is due to leakage from broken or malfunctioning cell membranes. Normally these enzymes escape slowly and continuously into the extracellular space, giving a normal range of serum enzyme levels in the blood. The enzymes are cleared from the extracellular space and blood by the reticuloendothelial system and, to a lesser extent, by renal excretion (Lang 1981).

Skeletal muscle has the highest CPK content of any body tissue, more than three times as much as heart and brain. Considerably smaller concentrations of CPK are found in muscular organs like the urinary bladder, uterus, gall bladder, colon, and stomach, and also in the adrenal and thyroid glands, kidneys, lungs, and prostate (Lang 1981). Consequently, nearly all the CPK activity in normal serum is derived from skeletal muscle, and elevated serum CPK levels are more specific for muscle disease than other serum enzyme elevations. The CPK test is also more frequently abnormal than other enzyme tests in neuromuscular disorders, and the range of abnormal values is much greater. For example, in early Duchenne's muscular dystrophy, the mean increase of serum CPK activity is five times as great as for aldolase, lactate dehydrogenase, and the transaminases (Munsat et al. 1973). The CPK test is not influenced by hemolysis, since there is no CPK in red blood cells. Since no additional diagnostic information is provided by the other enzyme tests, *it is rarely necessary to order multiple enzyme tests for neuromuscular diagnosis; the CPK test suffices.*

CPK Levels in Neuromuscular Diseases

Serum CPK elevations can be arbitrarily classified as mild (less than 4 times the upper level of normal), moderate (4 to 10 times normal), or marked (over 10 times normal). Despite its great sensitivity to muscle damage, the CPK test is not always abnormal in muscle disease. Among the acquired myopathies, serum CPK levels are consistently elevated in diseases characterized by muscle fiber necrosis. Marked elevations are recorded in severe necrotizing myopathies such as severe polymyositis and myoglobinuria, while only mild elevations are found in diseases with sparse necrosis like indolent polymyositis and mild hypokalemic myopathy. In contrast, CPK levels are normal in the atrophic myopathies and are normal or mildly elevated in the degenerative and infiltrative myopathies. Even in the muscular dystrophies there is a broad range of CPK values, from the marked elevations characteristic of early Duchenne's muscular dystrophy to the mild elevations found in facioscapulohumeral and myotonic muscular dystrophies.

Unfortunately, the CPK test is not always normal in motor nerve diseases. CPK levels are usually normal in the acute neurogenic disorders, but mild or moderate CPK elevations occur in many patients with chronic anterior horn cell diseases such as amyotrophic lateral sclerosis, old polio, and spinal muscular atrophy. Mild CPK elevations also occur occasionally in patients with chronic polyneuropathy. CPK levels are consistently normal in disorders of neuromuscular transmission.

Thus, in the appropriate clinical setting, a very high CPK level suggests a necrotic myopathy, and mild to moderate elevations suggest a nonatrophic myopathy or a chronic motor neuron disease. However, there are many incidental causes of CPK elevation that need to be considered in evaluating the significance of a high CPK value.

Other Causes of CPK Elevation

A glance at Table 17 might discourage many physicians from ordering a test with as many interpretive pitfalls as the CPK. Most of these conditions, however, cause a short-lived CPK elevation that would not interfere with the diagnosis of subacute and chronic neuromuscular disorders. The causes of *persistent* CPK elevation (lasting weeks or months) include frequent muscle cramps, tetanus, alcoholism, mediastinal radiation therapy, hypothyroidism, and rare cases of metastatic cancer.

TABLE 17. Misleading Causes of Serum CPK Elevation

A. Probably of muscle origin
   1. Trauma
   2. Surgical operations
   3. Severe burns
   4. Muscle hemorrhage
   5. Intramuscular injections
   6. Strenuous exercise
   7. Involuntary spasms or rigidity*
   8. Hypothermia
   9. Hyperthermia
   10. Alcoholism
   11. Electric shock, lightning stroke
   12. Large muscle mass*
   13. Malignant hyperthermia trait*
   14. Chronic idiopathic CPK elevation*

B. Central nervous system disease
   1. Cerebral infarction
   2. Subarachnoid hemorrhage
   3. Bacterial meningitis
   4. Head injury

C. Cardiac injury
   1. Acute myocardial infarction
   2. Electrical cardioversion
   3. Mediastinal radiation therapy*

D. Disease of other organs
   1. Pneumonia, pulmonary infarction
   2. Colonic infarction
   3. Metastatic carcinoma of lung or colon*

E. Miscellaneous disorders
   1. Sepsis
   2. Shock
   3. Acute psychosis
   4. Hypothyroidism
   5. Bee and wasp stings
   6. Acute asthmatic attack
   7. McLeod syndrome*

*May cause persistent CPK elevation.

People who appear entirely healthy sometimes have persistently elevated CPK levels in the mild or moderate range. Some of them may have the trait of malignant hyperthermia, and women could be carriers of X-linked muscular dystrophy. Persons with very large muscles may have mildly elevated CPK levels on that basis (Garcia 1974). Men with the McLeod syndrome (X-linked acanthocytosis) have high CPK levels without clinical evidence of myopathy (Marsh et al. 1981; Zyskowski et al. 1983). In many cases, however, there is no obvious explanation for the CPK elevation. Since these persons are asymptomatic, there is no need to launch a diagnostic workup merely to account for the abnormal laboratory finding.

Low CPK Activity

Although of little clinical importance, "subnormal" serum CPK activities have been reported in certain disease states. The best-documented associations are with hyperthyroidism (Chapter 3), lupus erythematosus, and rheumatoid arthritis (Wei et al. 1981). Other conditions claimed to have low CPK levels are steroid therapy (Hinderks and Frohlich 1979), prolonged bedridden states (Frohlich 1975), and alcoholic liver disease (Nanji and Blank

1981). The presence of heparin in the serum interferes with the CPK assay, giving a falsely low value. Some patients with metastatic carcinoma have an inactive form of serum CPK with low apparent activity that can be restored by incubating the serum with a sulfhydryl agent (Bruns et al. 1976).

CPK Isoenzymes

The main application of CPK isoenzyme determinations is in the diagnosis of acute myocardial infarction. More recently there has been interest in CPK-BB as an aid to the diagnosis and management of neoplasms (Nanji 1983). *There is practically no use for CPK isoenzyme measurements in neuromuscular diagnosis.* A brief review of this subject is appropriate, however, because muscle abnormalities interfere with the use of CPK isoenzymes for the diagnosis of myocardial infarction.

There are three cytoplasmic forms of CPK: CPK-MM, CPK-MB, and CPK-BB, formed by the combination of two nonidentical subunits, M (muscle type) and B (brain type). Skeletal muscle contains mostly CPK-MM with a small amount of CPK-MB; the proportion of total enzyme activity caused by CPK-MB ranges from 0.2 to 15 percent, with a mean value of 5 or 6 percent. The proportion of CPK-MB activity is higher in type 1 than in type 2 muscle fibers. Regenerating skeletal muscle fibers revert to an embryonic isoenzyme pattern with 10 to 50 percent CPK-MB. Heart muscle CPK is about 40 percent CPK-MB, the remainder being CPK-MM; the CPK-MB fraction ranges from 17 to 59 percent. Brain contains only CPK-BB. The CPK in other tissues is mainly CPK-BB with 5 to 20 percent CPK-MB (Lang 1981).

Normal adult serum contains no detectable CPK-MB; the CPK activity is due entirely to CPK-MM. In normal people, acute injury of skeletal muscle raises the total serum CPK activity and may increase the CPK-MB level slightly, but the CPK-MB fraction does not ordinarily exceed 6 percent of the total activity. Therefore, high serum CPK levels with a CPK-MB fraction greater than 6 percent are taken to confirm a clinical suspicion of acute myocardial infarction (Lang and Wurzburg 1982).

There are several pitfalls, however, in the interpretation of the isoenzyme results.

1. In normal children up to age 14, CPK-MB constitutes 14 to 26 percent of the serum CPK activity (Lang and Wurzburg 1982). Of course, this does not affect the diagnosis of myocardial infarction in adults.

2. The CPK-MB fraction tends to be elevated in patients with chronic neuromuscular diseases such as muscular dystrophy, alcoholic myopathy, polymyositis, and motor neuron disease (Brownlow and Elevitch 1974; Jockers-Wretou et al. 1976; Larca et al. 1981; Siegel and Dawson 1980; Somer et al. 1976). Continuing muscle breakdown and regeneration shifts the skeletal muscle isoenzymes toward a fetal pattern, and the serum isoenzyme pattern changes accordingly. This is not usually misleading, since CPK-MB levels rise and fall in acute myocardial infarction but remain steady in chronic neuromuscular disease. An acute muscle injury in a myopathic patient could cause confusion, however.

3. Acute muscle injury and surgical operations may raise the serum CPK-MB fraction above 6 percent in normal people. Misleading results of this kind have been reported in acute myoglobinuria (Russell et al. 1976), in marathon runners (Siegel et al. 1981), and after gastrointestinal resection, cesarian section, prostate resection, and neurosurgical procedures (Tsung 1981).

Recently, variant forms of CPK ("macro CPK") have caused occasional diagnostic confusion. One of these is an immune complex containing immunoglobulin and CPK-BB; another is an aggregate of mitochondrial CPK. The former tends to persist in the serum for long periods of time and has not been linked to any disease state, while the latter has mainly been found in seriously ill patients with widespread tissue damage. With electrophoretic methods of isoenzyme analysis, macro CPK-BB may be confused with CPK-MB, while immunologic methods tend to report both macro types as CPK-MB. Both of the macro forms can be distinguished from CPK-MB by their greater heat stability (Lang and Wurzburg 1982).

To summarize, the sequential measurement of CPK isoenzymes is a useful aid to the diagnosis of acute myocardial damage, provided that the above caveats are kept in mind. Without independent clinical or laboratory evidence of myocardial damage, however, a raised CPK activity with a CPK-MB portion greater than 6 percent should not be taken as incontrovertible evidence of myocardial damage.

Serum Myoglobin Levels

In the past several years there have been many publications reporting serum myoglobin levels in health and disease, but so far the results have been disappointing (Norregaard-Hansen and Hein-Sorensen 1982). Both serum CPK and myoglobin levels are elevated in acute and chronic diseases such as hypothyroidism (Kasai 1979), myoglobinuria (Olerud et al. 1975), and polymyositis (Kiessling et al. 1981), but the serum myoglobin test does not appear to be more sensitive or specific than the CPK test. Since the CPK test is a great deal less expensive to perform, I cannot see any clinical use for serum myoglobin measurements at present.

Electrodiagnostic Tests

The principal use of electrodiagnostic tests is to localize a neuromuscular abnormality within the motor unit. In the hands of a skillful operator, electrodiagnosis is unexcelled at distinguishing between myopathic and neurogenic weakness; defining a disorder of neuromuscular transmission; identifying and characterizing a peripheral neuropathy; and determining the location of a focal nerve lesion. To accomplish these tasks, the electrodiagnostician must be familiar with the patient's problem and have a clear idea of the specific anatomic questions that are to be addressed. When electrodiagnostic test results are unhelpful or misleading, it may be because the referring physician has failed to provide the necessary clinical information and guidance. The skill and knowledge of the electrodiagnostician are also very important, particularly for electromyography, which has a large subjective component.

Electromyography

TECHNIQUE. An oscilloscope displays electrical potential changes registered by a needle electrode inserted within the belly of a muscle. The potential changes are also made audible by the inclusion of a loudspeaker in the circuit. The tip of the needle electrode records from a sphere of tissue with a radius of about 0.5 mm. A standard test examines the electrical activity at rest (normally there is none), the electrical activity provoked by needle insertion and movement, the form of the motor unit potentials activated by weak effort, and the number and firing rate of motor unit potentials activated by weak, moderate, and full effort (Aminoff 1980; Kimura 1983).

INTERPRETATION. Each time a motor nerve discharges, it activates all of the muscle fibers in that motor unit. The EMG electrode registers the nearly simultaneous excitation of these muscle fibers as a single *motor unit potential.* During weak effort only a few motor nerves are activated, and the EMG displays a rhythmic discharge of a few motor unit potentials, each of which has a different appearance and firing rate. Maximal effort recruits a large number of motor units, which tend to fire rapidly; the EMG then displays a crowd of many different motor unit potentials that are difficult to distinguish from each other (the "interference pattern").

In *neurogenic disorders,* the EMG findings depend on the type and duration of the nerve disease. In acute nerve lesions the only EMG finding within the first week or two is a reduction in the number of motor unit potentials that can be activated by maximal effort. This reduced interference pattern is a direct consequence of a reduction in the number of functioning motor nerves. (A similar reduction occurs in upper motor neuron weakness and in poor effort, but in those conditions the motor units fire at a slow rate, while in lower motor neuron disorders the motor units discharge rapidly.)

If the nerve fibers degenerate, spontaneous discharges of single, denervated muscle fibers begin to occur after 1 to 3 weeks. On EMG these discharges are detected as fibrillations and positive waves occurring at rest. At this time, nearby nerve terminals belonging to surviving motor nerves begin to sprout, and during the next few months these new nerve terminals reinnervate the denervated muscle fibers. The result is a reduced number of motor nerves, many of which control a larger-than-normal number of muscle fibers. This anatomic alteration produces the characteristic EMG pattern of *chronic partial denervation and reinnervation:* large, polyphasic, prolonged motor unit potentials, and a reduced number of potentials activated by maximal effort (Fig. 4). This picture is typical of motor neuron diseases and also occurs in some axonal neuropathies.

A second type of reinnervation occurs only in peripheral nerve diseases. Nerve fibers whose distal segment has degenerated begin to regenerate from the healthy proximal "stump," growing toward the muscle at a rate of about an inch per month. On reaching the muscle, the regenerating nerve fibers form terminal branches that reinnervate any muscle fibers that are still without a nerve supply. Nerve fiber regeneration thus restores, to some extent, the complement of motor unit potentials that can be activated by maximal effort.

Nerve conduction block does not cause denervation changes in muscle fibers; fibrillations do not occur, and the EMG picture associated with distal nerve sprouting is not seen. Thus, in pure demyelinative polyneuropathies the EMG will show only a reduced interference pattern during maximal effort. However, most demyelinative neuropathies cause some degree of axonal degeneration and regeneration.

Fasciculations are spontaneous discharges of motor nerve fibers, evident on EMG as isolated motor unit potentials arising at rest, and sometimes evident clinically as muscle twitches. Fasciculations are not by themselves indicative of a neuromuscular disorder, since they often occur in healthy people. When associated with a neuromuscular disease, however, fasciculations are specific for lower motor neuron disorders, and they are encoun-

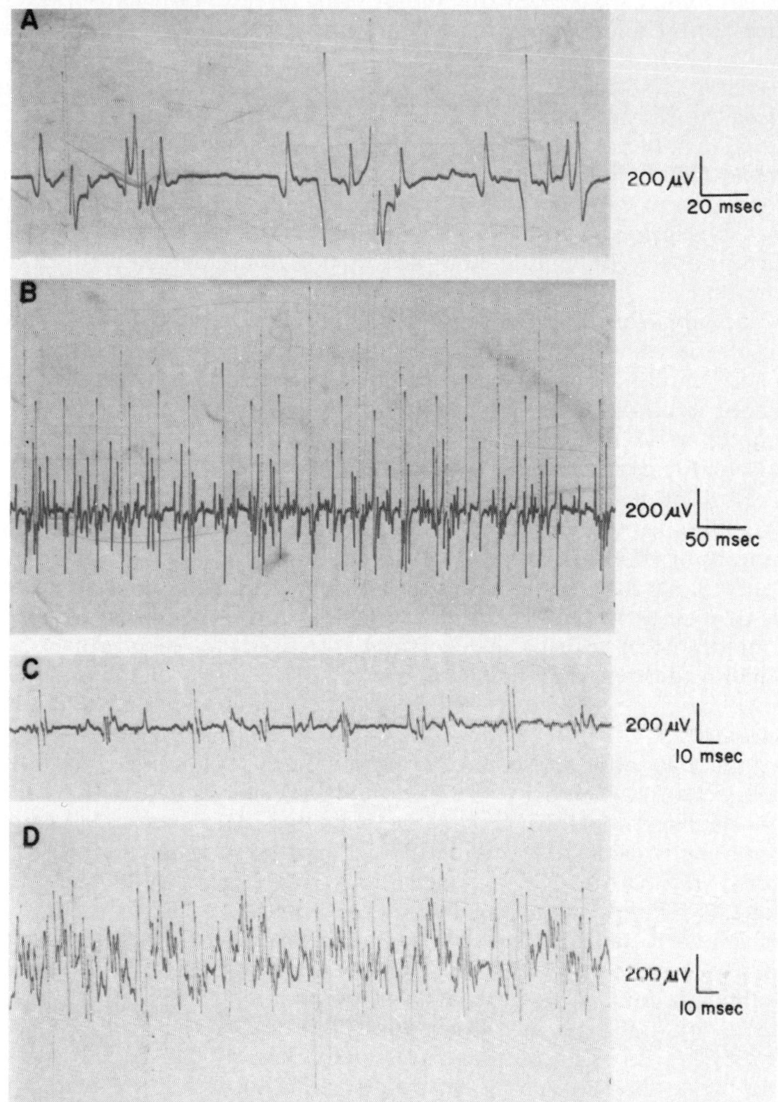

FIGURE 4. EMG findings in chronic neuromuscular disease. (*A*, *B*) Neurogenic disease. With weak effort (*A*), individual motor unit potentials can be seen, many of which are highly polyphasic and of long duration. Maximal effort (*B*) shows only a few different motor unit potentials firing repetitively. (*C*, *D*) Myopathy. With minimal effort (*C*), individual motor unit potentials are seen to be small, polyphasic, and of short duration. Weak effort (*D*) produces a full interference pattern because of the large number of motor unit potentials that fire repetitively.

tered more often in anterior horn cell diseases than in peripheral neuropathies. Physiologic investigations suggest that most fasciculations arise in the distal portion of motor nerves, probably within the terminal branches (Conradi et al. 1982; Roth 1982).

Myopathic disorders present two characteristic EMG abnormalities. First, the number of motor unit potentials activated during a weak contraction is larger than normal; the recruitment pattern is said to be "early" or "full for effort." Second, the motor unit potentials themselves have a reduced duration, are polyphasic, and may have a reduced amplitude (Fig. 4).

These EMG findings are thought to result from the fact that myopathy reduces the number of active muscle fibers within each motor unit, while the total number of active motor units remains normal. In order to generate a certain force, the patient must activate a greater-than-normal number of motor units, to compensate for the fact that each motor unit is weak. The altered configuration of the motor unit potentials has been attributed to the reduced density of muscle fiber action potentials detected by the needle electrode.

It is apparent that the same explanations would apply to disorders of the motor nerve terminals or neuromuscular junctions that result in "fractionated" motor units. Myopathic EMG abnormalities have, in fact, been observed in carcinomatous neuromyopathy, a disorder thought to involve the motor nerve terminals, and in botulism, a presynaptic disorder of neuromuscular transmission.

Fibrillations and irritability to needle movement can occur in myopathies, especially in necrotic and degenerative types. Fibrillation is due to an instability of the muscle fiber membrane potential (Layzer 1979), and it is not surprising that this electrical irritability occurs in primary muscle diseases as well as in denervation. A practical consequence, however, is that the presence of fibrillations cannot be used to distinguish between myopathic and neurogenic disorders.

APPLICATION. Table 18 summarizes the EMG findings in the motor unit disorders that cause subacute or chronic muscle weakness. (The EMG findings in acute weakness are listed in Table 4.) The ability of EMG to distinguish neurogenic from myopathic weakness is impressive. Among 57 patients with acquired myopathies, Buchthal and Kamieniecka (1982) detected myopathic EMG abnormalities in 82 percent of the cases; the remaining patients had normal results or nonspecific abnormalities, and no cases were erroneously classified as neurogenic. An even larger proportion of correct results was obtained in patients with chronic, nonhereditary neurogenic disorders; in 91 percent of these patients the EMG was diagnostic of neurogenic disease, and there were no myopathic results. Other investigators have reported similar success (Black et al. 1974). However, these results were obtained using quantitative methods that are not in routine use; the standard clinical technique is somewhat less accurate and is more dependent on the examiner's skill.

EMG is useful for the localization of focal nerve lesions. For example, a root lesion can be distinguished from a peripheral nerve lesion by the presence of fibrillations in the regional paraspinal muscles. EMG is also used for the differential diagnosis of motor unit hyperactivity states.

Nerve Conduction Tests

TECHNIQUE. A peripheral nerve is stimulated electrically at one point and a motor or sensory response is detected at a distant point. Both the amplitude of the response and its latency (the time between stimulus and response) are registered on an oscilloscope or on paper.

Motor nerve conduction is tested by stimulating a nerve trunk and recording the size and latency of the compound *muscle* action potential, which is ordinarily recorded from electrodes placed on the skin overlying

TABLE 18. Electromyographic Findings in Subacute and Chronic Neuromuscular Disorders

Type of Disorder	Activity at Rest	Form of Motor Unit Potentials	Recruitment Pattern*	
			Weak Contraction	Maximal Effort
Myopathy	None, or fibrillations and irritability	Reduced duration† Reduced amplitude Increased number of polyphasic potentials	Full for effort†	Full pattern in weak muscles† Reduced amplitude†
Disorders of neuromuscular transmission:				
Mild	None	Normal	Normal	Normal
Severe	None	May be myopathic	May be myopathic	May be myopathic
Neurogenic disorders	Fibrillations, fasciculations	Increased amplitude† Increased duration† Increased number of polyphasic potentials	Rapid firing	Reduced numbers† Increased amplitude† Rapid firing

*Number of motor unit potentials activated by voluntary contraction.
†Reliable features for distinguishing between myopathic and neurogenic weakness.

the muscle. When a distal segment of nerve is stimulated at a standard location, the distal motor latency is reported rather than a conduction velocity, because of the unknown delay in the nerve terminals and neuromuscular junctions. The motor nerve conduction velocity is determined by stimulating the nerve trunk at two different points and subtracting the distal latency from the proximal latency, to obtain the conduction time. The conduction velocity is calculated by dividing the distance between the stimulating electrodes by this conduction time.

For sensory nerve tests, a cutaneous nerve (e.g., a digital nerve in the hand, the superficial radial nerve at the wrist, or the sural nerve near the ankle) is stimulated and the amplitude and latency of the compound *nerve* action potential are recorded at a standard distance. Usually the latency of the response is reported rather than a conduction velocity, though a conduction velocity can be determined by recording the latencies at two separate points along the nerve.

The upper extremity nerve trunks can be stimulated as high up as the supraclavicular area (Erb's point); the femoral nerve can be stimulated at the groin; and the sciatic nerve can be stimulated as high as the gluteal fold. Information about conduction in proximal nerve segments, including the spinal nerve roots, can be obtained from two other electrophysiologic responses, the F response and the H reflex. The methods for obtaining these responses are described in standard textbooks (Daube 1980; Kimura 1983).

APPLICATION. 1. Subacute and chronic generalized weakness. (The nerve conduction findings in acute generalized weakness were described earlier in this chapter.)

In myopathies, disorders of neuromuscular transmission, and motor neuron diseases the amplitude of motor responses may be reduced in weak muscles. Motor nerve conduction velocity is normal except in severe motor neuron disease, in which conduction velocity may be mildly reduced owing to loss of the fastest-conducting nerve fibers. Sensory nerve conduction is normal.

In axonal polyneuropathies, motor and sensory responses are usually small and may be completely absent. If a motor response can be measured, motor nerve conduction velocity is normal or is reduced to a mild or moderate degree. The degree of nerve conduction slowing is roughly proportional to the clinical severity of the neuropathy.

In nonhereditary demyelinative polyneuropathies, the pathologic process tends to be multifocal; consequently the nerve conduction findings depend on whether there are lesions within the segment of nerve being tested. Sensory nerve responses may be normal or they may be small and have a prolonged latency. If several nerves are tested, at least one will show moderate to marked slowing of motor nerve conduction velocity (less than 70 percent of the lower limit of normal). Distal motor and sensory latencies are often prolonged as well. The amplitude of the motor and sensory responses may be normal or reduced, and the potentials may have a prolonged, irregular form owing to the broad range of conduction velocities in the component nerve fibers (Fig. 5). Focal areas of conduction block may be identified, within which nerve conduction is slowed or totally blocked, so that the muscle response to stimulation of the nerve at a site proximal to the block is considerably smaller than the response to distal stimulation.

2. Focal weakness. When tested within a few days of onset, an acute nerve lesion has the electrophysiologic characteristics of a conduction block, whether the nerve is irreversibly damaged or only functionally

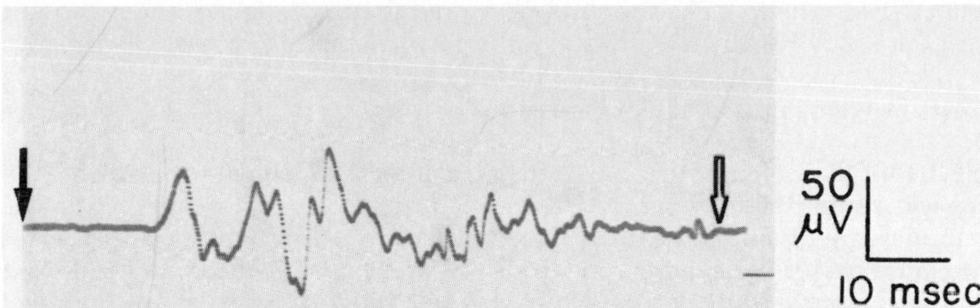

FIGURE 5. A dispersed muscle response in demyelinative neuropathy. The averaged compound muscle action potential was recorded with surface electrodes following supramaximal stimulation of the motor nerve. Arrows indicate the nerve stimulus *(left)* and the end of the response *(right)*. The complex, prolonged action potential reflects a broad range of conduction velocities among the motor nerve fibers.

blocked. Distal to the lesion, electrical stimulation and recording give normal results; stimulation of the nerve proximal to the lesion gives a distal response of diminished amplitude, or no response at all. Over the next 1 to 3 weeks, the irreversibly damaged nerve fibers degenerate distal to the lesion, reducing the amplitude of motor and sensory responses. (At the same time the EMG begins to show fibrillations.) In nerve fibers that are not irreversibly damaged, conduction block ordinarily resolves in less than 3 months. Many acute nerve lesions caused by trauma, compression, or ischemia show a mixture of conduction block and Wallerian degeneration.

Chronic nerve lesions give similar findings, except that the initial ambiguity is not present. Thus, the presence of conduction block, with good-sized motor and sensory responses to stimulation of the nerve distal to the block, indicates that most of the axons are intact and implies a good prognosis. In contrast, absent or markedly reduced motor and sensory responses in distal nerve segments imply that nerve degeneration has taken place; nerve regeneration will be necessary for recovery to occur.

RELIABILITY. Nerve conduction tests are objective and are generally quite reliable, but there are a few pitfalls.

1. Motor conduction is slow in infants, reaching adult values by around 5 years of age.

2. Conduction velocity is significantly reduced in cool limbs, and distal latencies are particularly vulnerable to this effect. It may be necessary to warm the limb with a heat lamp and to check the internal or surface temperature with a thermistor, particularly in patients with wasted muscles or poor circulation.

3. Motor conduction velocity is reported only for the fastest-conducting nerve fibers. If a nerve disease predominantly affects small-diameter, slowly conducting nerve fibers, the conduction velocity may be normal. In some cases of demyelinative neuropathy the fastest motor nerve conduction velocity is only mildly reduced but the range of velocities is abnormally broad, as indicated by dispersion of the muscle response. In such cases, reporting only the fastest motor nerve conduction velocity would be misleading.

4. Sensory nerve conduction tests are more difficult to perform than motor conduction tests. The amplitude of sensory nerve potentials, which is measured in microvolts, is about 0.2 percent of the amplitude of muscle responses, and baseline electrical noise may obscure the response. Locating

pure sensory nerves like the sural nerve requires experience, and an absent response may be due to technical failure rather than to disease.

Tests of Neuromuscular Transmission

TECHNIQUE. Neuromuscular transmission is evaluated by recording the muscle responses to repetitive nerve stimulation. A motor nerve trunk is stimulated with supramaximal intensity at various frequencies, and a series of compound muscle action potentials (M waves) is recorded, in order that changes in amplitude can be detected. The stimulating and recording electrodes must be prevented from moving so as to avoid artifactual changes in the amplitude of the responses.

At a slow rate of stimulation (2 to 3 Hz), a decline of 10 percent or more in the amplitude of the fifth response (compared with the first) is abnormal and usually indicates a disorder of neuromuscular transmission (Fig. 6). Stimulation at a faster rate (10 to 30 Hz) for 10 seconds is used to look for abnormal facilitation of neuromuscular transmission; an increment of greater than 10 to 15 percent is probably abnormal (see Fig. 6).

The muscle response to nerve stimulation can also be studied before and after a 10-second period of strong voluntary contraction, using either single stimuli or short trains of three shocks delivered at 2 or 3 Hz. In disorders of neuromuscular transmission, an abnormal increase in amplitude of the response to a single stimulus may be found a few seconds after exercise (post-tetanic facilitation). This increase persists for a few seconds or for several minutes, depending on the type of disorder, and it may be followed by a long period of post-tetanic depression or exhaustion, during which the muscle response to single nerve stimuli is reduced, or there is an abnormal decrement during repetitive stimulation at 2 to 3 Hz.

INTERPRETATION. The compound muscle action potential evoked by nerve stimulation reflects the *sum* of the individual muscle fiber action potentials. In a normal muscle (Fig. 7A), all the muscle fibers are excited by a nerve stimulus, and the number of muscle fibers excited does not change during nerve stimulation at rates up to 50 Hz.

In postsynaptic disorders of neuromuscular transmission (Fig. 7B), the muscle response to acetylcholine is diminished; a few of the neuromuscular junctions are blocked, and many have a reduced margin of safety. The initial muscle response will be nearly normal, however, since most of the neuromuscular junctions are still working. During repetitive nerve activity at 2 Hz, the amount of acetylcholine released by the nerve terminals actually declines; as a result, more neuromuscular junctions become blocked, fewer muscle fibers are excited by each nerve stimulus, and the amplitude of the compound muscle action potential declines (Pickett 1980).

In presynaptic disorders (Fig. 7C), the amount of acetylcholine released by a single nerve impulse is so small that neuromuscular transmission is blocked in a large proportion of the muscle fibers. As a result, the initial compound muscle action potential has a small amplitude. High-frequency repetitive nerve activity increases the amount of acetylcholine released by each nerve impulse, and this increase may overcome the block at some neuromuscular junctions. As a result, the number of muscle fibers activated by each nerve impulse increases during high-frequency nerve stimulation, and the compound muscle action potential increases accordingly (Pickett 1980).

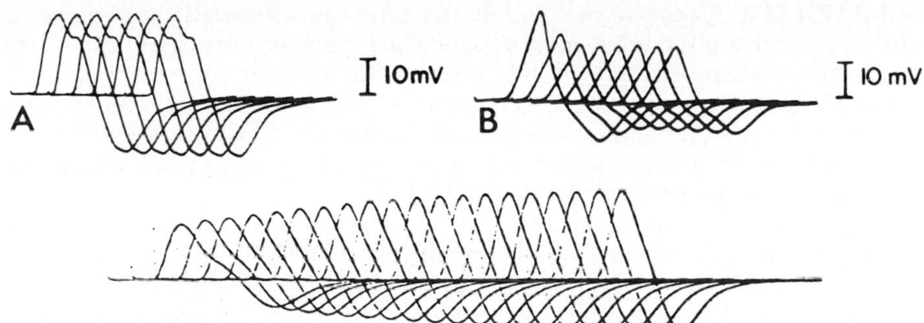

FIGURE 6. Repetitive stimulation test in disorders of neuromuscular transmission. The compound muscle action potentials were recorded with surface electrodes from a small hand muscle during repetitive stimulation of its motor nerve. *(Upper tracings)* Repetitive stimulation at 3 Hz: (*A*) normal response, (*B*) decrementing response in patient with myasthenia gravis. *(Lower tracing)* Repetitive stimulation at 20 Hz: this incrementing response is in a patient with botulism. (Upper tracings from Lisak, R. P., and Barchi, R. L.: *Myasthenia Gravis.* W. B. Saunders Co., Philadelphia, 1982, with permission.)

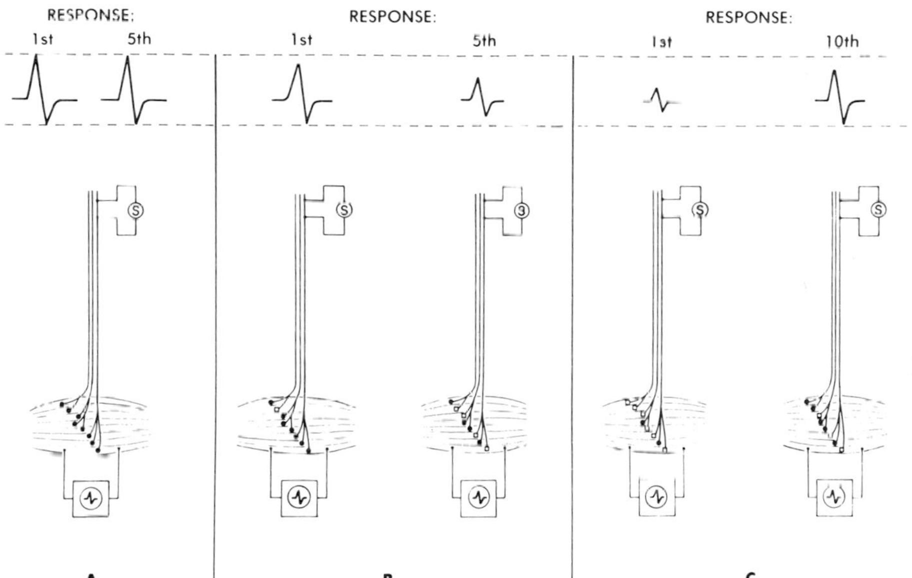

FIGURE 7. Mechanism of decrement and increment during repetitive stimulation. The filled circles represent neuromuscular junctions with intact transmission; the open squares represent blocked neuromuscular transmission. (*A*) In a normal subject, all neuromuscular junctions transmit impulses at nerve stimulation rates up to 50 Hz. (*B*) With a postsynaptic disorder, during nerve stimulation at 3 Hz, transmission block develops at some of the neuromuscular junctions, and causes a decline in the number of muscle fibers excited by each nerve impulse. The summated electrical response recorded from the muscle surface declines accordingly. (*C*) With a presynaptic disorder, initially, most of the neuromuscular junctions are blocked. During repetitive stimulation at 20 Hz, transmission is restored at some of the blocked junctions; the number of muscle fibers excited by each nerve impulse increases, and the amplitude of the compound muscle action potential grows larger.

RELIABILITY. Electrode movement can cause an artifactual increment or decrement in the recorded muscle potentials. Furthermore, a genuine decrementing response is not entirely specific for disorders of neuromuscular transmission; decrement can also occur in amyotrophic lateral sclerosis and in myotonic disorders. In the former condition the findings are similar to those seen in myasthenia gravis, but in myotonia the amount of decrement increases with increasing rates of stimulation.

Normal electrophysiologic findings are not unusual in myasthenia gravis and thus do not exclude that diagnosis. The likelihood of finding an abnormality increases when several muscles are tested, especially if weak muscles are included. The diagnostic sensitivity is also increased by testing for post-tetanic depression and by warming the limb to heighten the myasthenic defect. As a practical matter, however, the diagnosis of myasthenia gravis can nearly always be made by clinical, pharmacologic, and immunologic findings, so a negative electrophysiologic test is of little consequence.

The diagnosis of Lambert-Eaton syndrome, by contrast, can always be confirmed by tests of neuromuscular transmission, and abnormalities are present in nearly every muscle tested. The findings in botulism are less predictable; failure to demonstrate facilitation during repetitive stimulation or after voluntary contraction does not exclude that diagnosis.

Selection of Electrodiagnostic Tests

In the diagnostic scheme proposed earlier (see Fig. 2), localizing conjectures derived from the history and physical examination are tested and refined by basic laboratory aids. Table 19 lists the preliminary diagnoses that are likely to arise from clinical evaluation of a patient with subacute or chronic weakness, together with the electrodiagnostic tests that will help to answer the localizing questions. In some circumstances, electrodiagnosis will offer little new information. Thus, in the case of a patient with the typical clinical features of dermatomyositis and a high serum CPK activity, or a patient with typical myasthenia gravis and a positive response to anticholinesterase drugs, the experienced clinician may well do without electrodiagnostic tests.

TABLE 19. Most Useful Electrodiagnostic Tests in Localization of Subacute and Chronic Weakness

Clinical Problem	EMG	Nerve Conduction	Repetitive Stimulation
1. Myopathy versus neurogenic disorder	+	(+)*	
2. Weakness of uncertain type	+	+	+
3. Motor neuron disease versus peripheral neuropathy	+	+	
4. Demyelinative versus axonal neuropathy	+	+	
5. Disorder of neuromuscular transmission?			+
6. Localization of focal nerve lesion	+	+	

*To be performed if EMG is normal or neurogenic.

Imaging Procedures

These tests are not often used for neuromuscular diagnosis, but rapid advances in this field may soon make them much more important. Imaging can assist in the localization of focal muscle and nerve lesions and in some cases can provide important information about the underlying pathology.

Ultrasound Imaging

This technique has been used to identify muscle hematomas and abscesses in inaccessible locations such as the retroperitoneal space. It provides information about muscle size and about fatty replacement of muscle tissue in patients with generalized neuromuscular disorders (Heckmatt et al. 1980). However, the superior definition and pathologic insight provided by CT radiography and NMR imaging are rapidly making ultrasound imaging outmoded.

CT Radiography

This procedure gives excellent anatomic definition of muscle outlines, revealing muscle atrophy and hypertrophy and the presence of focal mass lesions (Genant et al. 1980). A fresh hematoma may show normal or increased attenuation, while areas of muscle necrosis or inflammation have reduced density. Following intravenous administration of contrast medium, areas of muscle necrosis show reduced enhancement in comparison with normal muscle. Calcification, fluid-filled cysts, and fatty tumors are easily identified. Malignant muscle neoplasms may have low, high, or mottled density and may contain areas of contrast enhancement (Laursen and Reiter 1980). A diffuse reduction of radiodensity in affected muscles occurs in chronic myopathies characterized by fatty replacement of muscle tissue, such as muscular dystrophies and polymyositis (Termote et al. 1980).

NMR Imaging

This procedure provides excellent definition of muscle structures; fat, muscle, fluid-filled cysts, tendons, nerves, and blood vessels each have different spin-echo intensity characteristics. The boundaries of malignant tumors may be better defined by NMR images than by CT radiography. NMR can also distinguish fibrous from nonfibrous tissue (Moon et al. 1983). It remains to be determined whether this technique will help to distinguish muscle necrosis from inflammation and tumor.

Radionuclide Scanning

^{67}Gallium scintigraphy is useful for detecting multiple muscle abscesses in patients with pyomyositis. ^{99m}Technetium diphosphonate uptake is increased in areas of muscle necrosis and injury (Vita and Harris 1981; Siegel et al. 1977), and this property may be useful in the evaluation of patients with acute necrotic myopathies (Chaikin 1980). Increased muscle uptake of technetium diphosphonate or pyrophosphate has also been demonstrated in patients with polymyositis, but uptake is not increased in regenerating, atrophic, or dystrophic muscle (Kula et al. 1976). Some authors have concluded that abnormal uptake of technetium diphosphonate is due to binding of the diphosphonate molecule to calcium, which is taken up by damaged muscle cells. Vita and Harris (1981) have argued, however, that the increased uptake is a consequence of increased capillary permeability, active endocytosis by invading inflammatory cells, and nonspecific entry of diphosphonate into muscle cells with damaged plasma membranes.

Biopsy of Muscle and Nerve

Muscle and nerve biopsy are performed more often than necessary, especially in patients with nonhereditary neuromuscular diseases, few of which require a biopsy for diagnosis. Even when the clinical indications for biopsy are appropriate, the tissue samples are sometimes handled so poorly that they provide little information and have to be repeated by another consultant. *If muscle or nerve biopsy samples cannot be processed and analyzed effectively, the patient should be referred to a specialty clinic for this purpose.*

Muscle Biopsy

TECHNIQUE. The muscle selected for biopsy should be weak but not severely weak or atrophic, since end-stage disease is difficult to interpret. The muscle must be free of recent trauma, such as EMG needling within the past month.

Muscle contracts when it is put into a fixative solution, and the resulting artifacts may render the specimen useless for pathologic interpretation. A simple way to avoid this is to pin the two ends of the muscle sample, under slight stretch, onto a piece of cardboard and cover it with a saline-moistened gauze sponge for 15 minutes, in order to let the muscle relax before placing it in the fixative solution. For histochemistry, a fresh segment of muscle is frozen in isopentane cooled by liquid nitrogen, prior to mounting for sectioning in the cryotome. For electron microscopy a long, thin strip of muscle is dropped into glutaraldehyde. The technique of muscle biopsy and the subsequent handling of the tissue samples is described in detail in a monograph by Dubowitz and Brooke (1973).

Open muscle biopsy is suitable for general use, but needle biopsy, if available, has several advantages. Samples can be obtained from more than one muscle, the procedure can be done in children without anesthesia, and the biopsy can easily be repeated (Dubowitz 1978). The disadvantages are that a special instrument is needed, the procedure requires practice, the samples are small and may not be representative, and longitudinal sections are not available. For nonhereditary diseases, open biopsy is generally preferable.

The fixed, paraffin-embedded tissue is sliced in longitudinal and transverse sections, mounted, and stained with hematoxylin and eosin. For histochemistry, frozen sections are stained with hematoxylin-eosin, a modified Gomori's trichrome stain, and several enzyme stains including one or two myosin ATPase stains and an oxidative stain such as NADH-tetrazolium reductase.

A separate specimen of muscle should be placed in glutaraldehyde and saved in case electron microscopy is needed. This is unlikely to be the case in nonhereditary muscular diseases, but the initial diagnostic premise may turn out to be mistaken.

INDICATIONS. As already pointed out, muscle biopsy is not diagnostically useful in cases of acute generalized weakness. It is also not useful for the evaluation of subacute or chronic neurogenic weakness; the histologic findings will probably confirm the neurogenic character of the disorder, but they will not reveal the cause.

Occasionally, the clinical and EMG findings are ambiguous and muscle biopsy is needed to decide whether the weakness is neurogenic or myopathic. In subacute neurogenic disorders, the characteristic abnormality is the presence of scattered atrophic muscle fibers, both type 1 and type 2, often clustered in small groups of 2 to 10 fibers of a single histochemical type (Fig. 8A). In some chronic neurogenic diseases, the continuing evolution of denervation and reinnervation produces large groups of muscle fibers of a single histochemical type. Some of these groups consist of normal-sized muscle fibers, while other groups consist entirely of atrophic fibers (Fig. 8B).

In subacute and chronic myopathies, the clinical features, EMG findings, and serum CPK levels usually permit a tentative classification of the myopathy as necrotic, atrophic, degenerative, or infiltrative. A muscle biopsy will define the pathologic category with greater certainty, and in some cases will provide a specific pathologic diagnosis (Figs. 8C–8F).

The question of whether to biopsy a focal muscle mass or to excise it entirely depends on the diagnosis being considered and the findings obtained with an imaging procedure. A suspected tumor should be excised, but if an inflammatory pseudotumor is more likely, simple biopsy is appropriate. Hematoma, infarction, and toxic necrosis can usually be diagnosed without a muscle biopsy, and in such cases surgical intervention may be inadvisable. Low-grade bacterial infections like pyomyositis are usually diagnosed without resorting to muscle biopsy, although needle aspiration may be done for bacteriologic diagnosis. Gram-negative necrotizing infections (gas gangrene) require surgical therapy rather than biopsy.

Sometimes a diagnostic muscle biopsy is performed in patients without clinical signs of myopathy who are suspected of having a systemic illness such as polyarteritis nodosa or sarcoidosis. Any convenient muscle can be chosen for this purpose.

Cutaneous Nerve Biopsy

TECHNIQUE. The processing and interpretation of a nerve biopsy specimen are even more specialized than the workup of a muscle biopsy, and this service is rarely available outside of a few university centers. Ordinarily, a segment of sural nerve is taken in the lower leg; the superficial radial nerve can also be biopsied at the wrist. Asbury and Johnson (1978) and Schaumburg and colleagues (1983) have described the technique of nerve biopsy and the methods of processing the tissue.

The paraffin-embedded sample of nerve is examined in transverse and longitudinal sections, looking for abnormalities of the connective tissue and blood vessels, signs of active nerve fiber degeneration, and qualitative evidence of selective myelin loss with preservation of axons.

Examination of cross-sections of plastic-embedded semithin sections allows the myelinated and unmyelinated nerve fibers to be counted, documenting any loss of large or small nerve fibers. Remyelination can be detected by the presence of abnormally thin myelin sheaths, and nerve fiber regeneration is revealed by the presence of small clusters of thinly myelinated axons.

Segmental demyelination and remyelination are most convincingly demonstrated by the laborious technique of examining single "teased"

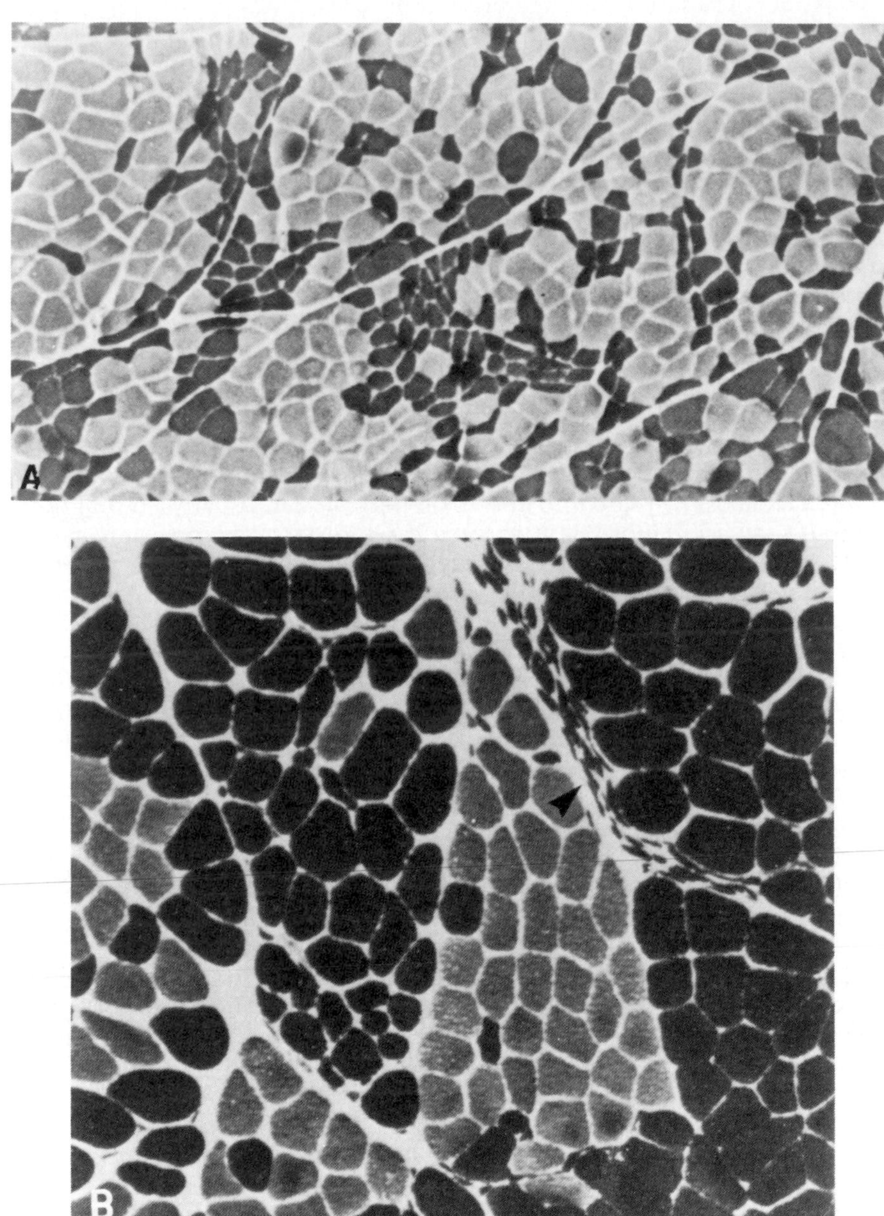

FIGURE 8. Photomicrographs of muscle pathology in subacute and chronic neuromuscular disorders. (*A*) In subacute neurogenic atrophy, mild fiber-type grouping and small-group atrophy occur, involving both type 1 and type 2 fibers (routine ATPase stain). (*B*) With chronic neurogenic atrophy, fiber-type grouping involving both type 1 and type 2 fibers occurs. A group of atrophic type 2 fibers is shown by the arrowhead (routine ATPase stain).

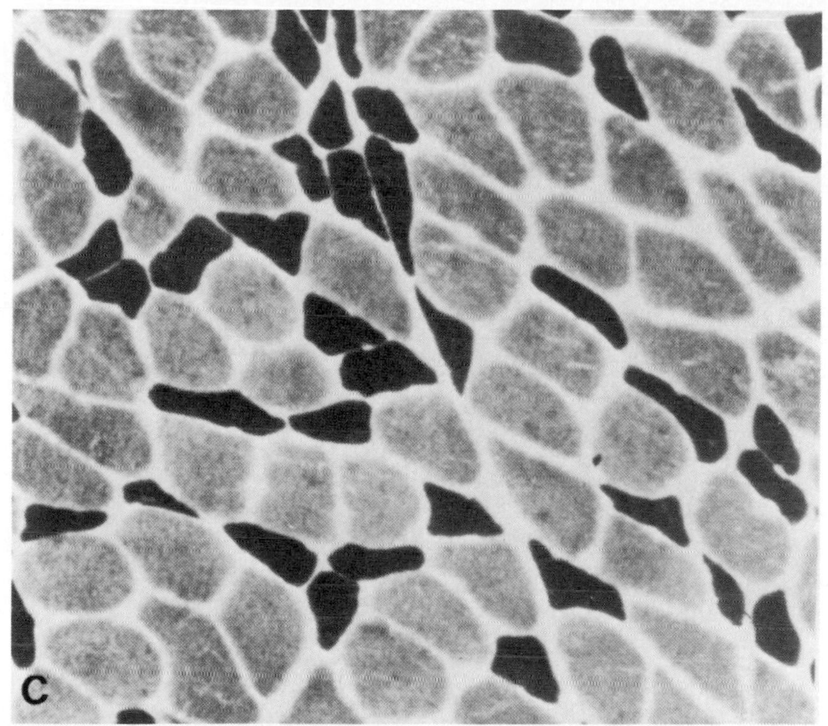

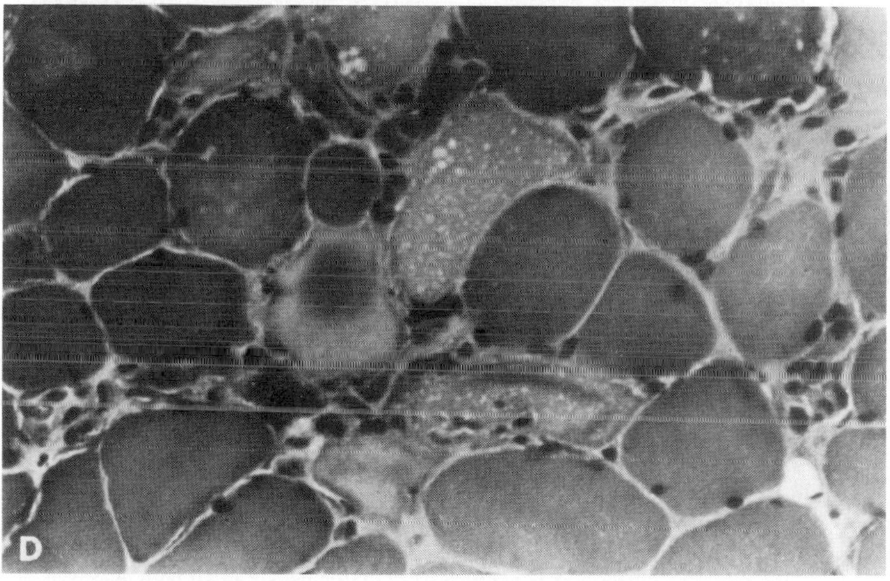

FIGURE 8 *continued.* (*C*) In atrophic myopathy (steroid therapy), selective atrophy of type 2 fibers is apparent (routine ATPase stain). (*D*) With subacute necrotic myopathy (potassium deficiency), there are vacuolar changes in several muscle fibers, and scattered degeneration of muscle fibers, some of which are undergoing phagocytosis (hematoxylin and eosin). *(Figure 8 continues.)*

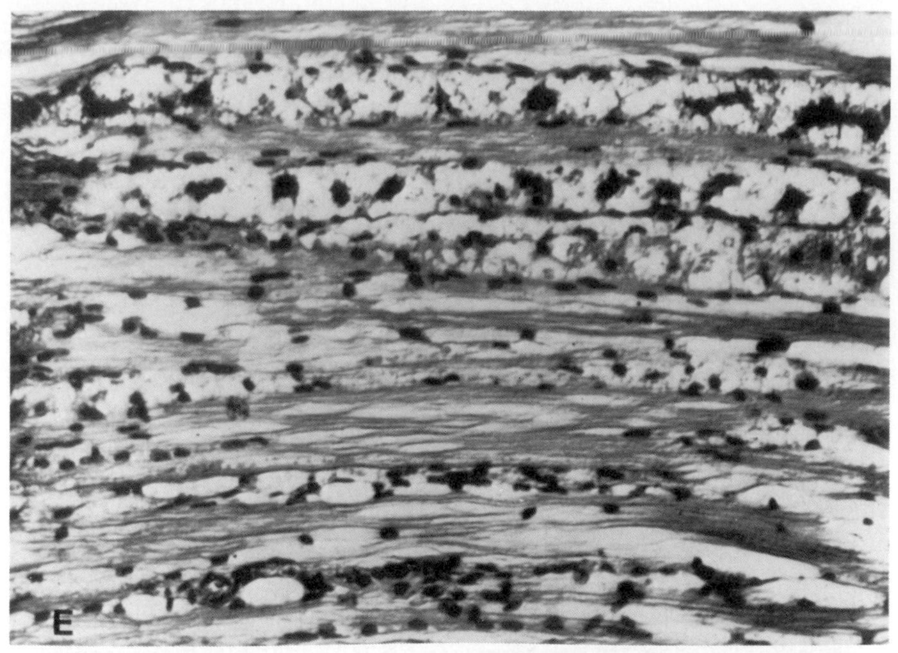

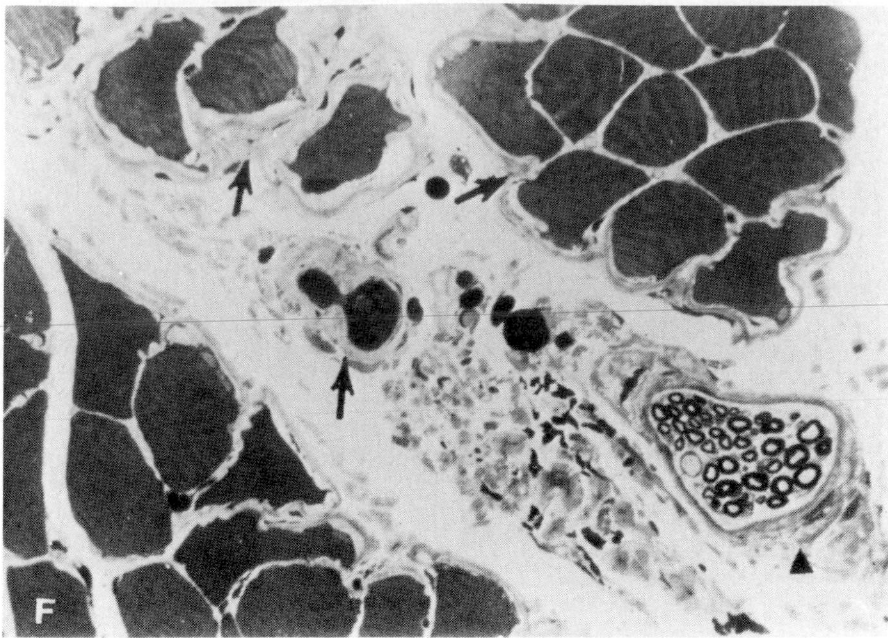

FIGURE 8 *continued.* (*E*) In degenerative myopathy (chloroquine therapy), a longitudinal section of paraffin-embedded muscle shows muscle fibers that are filled with large vacuoles, with many of the fibers degenerating (hematoxylin and eosin). (*F*) With infiltrative myopathy (amyloidosis), dense collections of amyloid surround and compress individual muscle fibers *(large arrows)* and a nerve fascicle *(arrowhead)* (methylene blue). (*A*, *B*, and *C* from Dubowitz and Brooke 1973, with permission. *D* from Atsumi, T., et al.: Neurology 29:1348, 1979, with permission. *E* from Hughes, J. T., et al.: Q. J. Med. 40:85, 1971, with permission. *F* from Ringel, S. P. and Claman, H. N.: Arch. Neurol. 39:413, 1982, with permission.)

nerve fibers mounted in longitudinal segments. In addition, the relation between mean internodal length (the distance between nodes of Ranvier) and nerve fiber diameter can be graphed. By this means, axonal degeneration with subsequent regeneration can be distinguished from chronic demyelination and remyelination.

APPLICATION. There are few indications for diagnostic nerve biopsy in patients with nonhereditary neuropathies. For polyneuropathies, the major indication is a clinical suspicion of subacute or chronic inflammatory polyneuropathy, especially when the clinical picture, nerve conduction results, or spinal fluid findings are ambiguous. (In unambiguous cases, nerve biopsy may be done for investigative purposes such as immunologic studies.) The pathology of purely axonal polyneuropathies is rarely informative except in the few diseases with specific findings, such as amyloidosis, sarcoidosis, and leprosy.

Sural nerve biopsies are sometimes performed to search for vasculitis in patients with mononeuropathy multiplex, but nerve biopsy is often superfluous in such cases. The diagnosis of ischemic mononeuropathy multiplex can usually be made on purely clinical grounds, and this syndrome is nearly always caused by either vasculitis or diabetes mellitus. A sural nerve biopsy will often confirm a strong clinical suspicion of vasculitis; however, a negative biopsy does not exclude vasculitis, since the vascular changes are distributed in a patchy, random fashion. When the clinical diagnosis of vasculitis is unclear, the diagnostic yield of nerve biopsy is quite low (Parry et al. 1980). It has been claimed that sural nerve conduction abnormalities can predict whether the biopsied nerve will show vasculitis (Wees et al. 1981). The published data are not convincing, however, and nerve conduction abnormalities in angiopathic neuropathy are usually due to Wallerian degeneration caused by much more proximal lesions.

REFERENCES

AMINOFF, MJ: *Electromyography.* In AMINOFF, MJ (ED): *Electrodiagnosis in Clinical Neurology.* Churchill Livingstone, New York, 1980, pp 197–228.

ASBURY, AK AND JOHNSON, PC: *Pathology of Peripheral Nerve.* WB Saunders, Philadelphia, 1978, pp 43–47, 268–281.

BLACK, JT, BHATT, GP, DEJESUS, PV, ET AL: *Diagnostic accuracy of clinical data, quantitative electromyography and histochemistry in neuromuscular diagnosis.* J Neurol Sci 21:59–70, 1974.

BROWNLOW, K AND ELEVITCH, FR: *Serum creatinine phosphokinase isoenzyme (CPK_2) in myositis. A report of six cases.* JAMA 230:1141–1144, 1974.

BRUNS, DE, MORGAN, WS, DAVIS, JE, ET AL: *Low apparent creatine kinase activity and prolonged lag phases in serum of patients with metastatic disease: Elimination by treatment of sera with sulfhydryl agents.* Clin Chem 22:1889–1895, 1976.

BUCHTHAL, F AND KAMIENIECKA, Z: *The diagnostic yield of quantified electromyography and quantified muscle biopsy in neuromuscular disorders.* Muscle Nerve 5:265–280, 1982.

CADNAPAPHORNCHAI, P, TAHER, S AND MCDONALD, FD: *Acute drug-associated rhabdomyolysis: An examination of its diverse renal manifestations and complications.* Am J Med Sci 280:66–72, 1980.

CHAIKIN, HL: *Rhabdomyolysis secondary to drug overdose and prolonged coma.* South Med J 73:990–994, 1980.

CLARK, JG, SUMERLING, MD, SEGAR, WE, ET AL: *Muscle necrosis and calcification in acute renal failure due to barbiturate intoxication.* Br Med J 2:214–215, 1966.

CONRADI, S, GRIMBY, L AND LUNDEMO, G: *Pathophysiology of fasciculations in ALS as studied by electromyography of single motor units.* Muscle Nerve 5:202–208, 1982.

DAUBE, JR: *Nerve conduction studies.* In AMINOFF, MJ (ED): *Electrodiagnosis in Clinical Neurology.* Churchill Livingstone, New York, 1980, pp 229–264.

DENNY-BROWN, D: *Clinical problems in neuromuscular physiology.* Am J Med 15:368–390, 1953.

DUBOWITZ, V: *Muscle Disorders in Childhood.* WB Saunders, Philadelphia, 1978, pp 14–17.

DUBOWITZ, V AND BROOKE, MH: *Muscle Biopsy: A Modern Approach.* WB Saunders, Philadelphia, 1973.

EKBOM, KA: *Restless legs.* In VINKEN, PJ and BRUYN, GW (EDS): *Handbook of Clinical Neurology, Vol 8.* North-Holland Publishing, Amsterdam, 1970, pp 311–320.

FROHLICH, J: *Prolonged illness and creatine kinase activity.* Clin Chem 21:1343–1344, 1975.

FROST, FA, JESSEN, B AND SIGGAARD-ANDERSEN, J: *A control, double-blind comparison of mepivacaine versus saline injections for myofascial pain.* Lancet i:499–501, 1980.

GARCIA, W: *Elevated creatine phosphokinase levels associated with large muscle mass. Another pitfall in evaluating the clinical significance of total serum CPK activity.* JAMA 228:1396, 1974.

GENANT, HK, WILSON, JS, BOVILL, EG, ET AL: *Computed tomography of the musculoskeletal system.* J Bone Joint Surg 62-A:1088–1101, 1980.

HECKMATT, JZ, DUBOWITZ, V AND LEEMAN, S: *Detection of pathological change in dystrophic muscle with B-scan ultrasound imaging.* Lancet i:1389–1390, 1980.

HINDERKS, GJ AND FROHLICH, J: *Low serum creatine kinase values associated with administration of steroids.* Clin Chem 25:2050–2051, 1979.

JOCKERS-WRETOU, E, GRABERT, K, MULLER, E, ET AL: *Serum creatine kinase isoenzyme pattern in nervous system atrophies and neuromuscular disorders.* Clin Chim Acta 73:183–186, 1976.

KASAI, K: *Serum myoglobin level in altered thyroid states.* J Clin Endocrinol Metab 48:1–4, 1979.

KIESSLING, WR, RICKER, K, PFLUGHAUPT, KW, ET AL: *Serum myoglobin in primary and secondary skeletal muscle disorders.* J Neurol 224:229–233, 1981.

KIMURA, J: *Electrodiagnosis in Diseases of Nerve and Muscle: Principles and Practice.* FA Davis, Philadelphia, 1983.

KNOCHEL, JP: *Rhabdomyolysis and myoglobinuria.* Ann Rev Med 33:435–443, 1982.

KULA, R, LINE, BR, SIEGEL, BA, ET AL: *^{99m}Tc-diphosphonate scanning of soft tissue in neuromuscular diseases.* Neurology 26:370, 1976.

LANG, H (ED): *Creatine Kinase Isoenzymes: Pathophysiology and Clinical Application.* Springer-Verlag, Berlin, 1981.

LANG, H AND WURZBURG, U: *Creatine kinase, an enzyme of many forms.* Clin Chem 28:1439–1447, 1982.

LARCA, LJ, COPPOLA, JT AND HONIG, S: *Creatine kinase MB isoenzyme in dermatomyositis: A noncardiac source.* Ann Intern Med 94:341–343, 1981.

LAURSEN, K AND REITER, S: *Computed tomography in soft tissue disorders of the lower extremities.* Acta Orthop Scand 51:881–885, 1980.

LAYZER, RB: *Motor unit hyperactivity states.* In VINKEN, PJ AND BRUYN, GW (EDS): *Handbook of Clinical Neurology, Vol. 41.* North-Holland Publishing, Amsterdam, 1979, pp 295–316.

LAYZER, RB: *Muscle pain, cramps and fatigue.* In ENGEL, AG AND BANKER, BQ (EDS): *Myology.* McGraw-Hill, New York, 1984 (in press).

LEWIT, K: *The needle effect in the relief of myofascial pain.* Pain 6:83–90, 1979.

MARSH, WC, MARSH, NJ, MOORE, A, ET AL: *Elevated serum creatine phosphokinase in subjects with McLeod syndrome.* Vox Sang 40:403–411, 1981.

MATTHEWS, WB: *Treatment of the restless legs syndrome with clonazepam.* Br Med J 1:751, 1979.

MELAMED, I, ROMEM, Y, KEREN, G, ET AL: March myoglobinemia: A hazard to renal function. Arch Intern Med 142:1277–1279, 1982.

MERONEY, WH, AVERY, GK, SEGAR, WE, ET AL: *The acute calcification of traumatized muscle with particular reference to acute posttraumatic renal insufficiency.* J Clin Invest 36:825–832, 1957.

MOON, KL JR, GENANT, HK, HELMS, CA, ET AL: *Musculoskeletal applications of nuclear magnetic resonance.* Radiology 147:161–171, 1983.

MUNSAT, TL, BALOH, R, PEARSON, CM, ET AL: *Serum enzyme alterations in neuromuscular disorders.* JAMA 226:1536–1543, 1973.

NANJI, AA: *Serum creatine kinase isoenzymes: A review.* Muscle Nerve 6:83–90, 1983.

NANJI, AA AND BLANK, D: *Low serum creatine kinase activity in patients with alcoholic liver disease.* Clin Chem 27:1954, 1981.

NOEBELS, JL AND PRINCE, DA: *Presynaptic origin of penicillin after-discharges at mammalian nerve terminals.* Brain Res 138:59–74, 1977.

NORREGAARD-HANSEN, K AND HEIN-SORENSEN, O: *Significance of serum myoglobin in neuromuscular diseases and in carrier detection of Duchenne muscular dystrophy.* Acta Neurol Scand 66:259–266, 1982.

NORRIS, FH, JR, GASTEIGER, EL AND CHATFIELD, PO: *An electromyographic study of induced and spontaneous muscle cramps.* Electroencephalogr Clin Neurophysiol 9:139–147, 1957.

OLERUD, JE, HOMER, LD AND CARROLL, HW: *Serum myoglobin levels predicted from serum enzyme values.* JAMA 293:483–485, 1975.

OSTER, J: *Growing pain: A symptom and its significance.* Dan Med Bull 19:72–79, 1972.

PARRY, GJ, BROWN, MJ AND ASBURY, AK: *Diagnostic value of nerve biopsy in mononeuritis multiplex.* Neurology 31(2):129–130, 1980.

PEIFFER, J AND BUNDSCHU, HD: *Umkehrbar Muskelverkalkungen bei akutem Nierenversagen.* Klin Wochenschr 56:1125–1131, 1978.

PETERSON, HA: *Leg aches.* Pediatr Clin North Am 24:731–736, 1977.

PICKETT, JB: *Neuromuscular transmission.* In SUMNER, AJ (ED): *The Physiology of Peripheral Nerve Disease.* WB Saunders, Philadelphia, 1980, pp 238–264.

PRINEAS, J: *Polyneuropathies of undetermined cause.* Acta Neurol Scand 46(suppl 44):1–72, 1970.

ROTH, G: *The origin of fasciculations.* Ann Neurol 12:542–547, 1982.

RUSSELL, SM, BLEIWEISS, S, BROWNLOW, K ET AL: *Ischemic rhabdomyolysis and creatine phosphokinase isoenzymes. A diagnostic pitfall.* JAMA 235:632–633, 1976.

SCHAUMBURG, HH, SPENCER, PS AND THOMAS, PK: *Disorders of Peripheral Nerves.* FA Davis, Philadelphia, 1983.

SIEGEL, AJ AND DAWSON, DM: *Peripheral source of MB band of creatine kinase in alcoholic rhabdomyolysis. Nonspecificity of MB isoenzyme for myocardial injury in undiluted serum samples.* JAMA 244:580–582, 1980.

SIEGEL, AJ, SILVERMAN, LM AND HOLMAN, L: *Elevated creatine kinase MB isoenzyme levels in marathon runners. Normal myocardial scintigrams suggest noncardiac source.* JAMA 246:2049–2051, 1981.

SIEGEL, BA, ENGEL, WK AND DERRER, EC: *Localization of technetium-99m diphosphonate in acutely injured muscle.* Neurology 27:230–238, 1977.

SOMER, H, DUBOWITZ, V AND DONNER, M: *Creatine kinase isoenzymes in neuromuscular diseases.* J Neurol Sci 29:129–136, 1976.

STANDAERT, FG: *Post-tetanic repetitive activity in the cat soleus nerve. Its origin, course, and mechanism of generation.* J Gen Physiol 47:53–70, 1963.

TERMOTE, JL, BAERT, A, CROLLA, D, ET AL: *Computed tomography of the normal and pathologic muscular system.* Radiology 137:439–444, 1980.

TSUNG, SH: *Several conditions causing elevation of serum CK-MB and CK-BB.* Am J Clin Pathol 75:711–715, 1981.

VITA, G AND HARRIS, JB: *The uptake of 99m technetium diphosphonate into degenerating and regenerating muscle.* J Neurol Sci 51:339–354, 1981.

VUKANOVIC, S, HAUSER, H AND WETTSTEIN, P: *CT localization of myonecrosis for surgical decompression.* AJR 135:1298–1299, 1980.

WEES, SJ, SUNWOO, IN AND OH, SJ: *Sural nerve biopsy in systemic necrotizing vasculitis.* Am J Med 71:525–532, 1981.

WEI, N, PAVLIDIS, N, TSOKOS, G, ET AL: *Clinical significance of low creatine phosphokinase values in patients with connective tissue diseases.* JAMA 246:1921–1923, 1981.

WELCH, KMA AND GOLDBERG, DM: *Serum creatine phosphokinase in motor neurone disease.* Neurology 22:697–702, 1972.

YUNUS, M, MASI, AT, CALABRO, JJ, ET AL: *Primary* fibromyalgia *(fibrositis): Clinical study of 50 patients with matched normal controls.* Semin Arthritis Rheum 11:151–171, 1981.

ZYSKOWSKI, LP, BUNCH, TW, HOAGLUND, HC, ET AL: *McLeod syndrome (hemolysis, acanthocytosis, and increased serum creatine kinase): Potential confusion with polymyositis.* Arthritis Rheum 26:806–808, 1983.

Chapter 2

MINERAL AND ELECTROLYTE DISORDERS

POTASSIUM DISORDERS

Hypokalemia

Acute Hypokalemic Paralysis

The phenomenon of acute hypokalemic paralysis came to general notice in the late 1940s, beginning with a report of recurrent paralysis in patients with potassium-losing nephritis (Brown et al. 1944). This was followed by several articles describing hypokalemic paralysis during treatment of diabetic ketoacidosis (Holler 1946; Nicholson and Branning 1947; Tuynman and Wilhelm 1948; Danowski et al. 1949; Stephens 1949). In time, transient or episodic paralysis was described in every major variety of potassium depletion: chronic diarrhea (Perkins et al. 1950), ammonium chloride therapy (Goulon et al. 1962), renal tubular acidosis (Owen and Verner 1960), ureterosigmoidostomy (Angeloni and Scott 1960), primary aldosteronism (Conn 1963), Bartter's syndrome (Cannon et al. 1968), licorice toxicity (Conn et al. 1968), treatment with amphotericin B (McChesney and Marquardt 1964), and hemodialysis for chronic renal failure (Wiegand et al. 1981). Paralysis seems to occur in patients with metabolic acidosis as readily as in those with alkalosis. In all these cases, however, there has been a background of chronic potassium deficiency; paralysis does not seem to occur from acute hypokalemia alone.

CLINICAL FEATURES. Muscle weakness develops over the course of several hours or days, often beginning slowly and then accelerating rapidly. In mild cases only the legs are weak; as weakness increases it involves the arms, trunk, neck, and even the thoracic and diaphragmatic muscles. Bulbar weakness occurs in very severe cases, but ocular movements are always spared. The sequence in which muscle weakness develops is unpredictable;

in patients being treated for diabetic acidosis, for example, respiratory weakness is often the first sign of paralysis, and though ascending paralysis is common, the arms can become weak before the legs. Generally the proximal limb muscles are weaker than the distal muscles. The tendon reflexes are reduced and then abolished, but there are no sensory symptoms or signs, and pain is mild or absent. The patient remains completely alert unless there is an additional metabolic disturbance such as severe acidosis or alkalosis.

The serum potassium concentration is always low at the time of paralysis and is usually well below 3.0 mEq per liter. The serum creatine phosphokinase (CPK) activity may be normal or elevated. Electrophysiologic tests have not been reported, but animal experiments suggest that the electromyogram (EMG) would probably show myopathic changes in weak muscles, and the results of motor nerve stimulation would be normal except for a low amplitude of the evoked muscle response.

TREATMENT. Administration of potassium salts, such as potassium chloride, usually brings about an improvement in muscle power in an hour or two, and complete recovery takes place over a period of a few hours or days. In some cases recovery takes longer because of the presence of necrosis in muscle fibers. Although oral administration of potassium salts may suffice, most patients need to be given intravenous potassium chloride. The appropriate rate of infusion will depend on the estimated potassium deficit, the degree of hypokalemia, the integrity of renal function, and the clinical response. The usual recommendation is for dosages not to exceed 20 mEq potassium per hour, but rates as high as 80 mEq per hour have been given for short periods of time (Pullen et al. 1967) and a few patients require as much as 800 mEq potassium in 24 hours.

PATHOPHYSIOLOGY. The explanation found in most textbooks is that a low serum potassium level renders muscle fibers inexcitable by hyperpolarizing the muscle membrane. This explanation, plausible as it seems, is clearly erroneous, but the true mechanism is still not known.

The traditional reasoning is based on the fact that the resting membrane potential of nerve and muscle is mainly determined by the ratio of intracellular to extracellular potassium concentrations, as expressed in the Nernst equation:

$$E_m = -\frac{RT}{F} \ln \frac{[K]_i}{[K]_o} = -61.5 \log \frac{[K]_i}{[K]_o}$$

Thus, if the intracellular potassium concentration, $[K]_i$ is 140 mEq per liter, the calculated membrane potential, E_m, is −94 mV for a serum potassium of 4.1 mEq per liter and −119 mV for a serum potassium of 1.6 mEq per liter.*

The hyperpolarization caused by hypokalemia is instantaneous, however, and this fact raises two difficulties. In the first place, if the paralysis were due to hyper-

*The measured E_m is smaller than this because the Nernst equation does not take into account the small permeability to sodium. A more accurate prediction is given by a simplified Goldman equation:

$$E_m = -61.5 \log \frac{[K]_i}{[K]_o + P_{Na}/P_K \cdot [Na]_o}$$

where P_{Na}/P_K is the ratio of sodium permeability to potassium permeability. This ratio normally has a value of 0.01 to 0.02.

polarization it would come and go abruptly, but actually it does so very gradually. In the second place, at the same serum potassium concentration normal muscle would be more hyperpolarized than potassium-depleted muscle; consequently it should be easier to induce hypokalemic paralysis in a normal person than in a potassium-deficient subject. In fact, however, the reverse is the case.*

Experimental data show that the muscle membrane is indeed hyperpolarized in early potassium deficiency, but weakness does not result. Riecker and associates (1964) measured the muscle resting potential in five potassium-deficient patients with serum potassium concentrations between 2.25 and 3.1 mEq per liter; the mean membrane potential was −102 mV compared with a normal mean of −87.2 mV. In potassium-deficient rats, the mean membrane potential rose from −89.1 mV to −94.9 mV (Bilbrey et al. 1973). Neither the patients nor the animals were weak, however. In a rat diaphragm preparation, the twitch tension evoked by indirect or direct muscle stimulation was the same for extracellular potassium concentrations between 0.5 mM and 8 mM, even though the muscle resting potential was 32 percent higher in the low-potassium concentration (Otsuka and Ohtsuki 1970). Thus, a moderate degree of hyperpolarization does not impair muscle excitability, and some other explanation must be sought for the paralysis.

Early speculation about familial hypokalemic periodic paralysis also attributed this paralysis to hyperpolarization, until actual measurements of the membrane potential during paralysis revealed *depolarization,* which was of sufficient degree to render the muscle fibers electrically inexcitable (Riecker and Bolte 1966; Creutzfeldt et al. 1963). Muscle fibers from patients with familial periodic paralysis are depolarized by insulin, whereas normal muscle fibers are hyperpolarized; the depolarization depends on the presence of extracellular sodium and may thus reflect either an increased permeability to sodium or a decreased permeability to potassium, giving sodium permeability a greater influence on the membrane potential (Hofmann and Smith 1970). A similar phenomenon has been observed in experimental potassium depletion. When muscle from potassium-deficient rats is placed in a medium very low in potassium (0.5 mM), a slight hyperpolarization occurs; when insulin is added the membrane potential and the twitch tension decline gradually over the course of 30 to 60 minutes. The depolarization produced by insulin can be prevented by replacing external sodium ions with choline, an impermeant cation (Offerijns et al. 1958; Otsuka and Ohtsuki 1970; Kao and Gordon 1975).

The rat is actually a poor model for potassium-deficient paralysis because even severe potassium depletion does not produce noticeable weakness in the intact animal (Smith et al. 1950; Bilbrey et al. 1973). Dogs are better experimental subjects. Whether potassium deficiency is produced by administration of deoxycorticosterone (Ferrebee et al. 1940) or by dietary deprivation (Smith et al. 1950), dogs develop spontaneous attacks of hypokalemic weakness, which can be reversed by administration of potassium, and paralytic attacks can be provoked by shrill noise or by injection of adrenaline (Smith et al. 1950). Bilbrey and colleagues (1973) compared the effects of progressive potassium depletion in rats and dogs. In rats, the mean membrane potential rose from −89 mV to −95 mV after severe potassium depletion, and the animals did not appear weak. In dogs, a loss of 10 to 14 percent of the total body potassium increased the mean membrane potential from −90 mV to −92 mV, but when the potassium deficit reached 20 to 25 percent, the dogs developed severe muscular weakness, and the mean membrane potential fell to −55 mV.

Thus, it is probable that the paralysis of potassium-deficient muscle results from depolarization of the muscle membrane, which renders the muscle fiber inexcitable. In fact, excitability can be temporarily restored by electrically hyperpolarizing the fiber with an intracellular microelectrode (Kao and Gordon 1975). But why is the membrane depolarized, and why does insulin depolarize potassium-deficient muscle fibers when it hyperpolarizes normal muscle fibers? To answer these ques-

*With a serum sodium of 140 mEq per liter, the E_m calculated by the modified Goldman equation is −86 mV in a normal person with $[K]_i$ = 140 and $[K]_o$ = 4.1. With $[K]_i$ = 140 and $[K]_o$ = 1.6, E_m = 102 mV. With $[K]_i$ = 105 and $[K]_o$ = 1.6, E_m = −95 mV.

tions it is necessary to examine the permeability changes that take place in skeletal muscle during chronic potassium depletion.

During the induction of potassium deficiency, muscle loses potassium and gains sodium; as this happens, the membrane sodium-potassium pump ought to be stimulated by the elevated internal sodium concentration (Sjodin and Ortiz 1975). The pump is electrogenic (i.e., hyperpolarizing), so that the membrane potential would be equal to the sum of the ionic diffusion potential (calculated by the Goldman equation) and the electrogenic pump potential (Akaike 1979). Actually, the membrane potential of potassium-deficient rat muscle in vivo closely approximates the ionic diffusion potential; only when the muscle is removed from the body and studied in vitro is substantial hyperpolarization observed (Akaike 1979). Recently Akaike (1981) showed that, during chronic potassium depletion, pump electrogenesis is inhibited by the central nervous system via α-adrenergic innervation, forcing muscle to give up potassium in exchange for sodium. The potassium lost by skeletal muscle presumably helps to maintain the brain potassium concentration while the total body content of potassium gradually falls. Rats are able to suppress the muscle sodium-potassium pump even when 40 percent of the muscle potassium has been replaced by sodium; the membrane is only mildly hyperpolarized, and muscle excitability remains normal. Without this inhibitory mechanism, the stimulated sodium-potassium pump would draw a large amount of extracellular potassium into muscle, greatly reducing the serum potassium concentration and hyperpolarizing the muscle membrane.

In dogs (and presumably in humans) the adaptation of skeletal muscle to prolonged potassium depletion must be different from that in rats because severe potassium depletion causes membrane depolarization and paralysis. At that point the measured membrane potential is 40 percent lower than the calculated ionic diffusion potential, suggesting that the ratio of sodium permeability to potassium permeability is about eight times normal (Bilbrey et al. 1973). The membrane permeability to these ions has not been measured, so it is not known whether sodium conductance is increased or potassium conductance is decreased. Whichever is the cause, the altered permeability ratio could be a membrane adaptation to chronic potassium deficiency. As the permeability ratio (P_{Na}/P_K) rises, the ionic diffusion potential falls, and the membrane potential will also decline unless there is a corresponding rise in the electrogenic pump potential.

Based on these considerations, I have suggested a hypothetical sequence of events to account for attacks of hypokalemic paralysis in dogs and humans with chronic potassium deficiency (Layzer 1982). (1) In the early stage of potassium depletion, the muscle behaves like rat muscle: membrane permeabilities are unchanged, the sodium-potassium pump is inhibited, muscle potassium is gradually exchanged for sodium, and the membrane potential rises slightly (Bilbrey et al. 1973). (2) As potassium depletion continues, the membrane permeability ratio (P_{Na}/P_K) increases so that the ionic diffusion potential falls. At the same time the sodium-potassium pump begins to escape from α-adrenergic inhibition and to respond to the high internal sodium concentration, contributing a growing pump potential that offsets the declining diffusion potential. (3) The sodium-potassium pump, released from α-adrenergic inhibition, is susceptible to sudden surges of activity caused by the stimulating influences of adrenalin (Clausen and Flatman 1977) and insulin (Clausen and Kohn 1977). During one of these surges a large amount of extracellular potassium is pumped into muscle over a period of several hours, so that the serum potassium concentration falls acutely. (4) The low extracellular potassium concentration "turns off" the pump.* This event eliminates the pump potential, leaving only the reduced ionic diffusion potential, and the membrane potential therefore falls to about −55 mV, rendering the muscle inexcitable.

*In animal experiments, the sodium-potassium pump activity declines steeply when the extracellular potassium concentration is very low (Sjodin and Ortiz 1975). Another factor that may shut off the sodium-potassium pump is a defect of cellular energy metabolism, which is discussed in the next section.

Hypokalemic Myopathy

The first report of myoglobinuria in a patient with potassium depletion was published in 1955 (Achor and Smith 1955), but 15 years earlier Ferrebee and colleagues (1940) described patchy necrosis of muscle fibers in dogs dying from hypokalemic paralysis induced by administration of deoxycorticosterone. The dogs often had episodes of mild, transient weakness before the terminal episode of severe, generalized paralysis. From 1950 to 1970 there were many reports of hypokalemic myopathy or myoglobinuria resulting from the medical use of licorice and its derivatives, which were popular remedies for dyspepsia in Great Britain and France. (The active principle of licorice, glycyrrhizic acid, has strong mineralocorticoid properties.) Nearly every known cause of potassium depletion has been reported with the complication of hypokalemic myopathy; the manifestations are the same regardless of the origin of the potassium deficiency. Although there has not been a systematic study of the causes of hypokalemic myopathy, the commonest reason for severe hypokalemia in hospitalized patients is drug therapy, especially the use of diuretics (Lawson et al. 1979).

CLINICAL FEATURES. Muscle weakness progresses over a few weeks or months, predominantly in the trunk and proximal limb muscles. Pain is usually absent, but sometimes the muscles ache or feel tender. Muscle stretch reflexes, cranial muscles, and sensation remain normal. The serum enzymes are usually elevated to a moderate or marked degree. The electromyogram shows myopathic abnormalities that are often accompanied by fibrillations and other signs of muscle fiber irritability. Muscle biopsy shows necrosis and degeneration of scattered muscle fibers, scattered muscle fiber regeneration, and multiple vacuoles in some muscle fibers (Van Horn et al. 1970; Oh et al. 1971). This cluster of laboratory abnormalities has sometimes led to an erroneous diagnosis of polymyositis, especially when invasion of necrotic muscle fibers by inflammatory cells and phagocytes is mistaken for primary inflammation. Electron microscopy shows that the vacuoles within myofibers are derived from dilated portions of the longitudinal and transverse tubular systems (Atsumi et al. 1979).

In patients with myoglobinuria the history is similar except that the course is more fulminating, and muscle pain and tenderness are more likely to be present. Weakness may be quite severe, with areflexia and respiratory failure (Campion et al. 1972; Drutz et al. 1970; Mitchell 1971; Barnes and Leonard 1971).

With potassium replenishment, muscle power returns fairly rapidly even when myoglobinuria has occurred. Complete recovery occurs in 1 to 2 weeks in mild cases and in 3 to 4 weeks in more severe cases.

PATHOPHYSIOLOGY. The mechanism of muscle necrosis in hypokalemic myopathy is unknown. It is intriguing that patients with acute hypokalemic paralysis often have high serum enzymes at the time of admission to the hospital, suggesting that muscle necrosis begins around the same time that the membrane potential begins to fall. Could these events be related to a critical deficiency of cellular energy stores? Based on experiments with dogs, Knochel and Schlein (1972) attributed the muscle necrosis to an absence of exercise-induced hyperemia, which they ascribed to a reduced efflux of potassium from potassium-deficient muscle during exercise. In their view, muscle necrosis results from energy depletion caused by relative ischemia during exercise. However, Hazeyama and Sparks (1979) showed that potassium-deficient muscle produces very little tension and consumes little oxygen during exercise, suggesting that the muscle simply could not work hard enough to cause much vasodilatation. As yet, the dynamic properties and energy metabolism of potassium-deficient muscle have not been carefully evaluated. In two patients without overt myopathy, the muscle content of adenine nucleotides, creatine phosphate, glycogen, pyruvate, and lactate was normal (Bergström et al. 1976). However, adenosine triphosphate (ATP) generation is reduced in mitochondria obtained from heart and kidney of potassium-deficient animals (Aithal et al. 1977; Aithal and Toback 1978), and the normal aerobic inhibition of glycolysis (Pasteur effect) is depressed in the renal medulla (Toback et al. 1979). These organs are the other prime targets of tissue damage in chronic potassium deficiency. Clearly there is a need for more information about the state of muscle energy metabolism in potassium deficiency.

Tetany

Tetany is a common symptom in patients with hypokalemic alkalosis, and latent tetany can often be demonstrated in asymptomatic patients. The combination of potassium deficiency and alkalosis is encountered in patients with intestinal potassium wastage, diuretic therapy, aldosteronism, Bartter's syndrome, and licorice intoxication (Parker et al. 1980). Paradoxically, hypokalemia seems to protect patients against the clinical expression of hypocalcemic tetany, perhaps because hypokalemia has a stabilizing effect on nerve excitability (Fourman 1954). Thus, treatment of potassium deficiency with potassium salts may precipitate tetany in patients with hypocalcemia (Coërs et al. 1972) or even without hypocalcemia (Fourman and McCance 1955). (A more detailed discussion of tetany will be found later in this chapter.)

Hyperkalemia

Acute Hyperkalemic Paralysis

Generalized, flaccid paralysis is a rare complication of hyperkalemia, but more than 30 cases have been reported since the original article by Finch and Marchand (1943). Most of the cases have involved patients with chronic hyperkalemia caused by renal or adrenal insufficiency; acute hyperkalemia in a normokalemic patient is more likely to cause fatal cardiac arrhythmia than muscle weakness.

CLINICAL FEATURES. The clinical features of hyperkalemic paralysis have been carefully described by Bull and associates (1953) and by Mollaret and colleagues (1958a, 1958b). Typically a patient with chronic hyperkalemia becomes weak in the legs, and paralysis ascends and becomes generalized in the course of a few hours or days. Several authors have noted that during this state of flaccid paralysis, the muscles react readily—in fact, excessively—to pinching or percussion. The patient may be mentally alert, confused, or somnolent. Respiratory failure occurs in about half of the cases, and a few patients have exhibited unilateral or bilateral facial weakness or impaired swallowing. Rado and coworkers (1968) stated that lid lag was a characteristic feature. The muscle stretch reflexes are lost in the legs, and some patients are areflexic. Most patients complain of distal paresthesias; these may precede the onset of weakness and may have a painful, burning character that is more distressing than the paralysis. Distal loss of sensation is present in some of the patients with sensory symptoms.

The serum potassium level at the time of paralysis can be as low as 5.4 mEq per liter (Mollaret et al. 1958b), but in most of the cases the values were between 7.5 and 11.5 mEq per liter. After treatment to lower the serum potassium level, the weakness and paresthesias usually resolve within a few hours, even though the serum potassium level is still elevated. Sensation and reflexes may not return to normal for several days after muscle power is restored.

In patients with chronic renal or adrenal insufficiency, paralytic attacks have been precipitated by ingestion of potassium salts or fruit juices, transfusion of old blood, or treatment with triamterene (Cohen 1966) or spironolactone (Rado et al. 1968). Acidosis aggravates hyperkalemia by promoting efflux of potassium ions from cells in exchange for hydrogen ions. A few patients have intermittent attacks of weakness with spontaneous recovery (Rado et al. 1968; Van Dellen and Purnell 1969), but usually the hyperkalemic crisis ends in death unless treated vigorously.

TREATMENT. The treatment of acute hyperkalemic paralysis depends on the underlying cause of chronic hyperkalemia, the magnitude of the hyperkalemia, and the electrocardiographic findings. The immediate object is to prevent ventricular asystole or fibrillation; arrhythmia is unlikely to occur if the serum potassium is under 8 mEq per liter, but the serum potassium is usually above this level. For a rapid effect, 10-percent calcium gluconate should be injected intravenously under continuous cardiac monitoring at a rate of 2 ml per minute, to a total of 10 to 30 ml, depending on the electrocardiographic response. Calcium protects the cardiac conduction system but does not lower the serum potassium or improve muscle power. Next, one or two ampules of sodium bicarbonate (44 mEq per ampule) can be given intravenously to promote the intracellular shift of potassium. A rapid infusion of 200 to 500 ml of 10-percent glucose, with 10 to 15 units of regular insulin and perhaps additional sodium bicarbonate, will take effect in an hour and reduce the serum potassium concentration by 1 to 2 mEq per liter for several hours. To remove potassium from the body, Kayexalate (sodium polystyrene sulfonate resin) can be given by mouth or by retention enema, or the patient can be subjected to hemodialysis or peritoneal dialysis (Conglione 1978; Levinsky 1966). If the serum potassium is below 8 mEq per liter, more leisurely measures may be adequate. A hypoadrenal patient should, of course, be given 100 mg hydrocortisone intravenously at once, and the initial intravenous fluid should contain isotonic saline in addition to glucose, insulin, and sodium bicarbonate. Patients with diabetes mellitus should not be given intravenous glucose without insulin, because hyperglycemia produces paradoxical hyperkalemia in insulin-deficient patients (Goldfarb et al. 1976; Nicolis et al. 1981).

Pathophysiology. Despite its resemblance to hypokalemic paralysis, acute hyperkalemic paralysis does not seem to be caused by muscular inexcitability. Although electrophysiologic tests have not been performed during a paralytic attack, the mechanical irritability of the paralyzed muscles is incompatible with the electrical inexcitability found in acquired hypokalemic paralysis and in hereditary hypokalemic and hyperkalemic periodic paralysis. Furthermore, there are many indications of peripheral nerve involvement: painful distal paresthesias, sensory loss, areflexia, and a peripheral type of facial weakness. These clinical features strongly suggest that hyperkalemic paralysis is a peripheral nerve disorder. Of course it is possible that both muscles and nerves are paralyzed in some cases, but this has not been demonstrated.

In laboratory experiments, increasing the extracellular potassium concentration reduces the resting membrane potential of both muscle and nerve. In a rat nerve-diaphragm preparation, raising the extracellular potassium concentration from 4.0 to 8.0 mEq per liter reduced the muscle membrane potential by 9 percent and *increased* the muscle twitch tension by 25 percent; at 16 mM potassium the membrane potential fell by 24 percent and the muscle became inexcitable to indirect or direct stimulation (Otsuka and Ohtsuki 1970).

Recently Troni (1978) carried out electrophysiologic studies in rabbits made hyperkalemic by the continuous intravenous infusion of potassium chloride. The animals became moderately weak 60 to 90 minutes after the start of the infusion, when the serum potassium concentration was in the range of 8.2 to 9.4 mEq per liter, but at that time there was no significant reduction of muscle or nerve excitability, and the muscle response to nerve stimulation was preserved, although there was a decreasing response at high rates of nerve stimulation. However, as weakness increased there was a progressive decline in the number of voluntary motor unit potentials recorded in postural muscles of the neck, and the H-reflex response declined markedly. The findings suggested an impairment of reflex excitability of motor neurons, perhaps caused by a failure of central synaptic transmission. These experiments were conducted with normal rabbits subjected to acute hyperkalemia, whereas the human syndrome of hyperkalemic paralysis usually occurs in patients with chronic hyperkalemia, in some of whom the serum potassium concentration is well below the level that would cause paralysis in a normal person. Perhaps some metabolic adaptation to chronic hyperkalemia plays a role in the development of paralysis, but this has not been studied.

SODIUM DISORDERS

Hypernatremia

Two patients with central neurogenic hypernatremia have been reported to have episodes of generalized weakness resembling periodic paralysis. Both patients had defective thirst function from lesions of the hypothalamus. In one patient the defect appeared after surgical treatment of a ruptured aneurysm of the anterior communicating artery (Pleasure and Goldberg 1966), while the other patient had the somatic features of Fröhlich's syndrome without evidence of a structural lesion (Maddy and Winternitz 1971). On many occasions the patients became weak when their serum sodium concentration rose to between 170 and 216 mEq per liter; muscle power returned over the course of several days as their water intake increased and serum sodium levels returned toward normal. During the periods of severe weakness the serum potassium level was slightly reduced (3.0 to 3.2 mEq per liter), and in one patient the ECG showed hypokalemic changes. Electrophysiologic studies were not performed during paralysis, and the mechanism of the muscular weakness was not elucidated.

BARIUM POISONING

Ingestion of soluble barium salts produces rapidly progressive, generalized paralysis accompanied by severe hypokalemia; death may ensue in a few hours from cardiac arrest or respiratory paralysis, unless vigorous therapy is given with intravenous potassium. Barium poisoning has resulted from suicidal ingestion of barium sulfide, which is used as a depilatory agent (Gould et al. 1973), and several large outbreaks of poisoning have been traced to the accidental contamination of foodstuffs with barium carbonate, which is used as a rat poison (Morton 1945; Lewis and Bar-Khayim 1964; Diengott et al. 1964). The most remarkable example of mass barium poisoning, however, came to light in 1943 in the Szechuan province of China, where an endemic form of periodic paralysis known as "Pa Ping" was traced to massive contamination of table salt by barium chloride. Chemical analysis of the salt, which was produced locally from brine wells, showed that it contained up to 25 percent barium chloride (Du and Dung 1943). Struck by the resemblance of these cases to familial periodic paralysis, Huang (1943) administered potassium citrate intravenously to two patients suffering from Pa Ping and observed rapid and complete recovery of muscle strength. Other Chinese physicians demonstrated that the same paralytic syndrome could be produced in dogs and rabbits by oral or parenteral administration of barium chloride (Ku et al. 1943; Chou and Chin 1943). It was not until 1964, however, that hypokalemia was documented in patients during an outbreak of food poisoning in Israel (Diengott et al. 1964).

The lethal dose of soluble barium salts taken by mouth is not well established, but 12 to 15 g can produce respiratory paralysis (Gould et al. 1973; Berning 1975). There is a fairly consistent sequence of toxic symptoms, though the rapidity and severity vary a good deal. Within 1 or 2 hours after ingestion of the poison, patients experience tingling around the mouth, diarrhea, vomiting, and colicky abdominal pain. Arterial hypertension is generally observed. In 2 or 3 hours the tingling moves from the face to the hands, the pupillary reactions are impaired, muscle stretch reflexes become depressed, muscle twitching is noticeable, and flaccid weakness begins to spread through the muscles of the upper and lower extremities. In some cases complete flaccid quadriplegia develops within a few hours, in other cases paralysis does not become severe until the second day of illness, and in mild cases the weakness remains confined to one or two limbs. In some patients reflexes are retained until severe weakness develops, and sensation is always preserved despite subjective paresthesias. In one case paralysis involved one hemidiaphragm, the face, and the oropharyngeal muscles (Gould et al. 1973), but usually the cranial muscles are spared.

The Chinese cases of Pa Ping included patients with the acute pattern of illness, but many other patients experienced recurrent episodes of paralysis during sleep, especially after having consumed a heavy meal or wine on the previous evening. The resemblance to periodic paralysis was thus quite striking. Those cases may have been examples of chronic barium poisoning.

Serum potassium levels during generalized paralysis have ranged from 1.2 to 2.7 mEq per liter (Berning 1975; Gould et al. 1973; Diengott et al. 1964; Wetherill et al. 1981). Except for ECG changes of hypokalemia there are no other significant laboratory abnormalities.

In mild poisoning, spontaneous improvement begins a few hours after the onset of symptoms and recovery is complete in 24 to 36 hours. Even quadriplegic patients have recovered without treatment, but those patients received potassium permanganate as a "gastric astringent" (Morton 1945). In severe cases, death results from respiratory paralysis or from cardiac asystole. Treatment consists of intravenous administration of large amounts of potassium chloride. It is not clear whether it is necessary to "flush out" the barium by forced diuresis. One patient was treated successfully simply by administration of potassium chloride, in a total dose of 100 mEq (Diengott et al. 1964); another was given 200 mEq potassium chloride over 8 hours, together with sodium sulfate, 30 g by mouth and 30 g IV (Berning 1975); and a third patient received 260 mEq potassium chloride, 6.5 liters of saline, and 160 mg of furosemide during the first 19 hours (Gould et al. 1973). Intravenous administration of sulfates may cause acute renal failure by precipitating barium sulfate in the renal collecting system, so it is safer to give only oral sulfates to precipitate unabsorbed barium (Wetherill et al. 1981).

PATHOPHYSIOLOGY. Clinical clues suggest that the paralysis affects muscles or neuromuscular transmission rather than nerves, although there may also be nerve involvement since paresthesias are common, and one patient had hemidiaphragmatic paralysis. The success of potassium therapy indicates that the muscle paralysis is related to the hypokalemia, and this has been verified in dog experiments (Roza and Berman 1971). When barium chloride was infused intravenously at a rate of 1 μmole per kg per minute, the plasma potassium concentration decreased by 0.3 to 2.1 mEq per liter over a period of 90 minutes. Simultaneous infusion of potassium chloride at a rate of 30 μmole per kg per minute maintained a stable plasma potassium concentration and prevented cardiac arrhythmias and skeletal muscle paralysis. (However, hypertension, diarrhea, skeletal muscle twitching, and premature ventricular contractions were not prevented and were presumed to be due to "direct stimulation" by barium.) Roza and Berman detected hypokalemia as early as three minutes following intravenous injection of a large amount of barium chloride. Since urinary excretion of potassium did not increase, it can be assumed that the hypokalemia results from a shift of extracellular potassium into intracellular compartments, and this was documented in the case of red blood cells.

Most of our information about the effect of barium on potassium fluxes comes from studies of isolated frog muscles, but the findings may well have more general application. Barium greatly reduces the passive permeability of muscle fibers to potassium ions but has little or no effect on permeability to sodium or chloride ions, or on active transport of sodium and potassium against their concentration gradients (Sperelakis et al. 1967; Henderson and Volle 1972; Sjodin and Ortiz 1975). Blocking the passive potassium channel should have two effects. First, the contribution of potassium ions to the diffusion potential (the membrane potential calculated by the Goldman equation) would be reduced, tending to depolarize the membrane. Second, since passive efflux and influx of potassium are reduced equally (Henderson and Volle 1972), the basal activity of the sodium-potassium pump would cause a net influx of potassium.

Actually, barium does not alter the resting membrane potential when the external potassium concentration is 2.5 mM, which is normal for the frog. However, if the sodium-potassium pump is blocked by the addition of a cardiac glycoside, barium produces about 30 mV of depolarization (Henderson 1974). Thus, the failure of barium to depolarize the muscle membrane in a normal-potassium medium is largely due to the electrogenic effect of the sodium-potassium pump. Furthermore, when the external potassium concentration is 0.5 mM, barium causes the membrane potential to fall from −110 mV to −60 mV, in the presence or absence of a cardiac glycoside (Henderson 1974). This large depolarization probably results from two factors. First, as a competitive inhibitor of potassium conductance, barium is more effective at low potassium concentrations (Henderson and Volle 1972). Second, the rate of active transport of potassium into muscle declines steeply as the external potassium concentration is reduced below 5 mM (Sjodin and Ortiz 1975). In other words, lowering the external potassium concentration reduces the hyperpolarizing effect of the electrogenic sodium-potassium pump, unmasking the depolarizing effect of the reduced potassium permeability.

On the basis of these observations it is possible to construct a speculative scheme of the events produced by barium poisoning in the intact mammal (Layzer 1982), while one must recognize that barium may not act identically in mammalian muscle. (1) Barium blocks the passive potassium conductance of muscle. The membrane potential remains normal at first, owing to the basal activity of the sodium-potassium pump. (2) Since barium inhibits passive efflux and influx of potassium equally, basal sodium-potassium pumping results in a net uptake of potassium. (3) Because the mass of skeletal muscle is very large (about 40 percent of body weight) the shift of extracellular potassium into muscle soon lowers the plasma potassium concentration. (4) As the plasma potassium concentration falls, barium blockade of potassium permeability becomes more effective and the ionic diffusion potential is increasingly dominated by the sodium conductance, which exerts a depolarizing influence on the membrane potential. At the same time the falling concentration of plasma potassium rapidly shuts off the sodium-potassium pump, so that the membrane potential is now determined by the ionic diffusion potential, which has fallen to less than −60 mV. At this membrane potential the muscle is inexcitable, and paralysis ensues.

In the reported cases of barium poisoning, the serum potassium level remained low until a very large amount of potassium chloride had been administered. Barium and potassium appear to compete in their interaction with the potassium conductance channels. Presumably the adminstered potassium continues to enter muscle until the serum potassium level rises high enough to displace barium from the potassium channels. Moreover, raising the serum potassium level may allow the muscle membrane to repolarize by increasing electrogenic sodium-potassium pumping. Administration of a large volume of fluid also allows barium to be "flushed out" by the resulting diuresis.

CALCIUM DISORDERS

Hypercalcemia

Neuromuscular symptoms are very common in patients with hypercalcemia, but it is difficult to find first-hand descriptions of genuine muscle weakness. In a hospital-based survey of patients with hypercalcemia caused by cancer or hyperparathyroidism, 67 to 73 percent of the patients complained of fatigue and 24 to 36 percent complained of weakness (Fisken et al. 1981). Bartter (1953) stated that weakness, hyporeflexia, hypotonia, and sensory hyposensitivity, "which occur with great regularity in hyperparathyroidism and hypercalcemia of other causes, represent, of course, the counterparts of the signs of peripheral nerve (and reflex arc) hypersensitivity in hypocalcemia." Henson (1966) recorded subjective weakness in 31 percent of patients with parathyroid tumor, but did not specify how many of them had objective weakness; he evidently believed that hypercalcemia was responsible for the symptoms, but the neuromuscular signs that he described were identical to those described by Vicale (1949) in patients with chronic myopathy caused by osteomalacia or hyperparathyroidism, a muscle disorder not presently considered to be caused by hypercalcemia.

Profound muscle weakness is said to occur in severe hypercalcemic states, along with nausea, vomiting, constipation, polyuria, polydipsia, confusion, or coma (O'Dorisio 1978; Kelly and Zarconi 1981). Unfortunately, detailed clinical descriptions of this syndrome are lacking, and there are no electrophysiologic studies, so that it is impossible to state whether patients have asthenia, upper motor neuron weakness, or a motor unit disorder. A hyperparathyroid patient described by Murphy and associates (1960) became weak in the legs and arms over a period of 1 month until he was nearly paraplegic with a serum calcium concentration of 17 mg per dl. His limbs were flaccid but the reflexes were hyperactive and there were bilateral Babinski's signs. The patient recovered completely within a week after parathyroid surgery. Two patients with multiple myeloma (Merigan and Hayes 1961) presented with severe confusion, muscle rigidity, hyperactive reflexes with normal plantar reflexes, and asterixis. The serum calcium levels were 18.2 mg per dl and 19.8 mg per dl, respectively, and the neurologic disturbances resolved gradually as the calcium levels returned toward normal. These are the only well-described cases that I have been able to discover, and they suggest that dysfunction of the central nervous system is the principal cause of neuromuscular symptoms in hypercalcemic states.

Recently, Frame and colleagues (1981) reported a patient with self-induced hypercalcemia that resulted from oral ingestion of calcium. With a serum calcium concentration of over 20 mg per dl, the patient was described as "most cooperative," but there was no mention of muscle weakness. This case suggests that even severe hypercalcemia may not have any important neuromuscular consequences.

Hypocalcemia

Tetany

The syndrome of hypocalcemic tetany has been recognized since 1815 (Isgren 1976), and in Western countries the disorder was very common in the nineteenth and early twentieth centuries because of a dietary deficiency of vitamin D. Today the full picture of hypocalcemic tetany is rarely seen, since even surgical (postoperative) hypoparathyroidism is uncommon, and treatment with vitamin D and calcium has largely eliminated the problem of chronic hypocalcemia. The peripheral manifestations of tetany fascinated clinicians for many decades, and as a result of their studies the clinical features of peripheral tetany are well defined and reasonably well understood.

CLINICAL FEATURES. Generalized tetany may occur spontaneously or may be provoked by hyperventilation. Kugelberg emphasized the regular sequence of symptoms in a typical attack:

> First of all, tingling sets in around the mouth and, peripherally, in the extremities. The tingling then increases in intensity, while it spreads proximally up over the extremities and over the face. Somewhat later a sensation of tension or spasm appears in the muscles of the mouth, the hands and the lower portion of the legs. This sensation of spasm increases in intensity and spreads the same way as the tingling. Somewhat later a tonic spasm sets in, commencing in the muscles in which the sensation of spasm first occurred. If the attack is aggravated, the spasms spread proximally up over the extremities to the trunk. Fasciculation in the muscles, verging on spasm, is common, though but little noticeable in man. Spasm in the laryngeal muscles may set in at an early stage, as may epileptic fits. (Kugelberg 1946)

The typical motor postures evoked by tetany (carpopedal spasm, main d'accoucheur) result from two factors: the intensity of spasm is greatest in the distal muscles, and the stronger muscles prevail over weaker antagonists. In the upper extremities one observes adduction of the thumb and fingers, extension of the interphalangeal joints, flexion of the metacarpal-phalangeal joints, and later flexion of the wrists and elbows (Fig. 9). In the lower extremities there is flexion of the foot and toes followed by equinovarus deviation at the ankles. If the spasms spread to the trunk the result is hyperextension of the back and neck (opisthotonus). The special susceptibility of the laryngeal muscles may be related to the length of the recurrent laryngeal nerves.

Latent Tetany. Latent tetany can be uncovered in several ways: by hyperventilation, which induces alkalosis; by ischemia, produced by compressing a limb with an inflated cuff or ligature; and by percussion or electrical stimulation of a nerve. These methods form the basis of the well-known diagnostic signs of latent tetany. The Trousseau's test is performed by inflating a pneumatic cuff, placed high up on the upper arm, about 20 torr above systolic pressure. In a patient with latent tetany, sensory symptoms and

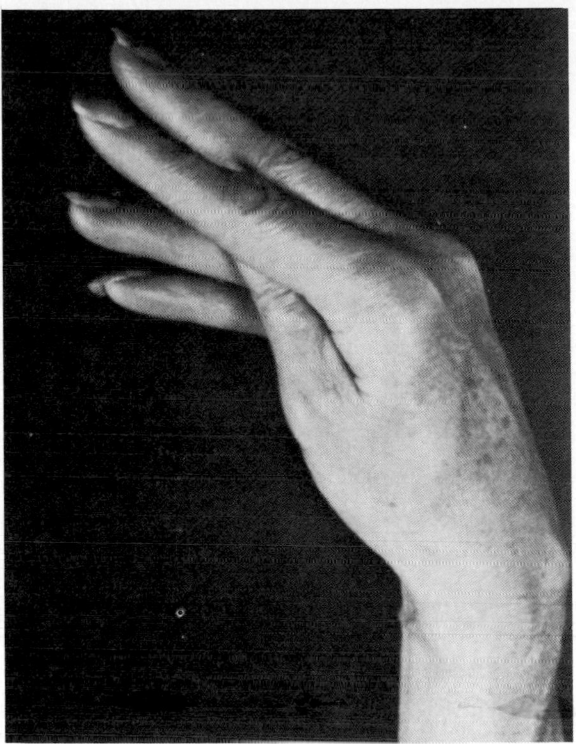

FIGURE 9. Appearance of the hand in tetany. This characteristic posture results from spasm of the intrinsic hand muscles. (From Spillane, JD: *An Atlas of Clinical Neurology*, ed 3. Oxford University Press, London, 1982, with permission.)

motor signs appear in the hand in the sequence described by Kugelberg, while in a negative test no signs appear within 3 minutes of ischemia. Chvostek's test, as originally described, requires sharp percussion of the facial nerve just anterior to the external auditory meatus; a positive response consists of a twitch of the muscles supplied by the middle branch of the facial nerve, but in strong responses the upper and lower facial muscles can also contract. A later modification by Schultze consisted of percussion over the cheek between the angle of the jaw and the zygoma; this response is more easily elicited than the former one.

Chvostek's and Schultze's signs are not very specific. The former is present in 8 percent and the latter in 36 percent of normal subjects (Schaff and Payne 1966). Electrophysiologic studies (Kugelberg 1951) show that Chvostek's sign is due to direct excitation of the facial nerve by mechanical stimulation. In 10 normal subjects who had Schultze's sign without Chvostek's sign, the muscle twitch was sometimes a reflex contraction, sometimes a response to direct excitation of a branch of the facial nerve, and sometimes a combination of the two.

Trousseau's sign, in contrast, is present in only 1 percent of normal subjects (Schaff and Payne 1966) and is nearly always present in symptomatic tetany. Furthermore, the amount of time that elapses before the onset of paresthesias or spasm in the fingers gives a rough indication of the severity of latent tetany, and the electrophysiologic changes can be monitored objectively by combining the test with an EMG of the hand muscles (Fig. 10). Indeed, the remarkable reproducibility of Trousseau's phenomenon in

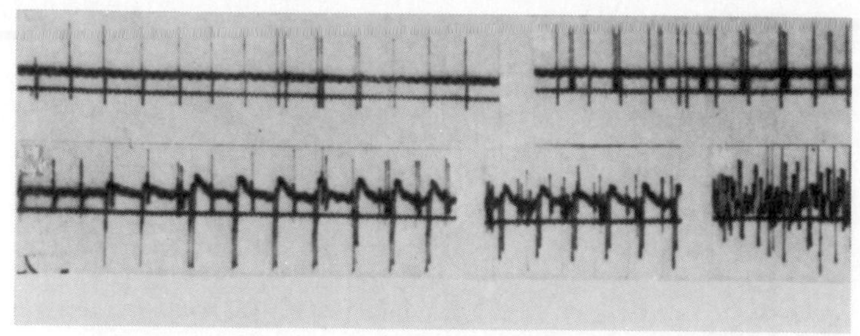

FIGURE 10. EMG of a hand muscle during induction of tetany by ischemic compression of its motor nerve above the elbow (Trousseau's test). Spontaneous repetitive discharges of a single motor unit are soon joined by discharges of other motor units with different configurations. The individual discharges consist of single, double, or multiple action potentials. (From Kugelberg, 1948a, with permission.)

a given subject enabled Lewis (1942) and Kugelberg (1946, 1948a, 1948b) to demonstrate the peripheral nerve origin of tetany by means of simple clinical experiments, which are discussed below.

Electromyography. Although Turpin and coworkers (1943) were the first to report electromyographic investigations of patients with tetany, Kugelberg (1948a, 1948b) has given the most authoritative account. He showed that the spasms of tetany are accompanied by irregular, repetitive action potentials that have the appearance of motor unit potentials. As tetany develops, a single motor unit potential begins to discharge spontaneously at a rate of 5 to 15 Hz. Often the potential is doubled; that is, there are repeating pairs of nearly identical potentials ("doublets"). The individual potentials in each pair are separated by an interval of 5 to 15 msec, and the second potential is usually slightly smaller than the first. Three or even more potentials may be grouped in the repetitive discharges. As tetany intensifies, new motor unit potentials appear and fire at a different frequency; the later units tend to have larger amplitudes and to fire at higher frequencies. Eventually the motor unit potentials are too numerous to distinguish from one another, but by this time the spasm is well developed. These EMG characteristics have not been found in any other state of motor unit hyperactivity (Layzer 1979).

Pathophysiology. Lewis (1942) demonstrated that Trousseau's test depends on ischemia rather than on nerve compression. The nerves under the pneumatic cuff tend to be activated earliest, because the threshold for nerve activation, whether it be ischemia or electrical stimulation, decreases as the activating stimulus moves proximally. Thus, Trousseau's sign is more easily elicited when the cuff is placed at the level of the axilla than at the elbow, and at the wrist it is very hard to elicit at all (Lewis 1942, Kugelberg 1946). While the proximal segments of nerves tend to be activated first, the longest nerves have the lowest threshold; this is why the sensory and motor symptoms always begin distally and spread proximally. Nerve fibers mediating the sensation of touch have the lowest threshold; consequently a tingling sensation always precedes the motor phenomena.

Kugelberg (1946) showed that ischemia lowers the electrical threshold of peripheral nerves in normal persons. The change begins after a few seconds of ischemia, and excitability is maximal at about 3 minutes, after which it returns to normal by 10 to 12 minutes even though ischemia is maintained. The excitability changes produced by ischemia in patients with tetany follow the same curve, but the absolute values for the electrical threshold are lower. This explains the clinical observation that Trousseau's test can be considered negative if no spasm appears after 3 minutes of ischemia.

Both Lewis (1942) and Kugelberg (1946, 1948a) were able to demonstrate, by using two pneumatic cuffs and anesthetic nerve blocks, that tetany does not require any participation of central reflexes and does not arise in the muscles or the neuromuscular junctions. This means that the mechanism of hypocalcemic tetany must be sought in the way calcium regulates peripheral nerve excitability.

In descriptive terms, a low extracellular calcium concentration reduces the amount of current needed to excite the nerves and reduces the accommodation of nerves to a depolarizing current (Kugelberg 1946). These effects stem from the ability of extracellular calcium to modify the relationship between membrane potential changes and membrane permeability to sodium and potassium. Normally, when the resting membrane is depolarized, sodium conductance increases until the threshold for spike activation is reached, whereupon sodium conductance increases sharply to a maximum. A high extracellular calcium concentration increases the amount of depolarization required to activate the sodium conductance mechanism, while a low calcium concentration has an opposite effect. If the calcium concentration is low enough, the sodium conductance mechanism will be activated at the normal resting membrane potential, and spontaneous rhythmic action potentials will result (Stein 1980). The molecular mechanism for this action of calcium on ionic conductance is not known with certainty, but it is thought that both calcium and magnesium ions affect the local electric field of the membrane near the ion channels, either by binding to negative charges or by screening charges (Hille 1968).

Relation of Plasma Calcium Levels to Tetany

Plasma levels of ionized calcium correlate with the occurrence of tetany more closely than do total calcium levels. In patients with hypoparathyroidism, Fanconi and Rose (1958) found that tetany occurred when the plasma ionized calcium level was below 4.3 mg per dl (their normal range was 5.9 to 6.5 mg per dl). When the plasma albumin concentration is low, as in the nephrotic syndrome, the ionized calcium level often remains normal when the total calcium concentration is low, and tetany does not occur. However, the absolute level of ionized calcium does not directly predict the presence or absence of tetany, since other factors may modify peripheral nerve excitability. Uremic patients with low plasma levels of ionized calcium do not ordinarily manifest tetany even when they are alkalotic; this discrepancy may be related to elevated magnesium levels in uremia (Fanconi and Rose 1958). Moreover, hypocalcemic tetany caused by hypoparathyroidism can be suppressed by standard doses of phenytoin (Schaff and Payne 1966).

Aside from the tetany of magnesium deficiency, which is discussed in the next section, cases of normocalcemic tetany without alkalosis are rare and poorly documented. The French and German literature abounds in reports of patients with "spasmophilia" who are said to have normocalcemic tetany (Durlach 1976), but to many readers these cases seem indistinguishable from the hyperventilation syndrome. Fourman and McCance (1955) described the occurrence of tetany during potassium replacement in a patient with potassium deficiency caused by renal tubular acidosis; total serum calcium levels were normal but the ionized fraction was not determined. The only EMG-documented example of idiopathic tetany was a patient with seizures and tetany since childhood, described by Isgren (1976); a sibling had seizures and latent tetany, and the mother had latent tetany as well, suggesting that this was a dominantly inherited abnormality of neural excitability.

Serum Enzyme Elevations

Serum enzyme elevations have been reported in a few patients with hypoparathyroidism and hypocalcemia. This syndrome is discussed in Chapter 3.

MAGNESIUM DISORDERS

Hypermagnesemia

Marked elevation of the plasma magnesium concentration causes generalized, flaccid paralysis, a complication rarely encountered in clinical practice. Although plasma levels of magnesium are almost as carefully regulated as those of calcium, no hormonal mechanisms are known to exist for maintaining the normal plasma concentration of 1.5 to 2.5 mEq per liter (2.0 to 3.0 mg per dl). The total body store of magnesium is 2000 mEq. Approximately half of this amount is contained in bone; liver, muscle, and brain also have a high content of magnesium, while only a small fraction of the total body content is contained in the extracellular fluid. The regulation of plasma magnesium levels occurs by movement of the ions into and out of bone and soft tissues, and by renal excretion; very little is known about how this regulation occurs. Normally only 3 to 5 percent of a filtered load of magnesium is excreted by the kidney, and on a magnesium-deficient diet there is nearly complete reabsorption of magnesium. Under normal circumstances, however, 80 percent of an oral load of magnesium is excreted in the urine within 48 hours (Mordes and Wacker 1977). Whatever the regulatory mechanisms may be, they are highly effective in preventing hypermagnesemia, which rarely reaches symptomatic proportions without some assistance from well-intentioned physicians. Thus, the usual antecedents of clinical magnesium toxicity are use of magnesium-containing antacids and cathartics in patients with chronic renal failure, absorption of magnesium from retained enemas, and magnesium sulfate therapy for hypertensive crisis.

CLINICAL FEATURES. The signs of magnesium toxicity can be roughly correlated with plasma levels, based on observations made during the treatment of eclampsia of pregnancy, as well as on data from animal experiments. The earliest effects, occurring at levels above 3 mEq per liter, consist of paralysis of smooth muscle and autonomic nerves, dry mouth, cutaneous flush, hypotension, nausea, and vomiting. As plasma levels rise from 5 to 10 mEq per liter the muscle stretch reflexes become depressed. Muscle weakness (including respiratory insufficiency) becomes apparent at levels greater than 9 to 10 mEq per liter, and heart block and cardiac arrest may appear with levels over 14 to 15 mEq per liter, although less serious cardiac conduction abnormalities are seen at lower levels.

Among these manifestations, cerebral symptoms are notable for their absence. There are highly efficient mechanisms for maintaining a narrow range of magnesium concentrations in the spinal fluid and central nervous system, even in the presence of extremely high plasma levels. In the published accounts of cerebral depression or coma owing to hypermagnesemia, the respiratory state was not monitored, and central depression may simply have been due to hypoxia from hypoventilation (Alfrey et al. 1970; Stevens and Wolff 1950). Somjen and colleagues (1966) induced severe hypermagnesemia in two volunteer subjects by slow intravenous infusion of magnesium sulfate, raising the plasma magnesium level to 15 mEq per liter (19 to 20 mg per dl). At this level the subjects exhibited complete paralysis of all the voluntary muscles except for the vocal cords, diaphragm, extraocular muscles, and some of the facial muscles; one subject had partial ptosis. Both subjects continued to breathe without assistance and remained completely alert and rational except for transient hypoxic clouding of consciousness in one subject. They felt pain and could hear and see normally, and afterward they remembered everything that had occurred. Thus, hypermagnesemia does not directly depress cerebral function in normal persons. However, cerebral depression may occur more readily in patients with defective function of the blood-brain barrier caused by uremia, stroke, or infection of the central nervous system.

TREATMENT. The paralyzing actions of magnesium are rapidly reversible on lowering the plasma magnesium level. In patients with normal renal function, renal excretion enables the clinician to "titrate" the rate of intravenous infusion of magnesium sulfate by following the activity of the muscle stretch reflexes, thus avoiding respiratory paralysis and cardiac toxicity (Fishman 1965). In patients who develop magnesium poisoning, however, renal excretion is often inadequate. Intravenous administration of 10 ml of 10-percent calcium gluconate will usually reverse the paralysis temporarily, but hemodialysis or peritoneal dialysis is the most effective means of reducing the magnesium overload.

PATHOPHYSIOLOGY. Like calcium, magnesium acts at several different sites in the central and peripheral nervous systems. However, hypermagnesemic paralysis is probably due entirely to neuromuscular blockade. The evidence for this is indirect. First, the clinical picture consists of a flaccid paralysis involving cranial, respiratory, and limb muscles, with normal sensation and alertness. Second, the paralysis is antagonized by calcium. Very high extracellular magnesium levels depress peripheral nerve conduction, but this effect would be increased rather than reversed by calcium, and the magnesium levels required for this effect are higher than are found clinically (Mordes and Wacker 1977).

The neuromuscular blocking action of magnesium has been extensively studied, and it has been an important experimental tool for investigating the physiology of neuromuscular transmission. The arrival of an action potential at the motor nerve terminals triggers the coordinated, simultaneous release of acetylcholine from a large number of synaptic vesicles. Calcium ions couple the electrical impulse with the release of acetylcholine. The higher the calcium concentration within the nerve terminals, the more "packets" of acetylcholine are released by a nerve impulse. Magnesium is a competitive inhibitor of this effect of calcium. Since the extracellular concentrations of calcium and magnesium directly influence the internal concentrations of these ions, acetylcholine release is reduced in a low-calcium medium and increased in a high-calcium medium, and high magnesium concentrations (8 to 15 mM) block the release of acetylcholine. The concentration ratio of magnesium to calcium determines the number of packets of acetylcholine that will be released and thus determines the amplitude of the end-plate potential. High magnesium concentrations do not impair the spontaneous release of individual packets of acetylcholine and thus the amplitude and frequency of miniature end-plate potentials (mepps) are unaltered. Magnesium blockade can be completely overcome by increasing the concentration of extracellular calcium.

Neuromuscular blockade by magnesium is very similar to that found in the Lambert-Eaton syndrome (Elmqvist and Lambert 1968). In both conditions the reflexes are depressed before the onset of profound weakness, probably because a single motor nerve volley, evoked by the monosynaptic stretch reflex, activates only a few muscle fibers, while repetitive nerve activity temporarily overcomes the defect in release of acetylcholine. During repetitive nerve activity at fast rates, calcium ions accumulate in the nerve terminals, opposing the inhibitory effect of magnesium. This phenomenon underlies the facilitation of neuromuscular transmission produced by repetitive nerve stimulation at 20 to 40 Hz, a feature of both magnesium intoxication and the Lambert-Eaton syndrome.

ELECTROPHYSIOLOGIC STUDIES. The only electrophysiologic study of a patient with paralysis attributed to magnesium poisoning was reported by Swift (1979), but the diagnosis in that patient is problematic, since the highest magnesium level was 3.7 mg per dl.* However, from experimental data and from clinical experience with other presynaptic disorders of neuromuscular transmission, one would predict that the findings would be similar to those of botulism (Chapter 4).

Magnesium Deficiency

Magnesium depletion is encountered in chronic alcoholism, in diabetic ketoacidosis, and in patients with poor dietary intake of magnesium, prolonged vomiting, intestinal malabsorption, or gastrointestinal fistulas. Tetany and muscular weakness occur in patients with magnesium deficiency, but there is controversy about whether magnesium plays a direct or an indirect role in producing these neuromuscular disturbances.

In the 1950s, when the central and peripheral nervous system symptoms of hypomagnesemia were first reported, there were several obstacles to accepting a causal connection between hypomagnesemia and the neurologic disturbances. In the first place, plasma levels of magnesium do not necessarily reflect tissue levels. Hypomagnesemia is often simply a transient result of hemodilution, and by the same token a tissue deficit of magnesium can exist with a normal plasma concentration. Secondly, patients with magnesium deficiency often have serious systemic diseases that could be the cause of the neurologic symptoms. Thirdly, magnesium deficiency tends to cause hypocalcemia, potassium deficiency, and phosphorus deficiency, and it is often difficult to know which metabolic disturbance is responsible for a given symptom. Fourthly, the clinical syndromes that some authors consider typical of magnesium deficiency are quite different from those delineated by other authorities. Not all these difficulties have been fully resolved, but there is general agreement that magnesium deficiency, directly or indirectly, does cause major cerebral and neuromuscular disorders, which may persist until the magnesium deficit is replaced.

CLINICAL FEATURES. Fishman (1965) described a distinctive syndrome of nervous system hyperirritability in five patients with magnesium deficiency unaccompanied by other overt metabolic disorders. There were mental symptoms (irritability, depression, negative behavior, and confusion); a coarse, generalized tremor accentuated by maintaining posture against gravity; multifocal myoclonus, and generalized myoclonic jerks or exaggerated startle responses; generalized or multifocal seizures; generalized hyperreflexia with normal plantar responses; generalized muscle twitching and hyperirritability of muscles to direct percussion; and Chvostek's sign without Trousseau's sign and without carpopedal spasm in response to

---

*The patient had increasing constipation for 5 days, received a magnesium citrate enema, became severely weak so as to require mechanical ventilation, and recovered very slowly even though treatment brought the serum magnesium level promptly down to 2.1 mg per dl. Electrophysiologic studies showed a presynaptic block. Could the patient have had a mild case of botulism, perhaps aggravated by magnesium therapy?

hyperventilation. The above symptoms responded rapidly to magnesium replacement, and in one patient (who suffered from malabsorption of magnesium) the symptoms returned whenever parenteral magnesium supplementation was omitted.

Hanna and associates (1960) described three patients with "pure" magnesium deficiency who differed from Fishman's patients in several respects. One patient had positional vertigo, ataxia of gait, confusion, convulsions, proximal muscle weakness and wasting, hyporeflexia, and Chvostek's sign without Trousseau's sign. The second patient exhibited depression and irritability, generalized weakness with normal reflexes, dysarthria, and a coarse tremor. The third patient had a convulsion, subjective weakness, hypoactive reflexes, and Chvostek's sign without Trousseau's sign. All three patients had low-voltage complexes on the ECG.

Other authors have described generalized muscular hypertonus, carpopedal spasm, positive Trousseau's signs, and athetoid movements, in the absence of significant hypocalcemia. These manifestations did not respond to calcium therapy but subsided promptly after magnesium was given (Back et al. 1962; Vallee et al. 1960; Wacker et al. 1962; Saul and Selhorst 1981). Other patients have had a syndrome resembling Wernicke's encephalopathy, with dysphagia, diplopia, vertical nystagmus, and vestibular ataxia that took several months to resolve even after magnesium replacement (Hamed and Lindeman 1978; Saul and Selhorst 1981).

In an attempt to determine the effects of pure magnesium deficiency, Shils (1969) excluded magnesium from the nasogastric tube feeding of seven cancer patients for periods of 40 to 266 days. Unfortunately the results were even harder to interpret than were the spontaneous cases of magnesium deficiency. Most of the patients went into negative potassium balance and became hypokalemic. Weakness occurred in several patients and responded to potassium treatment, but in two subjects hypokalemia persisted despite large potassium supplements. The six male patients became hypocalcemic, and in five of them Trousseau's sign was demonstrated; the female patient did not become hypocalcemic and did not have Trousseau's sign. Other neurologic signs observed were tremor, "fibrillations," "spasticity," and areflexia. Myopathic EMG abnormalities were present in several patients.

With such confusing accounts in the literature, is it possible to list the neurologic symptoms of "pure" magnesium deficiency? The cerebral symptoms almost certainly include mental depression and irritability, postural tremor, convulsions, multifocal seizures, myoclonus, and hyperactive reflexes. The peripheral nervous system signs include muscle twitching, muscle irritability to percussion, and (for what it is worth) Chvostek's sign. Muscle weakness and hyporeflexia occur in some patients, but it is difficult to know whether these signs are related to the magnesium deficit or to the deficits of potassium or phosphate that result from increased urinary excretion of those minerals in magnesium deficiency (Whang and Aikawa 1977).

HYPOMAGNESEMIA AND TETANY. There has been lively debate over whether magnesium deficiency causes carpopedal spasm in the absence of hypocalcemia. From the published cases it is clear that many patients with symptomatic magnesium deficiency do not have peripheral tetany. Some patients have tetany and hypocalcemia, both of which are resistant to calcium therapy but resolve with magnesium therapy. A few patients undoubtedly do have tetany without hypocalcemia, and the tetany responds to magnesium but not to calcium; it is this group that has engendered most of the controversy (Wacker et al. 1962).

The observations of Zimmet and colleagues (1968) may help to resolve these contradictions. They measured plasma ionized calcium concentrations in two magnesium-deficient patients with spontaneous tetany. Initially Trousseau's sign was present and plasma calcium levels were normal, but ionized calcium levels were 1.7 to 1.9 mEq per liter (normal 2.5 to 3.5 mEq per liter). Following treatment with magnesium the levels of plasma ionized calcium rose, and when the levels reached 2.4 to 2.5 mEq per liter, Trousseau's sign could no longer be elicited. Some hours later the plasma ionized calcium had risen to 3.5 mEq per liter and the total calcium level was elevated (7.2 to 7.5 mEq per liter). The authors concluded that magnesium repletion permitted mobilization of ionized calcium from tissue stores such as bone or muscle. In none of the other cases of normocalcemic, hypomagnesemic tetany have ionized calcium levels been measured.

Hypomagnesemia develops frequently during treatment of cancer with cisplatin. Among eight children who became hypomagnesemic during cisplatin therapy, the serum calcium concentration fell below 8.5 mg per dl in four children and remained normal in the others. Tetany with carpopedal spasm appeared in all of the hypocalcemic children, while none of the normocalcemic children had tetany (Hayes et al. 1979).

Thus, the occurrence of tetany in magnesium deficiency is probably related to hypocalcemia, and specifically to low plasma levels of ionized calcium. There is still no evidence that magnesium deficiency can cause tetany when the plasma level of ionized calcium is normal.

Experimental Myopathy. A necrotizing myopathy has been induced in rats and dogs by chronic magnesium depletion, but overt muscle weakness was not noticeable in these animals. In rats, both fast and slow muscles showed segmental necrosis of scattered muscle fibers; tetanic muscle tension was reduced when expressed in terms of muscle weight, but twitch tension was normal, although the rates of contraction and relaxation were slowed (Sarkar et al. 1981). The magnesium content of dog muscle was only slightly diminished, and although the sodium content was increased the potassium content was normal; the resting membrane potential was normal or even increased. There was a mild reduction of muscle phosphorus, but it seems unlikely that this could account for the muscle fiber necrosis, especially since the plasma phosphorus concentration remained normal (Cronin et al. 1982).

TREATMENT. In practice it does not matter what causes muscle weakness and tetany in magnesium deficiency, because the secondary disturbances of calcium and potassium metabolism are quite resistant to therapy unless magnesium is replaced, and the secondary deficiencies often respond to magnesium replacement alone. Magnesium sulfate can be administered by intramuscular injection (e.g., 2 ml [8.1 mEq] of a 50-percent solution), or by slow intravenous infusion (e.g., 16.2 mEq in 250 to 500 ml of 5-percent glucose or isotonic saline, over a period of 2 to 4 hours) (Fishman 1965). For patients with complex disturbances of mineral metabolism, potassium chloride and potassium phosphate can be added to the glucose or saline solution containing magnesium (Knochel 1981).

DISORDERS OF ACID-BASE METABOLISM

Acidosis

Although there are no direct effects of acidosis on neuromuscular function, there are indirect effects via disturbances of potassium metabolism. *Acute acidosis* tends to cause hyperkalemia, principally because potassium moves out of the intracellular compartment in exchange for extracellular hydrogen ions. By itself this hyperkalemia, which may reach levels of 6 to 7 mEq per liter, is not of sufficient magnitude to cause paralysis; in patients with renal insufficiency and chronic hyperkalemia, however, an acute acidotic shift may precipitate hyperkalemic paralysis.

Chronic metabolic acidosis is accompanied by renal potassium wasting, which may result in transient or periodic paralysis, subacute or chronic hypokalemic myopathy, or generalized muscle necrosis with myoglobinuria. Hypokalemic muscle weakness has been reported in patients with metabolic acidosis caused by renal tubular acidosis, diabetic ketoacidosis, severe diarrhea, intestinal malabsorption, ammonium chloride therapy, or ureteroenterostomy.

Alkalosis

The single neuromuscular manifestation of alkalosis is tetany. There are two mechanisms that might explain why alkalosis gives precisely the same electrophysiologic abnormality as hypocalcemia.

First, acute alkalosis reduces the plasma ionized calcium concentration by increasing both the protein-bound and the complexed fractions of calcium. Fanconi and Rose (1958) reported that hyperventilation, when continued long enough to raise the plasma pH by 0.3 to 0.5 units, reduced the plasma ionized calcium concentration by about 1 mg per dl.

Second, alkalosis has a direct unstabilizing effect on peripheral nerve excitability. Reducing the concentration of either calcium or hydrogen ions in the extracellular fluid reduces the amount of depolarization needed to increase the sodium conductance and reduces the accommodation of conductance changes to a constant depolarizing stimulus (Hille 1968). Although the precise mechanism of this effect is not known, it seems likely that both cations are bound to fixed negative charges on the surface of the membrane, and that they affect ionic permeability by altering the local potential gradients around ion channels. From the data presented by Hille (1968), a pH increase of 0.5 units would have about the same effect as a 16-percent reduction of the ionized calcium concentration—that is, about 1 mg per dl. The combined effects, direct and indirect, would thus be sufficient to produce clinical tetany.

DISORDERS OF PHOSPHORUS METABOLISM

In the past decade several neuromuscular and cerebral disorders related to cellular phosphorus depletion have emerged. The clinical definition of these syndromes is still incomplete, but it appears that different etiologic settings tend to produce different syndromes. When chronic phosphorus depletion develops over months or years, it leads to osteomalacia, bone pain, and chronic proximal myopathy, while an acute disturbance of the central nervous system, peripheral nerves, and muscles is encountered in malnourished, phosphorus-depeleted patients who become acutely hypophosphatemic during nourishment. The former syndrome is discussed, along with other myopathies associated with osteomalacia, in Chapter 3. Here we are concerned with the neuromuscular disorders that accompany acute hypophosphatemia, which can be divided into two syndromes: acute, generalized paralysis resembling the Guillain-Barré syndrome, and generalized muscle necrosis with myoglobinuria.

Acute Areflexic Paralysis

Most cases of acute paralysis caused by hypophosphatemia have occurred in patients receiving intravenous hyperalimentation because of severe diarrhea, regional ileitis, ulcerative colitis, or chronic pancreatitis (Silvis and Paragas 1972; Furlan et al. 1975; Weintraub 1976; Finck et al. 1979; Chudley et al. 1981). A few examples have been described in malnourished alcoholic patients who were given intravenous or oral alimentation (Newman et al. 1977; Silvis et al. 1980), and one was a uremic patient treated with antacids and hemodialysis (Boelens et al. 1970).

The neurologic symptoms usually begin a few days after the institution of phosphate-free alimentation; the duration of hyperalimentation has ranged from 12 hours to several weeks. Often the first symptom is tingling paresthesia in the mouth, tongue, fingers, and feet; then, over a period of several days, there is a rapid onset of generalized limb weakness, areflexia, impairment of sensation in the distal portions of the limbs and over the trunk, and cranial nerve disturbances such as dysarthria, dysphagia, ptosis, oculomotor weakness, pupillomotor dysfunction, facial and oropharyngeal numbness, and loss of taste. Limb ataxia may be prominent, perhaps reflecting sensory impairment, and respiratory weakness may be severe enough to require tracheal intubation and mechanical support of ventilation.

In addition to these neurologic signs, which suggest a diffuse cranial and spinal polyneuropathy, there may be cerebral cortical disturbances such as irritability, apprehension, disorientation, confusion, somnolence, coma, convulsions, involuntary movements, and Babinski's signs. In a number of reports the cerebral manifestations were emphasized and weakness was not described, while in other reports the peripheral nerve manifestations were prominent and cerebral signs were inconspicuous or absent. A few patients have had hemolytic anemia, bleeding diathesis caused by platelet dysfunction, increased susceptibility to infection because of leukocyte dysfunction, or impaired myocardial contractility (Knochel 1981).

At the onset of neurologic symptoms the serum phosphorus level is almost always less than 1.0 mg per dl, and at the height of the disorder the level is usually less than 0.6 mg per dl (normal range 3.0 to 4.5 mg per dl). Other electrolyte derangements are often present, but the symptoms do not respond to administration of potassium or magnesium, without phosphate. Intravenous administration of phosphate brings striking improvement within a few hours, though complete recovery may not occur for up to 2 weeks. There are usually no permanent after-effects.

Although the clinical picture resembles a profound disturbance of peripheral nerve function, the published cases provide almost no confirmatory laboratory information such as serum enzyme values or muscle biopsy findings, and electrophysiologic testing has been reported only in one patient, who had chronic renal failure (Boelens et al. 1970). Experimental studies of acute paralysis in phosphate-depleted animals have focused on skeletal muscle metabolism, leaving unexamined the central and peripheral nervous systems. Until more information is available, therefore, it cannot be stated whether the syndrome of acute hypophosphatemic paralysis is a peripheral nerve disorder, a disorder of motor and sensory neurons, or a diffuse disturbance of the central and peripheral nervous systems and muscle.

Myoglobinuria, Hypophosphatemia, and Acute Alcoholic Myopathy

Knochel and associates (1975) were the first to incriminate phosphorus depletion in the pathogenesis of acute alcoholic rhabdomyolysis. Hed and colleagues (1962) had described the occasional occurrence of acute myoglobinuria in spree-drinkers following bouts of heavy alcohol consumption. Perkoff et al (1966) and Nygren (1966) noticed that milder degrees of acute muscle damage could be detected in the majority of alcoholic patients who entered the hospital following a drinking bout. Asymptomatic cases were detected by high serum CPK levels, and symptomatic patients had muscle pain, swelling, tenderness and weakness, mainly in the lower extremities. A curious but characteristic feature of this syndrome was the fact that muscle symptoms and CPK elevation tended to occur a few days after admission to the hospital (Nygren 1966; Lafair and Myerson 1968), suggesting that medical treatment might somehow be responsible.

Against this background, Knochel and associates (1975) noticed that the serum phosphorus levels of alcoholic patients, generally normal or slightly depressed at the time of admission, often fell precipitously 1 to 3 days later, returning to normal about a week after admission. The rise of serum CPK levels appeared to correspond to the nadir of serum phosphorus levels, and Knochel and his coworkers (Knochel et al. 1975; Knochel 1977) postulated that muscle cell injury resulted from an acute intracellular deficiency of high-energy phosphate compounds, caused by the unavailability of inorganic phosphate. They suggested that the muscle of malnourished, alcoholic patients is already depleted of high-energy phosphate compounds and inorganic phosphate at the time the patients enter the hospital. Nourishment with high-calorie, glucose-containing nutrients then causes rapid cellular uptake of extracellular phosphate, which is incorporated into glycolytic intermediates so that inorganic phosphorus becomes unavailable for maintaining glycolysis and for phosphorylating adenosine diphosphate (ADP). They also pointed out that myoglobinuria has occurred (rarely) during the treatment of diabetic acidosis (Rainey et al. 1963) and that serum CPK elevations occur commonly 24 to 72 hours after initiation of insulin treatment (Velez-Garcia et al. 1966; Knight et al. 1974).* Myoglobinuria has also been reported as a complication of hypophosphatemia during treatment of diabetic hyperosmolar coma (Rumpf et al. 1981).

In support of their hypothesis, Knochel and associates (1975) showed that the average muscle concentration of inorganic phosphate was half of normal in alcoholic patients with elevated serum CPK activities. The theoretical muscle membrane potential calculated from the intracellular and extracellular ion concentrations was normal, but the actual resting potential was well below normal in every patient. Borghi and coworkers (1981) showed a striking increase of muscle sodium content and a reduction of potassium content in phosphorus-depleted patients with acute hypophosphatemia. These findings suggest either an increased permeability to sodium or a reduced activity of the electrogenic sodium-potassium pump, which in turn could result from impairment of cellular energy metabolism.

The clinical relationship between alcoholism, hypophosphatemia, and muscle necrosis has not yet been confirmed. Curiously enough, none of the

*However, in a recent series, the serum CPK level was elevated *on admission* in 9 of 44 patients with diabetic ketoacidosis, and the CPK level rose during treatment in 3 other patients, whether or not phosphate replacement was provided (Wilson et al. 1982).

reports describing acute areflexic paralysis mention serum enzyme levels, while reports of patients with acute alcoholic myopathy do not mention sensory, cranial nerve, or cerebral symptoms (Anderson et al. 1980; Lafair and Myerson 1968).* Hyperphosphatemia is actually a more common finding than hypophosphatemia in hospitalized alcoholic patients (Ryback et al. 1980), but random tests are not likely to be informative if hypophosphatemia is transient, especially since muscle necrosis releases phosphate into the extracellular fluid (Knochel et al. 1975). In a later study (Anderson et al. 1980), Knochel and his colleagues studied muscle chemical composition in 13 patients with alcoholic myopathy, most of whom had frank rhabdomyolysis. There were multiple electrolyte abnormalities, including reduced phosphorus, magnesium, and potassium and increased calcium and sodium. The lowest serum phosphorus level ranged from 0.9 to 5.9 mg per dl and was below 1.0 mg per dl in only one patient. No prospective study of alcoholic patients has yet been performed to correlate serum phosphorus levels with evidence of muscle cell necrosis, or to compare the effects of nourishment with and without phosphate supplements.

A further discussion of alcoholic myopathy appears in Chapter 9.

Pathophysiology of Hypophosphatemic Complications. In experiments in dogs, chronic phosphorus depletion with a *normal* caloric intake produced a moderate decline in serum phosphorus concentration and in total muscle phosphorus. Muscle sodium concentration increased slightly and potassium decreased slightly, and the mean resting membrane potential fell by 15 mV (Fuller et al. 1976). Muscle concentrations of adenosine triphosphate (ATP), ADP, and inorganic phosphate were each reduced approximately 50 percent, so that the value of the "phosphorylation potential," $ATP/(ADP \times P_i)$, was twice normal (Fuller et al., cited by Knochel 1981).† Some of the animals appeared weak and lethargic, but serum CPK activities did not rise. These animals were not challenged with hyperalimentation.

In contrast, when dogs were simultaneously starved and depleted of phosphorus until they lost 30 percent of their initial weight, serum and muscle phosphorus levels fell very little, but nourishment with a high-calorie, high-carbohydrate, phosphorus-deficient diet caused a rapid drop in the serum phosphorus concentration, a moderate decline in total muscle phosphorus, a large rise in serum CPK activity, and marked necrosis of muscle as assessed by light microscopy. These animals appeared extremely weak and tremulous, some showed convulsive movements, and several animals died. In other animals, hyperalimentation with supplemental phosphate produced no ill effects, and the biochemical findings in these animals were normal (Knochel et al. 1978).

Starvation alone, with adequate phosphorus intake, produced no change in muscle biochemical composition, and when the starved dogs were hyperalimented without phosphorus, the serum CPK activity remained normal and there were no adverse clinical effects, even though hypophosphatemia occurred that was just as severe as in the phosphorus-depleted animals. The total muscle phosphorus content fell, but the muscle content of inorganic phosphate declined very little and the phosphorylation potential remained normal (Knochel et al. 1979). Thus, hypophospha-

*In a brief communication, Demarcq and colleagues (1981) mentioned eight hypophosphatemic patients with encephalopathy, six of whom also had difficulty breathing; signs of peripheral neuropathy were said to be absent, though no details were given. Serum CPK activity was apparently increased in some cases, but the normal range was not stated. A ninth patient had myoglobinuria, acute cardiac failure, and respiratory insufficiency, without cerebral symptoms.

†When the phosphorylation potential is high, mitochondrial respiration is slowed and the cell is unable to step up ATP synthesis in response to a sudden increase in energy expenditure, even though the ATP concentration is much reduced.

temia itself appears to have no immediate adverse effects unless the muscle is phosphorus-deficient.

Other workers showed that acute hypophosphatemia had no effect on muscle glucose uptake in normal rats, but in phosphorus-depleted rats glucose uptake fell in direct proportion to the decline of serum phosphorus concentration (Davis et al. 1979). These observations support Knochel's contention that cellular deficiency of inorganic phosphate is the crucial determinant of cellular dysfunction or injury in phosphorus depletion (Knochel 1981).

The pathophysiology of central and peripheral nervous system dysfunction in acute hypophosphatemia has not been studied, though it is possible that a similar biochemical mechanism operates in these tissues. It has been suggested that phosphorus deficiency may interfere with delivery of oxygen to the brain, because hemoglobin releases oxygen more reluctantly when erythrocyte levels of 2,3-diphosphoglycerate are low, as they are in phosphorus deficiency (Travis et al. 1971). This hypothetical mechanism for hypophosphatemic encephalopathy has not been investigated directly.

Differential Diagnosis

There are a number of similarities between the clinical effects of hypokalemia and of hypophosphatemia. In both conditions, the low plasma electrolyte level itself has little or no adverse effect unless there is a pre-existing chronic deficiency of the mineral; acute muscle paralysis results from a sudden shift of the mineral from plasma into muscle; the paralysis is often accompanied by evidence of muscle necrosis in the form of high CPK levels or frank myoglobinuria; and mineral deficiency tends to occur in alcoholic patients and in patients with chronic gastrointestinal fluid loss. The most notable difference is the fact that sensory, cranial nerve, and cerebral manifestations are peculiar to hypophosphatemia; the hypophosphatemic syndrome of acute areflexic paralysis is not likely to be confused with acute hypokalemic paralysis. The distinction between hypokalemic and hypophosphatemic muscle necrosis, however, is much more difficult to make.

Acute hypokalemic paralysis has been reported in alcoholic patients, but those patients did not have painful, swollen muscles or myoglobinuria (Martin et al. 1971). Many patients who develop myoglobinuria are severely depleted of both potassium and phosphorus. The diagnostic confusion is illustrated by a recent report of rhabdomyolysis in a patient receiving total parenteral nutrition for pyloric obstruction. The authors attributed the complication to potassium deficiency, but serum phosphorus levels were not measured until the onset of acute renal failure, by which time hyperphosphatemia was present (Nadel et al. 1979).

Treatment

Rapid replacement of phosphorus is difficult to achieve because intravenous administration can precipitate calcium phosphate, which results in hypocalcemia and metastatic calcification. Hypocalcemia is especially likely to occur in magnesium-deficient patients, whose parathyroid glands respond sluggishly to low blood levels of calcium. Knochel (1981) recommends giving adult patients about 20 mM phosphate every 8 hours, adding 40 mEq potassium and 16 mEq magnesium to 1 liter of solution in cases of multiple electrolyte deficiencies. In severe phosphorus deficiency, Fitzgerald (1978) recommends giving 60 mEq potassium phosphate every 8 hours, while closely monitoring serum levels of calcium, phosphorus, and potassium. Patients who are able to tolerate oral phosphate supplements can be given dairy products, which contain large amounts of calcium and phosphorus, or buffered sodium phosphate (Phospho-Soda), 15 to 30 ml three times a day (though this preparation may cause diarrhea).

REFERENCES

Achor, RWP and Smith, LA: *Nutritional deficiency syndrome with diarrhea resulting in hypopotassemia, muscle degeneration and renal insufficiency. Report of a case with recovery.* Mayo Clin Proc 30:207–215, 1955.

Aithal, HN and Toback, FG: *Defective mitochondrial energy production during potassium depletion nephropathy.* Lab Invest 39:186–293, 1978.

Aithal, HN, Toback, FG, Ordonez, NG, et al: *Functional defects in mitochondria from renal inner red medulla during potassium depletion nephropathy.* Lab Invest 37:423–429, 1977.

Akaike, N: *Development of pump electrogenesis in hypokalemic rat muscle.* Pflugers Arch 379:215–218, 1979.

Akaike, N: *Sodium pump in skeletal muscle: Central nervous system-induced suppression by α-adrenoreceptors.* Science 213:1252–1254, 1981.

Alfrey, AC, Terman, DS, Brettschneider, L, et al: *Hypermagnesemia after renal homotransplantation.* Ann Intern Med 73:367–371, 1970.

Anderson, R, Cohen, M, Haller, R, et al: *Skeletal muscle phosphorus and magnesium deficiency in alcoholic myopathy.* Mineral Electrolyte Metab. 4:106–112, 1980.

Angeloni, JM and Scott, GW: *Flaccid quadriplegia following ureteric transplant.* Lancet i:1005–1006, 1960.

Atsumi, T, Ishikawa, S, Miyatake, T, et al: *Myopathy and primary aldosteronism: Electron microscopic study.* Neurology 29:1348–1353, 1979.

Back, EH, Montgomery, RD and Ward, EE: *Neurological manifestations of magnesium deficiency in infantile gastroenteritis and malnutrition.* Arch Dis Child 37:106–109, 1962.

Barnes, PC and Leonard, JHC: *Hypokalaemic myopathy and myoglobinuria due to carbenoxolone sodium.* Postgrad Med J 47:813–814, 1971.

Bartter, FC: *The parathyroid gland and its relationship to diseases of the nervous system.* Proc Assoc Res Nerv Ment Dis 32:1–20, 1953.

Bergström, J, Alvestrand, A, Furst, P, et al: *Influence of severe potassium depletion and subsequent repletion with potassium on muscle electrolytes, metabolites and amino acids in man.* Clin Sci Molec Med 51:589–599, 1976.

Berning, J: *Hypokalaemia of barium poisoning.* Lancet i:110, 1975.

Bilbrey, GL, Herbin, L, Carter, NW, et al: *Skeletal muscle resting membrane potential in potassium deficiency.* J Clin Invest 52:3011–3018, 1973.

Boelens, PA, Norwood, W, Kjellstrand, C, et al: *Hypophosphatemia with muscle weakness due to antacids and hemodialysis.* Am J Dis Child 120:350–353, 1970.

Borghi, L, Curti, A, Canali, M, et al: *Relationships between muscle K, Mg and Na and acute hypophosphatemia (AH) with and without phosphate depletion in man.* Magnesium-Bulletin 3:154–159, 1981.

Brown, MR, Currens, JH and Marchand, JF: *Muscular paralysis and electrocardiographic abnormalities resulting from potassium loss in chronic nephritis.* JAMA 124:545–549, 1944.

Bull, GM, Carter, AB and Lowe, KG: *Hyperpotassaemic paralysis.* Lancet ii:60–63, 1953.

Campion, DS, Arias, JM and Carter, NW: *Rhabdomyolysis and myoglobinuria. Association with hypokalemia of renal tubular acidosis.* JAMA 220:967–969, 1972.

Cannon, PJ, Leeming, JM, Sommers, SC, et al: *Juxtaglomerular cell hyperplasia and secondary hyperaldosteronism (Bartter's syndrome): A reevaluation of the pathophysiology.* Medicine 47:107–131, 1968.

Chou, C and Chin, YC: *The absorption, fate and concentration in serum of barium in acute experimental poisoning.* Chin Med J (Engl) 51:313–322, 1943.

Chudley, AE, Ninan, A and Young, GB: *Neurologic signs and hypophosphatemia with total parenteral nutrition.* J Can Med Assoc 125:604–607, 1981.

Clausen, T and Flatman, JA: *The effect of catecholamines on Na-K transport and membrane potential in rat soleus muscle.* J Physiol 270:383–414, 1977.

Clausen, T and Kohn, PG: *The effect of insulin on the transport of sodium and potassium in rat soleus muscle.* J Physiol 265:19–42, 1977.

COËRS, C, TELERMAN-TOPPET, N AND CREMER, M: *Acute quadriparesis with muscle spasms related to electrolyte disturbances in steatorrhea. Clinical and biochemical data.* Am J Med 52:849–856, 1972.

COHEN, AB: *Hyperkalemic effects of triameterene.* Ann Intern Med 65:521–527, 1966.

CONIGLIONE, TC: *Treatment of hypercalcemia and hyperkalemia.* Med Times 106(7):69–75, 1978.

CONN, JW: *Aldosteronism in man. Some clinical and climatological aspects, Part II.* JAMA 183:871–878, 1963.

CONN, JW, ROONER, DR AND COHEN, EL: *Licorice-induced pseudoaldosteronism. Hypertension, hypokalemia, aldosteronopenia, and suppressed plasma renin activity.* JAMA 205:492–496, 1968.

CREUTZFELDT, OH, ABBOTT, BC, FOWLER, WM, ET AL: *Muscle membrane potentials in episodic adynamia.* Electroencephalogr Clin Neurophysiol 15:508–519, 1963.

CRONIN, RE, FERGUSON, ER, SHANNON, WE, JR, ET AL: *Skeletal muscle injury after magnesium depletion in the dog.* Am J Physiol 243:F113–F120, 1982.

DANOWSKI, TS, PETERS, JH, RATHBUN, JC, ET AL: *Studies in diabetic acidosis and coma, with particular emphasis on the retention of administered potassium.* J Clin Invest 28:1–9, 1949.

DAVIS, JL, LEWIS, SB, SCHULTZ, TA, ET AL: *Acute and chronic phosphate depletion as a modulator of glucose uptake in rat skeletal muscle.* Life Sci 24:629–632, 1979.

DEMARCQ, JM, LAMBERT, P, DELBAR, M, ET AL: *Encêphalopathie fonctionnelle et dêtresse respiratoire avec hypophosphorêmie.* Nouv Presse Med 10:431–432, 1981.

DIENGOTT, D, ROSZA, O AND LEVY, N: *Hypokalemia in barium poisoning.* Lancet ii:343–344, 1964.

DRUTZ, DJ, FAN, JH, TAI, TY, ET AL: *Hypokalemic rhabdomyolysis and myoglobinuria following amphotericin B therapy.* JAMA 211:824–826, 1970.

DU, KT AND DUNG, CL: *"Pa" disease.* Chin Med J (Engl) 51:302, 1943.

DURLACH, J: *Neurological manifestations of magnesium imbalance.* In VINKEN, PJ AND BRUYN, GW (EDS): *Handbook of Clinical Neurology, Vol 28.* North-Holland Publishing, Amsterdam, 1976, pp 545–579.

ELMQVIST, D AND LAMBERT, EH: *Detailed analysis of neuromuscular transmission in a patient with the myasthenic syndrome sometimes associated with bronchogenic carcinoma.* Mayo Clin Proc 43:689–713, 1968.

FANCONI, A AND ROSE, GA: *The ionized, complexed, and protein-bound fractions of calcium in plasma.* Q J Med 27:463–494, 1958.

FERREBEE, JW, PARKER, D, CARNES, WH, ET AL: *Certain effects of desoxycorticosterone. The development of "diabetes insipidus" and the replacement of muscle potassium by sodium in normal dogs.* Am J Physiol 135:230–237, 1940.

FINCH, CA AND MARCHAND, JF: *Cardiac arrest by the action of potassium.* Am J Med Sci 206:507–520, 1943.

FINCK, GA, MAI, C AND GREGOR, M: *Passagere polyneuropathie mit Hirnnervenbeteilegung durch Hypophosphatamie.* Nervenarzt 50:778–782, 1979.

FISHMAN, RA: *Neurological aspects of magnesium metabolism.* Arch Neurol 12:562–565, 1965.

FISKEN, RA, HEATH, DA, SOMERS, S, ET AL: *Hypercalcaemia in hospital patients. Clinical and diagnostic aspects.* Lancet i:202–207, 1981.

FITZGERALD, F: *Clinical hypophosphatemia.* Ann Rev Med 29:177–189, 1978.

FOURMAN, P: *Experimental observations on the tetany of potassium deficiency.* Lancet ii:525–528, 1954.

FOURMAN, P AND MCCANCE, RA: *Tetany complicating the treatment of potassium deficiency in renal acidosis.* Lancet i:329–331, 1955.

FRAME, B, HEINZE, EG, BLOCK, MA, ET AL: *Myopathy in primary hyperparathyroidism. Observations in three patients.* Ann Intern Med 68:1022–1027, 1968.

FRAME, B, JACKSON, GM, KLEEREKOPER, M, ET AL: *Acute severe hypercalcemia a la Munchausen.* Am J Med 70:316–319, 1981.

FULLER, TJ, CARTER, NW, BARCENAS, C, ET AL: *Reversible changes of the muscle cell in experimental phosphorous deficiency.* J Clin Invest 57:1019–1024, 1976.

FURLAN, AJ, HANSON, M, COOPERMAN, A, ET AL: *Acute areflexic paralysis. Association with hyperalimentation and hypophosphatemia.* Arch Neurol 32:706–707, 1975.

GOLDFARB, S, COX, M, SINGER, I, ET AL: *Acute hyperkalemia induced by hyperglycemia: Hormonal mechanisms.* Ann Intern Med 84:426–432, 1976.

GOULD, DB, SORRELL, MR AND LUPARIELLO, AD: *Barium sulfide poisoning. Some factors contributing to survival.* Arch Intern Med 132:891–894, 1973.

GOULON, M, RAPIN, M, LISSAC, J, ET AL: *Quadriplêgie avec hypokaliêmie et acidose hyperchlorêmique secondaire à l'absorption pendant trois années de chlorure de l'ammonium.* Bull Soc Med Hop Paris 113:986–995, 1962.

HAMED, IA AND LINDEMAN, RD: *Dysphagia and vertical nystagmus in magnesium deficiency.* Ann Intern Med 89:222–223, 1978.

HANNA, S, MACINTYRE, I, HARRISON, M, ET AL: *The syndrome of magnesium deficiency in man.* Lancet ii:172–176, 1960.

HAYES, FA, GREEN, AA, SENZER, N, ET AL: *Tetany: A complication of* cis-*dichlorodiammineplatinum (II) therapy.* Cancer Treat Rep 63:547–548, 1979.

HAZEYAMA, Y AND SPARKS, HV: *Exercise hyperemia in potassium-depleted dogs.* Am J Physiol 236(3):H480–H486, 1979.

HED, R, LUNDMARK, C, FAHLGREN, H, ET AL: *Acute muscular syndrome in chronic alcoholism.* Acta Med Scand 171:585–599, 1962.

HENDERSON, EG: *Strophanthidin sensitive electrogenic mechanisms in frog sartorius muscles exposed to barium.* Pflugers Arch 350:81–95, 1974.

HENDERSON, EG AND VOLLE, RL: *Ion exchange in frog sartorius muscle treated with 9-aminoacridine or barium.* J Pharmacol Exp Ther 183:356–369, 1972.

HENSON, RA: *The neurological aspects of hypercalcaemia, with special reference to primary hyperparathyroidism.* J R Coll Physicians Lond 1:41–50, 1966.

HILLE, B: *Charges and potentials at the nerve surface. Divalent ions and pH.* J Gen Physiol 51:221–236, 1968.

HOFMANN, WW AND SMITH, RA: *Hypokalemic periodic paralysis studied in vitro.* Brain 93:455–474, 1970.

HOLLER, JW: *Potassium deficiency occurring during the treatment of diabetic acidosis.* JAMA 131:1186–1189, 1946.

HUANG, KW: *Pa Ping (transient paralysis simulating family periodic paralysis).* Chin Med J (Engl) 51:305–312, 1943.

ISGREN, WP: *Normocalcemic tetany. A problem of erethism.* Neurology 26:825–834, 1976.

KAO, L AND GORDON, AM: *Mechanisms of insulin-induced paralysis of muscles from potassium-depleted rats.* Science 188:740–741, 1975.

KELLY, TR AND ZARCONI, J: *Primary hyperparathyroidism: Hyperparathyroid crisis.* Am J Surg 142:539–542, 1981.

KNIGHT, AH, WILLIAMS, DN, SPOONER, RJ, ET AL: *Serum enzyme changes in diabetic ketoacidosis.* Diabetes 23:126–131, 1974.

KNOCHEL, JP: *The pathophysiology and clinical characteristics of severe hypophosphatemia.* Arch Intern Med 137:203–220, 1977.

KNOCHEL, JP: *Hypophosphatemia (Nutrition in Medicine).* West J Med 134:15–26, 1981.

KNOCHEL, JP, BARCENAS, C, COTTON, JR, ET AL: *Hypophosphatemia and rhabdomyolysis.* J Clin Invest 62:1240–1246, 1978.

KNOCHEL, JP, BILBREY, GL, FULLER, TJ, ET AL: *The muscle cell in chronic alcoholism: The possible role of phosphate depletion in alcoholic myopathy.* Ann NY Acad Sci 252:274–286, 1975.

KNOCHEL, JP, HALLER, R AND FERGUSON, E: *Selective phosphorus deficiency in the hyperalimented hypophosphatemic dog and phosphorylation potentials in the muscle cell.* Adv Exp Med Biol 128:324–334, 1979.

KNOCHEL, JP AND SCHLEIN, EM: *On the mechanism of rhabdomyolysis in potassium depletion.* J Clin Invest 51:1750–1758, 1972.

KU, DY, YEN, CK AND LI, CC: *Acute poisoning by common salt containing barium chloride.* Chin Med J (Engl) 51:303–304, 1943.

KUGELBERG, E: *Neurologic mechanism for certain phenomena in tetany.* Arch Neurol Psychiatry 56:507–521, 1946.

KUGELBERG, E: *Activation of human nerves by ischemia. Trousseau's phenomenon in tetany.* Arch Neurol Psychiatry 60:140–152, 1948a.

KUGELBERG, E: *Activation of human nerves by hyperventilation and hypocalcemia. Neurologic mechanism of symptoms of irritation in tetany.* Arch Neurol Psychiatry 60:153–164, 1948b.

KUGELBERG, E: *The mechanism of Chvostek's sign.* Arch Neurol Psychiatry 65:511–517, 1951.

LAFAIR, JS AND MYERSON, RM: *Alcoholic myopathy, with special reference to the significance of creatine phosphokinase.* Arch Intern Med 122:417–422, 1968.

LAWSON, DH, HENRY, DA, LOWE, JM, ET AL: *Severe hypokalemia in hospitalized patients.* Arch Intern Med 139:978–980, 1979.

LAYZER, RB: *Motor unit hyperactivity states.* In VINKEN, PJ AND BRUYN, GW (EDS): *Handbook of Clinical Neurology, Vol 41.* North-Holland Publishing, Amsterdam, 1979, pp 295–316.

LAYZER, RB: *Neurological progress: Periodic paralysis and the Na-K pump.* Ann Neurol 11:547–552, 1982.

LEVINSKY, NG: *Management of emergencies. VI. Hyperkalemia.* N Engl J Med 274:1076–1077, 1966.

LEWIS, T: *Trousseau's phenomenon in tetany.* Clin Sci 4:361–364, 1942.

LEWIS, Z AND BAR-KHAYIM, Y: *Food poisoning from barium carbonate.* Lancet ii:342–343, 1964.

MADDY, JA AND WINTERNITZ, WW: *Hypothalmic syndrome with hypernatremia and muscular paralysis.* Am J Med 51:394–402, 1971.

MARTIN, JB, CRAIG, JW, ECKEL, RE, ET AL: *Hypokalemic myopathy in chronic alcoholism.* Neurology 21:1160–1168, 1971.

MCCHESNEY, JA AND MARQUARDT, JF: *Hypokalemic paralysis induced by amphotericin B.* JAMA 189:1029–1031, 1964.

MERIGAN, TC, JR AND HAYES, RE: *Treatment of hypercalcemia in multiple myeloma.* Arch Intern Med 107:389–394, 1961.

MITCHELL, ABS: *Duogastrone-induced hypokalaemic nephropathy and myopathy with myoglobinuria.* Postgrad Med J 47:806–813, 1971.

MOLLARET, P, GOULON, M AND TOURNILHAC, M: *Contribution à l'étude des paralysies avec hyperkaliémie. I. Role de l'insuffisance corticosurrénalienne.* Rev Neurol (Paris) 98:341–357, 1958a.

MOLLARET, P, GOULON, M AND TOURNILHAC, M: *Contribution à l'étude des paralysies avec hyperkaliémie. II. Les paralysies avec hyperkaliémie au cours de l'insuffisance rénale.* Rev Neurol (Paris) 99:241–263, 1958b.

MORDES, JP AND WACKER, WEC: *Excess magnesium.* Pharmacol Rev 29:273–300, 1977.

MORTON, W: *Poisoning by barium carbonate.* Lancet ii:738–739, 1945.

MURPHY, TR, REMINE, WH AND BURBANK, MK: *Hyperparathyroidism: Report of a case in which parathyroid adenoma presented primarily with profound muscular weakness.* Proc Mayo Clin 35:629–640, 1960.

NADEL, SM, JACKSON, JW AND PLOTH, DW: *Hypokalemic rhabdomyolysis and acute renal failure. Occurrence following total parenteral nutrition.* JAMA 241:2294–2296, 1979.

NEWMAN, JH, NEFF, TA AND ZIPORIN, P: *Acute respiratory failure associated with hypophosphatemia.* N Engl J Med 296:1101–1103, 1977.

NICHOLSON, WM AND BRANNING, WS: *Potassium deficiency in diabetic acidosis.* JAMA 134:1292–1294, 1947.

NICOLIS, GL, KAHN, T, SANCHEZ, A, ET AL: *Glucose-induced hyperkalemia in diabetic subjects.* Arch Intern Med 141:49–53, 1981.

NYGREN, A: *Serum creatine phosphokinase activity in chronic alcoholism, in connection with acute alcohol intoxication.* Acta Med Scand 179:623–630, 1966.

O'DORISIO, TM: *Hypercalcemic crisis.* Heart Lung 7:425–434, 1978.

OFFERIJNS, FGJ, WESTERINK, D AND WILLEBRANDS, AF: *The relation of potassium deficiency to muscular paralysis by insulin.* J Physiol 141:377–384, 1958.

OH, SJ, DOUGLAS, JE AND BROWN, RA: *Hypokalemic vacuolar myopathy associated with chlorthalidone treatment.* JAMA 216:1858–1859, 1971.

OTSUKA, M AND OHTSUKI, I: *Mechanism of muscular paralysis by insulin with special reference to periodic paralysis.* Am J Physiol 219:1178–1182, 1970.

OWEN, EE AND VERNER, JW, JR: *Renal tubular disease with muscle paralysis and hypokalemia.* Am J Med 28:8–21, 1960.

PARKER, MS, OSTER, JR, PEREZ, GO, ET AL: *Chronic hypokalemia and alkalosis. Approach to diagnosis.* Arch Intern Med 140:1336–1337, 1980.

PERKINS, JG, PETERSEN, AB AND RILEY, JA: *Renal and cardiac lesions in potassium deficiency due to chronic diarrhea.* Am J Med 8:115–123, 1950.

PERKOFF, GT, DIOSO, MM, BLEISCH, V, ET AL: *A spectrum of myopathy associated with alcoholism. I. Clinical and laboratory features.* Ann Intern Med 67:481–492, 1966.

PLEASURE, D AND GOLDBERG, M: *Neurogenic hypernatremia.* Arch Neurol 15:78–87, 1966.

PULLEN, H, DOIG, A AND LAMBIE, AT: *Intensive intravenous potassium replacement therapy.* Lancet ii:809–811, 1967.

RADO, J, MAROSI, J, TAKO, J, ET AL: *Hyperkalemic intermittent paralysis associated with spironolactone in a patient with cardiac cirrhosis.* Am Heart J 76:393–398, 1968.

RAINEY, RL, ESTES, PW, NEELEY, CL, ET AL: *Myoglobinuria following diabetic acidosis with electromyographic evaluation.* Arch Intern Med 111:564–571, 1963.

RIECKER, G AND BOLTE, HD: *Membranpotentiale einzelner Skeletmuskelzellen bei hypokaliamischer periodischer Muskelparalyse.* Klin Wochenschr 44:804–807, 1966.

Riecker, G, Bolte, HD and Röhl, D: *Hypokaliämie und Membranpotential. Mikropunktionen einzelner Muskelzellen beim Menschen.* Reanim Org Artif 1:41–50, 1964.

Roza, O and Berman, LB: *The pathophysiology of barium: Hypokalemic and cardiovascular effects.* J Pharmacol Exp Therap 177:433–439, 1971.

Rumpf, KW, Kaiser, H, Gröne, HJ, et al: *Myoglobinurisches Nierenversagen bei hyperosmolarem diabetischem Koma.* Dtsch Med Wochenschr 106:708–711, 1981.

Ryback, RS, Eckardt, MJ and Pautler, CP: *Clinical relationships between serum phosphorus and other blood chemistry values in alcoholics.* Arch Intern Med 140:673–677, 1980.

Sarkar, K, Parry, DJ and Heggtveit, HA: *Skeletal myopathy in chronic magnesium depletion.* Magnesium-Bulletin 3:108–113, 1981.

Saul, RF and Selhorst, JB: *Downbeat nystagmus with magnesium depletion.* Arch Neurol 38:650–652, 1981.

Schaff, M and Payne, CA: *Diphenylhydantoin and phenobarbital in overt and latent tetany.* N Engl J Med 274:1228–1232, 1966.

Shils, ME: *Experimental human magnesium depletion.* Medicine 48:61–85, 1969.

Silvis, SE, DiBartolomeo, AG and Aaker, HM: *Hypophosphatemia and neurological changes secondary to oral caloric intake. A variant of hyperalimentation syndrome.* Am J Gastroenterol 73:215–222, 1980.

Silvis, SE and Paragas, PD, Jr: *Paresthesias, weakness, seizures, and hypophosphatemia in patients receiving hyperalimentation.* Gastroenterology 62:513–520, 1972.

Sjodin, RA and Ortiz, O: *Resolution of the potassium ion pump in muscle fibers using barium ions.* J Gen Physiol 66:269–286, 1975.

Smith, SG, Black-Schaffer, B and Lasater, TE: *Potassium deficiency symdrome in the rat and the dog.* Arch Pathol 49:185–199, 1950.

Somjen, G, Hilmy, M and Stephen, CR: *Failure to anesthetize human subjects by intravenous administration of magnesium sulfate.* J Pharmacol Exp Ther 154:652–659, 1966.

Sperelakis, N, Schneider, MF and Harris, EJ: *Decreased K^+ conductance produced by Ba^{++} in frog sartorius fibers.* J Gen Physiol 50:1565–1583, 1967.

Stein, RB: *Nerve and Muscle. Membranes, Cells and Systems.* Plenum Press, New York, 1980, pp 56–59.

Stephens, FI: *Paralysis due to reduced serum potassium concentration during treatment of diabetic acidosis: Report of a case treated with 33 grams of potassium chloride intravenously.* Ann Intern Med 30:1272–1286, 1949.

Stevens, AR, Jr and Wolff, HG: *Magnesium intoxication. Absorption from the intact gastrointestinal tract.* Arch Neurol Psychiatry 63:749–759, 1950.

Swift, TR: *Weakness from magnesium-containing cathartics: Electrophysiologic studies.* Muscle Nerve 2:295–298, 1979.

Toback, FG, Aithal, HN, Ordonez, NG, et al: *Altered bioenergetics in proliferating renal cells during potassium depletion.* Lab Invest 4:265–267, 1979.

Travis, SF, Sugerman, HJ and Ruberg, RL: *Alterations of red cell glycolytic intermediates and oxygen transport as a consequence of hypophosphatemia in patients receiving intravenous hyperalimentation.* N Engl J Med 285:763–768, 1971.

Troni, W: *Electromyographic study on experimental hyperkalemia.* Acta Neurol (Napoli) 33:381–389, 390–398, 399–407, 1978.

Turpin, R, Lefebvre, J and Lérique, J: *Modifications de l'électromyogramme élémentaire et trouble de la transmission neuro-musculaire dans la tétanie.* C R Acad Sci [D] (Paris) 25:579–580, 1943.

Tuynman, PE and Wilhelm, SK: *Potassium deficiency associated with diabetic acidosis.* Ann Intern Med 29:356–361, 1948.

Vallee, BL, Wacker, WEC and Ulmer, DD: *The magnesium deficiency tetany syndrome in man.* N Engl J Med 262:155–161, 1960.

Van Dellen, RG and Purnell, DC: *Hyperkalemic paralysis in Addison's disease.* Mayo Clin Proc 44:904–914, 1969.

Van Horn, G, Drori, JB and Schwartz, FD: *Hypokalemic myopathy and elevation of serum enzymes.* Arch Neurol 22:335–341, 1970.

Velez-Garcia, E, Hardy, P, Dioso, M, et al: *Cysteine-stimulated serum creatine phosphokinase. Unexpected results.* J Lab Clin Med 68:636–645, 1966.

Vicale, CT: *The diagnostic features of a muscular syndrome resulting from hyperparathyroidism, osteomalacia owing to renal tubular acidosis, and perhaps to related disorders of calcium metabolism.* Trans Am Neurol Assoc 74:143–147, 1949.

Wacker, WEC, Moore, FD, Ulmer, DD, et al: *Normocalcemic magnesium deficiency tetany.* JAMA 180:161–163, 1962.

Weintraub, MI: *Hypophosphatemia mimicking acute Guillain-Barre-Strohl syndrome. A complication of parenteral hyperalimentation.* JAMA 235:1040–1041, 1976.

Wetherill, SF, Guarino, MJ and Cox, RW: *Acute renal failure associated with barium chloride poisoning.* Ann Intern Med 95:187–188, 1981.

Whang, R and Aikawa, JK: *Magnesium deficiency and refractoriness to potassium repletion.* J Chronic Dis 30:65–68, 1977.

Wiegand, CF, Davin, TD, Raij, L, et al: *Severe hypokalemia induced by hemodialysis.* Arch Intern Med 141:167–170, 1981.

Wilson, HK, Keuer, SP, Lea, AS, et al: *Phosphate therapy in diabetic ketoacidosis.* Arch Intern Med 142:517–520, 1982.

Zimmet, P, Breidahl, HD and Nayler, WG: *Plasma ionized calcium in hypomagnesemia.* Br Med J 1:622–623, 1968.

Chapter 3

ENDOCRINE DISORDERS

THYROID DISORDERS

Hypothyroidism

Neuromuscular symptoms are among the most frequent manifestations of hypothyroidism (Table 20). The high incidence of these complaints is attested to by both retrospective (Collins et al. 1964) and prospective studies (Nickel et al. 1961; Rao et al. 1980). Between 44 and 100 percent of hypothyroid patients complain of muscle weakness; 49 to 56 percent have muscle pain or cramps; and 24 to 100 percent report paresthesias. Unfortunately, none of these surveys distinguished between spontaneous complaints and symptoms elicited by questioning.

Symptoms of Disordered Contraction

Slowness of the muscle stretch reflexes was recognized as a sign of myxedema by Ord in 1884. Chaney in 1924 devised the first graphic instrument for measuring the Achilles reflex time. After Lambert and associates (1951), using an isometric device with a strain gauge, established that the contraction and relaxation phases of the ankle jerk were prolonged in hypothyroidism and abbreviated in hyperthyroidism, measurement of the reflex time of the ankle jerk became available as an office procedure for the diagnosis of hypothyroidism. Lawson (1958) used an electromagnetic device called a Kinemometer to record the contraction time of the free, isotonic Achilles reflex, while Sherman and colleagues (1963) reported good diagnostic results with a photoelectric device known as the Photomotograph. With either device, a high detection rate and a low incidence of false positive results were claimed by the proponents.

However, many investigators were unable to duplicate these good results. For example, Rives and coworkers (1965) compared 116 hypothy-

TABLE 20. Neuromuscular Manifestations of Hypothyroidism

Symptoms	Signs
Weakness	Slow reflexes
Muscle aches	Myoedema
Stiffness and slowness of movement	Muscular enlargement
Cramps	Myopathy
Acroparesthesias	Carpal tunnel syndrome
	Peripheral neuropathy

roid patients with 510 euthyroid subjects, using both the Kinemometer and the Photomotograph and correlating the results with four tests of thyroid function. When the upper limit of normal was set at 2 standard deviations above the mean, only 62 percent of patients had a prolonged reflex time with the Kinemometer and 66 percent with the Photomotograph. With the upper limit of normal at 1.5 standard deviations above the mean, the proportion of false positives was larger, but only 75 percent of hypothyroid patients were detected by reflex measurements compared with 92 percent by protein-bound iodine levels. Of course, the diagnostic accuracy of these instruments is probably lower in the physician's office than in the laboratory, and clinical evaluation of "hung-up reflexes" is even less likely to be reliable.

Furthermore, the reflex time may be lengthened by drugs (such as propranolol, procainamide, quinidine, and reserpine), cooling, local edema, diabetes, and other factors (Waal-Manning 1969). Serial measurements of the reflex time may be a convenient means of following the response of individual hypothyroid patients to replacement therapy, but the availability of inexpensive and accurate radioimmunoassays has made this office apparatus obsolete.

Myoedema is a localized knot of contracting muscle induced by direct percussion or by some other form of mechanical irritation of the muscle. Local contractions lasting up to 5 seconds can be elicited in normal persons, but the response is larger and of longer duration in cachectic patients, and it is especially pronounced in some hypothyroid patients. Nickel and associates (1961) found myoedema in 8 of 25 hypothyroid patients.

The EMG electrode records an initial, brief burst of action potentials at the site of percussion, followed by brief tightening of the whole muscle fascicle as the action potentials spread down the length of the muscle; immediately afterward, a knot of electrically silent contraction remains at the site of impact (Denny-Brown and Pennybacker, 1938). In a hypothyroid patient studied by Salick and Pearson (1967), the mounding persisted for 30 to 60 seconds and receded slowly. This type of electrically silent contraction, which is termed a contracture, probably results from local prolongation of the active state, a phenomenon that is explained by the anatomic arrangements that underlie excitation-contraction coupling (Fig. 11). While the surface muscle action potential is self-propagating, contraction itself is governed by events that are not propagated longitudinally, namely, the local release of calcium from the cisterns of the sarcoplasmic reticulum, and the combination of calcium with the troponin-tropomyosin complex, which causes myosin and actin to interact and generate tension. The active state persists until the local calcium concentration is reduced by transport of calcium back into the sarcoplasmic reticulum. Myoedema is not prevented by pharmacologic agents that block excitation of the muscle membrane or of the transverse tubular system, but it may result from excessive release or abnormally slow reaccumulation of calcium by the sarcoplasmic reticulum (Mizusawa et al. 1983).

Muscle pain, cramp, or stiffness occurs in 20 to 56 percent of hypothyroid patients, and these symptoms may be the chief reason for consulting a physician. Complaints of generalized aching may be present for several years before a diagnosis is reached. Often a rheumatic disorder is suspected because the pain affects joints as well as muscles, is worse in cold weather, and is accompanied by morning stiffness (Golding 1970). To add to the confusion, synovial thickening and joint effusions may be present (Frymoyer and Bland 1973).

The term "stiffness" also applies to a peculiar slowness of muscular contraction and relaxation experienced by hypothyroid patients. During activity the muscles may become increasingly stiff, firm, and painful, so that the patient is forced to rest briefly before resuming activity. These "myotonoid" features, which bear the eponym of Hoffmann's syndrome, are prob-

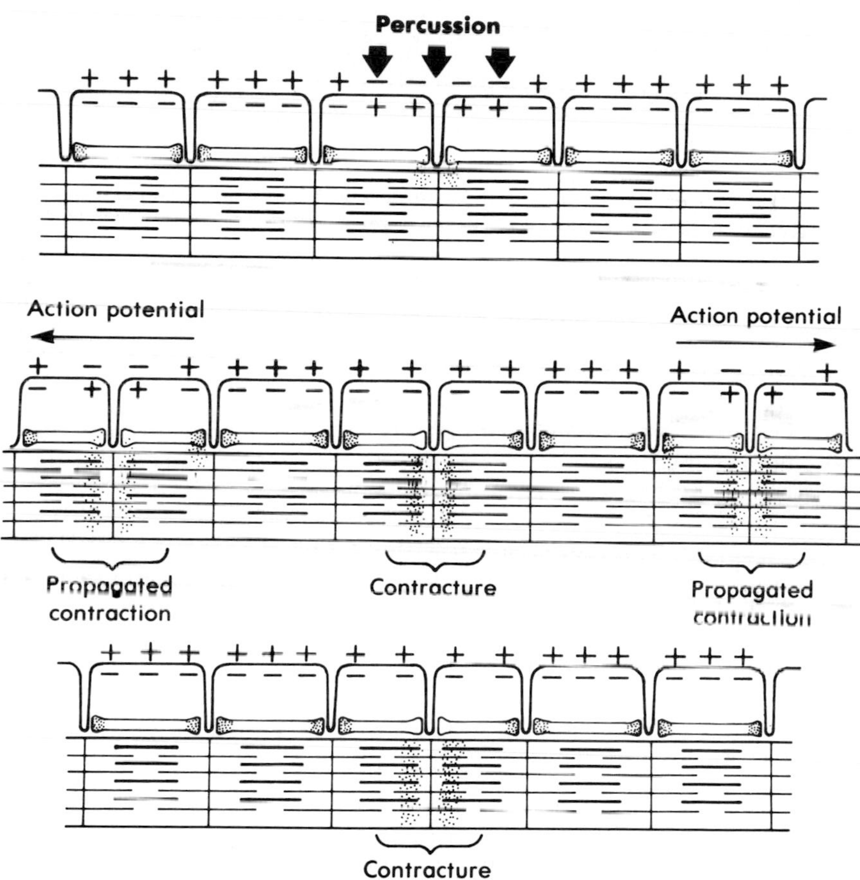

FIGURE 11. Pathophysiology of myoedema. (*Top*) Percussion of the muscle causes localized depolarization of the plasma membrane and T-tubules, with localized release of calcium (shown by small dots) from the sarcoplasmic reticulum. (*Middle*) A propagated action potential travels along the muscle fiber membrane in both directions away from the site of percussion, causing the muscle fiber to twitch. The site of percussion remains in a state of contracture despite repolarization of the plasma membrane and T-tubules. (*Bottom*) The entire plasma membrane has repolarized, but a local contracture (myoedema) persists, owing to slow reuptake of calcium by the sarcoplasmic reticulum.

ably related to the slow contraction and relaxation exhibited by the muscle stretch reflexes. True myotonia does not occur, though in one recent case subclinical myotonia was apparently uncovered by hypothyroidism (Venables et al. 1978).

Muscle pain, slowness, and stiffness, are sometimes loosely referred to as "cramps," but true cramps—sudden, painful muscle spasms—also occur frequently in hypothyroidism. The EMG of a muscle cramp in a hypothyroid patient showed an abundance of motor unit potentials (Hurwitz et al. 1970), the same as in ordinary cramps. It seems probable that electrically silent muscle spasms also occur in some patients; Takamori and coworkers (1972) demonstrated a transient muscle contracture following repetitive nerve stimulation at 15 Hz for 15 seconds. Carpopedal spasms resembling tetany have also been described, and in one case (Wilson and Walton 1959) the spasms were accompanied by paresthesias and a Trousseau's sign, suggesting a neural mechanism.

Muscle Enlargement

Myxedema can lead to gradual enlargement of the muscles over a period of months or years, especially in patients with muscle stiffness and pain (Wilson and Walton 1959; Norris and Panner 1966; Salick and Pearson 1967). The enlarged muscles are unusually firm, and a few patients take on the appearance of a weightlifter (Hurwitz et al. 1970). Muscle enlargement seems to be uncommon in adults, but it has been very striking in some hypothyroid children, whose "infant Hercules" appearance bears the eponym, Kocher-Debré-Sémélaigne syndrome. Najjar (1974) observed muscular enlargement in 23 (19 percent) of 118 hypothyroid children whose ages ranged from 18 months to 10 years. The syndrome seems to develop more readily in boys and in children with long-standing hypothyroidism.

The reason for the muscle enlargement is unknown. Mucopolysaccharide deposition in muscle has been noted in some cases but not in others; with light microscopy some authors observed large or rounded muscle fibers, but others found mainly atrophy. Afifi and associates (1974) found no distinctive light- or electron-microscopic features in muscle samples from children with Kocher-Debré-Sémélaigne syndrome compared with samples from hypothyroid children without muscle enlargement.

Muscle enlargement in childhood is also a feature of myotonia congenita and of Schwartz-Jampel syndrome (chondrodystrophic myotonia), conditions in which overactivity of muscle fibers may contribute to the muscle hypertrophy. It is possible that in myxedema the prolonged contraction time and frequent spasms are the cause of muscle enlargement, which subsides within a few months following the institution of replacement therapy.

Hypothyroid Myopathy

Proximal muscle weakness develops in about one fourth of hypothyroid patients (Rao et al. 1980; Nickel et al. 1961). The weakness is usually mild and develops slowly over a period of months or years. The muscles may be normal in size, enlarged, or even atrophic (Bergouignan et al. 1967). Wilson and Walton (1959) considered muscular atrophy an unusual feature, but Rao and colleagues (1980) observed muscle wasting in three out of four weak patients. Most weak patients also complain of pain, slowness, or stiffness.

During treatment the weakness resolves gradually within a period of several months.

A few patients have had unusual myopathic syndromes. Katz and Pate (1980) described a patient with weakness restricted to the neck muscles, so severe that she could not hold up her head. They pointed out that the first recorded case of muscle weakness in myxedema, published by Ord in 1879, was very similar. A case of myoglobinuria accompanying myxedema may have been a coincidental association, since extensive muscle inflammation was said to be present in the muscle biopsy (Halverson et al. 1979). A hypothyroid patient with muscle pain, slowness, and fatigue had two episodes of normokalemic periodic paralysis following anesthesia (Wilson and Walton 1959). There are several reports of a coincidental association of hypothyroidism with myotonic disorders and with other myopathies. An association with myasthenia gravis is more than coincidental; this is discussed later in this chapter.

ELECTROPHYSIOLOGY. EMG abnormalities are common in myxedema, even in the absence of overt weakness. Rao and colleagues (1980) studied 20 unselected patients by quantitative EMG techniques. There were no fibrillations or other signs of muscle fiber irritability. The mean duration of motor unit potentials was reduced in proximal muscles in 70 percent of patients, the mean amplitude of motor unit potentials was reduced in 40 percent of patients, and the proportion of polyphasic motor unit potentials was increased in 90 percent of patients. Only 4 of the 20 patients had detectable weakness.

Ramsay (1974) reviewed the EMG studies published between 1955 and 1970, none of which used quantitative techniques for measuring individual motor unit potentials. Features of hyperirritability (increased insertional activity, fibrillations, positive waves, and repetitive discharges) were prominent in two series but not in the others. Scarpalezos and associates (1973) also failed to detect hyperirritability in a quantitative EMG study of 15 hypothyroid patients.

MUSCLE PATHOLOGY. The most consistent pathologic change is a reduction in the proportion and size of type-2 muscle fibers, which contain increased numbers of central nuclei (McKeran et al. 1975 and 1979; Wiles et al. 1979). The contribution of type-2 fibers to the overall cross-sectional area of muscle is reduced to one half of normal in men and to one third of normal in women.

Ramsay (1974) collated the light-microscopic abnormalities in 33 patients reported in 15 articles published between 1940 and 1970. The most frequent changes were muscle fiber degeneration and regeneration, increased numbers of central nuclei, and deposition of mucopolysaccharides. The muscle fiber degeneration was usually confined to a few, scattered fibers, and in general the paucity of abnormalities was striking compared with the prominence of clinical symptoms. Electron-microscopic studies have revealed a variety of nonspecific degenerative changes and mitochondrial abnormalities.

SERUM ENZYMES. The serum CPK level is increased in about 90 percent of hypothyroid patients, most of whom do not have overt myopathy (Graig and Smith 1965; Griffiths 1965). Although this finding might be indicative of a subtle myopathic abnormality, the fact that serum CPK levels are often *below* normal in hyperthyroidism suggests another explanation. In fact, the protein-bound iodine (PBI) level bears an inverse relation to the logarithm of the CPK level (Fig. 12) (Graig and Smith 1965). According to recent experiments by Karlsberg and Roberts (1978), these changes in the level of serum CPK can be accounted for by changes in the rate of clearance of the enzyme from the plasma. They prepared purified CPK from dog muscle and measured its rate of disappearance from the plasma of dogs following intravenous injection. The normal half-time for disappearance was about 2 hours; in hypothyroid dogs the rate of clearance was decreased by 31 percent and the baseline CPK level increased by 65 percent, while in hyperthyroid dogs the rate of clearance was increased by 56 percent and the baseline CPK level was reduced by 46 percent. Thus, the serum CPK level cannot be used as an indication of myopathy in hypothyroidism. During the treatment of hypothyroid patients, the CPK level returns to normal at a fairly constant rate, with a half-time of 10 to 12 days (Klein et al. 1980).

Carpal Tunnel Syndrome

Murray and Simpson (1958) were the first to point out that the acroparesthesias of myxedema are usually due to median nerve compression at the

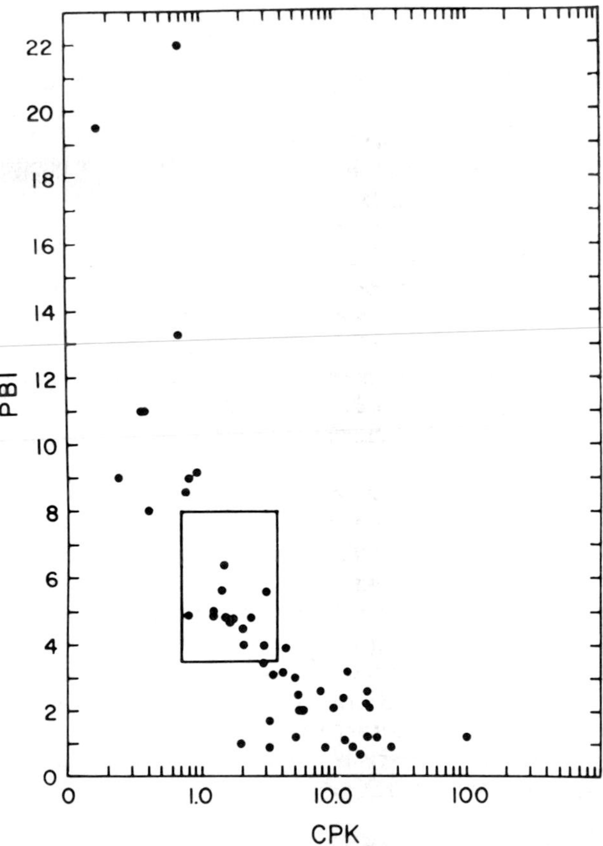

FIGURE 12. Semi-logarithmic plot of serum CPK activity versus serum protein-bound iodine (PBI) in euthyroid, hyperthyroid, and hypothyroid patients. The enclosed area represents the range of normal values. CPK levels tend to be elevated in hypothyroid patients and low in hyperthyroid patients. (From Graig and Smith [1965], with permission.)

wrist—the carpal tunnel syndrome. They found that paresthesias were almost always located in the hands and were usually bilateral. They made a clinical diagnosis of carpal tunnel syndrome in 10 (29 percent) of 35 unselected hypothyroid patients, and reported prolongation of motor nerve conduction in the median nerve across the wrist. Rao and associates (1980) detected clinical signs of the carpal tunnel syndrome in 3 (15 percent) of 20 unselected patients, and they found distal abnormalities of median nerve conduction in 6 more patients, though they did not test ulnar nerve conduction to rule out a generalized slowing of distal nerve conduction.

In two large retrospective studies of patients with carpal tunnel syndrome, the incidence of hypothyroidism ranged from 0.7 percent (Phalen 1966) to 10 percent (Frymoyer and Bland 1973). A recent prospective study of 41 consecutive patients with carpal tunnel syndrome yielded 5 hypothyroid patients, an incidence of 12 percent (Gelberman et al. 1980).

Several authors have speculated that deposition of mucopolysaccharides in the soft tissues of the carpal tunnel might be responsible for the nerve compression. However, in two surgical specimens only edema, fat, and fibrous tissue were seen (Purnell et al. 1961). Most patients do not require surgical treatment because the symptoms respond to thyroid replacement, but in long-standing cases the presence of fat and fibrosis might require surgical treatment (Frymoyer and Bland 1973; Purnell et al. 1961).

Polyneuropathy

A distal, symmetrical, sensorimotor polyneuropathy is an uncommon complication of hypothyroidism. Scarpalezos and colleagues (1973) found absent ankle jerks in 4 out of 51 hypothyroid patients, and Rao and associates (1980) noted signs of polyneuropathy in 2 of their 20 patients, an incidence of 10 percent. In most of the reported cases, the rather mild deficits were confined to the lower extremities, and sensory impairment was greater than motor. The muscle stretch reflexes were diminished or absent at the ankles and were sometimes diminished at the knees. The symptoms and signs improved during treatment, but improvement was slow and in one case there were residual abnormalities 18 months later (Shirabe et al. 1975; Meier and Bischoff 1977; Dyck and Lambert 1970; Nickel et al. 1961; Pollard et al. 1982).

In patients with overt neuropathy, nerve conduction velocities are mildly or moderately slow, and sensory nerve action potentials are reduced or absent (Meier and Bischoff 1977; Shirabe et al. 1975; Pollard et al. 1982). Dyck and Lambert (1970) analyzed the compound action potential evoked by *in-vitro* stimulation of segments of biopsied sural nerves. There was a marked reduction in evoked amplitude and conduction velocity of the large myelinated nerve fibers, while small and unmyelinated fibers were much less affected. Studies of unselected patients, most of whom do not have overt neuropathy, show mild slowing of motor and sensory nerve conduction, more so in the upper than in the lower extremities and more marked in sensory than in motor nerves (Rao et al. 1980; Scarpalezos et al. 1973; Fincham and Cape 1968).

A quantitative histopathologic study of biopsy specimens of sural nerve revealed a loss of myelinated nerve fibers as well as evidence of segmental demyelination and remyelination, suggesting that segmental demyelination was the main pathologic mechanism (Dyck and Lambert

1970). Other investigators (Meier and Bischoff 1977; Pollard et al. 1982) confirmed the preponderant loss of myelinated fibers, especially those of large diameter, but they observed degenerative changes in axons of all sizes, including some with well-preserved myelin sheaths and even some small unmyelinated axons. There were clusters of unmyelinated or thinly myelinated axons, which suggested axonal regeneration. These authors concluded that axonal degeneration was the primary pathologic mechanism, and they postulated that segmental demyelination was secondary to axonal degeneration. This conclusion is consonant with the results of nerve conduction studies and with the slow improvement observed in some cases. An earlier report (Nickel et al. 1961) of deposits of mucoid material in the nerve has not been confirmed by recent pathologic studies.

Myasthenic Syndromes

Norris (1966) described three hypothyroid patients with limb girdle and trunk muscle weakness characterized by unusual fatigability. Two of the patients also had weakness of chewing and speech. Repetitive nerve stimulation at fast rates (10 to 30 Hz) resulted in abnormal decrement of the muscle response; presumably there was no decrement at slow rates of stimulation, though that was not stated. Edrophonium partly counteracted the decrement in the two patients with bulbar muscle weakness. In another patient with a similar abnormality, the degree of decrement increased in proportion to the rate of repetitive nerve stimulation (Takamori et al. 1972). The clinical and electrophysiologic abnormalities resolved after treatment with thyroid hormone. The abnormality of neuromuscular transmission in these patients was different from that seen in myasthenia gravis. Takamori and coworkers (1972) postulated that it was due either to desensitization block at the postsynaptic membrane or to conduction block in the motor nerve terminals.

Hyperthyroidism

The neuromuscular disorders in hyperthyroidism include the following:

1. Myopathy
2. Myokymia
3. Acute bulbar myopathy
4. Hypokalemic periodic paralysis
5. Motor polyneuropathy(?)
6. Ocular myopathy

Thyrotoxic Myopathy

Proximal muscle weakness was once thought to be uncommon in thyrotoxicosis, but since 1955 several clinical and electromyographic surveys, most notably those of Ramsay (1965, 1966, 1974), have shown that weakness is a frequent complication. The weakness is conveniently referred to as a myopathy, although the pathogenesis of the weakness is still a subject of controversy (McComas et al. 1974; Feibel and Campa 1976).

DIAGNOSIS. In addition to the six series of unselected thyrotoxic patients tabulated by Ramsay in his 1974 monograph, there is a recent survey of 48 patients from Singapore (Puvanendran et al. 1979a). The combined results of these seven studies indicate that 33 to 64 percent of patients complain of weakness, while 61 to 82 percent have weakness on examination. The percentages are the same in men and women. Weakness is usually an early symptom, affects the proximal limb muscles, and is often accompanied by excessive liability to fatigue. Muscle pain, stiffness, and cramps are infrequent symptoms.

On physical examination, there is mild or moderate weakness in muscles of the shoulder girdle and upper arms; the lower extremities are less involved, and the iliopsoas is the only lower extremity muscle affected in more than half of the weak patients (Ramsay 1966). Muscle atrophy is usually evident and may be remarkably severe, especially in the shoulder girdles. Muscle twitches (fasciculations) were mentioned in 42 percent of the published cases of myopathy reviewed by Ramsay (1974) and were observed in 12 percent of the unselected thyrotoxic patients studied by Puvanendran and colleagues (1979a). The combination of muscle wasting and fasciculations has occasionally led to a mistaken diagnosis of amyotrophic lateral sclerosis. To compound the confusion, muscle stretch reflexes are often very brisk, and a few patients have even had spastic paraparesis and Babinski's signs, which reverted to normal after treatment of hyperthyroidism (Garcia and Fleming 1977).

In a few cases, muscle twitching assumes spectacular proportions. There is continuous, undulating myokymia of the face, tongue, limbs, and trunk, and muscle cramps may occur. After the thyrotoxicosis is controlled the muscle twitching subsides over the course of several months (McEachern and Ross 1942). In one case of this type (Harman and Richardson 1954), the EMG showed continuous, repetitive discharges consisting of groups of 2 to 6 motor unit potentials recurring at a frequency of 1 to 4 Hz, even during sleep. The abnormal muscle activity appeared to arise in the distal portions of the motor nerves, since it was not altered by spinal anesthesia or brachial plexus block but was abolished by curare. (This type of myokymia differs clinically and electromyographically from the syndrome of neuromyotonia, in which myokymia is associated with generalized muscle stiffness at rest and slow relaxation of muscles after voluntary contraction (Layzer 1979).

Achilles Reflex Recordings. Achilles reflex recordings in hyperthyroidism show a reduced duration of both contraction and relaxation, the opposite of the abnormalities produced by hypothyroidism. Since the degree of overlap with euthyroid values is even greater than that found in hypothyroidism, this finding has little diagnostic value (Lambert et al. 1951; Rives et al. 1965).

Serum Enzymes. The serum concentration of CPK and other myoplasmic enzymes is nearly always normal, and in fact the serum CPK activity tends to be low (Graig and Smith 1965), perhaps because of an increased rate of clearance from the plasma (Karlsberg and Roberts 1978).

Electromyography. Electromyography shows typical myopathic abnormalities in almost all patients, and the abnormalities tend to be more marked in patients who are weak. The mean duration of motor unit potentials is reduced, and an increased proportion of these are polyphasic (Ramsay 1965; Puvanendran et al. 1979a). The abnormalities are found more than twice as often in proximal as in distal upper extremity muscles (Ramsay 1965). Fibrillations and fasciculations are infrequent in proximal muscles; in distal lower extremity muscles, however, Ludin and coworkers (1969) found signs of neurogenic involvement.

Puvanendran and associates (1979b) evaluated neuromuscular transmission in a series of 48 unselected thyrotoxic patients, none of whom had clinical findings resembling myasthenia gravis. Eight patients showed significant decrement of the muscle response to nerve stimulation at low or intermediate frequencies, and in four of these patients edrophonium corrected the abnormality. In three other patients the amplitude of the initial response was small and there was modest facilitation both at 2 Hz and at 20 Hz, with long-lasting posttetanic facilitation. The findings in the first group of patients suggested a postsynaptic abnormality like that of myasthenia gravis, while the latter findings could indicate a presynaptic abnormality of neuromuscular transmission. Although serum levels of acetylcholine receptor antibodies were not measured, the electrophysiologic abnormalities were probably not due to latent myasthenia gravis, because neuromuscular transmission returned to normal after the patients became euthyroid. Similar findings have been described in a few earlier reports. Thus, it is possible that abnormalities of neuromuscular transmission contribute to the weakness and fatigability of hyperthyroid patients.

PATHOLOGY. The main abnormality encountered in muscle biopsies is a general reduction of muscle fiber diameter, without the angular shape that is characteristic of denervation atrophy (Ramsay 1974). Both of the main muscle fiber types are affected, and in one study the proportion of fiber types was within the normal range (Wiles et al. 1979). Other histologic abnormalities are infrequent. Ramsay (1966) found minor changes in less than one fourth of the biopsy samples from 30 patients; the abnormalities included scattered muscle fiber degeneration, lymphorrhages, and increased amounts of fat and connective tissue. An electron-microscopic study showed enlargement of mitochondria and focal dilatation of the transverse tubules (Engel 1966).

PATHOPHYSIOLOGY. In animal experiments, hyperthyroidism produces a large increase in the proportion of type-2 muscle fibers (Ianuzzo et al. 1977; Fitts et al. 1980), an effect opposite to that produced by hypothyroidism. In rat muscles the major histochemical change was an increase in the number of fast oxidative-glycolytic (FOG) fibers; in the soleus this occurred at the expense of slow-oxidative (SO) fibers, which comprised 88 percent of the muscle fibers, but in the fast extensor digitorum longus the number of FOG fibers increased, mainly at the expense of fast-glycolytic (FG) fibers (Bruce and Nicol 1981).

TREATMENT. Ramsay (1966) undertook careful follow-up during treatment of nearly all his 34 patients with proximal weakness. Muscle power and thyroid function returned to normal in about 2 months, while muscle wasting resolved a bit more slowly. In severe cases, normal strength may not be restored for many months.

Pimstone and colleagues (1968) made the intriguing observation that, even before specific treatment, propranolol (in a daily dose of 120 to 320 mg) substantially reduced proximal weakness within 1 to 4 weeks in five out of eight thyrotoxic patients. A similar effect of propranolol has been observed in thyrotoxic bulbar myopathy and in thyrotoxic periodic paralysis.

Thyrotoxic Bulbar and Respiratory Muscle Weakness

Dysphagia was mentioned in 16 percent of the 73 cases of thyrotoxic myopathy published before 1964 (Ramsay 1974), but the findings were so poorly documented that concomitant myasthenia gravis could not be excluded. Since 1967, however, 18 cases of thyrotoxic bulbar weakness have been reported in which myasthenia gravis was reasonably well excluded, and in every case the weakness resolved completely following correction of the hyperthyroidism (Gaan 1967; Joasoo et al. 1977; Kammer and Hamilton 1974; Weinstein et al. 1975). The 6 men and 12 women ranged in age from 21 to 83 years. All of them had dysphagia, often accompanied by aspiration of liquids, nasal voice, nasal regurgitation, hoarseness, and weak cough. In addition, some patients had weakness of chewing, myopathic facies, weakness of the tongue, or weakness of eye movements. Respiratory muscle weakness was documented by vital capacity measurements in one case (Gaan 1967). Most of the patients also had proximal limb weakness. In some patients the bulbar symptoms appeared gradually along with a generalized myopathy, but in other patients bulbar symptoms came on rapidly in 2 or 3 weeks. The response to testing with edrophonium chloride (nine patients) and repetitive nerve stimulation (five patients) was always negative.

All of the patients recovered completely after returning to the euthyroid state. Five patients were treated with propranolol in addition to antithyroid measures, and two of them began to improve so quickly (within 1 to 4 days) that it is reasonable to suppose that propranolol was responsible for the improvement (Kammer and Hamilton 1974; Weinstein et al. 1975).

Thyrotoxic Periodic Paralysis

This fascinating complication has been the subject of numerous articles since it was first described in 1902 (Rosenfeld 1902). It seems to be uncommon in non-Oriental populations; Ramsay (1966) apparently did not encounter the condition among 54 consecutive hyperthyroid patients in Belfast, and even in Singapore there was only 1 case among 48 consecutive patients with thyrotoxicosis (Puvanendran et al. 1979a). In Japanese and Chinese populations, however, periodic paralysis occurs in 8 to 34 percent of thyrotoxic males and in 0.2 percent of thyrotoxic females (Okinaka et al. 1957; Satoyoshi et al. 1963; McFadzean and Yeung 1967). There is some indication that persons of Mexican, American Indian, or Filipino ancestry also have an increased susceptibility (Bernard et al. 1972; Conway et al. 1974). There is a marked predominance of male patients, despite the fact that more than 70 percent of hyperthyroid patients are female. Regardless of race or ancestry, a man who begins to have attacks of periodic paralysis after the age of 20, without a positive family history, is very likely to have hyperthyroidism.

The clinical and laboratory features of this disorder are remarkably similar to those of familiar hypokalemic periodic paralysis, which are described in Chapter 1. As in the hereditary form, attacks tend to occur during sleep or during rest; precipitating factors include heavy exercise, ingestion of a meal rich in carbohydrate or salt, menstruation, cold weather, anesthesia, and surgery. During an attack the serum potassium level generally falls below normal, though rather less so than in the primary, hereditary variety. Between attacks the serum potassium level is usually normal.

DIAGNOSIS. In most cases the diagnosis can be confirmed by finding a low level of serum potassium during an attack of paralysis, together with laboratory evidence of hyperthyroidism. If this information is lacking, a glucose and insulin test can be performed. McFadzean and Yeung (1967) were able to induce attacks of weakness with carbohydrate and insulin in 18 out of 23 patients with thyrotoxic periodic paralysis; the other 5 patients became susceptible to this provocation after pretreatment with fludrocortisone, 0.6 mg daily for 3 to 5 days.

TREATMENT. Administration of potassium chloride (KCl) will usually hasten recovery from an attack of paralysis. Divided doses totalling 80 to 100 mEq can be given orally over 4 to 6 hours. If oral potassium is not tolerated because of gastric irritation, an intravenous infusion of 80 mEq of KCl in 1000 ml of 5-percent glucose can be given over 4 to 6 hours.

Although Resnick and colleagues (1969) found that administration of reserpine for 6 weeks did not curb attacks of paralysis in one patient, several subsequent reports indicate that propranolol, in a dose of 160 mg daily, completely or partially suppresses attacks in most patients (Yeung and Tse 1974; Conway et al. 1974; Payne et al. 1979). In one patient, a glucose challenge during propranolol treatment induced striking hypokalemia (serum potassium 1.6 mEq per liter) just as before treatment, but no weakness developed. Treatment with acetazolamide has had no consistent effect (Yeung and Tse 1974; Norris 1972), even though this drug is usually efficacious in primary hypokalemic periodic paralysis.

Attacks of paralysis cease entirely when the patient becomes euthyroid. An abnormal susceptibility persists, however; if hyperthyroidism recurs, or if exogenous thyroid hormone is given, the attacks will return (Okihiro and Nordyke 1966). Furthermore, a few persons without a prior history of periodic paralysis have had attacks of paralysis while taking thyroid medication in order to lose weight (Layzer and Goldfield 1974).

Polyneuropathy

Charcot (1889) recognized a syndrome of progressive weakness and areflexia of the lower extremities in Basedow's disease (Graves' disease), and he mentioned that bladder function and sensation were unexpectedly preserved in those cases. For decades "Basedow's paraplegia" was all but forgotten, but recently a few cases have been reported of patients with a subacute, mainly motor polyneuropathy, virtually restricted to the lower extremities (Chollet et al. 1971; Feibel and Campa 1976). Motor nerve conduction was slow, but the spinal fluid protein concentration was not reported, and the nerves were not biopsied. From the scanty data provided, a concomitant autoimmune polyneuritis may be as good an explanation as "thyrotoxic polyneuropathy." Indeed, acute and subacute Guillain-Barré syndromes have been reported in euthyroid patients recently treated for hyperthyroidism (Birket-Smith and Olivarius 1957; Bronsky et al. 1964).

Nevertheless, there is some evidence for the existence of an axonal polyneuropathy directly related to hyperthyroidism. Ludin and associates (1969) found EMG changes of denervation in distal leg muscles in 8 of 11 thyrotoxic patients, although signs of distal weakness were slight. Most of the patients had the usual myopathic EMG abnormalities in proximal muscles, and motor conduction velocity was normal in the peroneal nerves. More recently, two unselected series showed normal motor and sensory nerve conduction in hyperthyroidism (McComas et al. 1974; Puvanendran

1979a), but in one series the amplitudes of M-waves (compound action potentials recorded from the muscle surface) were reduced in the hands and feet in about half of the patients, a finding more compatible with neuropathy than with myopathy (McComas et al. 1974).

The available evidence suggests that a mild or subclinical motor axonopathy may occur in hyperthyroidism, but the proximal weakness probably has a different mechanism. McComas and colleagues (1974) speculated that thyrotoxic myopathy could be a motor neuron disorder, basing their view on estimates of motor unit numbers in distal nerves, but the validity of their electrophysiologic technique has been disputed by later investigators (Ballantyne and Hansen 1974a, 1974b).

Pathophysiology of Muscle Disorders in Thyroid Disease

Alterations of Contractile Function

The opposite alterations of Achilles reflex times in hypothyroidism and hyperthyroidism reflect alterations of the intrinsic contractile properties of skeletal muscle. Both in human subjects (Takamori et al. 1971) and in animals (Gold et al. 1970) the velocity of shortening during isotonic contractions, and the rate of rise and fall of tension during isometric contractions, are increased in hyperthyroidism and decreased in hypothyroidism.

Two factors determine these velocity measurements: the rate of formation and interruption of linkages between actin and myosin cross-bridges, which is directly proportional to myosin ATPase activity; and the rate of release and reaccumulation of calcium by the sarcoplasmic reticulum. Myosin ATPase activity correlates best with the velocity of shortening, while the rate of calcium reaccumulation is the main determinant of the relaxation time. Both rates are altered in thyroid disease.

In experimental hyperthyroidism, there is a marked increase of rat soleus myosin ATPase activity measured at alkaline pH (the ATPase activity found in fast-twitch (type-2) muscle fibers); in addition, the proportion of type-2 fibers in soleus muscle is doubled. The opposite change, a marked reduction in the proportion of type-2 fibers and of alkaline myosin ATPase activity, occurs in hypothyroid muscle (Ianuzzo et al. 1977). These changes account for the increased velocity of shortening in hyperthyroidism and the slowness of contraction in hypothyroidism.

In hyperthyroid rats, the yield of fragmented sarcoplasmic reticulum and its rate of calcium uptake are doubled, producing a fourfold increase in calcium uptake per unit weight of muscle. These changes could affect both release and uptake of calcium, increasing the rate of rise of isometric tension, shortening the duration of the active state, and hastening relaxation (Fitts et al. 1980). The rate of calcium uptake is substantially reduced in the sarcoplasmic reticulum of hypothyroid rats (Fanburg 1968).

The changes of myosin ATPase activity probably reflect new synthesis of different molecular species of myosin. Differences in the composition of heavy and light chains characterize the myosins isolated from fast and slow skeletal muscle, and from atrial and ventricular cardiac muscle. In cross-innervation experiments, in which fast and slow muscles are interconverted, the molecular species of myosin are altered along with the contraction velocities. Preliminary evidence indicates that hyperthyroidism alters the amino acid composition of rabbit cardiac myosin (Morkin 1979), and in hypothyroid rat soleus muscle there is a selective disappearance of the myosin light chains characteristic of fast-twitch muscle fibers (Johnson et al. 1980).

Denervation, which tends to convert slow muscle fibers to fast fibers, nullifies the "fast to slow" biochemical changes induced by hypothyroidism, but enhances the "slow to fast" changes in hyperthyroidism. This suggests that thyroidal effects on muscle fiber properties are independent of neural influence (Nwoye et al. 1982).

Alterations of Energy Metabolism

Hypothyroidism reduces the muscle's content of mitochondria (Janssen et al. 1978) and the muscle's ability to oxidize carbohydrate and lipid fuels (Baldwin et al. 1980a, 1980b). In the intact animal there is reduced mobilization of fatty acids from lipid stores, and blood levels of free fatty acids do not increase normally during exercise; as a result there is increased utilization of endogenous and exogenous carbohydrates during prolonged exercise. These metabolic alterations reduce the endurance of running animals (Baldwin et al. 1980a, 1980b). Paradoxically, lactate production of muscle is reduced in human subjects during ischemic exercise (McDaniel et al. 1977). Wiles and coworkers (1979) found that muscle hydrolysis of creatine phosphate and formation of lactate during ischemic exercise were both reduced in hypothyroid subjects. For the same amount of work, the ATP turnover was 25 percent of normal—that is, hypothyroid muscle worked *more* economically than normal muscle. Experiments with the perfused rat hindlimb gave very similar results (Everts et al. 1981). The muscle force generated by sciatic nerve stimulation at 3 Hz for 30 minutes was normal in hypothyroid animals, but oxygen consumption, glucose consumption, and lactate release were much lower than in euthyroid animals, again suggesting more efficient energy utilization in hypothyroid muscle. Wiles and coworkers (1979) suggested that a decreased utilization of ATP during exercise could be explained by the reduced myosin ATPase activity of hypothyroid muscle. By their view, the reduced oxidative and glycolytic capacity of hypothyroid muscle appears to be an adaptation to a reduced rate of energy expenditure, which is a consequence of increased work efficiency.

In *hyperthyroidism* the opposite changes occur. Mitochondrial protein and enzyme activities increase, more in red than in white muscle (Winder and Holloszy 1977; Janssen et al. 1978), and one hyperthyroid patient expended ATP abnormally rapidly (Wiles et al. 1979). These preliminary findings suggest that hyperthyroid muscle works less economically than normal muscle and consequently requires a greater oxidative capacity in order to generate ATP from metabolic fuels.

Mechanisms of Weakness

We still do not know the mechanisms of weakness in the dysthyroid myopathies. Attempts to account for the weakness on the basis of contractile alterations are probably misdirected because they do not explain the principal physiologic abnormality: the myopathic EMG. Brief, low-amplitude, polyphasic motor unit potentials result from a loss of many individual muscle fiber action potentials in each motor unit potential. This abnormality can result from degeneration of muscle fibers, as in muscular dystrophy; from a temporary inexcitability of muscle fibers, as in periodic paralysis; from blockade of neuromuscular transmission, as in botulism; or from blockade of transmission along nerve terminals, as in tick paralysis. It cannot be attributed to an alteration of contractile properties of muscle fibers.

From pathologic studies we know that muscle fiber degeneration is a very minor feature of the dysthyroid myopathies, but very little is known of the electrophysiologic properties of the neuromuscular junction and the muscle membrane. Hofmann and Denys (1972) performed microelectrode studies on phrenic nerve-diaphragm preparations from rats. In hyperthyroid rat diaphragm the resting muscle membrane potential was reduced by 31 percent and the amplitude of miniature endplate potential was reduced by 28 percent. Some muscle fibers did not respond to direct stimulation, implying an abnormality of the muscle membrane, but those action potentials that could be elicited appeared normal. There were no electrophysiologic abnormalities in hypothyroid animals.

So far, animal models of thyroid disease have been successful in elucidating the alterations of muscle contractile properties but have failed to provide convincing models of thyrotoxic or hypothyroid myopathy. It may be that experiments with other animal species, or more prolonged alterations of thyroid function, will be required to produce satisfactory animal models of the dysthyroid myopathies.

Thyrotoxic Periodic Paralysis

Shizume and coworkers (1966) showed that potassium ions shift into muscle during an attack of thyrotoxic periodic paralysis, just as in the familial hypokalemic form. There is now convincing evidence that the paralysis itself, both in the familial and thyrotoxic forms, results from temporary inexcitability of the muscle membrane, owing to partial depolarization (see Chapter 2). The mechanism of this depolarization and the reason for the potassium shift remain obscure. There is some evidence that depolarization may result from increased permeability to sodium or from reduced permeability to potassium, either of which would increase the ratio of sodium permeability to potassium permeability (Hofmann and Smith 1970). If this is true, the reason for this change is unknown. Shishiba and colleagues (1972) thought that elevations of plasma insulin might be an important factor triggering spontaneous attacks, but Yeung and Tse (1974) did not confirm this.

Several important clues remain uninvestigated. The beta-adrenergic blocking drug propranolol tends to prevent attacks of thyrotoxic periodic paralysis, and thyrotoxicosis produces a state of supersensitivity to catecholamines that may be mediated by an increased number of beta-adrenergic receptors in plasma membranes (Tse et al. 1980). Among their many actions, beta-adrenergic drugs promote potassium influx and sodium efflux by stimulating the sodium-potassium pump of muscle, an effect probably mediated by the membrane enzyme adenyl cyclase (Clausen and Flatman 1977). Thyrotoxicosis itself produces a substantial increase in the basal sodium-potassium ATPase activity of skeletal muscle and other tissues, perhaps by increasing the passive sodium permeability.

Based on these considerations I have suggested the following speculative sequence of events in thyrotoxic periodic paralysis (Layzer 1982). (1) The resting ionic diffusion potential of muscle is reduced because of an increased sodium permeability. However, the increased sodium leak stimulates the sodium-potassium pump, and the resulting pump potential offsets the reduced diffusion potential, so that the resting membrane potential remains stable. (2) Under the combined influence of increased sodium permeability and an expanded number of beta-adrenergic receptors, the sodium-potassium pump is highly susceptible to the actions of adrenalin and insulin, agents that stimulate the ouabain-sensitive sodium-potassium pump of muscle. (3) The extra stimulation produced by adrenalin or insulin causes a transient surge of inward potassium pumping in muscle, gradually lowering the serum potassium concentration. (4) When the extracellular potassium concentration falls to a critically low level, the sodium-potassium pump shuts off. This event permits the membrane potential to drop down to the level determined by the reduced ionic diffusion potential, which is below the level of electrical excitability.

This hypothetical mechanism accounts for the beneficial effect of propranolol, which opposes the catecholamine-mediated increase in membrane sodium permeability and sodium-potassium pump activity. It also explains the temporary efficacy of potassium therapy during a paralytic attack. Raising the extracellular K concentration allows the sodium-potassium pump to resume its electrogenic pumping, raising the membrane potential and restoring muscle excitability until the temporary effects of adrenalin or insulin subside. Potassium pumping can then decline to a basal level, allowing the large amount of potassium that has accumulated in muscle to pass gradually back into the extracellular space and thence back into the other body tissues.

Thyrotoxic Ocular Myopathy

In patients with Graves' disease, ocular myopathy is nearly always present. The same ocular disorder, however, sometimes occurs in patients without overt thyroid dysfunction. Furthermore, thyrotoxic ocular myopathy may be confused with other conditions that cause ocular paralysis or diplopia.

Clinical Features

The usual symptoms are an irritating sensation in the eye, retraction of the upper lid, redness and swelling of the conjunctiva and eyelids, exophthalmos, and restriction of eye movements. Both eyes are nearly always affected, though often asymmetrically. The clinical course may be fulminating or slow; in either case the active process eventually ceases spontaneously. There is inflammation of the orbital connective tissue and fat, but the most striking changes take place in the extraocular muscles, which swell to as much as eight times their normal size. The thickened, unyielding eye muscles restrict ocular excursion, especially upward movements, and deposition of fibrous tissue may permanently restrict the eye movements and cause strabismus.

Lid retraction is a hallmark of the disorder. When it is bilateral and the patient has active thyrotoxicosis, retraction may be due to sympathetic supersensitivity of the smooth muscle of the lids; conjunctival instillation of guanethidine will then abolish the retraction. However, retraction may be largely or entirely unilateral; moreover, a few patients are euthyroid or even hypothyroid, and guanethidine does not always abolish the lid retraction. In such cases it is likely that the levator muscle and Mueller's muscle, which arises from the undersurface of the levator, are directly involved by inflammation or fibrosis (Hodes et al. 1979).

Orbital Imaging Procedures

A-mode and B-mode ultrasonography (Hodes et al. 1979) and orbital computed tomography (Enzmann et al. 1979) demonstrate that in the great majority of cases multiple muscles are enlarged in both eyes. In a recent axial CT study of 116 patients with Graves' disease, 6 of the 12 patients with unilateral eye signs had bilateral enlargement of eye muscles on CT, and 5 of the 13 patients without eye signs had positive CT scans. Nine percent had normal CT scans and 5 percent had unilateral abnormalities; the remaining 85 percent had bilateral involvement, which was symmetrical in three fourths of the patients (Enzmann et al. 1979). The advent of high resolution CT, coronal scans, and coronal reformations of axial scans now gives even more precise information.

Differential Diagnosis

The diagnosis of Graves' ophthalmoplegia is rarely difficult. Uncertainty may arise in the case of patients with unilateral eye signs or when routine thyroid function tests are normal. Discrete neoplasms can now almost always be identified with orbital CT (Nikoskelainen et al. 1977). The differential diagnosis thus deals mainly with a group of poorly understood inflammatory processes of the orbit, known as orbital pseudotumor, nonspecific orbital granuloma, and orbital myositis (Fig. 13). There is still considerable confusion about the classification of these disorders, but recent CT data suggest that it may be useful to divide them into two groups: those in which inflammation arises in the connective tissue of the orbit (pseudotumor) and those in which the extraocular muscles are the principal site of inflammation (orbital myositis).

ORBITAL PSEUDOTUMOR. Orbital pseudotumor occurs at any age and affects the two sexes equally. The most common clinical features are pain in the eye, limitation of eye movement, proptosis, and swelling of the lids. Papilledema and optic nerve damage occur frequently, and the first division of the trigeminal nerve may also be affected (Jellinek 1969). Involvement is unilateral in about three fourths of the cases. The onset of symptoms can be acute, subacute, or slow. Spontaneous recovery is common, but the disorder may recur in the same eye or in the other eye (Blodi and Gass 1968).

The inflammatory process usually consists of lymphocytic infiltration but may feature lymphoid follicles, neutrophils, plasma cells, or granulomas with giant cells. It may be focal, multifocal, or diffuse and may involve any of the nonocular orbital structures. Some cases are probably etiologically related to inflammatory lesions of the superior orbital fissure (the syndrome of painful ophthalmoplegia) or the retro-orbital region and cavernous sinus (Tolosa-Hunt syndrome) (Levy et al. 1975).

Patients with orbital pseudotumor often feel unwell. The sedimentation rate may be raised, and spinal fluid abnormalities (increased protein concentration and lymphocytic pleocytosis) are found in half of the cases, which suggests that the inflammation has extended through the dura mater. The disorder has sometimes been associated with polyarteritis nodosa, Wegener's granulomatosis (Cassan et al. 1970), or the systemic fibrosclerotic syndromes—retroperitoneal fibrosis, sclerosing cholangitis, Riedel's thyroiditis, and mediastinal fibrosis (Comings et al. 1967).

Enzmann and coworkers (1976) reported that orbital CT scans in nine cases showed single or multiple soft tissue densities that often enhanced with contrast material and appeared to be separate from the optic nerve, globe, and muscles, though often extending into them. The CT abnormalities were bilateral in six of the nine cases. Nugent and colleagues (1981), however, found bilateral involvement by CT scan in only one of fourteen cases.

ORBITAL MYOSITIS. Orbital myositis is now defined as an acute inflammation of one or several eye muscles, manifest as orbital pain, redness of the conjunctiva adjacent to the muscle insertions, diplopia caused by restriction of ocular movement, lid edema, and little or no proptosis (Slavin and Glaser 1982; Keane 1977). There may be an antecedent upper respiratory tract infection (Purcell and Taulbee 1981). The patient may feel unwell and the sedimentation rate may be raised, but the signs and symptoms often resolve simultaneously within a few weeks or months. Orbital myositis accounts for about 13 percent of the cases of acute idiopathic orbital inflammation (Nugent et al. 1981).

A clinical diagnosis of orbital myositis has also been applied to patients with scleroderma (Arnett and Michels 1973) or dermatomyositis (Susac et al. 1973) who developed bilateral involvement of several eye muscles. Unfortunately, those cases were reported before the introduction of orbital CT; it is possible that the patients had orbital pseudotumor rather than orbital myositis. Enlargement of multiple eye muscles in both eyes has been considered pathognomonic of Graves' disease (Trokel and Hilal 1979; Enzmann et al. 1976, 1979), even in euthyroid patients, but the same CT

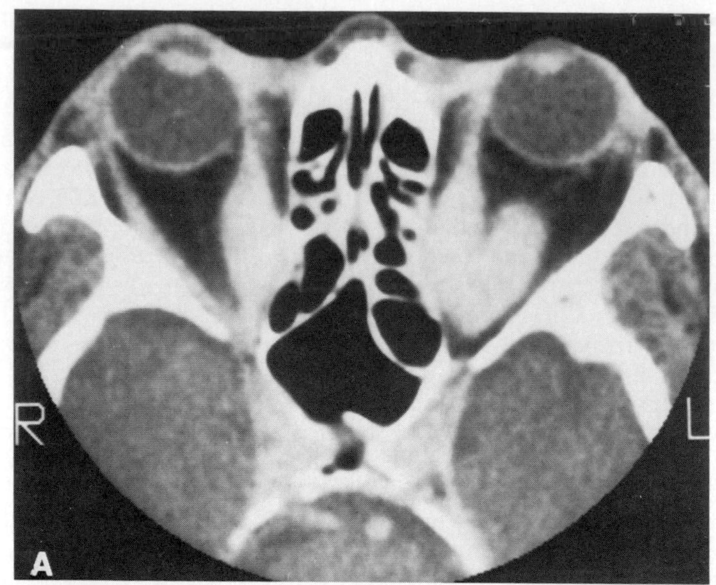
R
L
A

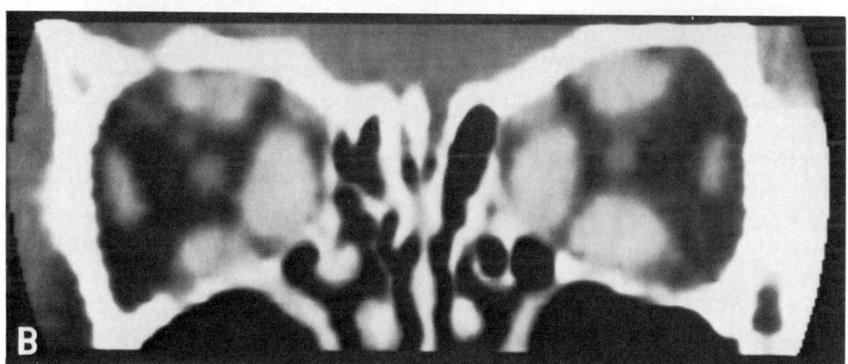
B

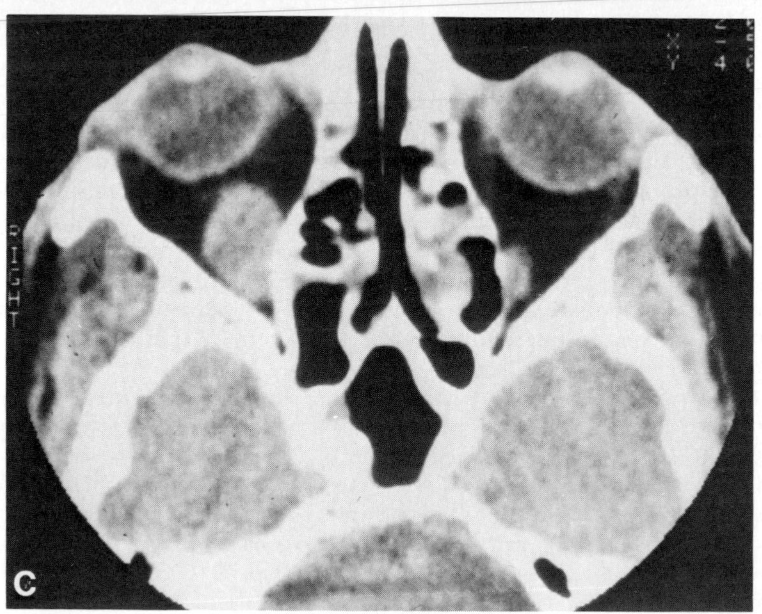
RIGHT
C

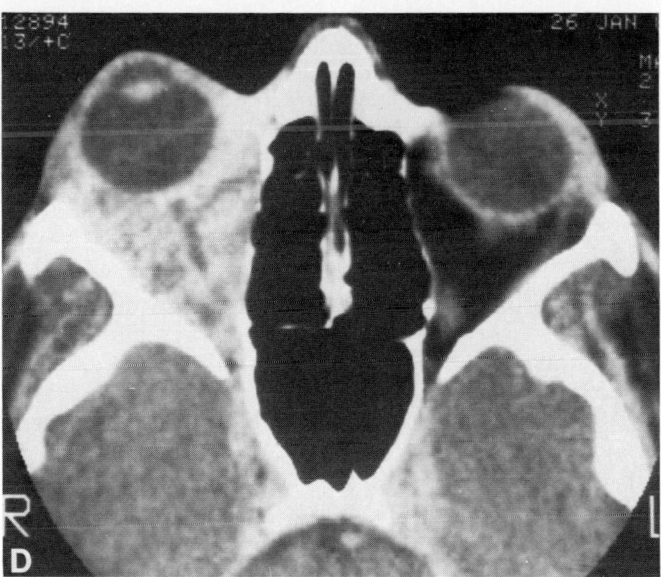

FIGURE 13. Post-contrast CT radiographs in orbital inflammatory diseases. (*A*) Axial view of orbits in patient with Graves' disease. There is enlargement of the left inferior rectus and of both medial rectus muscles. However coronal reformations (*B*) show more extensive involvement of the superior, medial, and inferior rectus muscles bilaterally. (C) Orbital myositis. There is enlargement of the right inferior rectus muscle that resembles a tumor in the orbital apex. (D) Orbital pseudotumor. There is a nonhomogeneous soft tissue density filling the retrobulbar space, with secondary proptosis. Note loss of the normal fat density (low attenuation) compared with the opposite side.

picture can occur in idiopathic orbital myositis (Slavin and Glaser 1982) and has recently been reported in a patient with leukemic infiltration of the orbits (Nikoskelainen et al. 1977). In another patient with unilateral proptosis, CT showed enlargement of one eye muscle that later proved to be due to infiltration by a malignant lymphoma (Burrows and Barnett 1981).

Fewer than 10 percent of patients with a clinical diagnosis of Graves' eye disease are euthyroid. About three fourths of these patients respond abnormally to either the T3 suppression test or the TRH stimulation test; the remainder could have idiopathic orbital myositis, but a follow-up study showed that overt or subclinical abnormalities of thyroid function developed later in about half of them (Tamai et al. 1980). From this it would seem that the clinical diagnosis of Graves' eye disease is remarkably accurate, but the published criteria for this diagnosis are rather ambiguous (Hall et al. 1970; Shammas et al. 1979). A long follow-up study is needed, including orbital CT scans and full thyroid function tests, of patients who raise the differential diagnosis of idiopathic orbital myositis, orbital pseudotumor, and euthyroid Graves' disease.

Pathogenesis. In Graves' disease, hyperthyroidism is probably due to the stimulating effect of autoantibodies that react with TSH receptors in the thyroid gland (Havard 1979). The pathogenesis of the extraocular myositis, however, remains uncertain, in part because an overabundance of autoimmune abnormalities has been demonstrated. Current views assign a major role to the deposition of thyroglobulin-antithyroglobulin complexes, which have an unusual affinity for eye muscles. Thyroglobulin may reach the orbit by retrograde lymphatic flow, since the orbital lymphatics communicate with those draining the thyroid gland. There is also evidence for cell-mediated autoimmunity against ocular muscle antigen (Havard 1979). The degree to which hyperthyroidism, hypothyroidism, and orbital myositis are clinically expressed in an individual patient may therefore depend on the intensity and interaction of several different autoimmune processes: thyroid stimulation, thyroid inflammation, and ocular muscle inflammation. Even so, while ocular myopathy is an almost constant feature of Graves' disease, it is rarely encountered in Hashimoto's disease (Amino et al. 1980).

Treatment

The management of Graves' eye disease remains difficult and unsatisfactory. Havard (1979) has reviewed current approaches to treating the small number of patients whose vision is threatened by severe exophthalmos. High-dose prednisone and surgical decompression of the orbit have established roles; plasmapheresis combined with immunosuppressive therapy appears promising. Supervoltage irradiation of the orbit has given inconsistent results (Tseng et al. 1980).

Orbital pseudotumor and idiopathic orbital myositis generally respond well to treatment with large doses of prednisone. In pseudotumor especially, the high risk of optic nerve damage justifies early and vigorous anti-inflammatory treatment. That condition may have a chronic relapsing course, so that steroid therapy may need to be continued at a lower maintenance dose (Jellinek 1969). In steroid-resistant cases, low-dose supervoltage radiation of the orbit may be beneficial (Sergott et al. 1981).

Myasthenia Gravis and Thyroid Disease

It was the association of myasthenia gravis with Graves' disease and other putative autoimmune disorders that led Simpson (1960) to formulate his prescient hypothesis of the autoimmune pathogenesis of myasthenia. The reason for this assocation is still unclear, but it may reside in genetic factors to which leukocyte HLA antigen patterns provide a clue. In animals these cell-surface components correlate with immune responses and resistance to viral infection, while in man certain HLA haplotypes have been found with increased frequency in patients with lymphoproliferative disorders and with diseases known or suspected to be of autoimmune etiology. Haplotype HLA-B8 is associated with myasthenia gravis, Graves' disease, Addison's disease, juvenile diabetes, and several other diseases. In myasthenia gravis the association is stronger with HLA-B8 than with HLA-DR3 (Behan 1980), but in Graves' disease the reverse is true, and Graves' eye disease is significantly associated only with HLA-D3 (Farid et al 1980). It is clear that haplotype HLA-B8 is neither essential nor sufficient to produce these autoimmune diseases, and the nature of any genetic predisposition to autoimmunity is still obscure.

Ramsay (1974) reviewed the published cases of myasthenia gravis associated with thyroid disease. Hyperthyroidism develops in about 5 percent of myasthenic patients. In half of them hyperthyroidism precedes myasthenia; in 20 to 30 percent of patients the two diseases appear simultaneously; and in the remainder myasthenia appears first. Since the incidence of hyperthyroidism is 10 to 20 times as great as that of myasthenia gravis, less than 0.1 percent of thyrotoxic patients become myasthenic. Serum levels of thyroid antibodies are increased more often in patients with myasthenia gravis than in normal subjects, and hypothyroidism has been found in up to 6 percent of myasthenic patients. Furthermore, at autopsy the thyroid glands of 12 to 19 percent of myasthenic patients show pathologic changes of Hashimoto's disease. Thus, the association of myasthenia gravis with autoimmune thyroiditis is stronger even than with Graves' disease.

It is sometimes difficult to distinguish between the eye signs of myasthenia and those of Graves' disease. Lid retraction and proptosis, of course, point to Graves' disease, while ptosis occurs only in myasthenia. Forced duction tests (gripping the bulbar conjunctiva with a forceps and moving the globe) and anticholinesterase drugs can usually distinguish ocular myositis from myasthenic weakness. However, when Graves' eye disease develops simultaneously with ocular myasthenia, some confusion can be expected. Nowadays orbital CT scans, the full battery of thyroid function tests, and measurement of antibodies to acetylcholine receptor can unravel these problems.

Both hyperthyroidism and hypothyroidism may aggravate the symptoms of myasthenia gravis, though probably to no greater degree than many other intercurrent illnesses. Both conditions are treated in the usual way, with a few precautions. Because of its neuromuscular blocking properties, propranolol should be used circumspectly in myasthenic patients, though in actual practice it does not seem to cause much difficulty. Thymectomy should be postponed until thyroid function has returned to normal, but steroid therapy and plasmapheresis can be used as needed.

ADRENAL DISORDERS

Hypoadrenalism

Asthenia

Nearly all hypoadrenal patients complain of weakness and easy fatigability (Nerup 1974), yet objective signs of neuromuscular dysfunction are rarely found. Addison mentioned "general languor and debility" as one of the characteristic features, and modern authors have usually applied the term *asthenia* to this peculiar state, which combines lack of physical endurance with a disinclination to physical or mental effort. Even the voice is soft, faint, and slurred. Other nonspecific symptoms are nausea, vomiting, and paresthesias in the hands and feet (Rowntree and Snell 1931). Since emotional disturbances are also frequent in hypoadrenalism, there is a real danger that physicians may attribute all the symptoms to neurosis or depression.

The classic monographs on Addison's disease provide almost no description of the neuromuscular examination (Rowntree and Snell 1931; Thorn et al. 1951). Mild, generalized muscular wasting is a frequent finding, but there is little or no weakness at rest (Forsham 1981). No abnormality of muscle histology has been observed (Adams et al. 1962), though histochemical studies have not been reported.

There are probably many different reasons for hypoadrenal asthenia. Low blood volume causes orthostatic hypotension, and there is a tendency to hypoglycemia that may be accentuated by muscular activity. When treatment with desoxycorticosterone was first introduced, it was observed that asthenia was much improved by the treatment, but lack of physical endurance remained a prominent complaint until the advent of cortisone therapy (Forsham 1981).

Myalgia, Cramps, and Contractures

In a recent retrospective survey of Addison's disease, only 6 percent of the patients complained of muscle or joint pain (Nerup 1974). Rowntree and Snell (1931), however, said that half of Addisonian patients complained of pain in the abdomen, back, or loins. Attacks of pain were sometimes so severe that patients would groan or scream, and the abdomen might become rigid.

A related problem is the occurrence of painful flexion contractures of the abdomen and lower extremities (Thorn et al. 1951; Adams et al. 1962; Aubertin and Bergouignan 1951; Leys et al. 1982). In some cases the contractures were preceded by violent muscle cramps in the thighs and lower trunk; between paroxysms the patients displayed continuous muscular rigidity in the lower extremities, back, and abdomen, and sometimes even in the neck or face. The patients were difficult to examine because manipulating the flexed lower limbs, or even stroking the skin, set off "atrociously painful" muscle spasms; however, there did not appear to be any abnormality of muscle power, reflexes, or sensation. The EMG was normal in two cases (Castaigne et al. 1959, 1974) and showed myopathic abnormalities in another (Cambier et al. 1970), but nobody has described the EMG findings in muscles involved by rigidity or spasm. Motor nerve conduction velocity, serum enzymes (Cambier et al. 1970), and muscle biopsies (Adams et al. 1962; Cambier et al. 1970) were also normal. Treatment with deoxycorticosterone may have made the contractures worse (Thorn et al. 1951; Aubertin and Bergouignan 1951), but glucocorticoid replacement brought rapid relief of the painful cramps and a gradual easing of the contractures.

Adams and colleagues (1962) attributed the flexion contractures to a disorder of the tendons and fascia, because there were no pathologic changes in the muscle. Apparently he did not observe the extraordinary muscle rigidity and spasms described by other authors, phenomena that strongly suggest a neural disorder. The clinical descriptions are reminiscent of the stiff-man syndrome, but without electrophysiologic data, speculation about the mechanism is useless. A recent case of neuromyotonia (muscle stiffness, slow relaxation, and myokymia) in an Addisonian patient (Vilchez et al. 1980) must be a different disorder, since that patient did not have flexion contractures of the legs, and none of the other patients had myokymia.

Acute Hyperkalemic Paralysis

Thirteen cases of this rare complication of untreated Addison's disease had been reported by 1969 (Van Dellen and Purnell 1969), and a few more examples have been recorded since then (Waron et al. 1970; Vilchez et al. 1980). The clinical features of acquired hyperkalemic periodic paralysis are discussed in Chapter 2. Curiously enough, periodic paralysis does not seem to occur in patients with isolated hyporeninemic hypoaldosteronism (Schambelan and Sebastian 1979), and muscular weakness is rarely mentioned in such cases (Perez et al. 1972), although chronic hyperkalemia is the main presenting feature. An exception is the patient reported by Posner and Jacobs (1964), a young man with an 8-year history of periodic paralysis, who had isolated aldosterone deficiency, metabolic acidosis, and serum-potassium levels ranging from 7.7 to 9.0 mEq per liter between attacks of paralysis. The aldosterone antagonist spironolactone has been responsible for a few cases of transient and periodic hyperkalemic paralysis, even in patients without azotemia (Rado et al. 1968).

Polyneuropathy

The association, in a few reported cases, of peripheral neuropathy with Addison's disease might be considered coincidental, except that the neuropathic and endocrine symptoms came on together, and the neuropathy resolved gradually following steroid replacement therapy. One patient had a pure motor polyneuropathy, most severe in the lower extremities; the spinal fluid protein was 168 mg per dl, and motor nerve conduction velocities were slightly reduced (Abbas et al. 1977). Another case was the patient with neuromyotonia and hyperkalemic periodic paralysis mentioned earlier; he had slight weakness and sensory loss in the distal lower extremities, slightly reduced nerve conduction velocity, and a normal spinal fluid protein concentration. A sural nerve biopsy showed vacuolation and splitting of myelin sheaths and paranodal demyelination (Vilchez et al. 1980).

Another Addisonian patient had no neuropathic symptoms until an attack of hyperkalemic paralysis, during which he experienced painful paresthesias and loss of sensation in the distal lower extremities. With steroid replacement he improved rapidly, but 1 week later he still had impaired sensation in the feet (Bull et al. 1953). This observation suggests that the peripheral nerves can be damaged by acute hyperkalemia.

Primary Aldosteronism

Aldosterone-producing adrenal adenomas, though uncommon, have received much medical attention as potentially curable causes of arterial hypertension. Three fourths of the patients are female. Aside from hypertension, muscular weakness is the most frequent symptom of aldosteronism, occurring in 73 percent of the 103 cases reviewed by Conn (1963); periodic hypokalemic paralysis and tetany each occurred in 20 percent of the cases. Chronic myopathic weakness and periodic paralysis are consequences of the chronic potassium deficiency typical of this condition, while tetany is caused by the associated alkalosis. These electrolyte syndromes are discussed in Chapter 2. Aldosterone-producing adenomas can be distinguished from idiopathic adrenal hyperplasia and from benign essential hypertension by means of aldosterone-suppression tests (Vaughn et al. 1981). The adenoma can be located by measuring aldosterone concentrations in adrenal vein samples, but computed tomography is much easier and has a high diagnostic yield (White et al. 1980).

Glucocorticoid Excess

Muscle weakness and wasting are among the cardinal signs of Cushing's syndrome; up to 90 percent of the patients complain of muscle weakness (Urbanic and George 1981; Ross et al. 1966), and myopathy is one of the most reliable signs that distinguish Cushing's syndrome from the more benign disorders resembling it (Ross and Linch 1982). Pituitary overproduction of adrenocorticotropic hormone (ACTH), caused by pituitary adenoma or microadenoma, accounts for about two thirds of the cases; 75 percent of these patients are women, usually of child-bearing age. The remaining one third of cases of Cushing's syndrome are caused by adrenal adenoma or carcinoma or by "ectopic" production of ACTH by nonpituitary tumors (Gold 1979). Whatever the cause, spontaneous Cushing's syndrome is an uncommon disease, but muscle weakness caused by corticosteroid therapy is one of the commonest muscular disorders encountered in medical practice. The clinical and laboratory features of spontaneous and iatrogenic steroid myopathy appear to be identical, but almost all the published information relates to corticosteroid therapy.

Clinical Features

The clinical picture is rather uniform (Afifi et al. 1968). Muscle weakness and wasting begin in the pelvifemoral muscles, especially the quadriceps, and spread to the trunk, anterior neck, shoulders, and upper arms. Eventually all the limb muscles become weak, though a proximal emphasis persists. The cranial muscles are not significantly affected. Patients may experience a mild aching in the thighs but severe muscle pain does not occur. The onset of weakness is usually subacute, causing important limitation of physical activity within a few weeks, and occasionally substantial weakness develops in only a few days. On examination the affected muscles are flabby and wasted enough to suggest a neurogenic disease, but there are no fasciculations and the tendon reflexes are well preserved.

Laboratory Findings

The serum activity of CPK and other cytoplasmic muscle enzymes is almost invariably normal. Recently, Kanayama and colleagues (1981) reported that serum lactic dehydrogenase (LDH) activity was selectively elevated in lupus patients with steroid myopathy; the validity of this observation has yet to be established. The EMG is commonly unrevealing but may show mild myopathic changes, without abnormal irritability or spontaneous activity. Motor nerve conduction is normal. Muscle biopsy shows few structural changes except for increased numbers of central nuclei and occasional degenerating muscle fibers. Much more impressive and constant is the atrophy of muscle fibers, which involves both type-1 and type-2 fibers but is more striking in type-2 fibers, which have an angulated, shrunken appearance resembling denervation atrophy (Pleasure et al. 1970). This change may be present in steroid-treated patients or animals lacking clinical symptoms or signs (Braund et al. 1980) and therefore does not by itself establish a diagnosis of steroid myopathy. Minor ultrastructural changes that have been seen by electron microscopy do not seem to be distinctive (Engel 1966).

Relationship to Steroid Therapy

It is necessary to distinguish between the generalized reduction of muscle bulk that accompanies long-standing steroid therapy, reflecting the catabolic effect of glucocorticoid hormones, and steroid myopathy, which tends to have a distinct onset and continues to worsen until the steroid dose is reduced. Myopathy has resulted from treatment with all the commonly used glucocorticoids, regardless of the medical condition being treated. It is difficult to find convincing support for the conventional statement that muscle weakness is more frequent after treatment with 9-alpha-fluorinated steroids (triamcinolone and dexamethasone) than with nonfluorinated steroids at equivalent doses (Afifi et al. 1968). There is a marked variation of individual susceptibility to steroid-induced weakness, and there seems to be a "myopathy threshold" in each patient. Some patients become weak after a few weeks of steroid treatment at a dosage that does not cause weakness in other patients even after months of treatment. The daily dose may be as low as 15 mg of prednisone, but in general larger doses are more likely to produce weakness and will do so sooner than small doses. The shortest recorded duration of treatment before onset of weakness is 1 week, and the interval is rarely less than 3 weeks. There is a general impression that alternate-day schedules of prednisone are less likely to cause myopathy than daily doses. Often a patient tolerates a stable maintenance dose but becomes weak when the dose is raised (Askari et al. 1976). Once weakness begins it tends to worsen at a rapid pace even though there was no weakness during previous months at the same dose.

Treatment

There are reports that weakness occurring during treatment with triamcinolone or dexamethasone improved when the drug was replaced by a nonfluorinated steroid in an equivalent dose. Usually it is safer to reduce the dose; a rough rule of thumb is to cut the dose in half and wait for the weakness to stabilize and improve—usually a matter of several weeks. Complete recovery after stopping steroid therapy can be expected within 2 to 3 months, but when treatment is continued at a reduced dose recovery may be much slower. There are no permanent muscular after-effects of steroid myopathy.

PATHOPHYSIOLOGY. Although much is known about the physiologic and biochemical effects of glucocorticoids on skeletal muscle, the relevance of this information to the pathogenesis of steroid myopathy is still uncertain. Glucocorticoid hormones mobilize muscle protein stores during fasting and starvation, providing the liver and kidneys with amino acids to be used for gluconeogenesis. These catabolic effects are achieved by both a reduction in the rate of protein synthesis and an increase in the rate of protein degradation. Red muscle is relatively resistant to the atrophy caused by starvation or by glucocorticoid hormone (Li and Goldberg 1976); the more vulnerable white muscle appears to be sacrificed early, in order to preserve the more fuel-efficient red muscle.

Glucocorticoid atrophy is enhanced by inactivity and diminished by exercise, as if the body wishes to preserve working muscle as long as possible during starvation (Goldberg and Goodman 1969; Gardiner et al. 1980a). In this regard it is interesting that immobilization of an extremity increases the number of cytoplasmic glucocorticoid "receptors" in the inactive muscle (DuBois and Almon 1980). Histochemical studies suggest that the pattern of muscle activity may influence which types of muscle fibers undergo steroid atrophy. In the cat, corticosteroids cause atrophy of the fast-glycolytic fibers in all muscles, but also affect slow-oxidative (SO) fibers in the fast-twitch vastus medialis muscle, while sparing SO fibers in the slow-twitch soleus muscle (Gardiner et al. 1978).

In the cat experiments, muscle power per unit of muscle weight was normal in the atrophic muscles, indicating that steroid atrophy is not necessarily the same as steroid myopathy. Similarly, in rats, glucocorticoid treatment *increased* contractile force per unit of muscle weight in both red and white muscles and did not alter the rates of contraction and relaxation, despite marked atrophy of the fast-twitch type-2 muscle fibers (Gardiner et al. 1980b). The concentrations of glycolytic and oxidative enzymes were reduced in white but not in red muscle, and white muscle became fatigued more rapidly than normal during repetitive stimulation, a result of its reduced oxidative capacity (Gardiner et al. 1978). However, the reduced energy-producing capacity of atrophic white muscle may simply be an adaptation to its reduced energy consumption, an explanation that could also account for a doubling of muscle glycogen content observed by Shoji and associates (1974).

There have been few experimental studies of muscle membrane properties during steroid treatment. In fast muscle of mice, Gruener and Stern (1972a) found a slight reduction of the resting potential and an upward shift of the excitation threshold, resulting in reduced excitability. This effect was selective, because soleus muscle was unchanged. In-vitro application of phenytoin reversed these abnormalities (Gruener and Stern 1972b). These experimental findings, which were confirmed by Grossie and Albuquerque (1978), suggest that glucocorticoids, by reducing the excitability of white muscle fibers, may produce a kind of disuse atrophy. However, Ruff and colleagues (1982) reported that glucocorticoid effects on muscle excitability could not be demonstrated in vivo, casting doubt on the importance of the previous in vitro observations. The ionic conductances and cable properties of muscle plasma membrane have not been studied in steroid myopathy, nor have standard tests of mechanical and electrical muscle function been applied to experimental animals with clear-cut weakness attributable to steroid treatment.

Other Complications of Steroid Therapy

An *acute hydrocortisone myopathy* has been reported in two patients with status asthmaticus treated with intravenous hydrocortisone in a dose of several grams per day. In contrast with ordinary steroid myopathy, muscle weakness was equally severe in distal and proximal muscles, the serum CPK levels were markedly elevated, and muscle biopsy revealed a vacuolar myopathy. Recovery occurred slowly over a period of several months (Van Marle and Woods 1980). *Tendon ruptures* may occur during chronic steroid treatment or after local injections of steroids. Most of the reported patients had lupus erythematosus, but a few patients had rheumatoid arthritis or disorders other than collagen-vascular diseases. A direct effect of the underlying disease may contribute to this complication (Halpern et al. 1977).

The well-known central fat deposition caused by glucocorticoid hormones may lead to *spinal epidural lipomatosis,* which can compress the spinal cord (Butcher and Sahn 1979) or cauda equina (Lipson et al. 1980). The latter complication could be mistaken for a peripheral neuropathy, delaying effective surgical treatment.

DISORDERS OF VITAMIN D AND PARATHYROID HORMONE

Muscle Weakness in Osteomalacia

Osteomalacia causes a distinctive syndrome of bone pain and muscle weakness that has been receiving increasing medical attention in recent years. Recognizable descriptions of the syndrome can be traced back many centuries. In ancient India, Vagbhatta mentioned a malady in which "there is excessive and constant pain of the hip bones, great loss of strength and above all increased porosity of the bones" (Skaria 1975). Muscle weakness was mentioned in seventeenth-century English accounts of rickets and in eighteenth-century writings on osteomalacia, but it was the brief report of Vicale (1949) that reacquainted contemporary neurologists with this syndrome. After delineating the typical picture of bone pain, reluctant gait, and limb weakness in patients with either hyperparathyroidism or osteomalacia, Vicale warned that these signs and symptoms could easily be mistaken for "the neurotic muscular disorders." Recent case reports confirm this diagnostic pitfall (Schott and Wills 1975); one patient attended over a period of 4 years eight separate hospitals, in each of which she received treatment for hysteria or depression, including two courses of electroconvulsive therapy (Marsden et al. 1973).

There is still considerable uncertainty about the pathogenesis of muscle weakness in the different metabolic bone disorders. To simplify matters,

I will begin by describing the least controversial entity: osteomalacia caused by simple dietary deficiency of vitamin D. Osteomalacia is the adult form of the bone disease that produces rickets in growing children. It consists of a defect of mineralization of bone matrix, leading to an accumulation of osteoid over bone surfaces.

Nutritional Osteomalacia

Only small amounts of vitamin D are present in unfortified foods like milk, butter, and eggs. Most of the body's requirements are met by synthesis of the vitamin in the skin, through photolytic action of sunlight. The conversion of 7-dehydrocholesterol to cholecalciferol (D_3) is brought about by ultraviolet irradiation in the range of 250 to 310 nm, and cholecalciferol is the precursor of the hydroxylated, biologically active forms of vitamin D_3.

In Western countries, osteomalacia and rickets are rarely seen except in northern latitudes with little sunlight, especially in cities where ultraviolet light is filtered out by smog. Dark skin pigmentation also reduces substantially the capacity to synthesize vitamin D_3 (Clemens et al. 1982). Routine fortification of milk with vitamin D can compensate for these handicaps, but vitamin-D deficiency may still occur in food faddists or vegetarians who eschew fatty foods and dairy products (Dent and Smith 1969). In India, where most contemporary cases originate, there is plenty of sunlight but the patients are dark-skinned women who eat poorly, spend most of the day out of the sun, and lose vitamin D through prolonged periods of lactation (Irani 1976; Dastur et al. 1975). The importance of sunlight is illustrated by the fact that Pakistani immigrants to Great Britain arrive with normal serum vitamin D levels, which decline to subnormal levels within the first year, although their diet remains the same (Preece et al. 1975). Vitamin D deficiency is also common among elderly whites in Great Britain because of poor diet and the fact that they are housebound (Preece et al. 1975).

CLINICAL FEATURES. In India, Skaria and associates (1975) evaluated neuromuscular function in 30 consecutive, unselected osteomalacic women, whose average age was 25 years. All were poor and badly nourished, and the cause of the osteomalacia was believed to be nutritional in every case except for one patient with renal tubular acidosis. All the patients complained of bone pain, and 93 percent complained of muscle weakness, which was the initial symptom in 30 percent of cases. The weakness was mainly noticed when the patient climbed stairs or got up from the ground. Examination disclosed weakness of the pelvic muscles and thighs in all but one patient (97 percent), proximal arm weakness in 57 percent, and muscle wasting proportionate to the weakness, without fasciculations or isolated distal weakness. More than half of the patients had a waddling gait and used the Gower maneuver to rise from recumbency. One fifth of the patients were unable to walk, and an equal proportion had a limping gait. There were no abnormalities of the cranial nerves, sensation, or reflexes, though other authors have described very brisk muscle stretch reflexes (Vicale 1949; Smith and Stern 1967, 1969).

In these patients it is sometimes difficult to distinguish genuine weakness from guarding or giving-way because of bone pain. Irani (1976) acknowledged this difficulty but gave convincing reasons for believing that the 15 patients whom he examined had real weakness: a waddling gait; pelvic girdle weakness in two patients with little pain; shoulder girdle weakness in seven patients who did not have pain in that region; and persistence of weakness after the pain subsided under treatment with vitamin D. The muscles themselves do not seem to be tender or painful to move; it is the bones that hurt when they are stressed by weight-bearing or muscle tension. Bone pain and tenderness are most prominent in the pelvis, the femurs, the spine, and the ribs, but some patients have "total body pain," a symptom that tends to provoke skepticism in many physicians. Spinal collapse with loss of height is a frequent outcome, and in advanced cases other skeletal deformities can occur.

LABORATORY DIAGNOSIS. The diagnosis of osteomalacia may be suggested by roentgenographic findings, but if nonspecific osteopenia is excluded, only about two thirds of patients have typical abnormalities such as pseudofractures and biconcave vertebrae. Serum calcium and phosphorus levels are reduced in about 40 percent of cases. The best screening tests for osteomalacia are the serum alkaline phosphatase activity, which is elevated in 80 to 93 percent of cases (Irani 1976; Skaria et al. 1975), and the urinary excretion of calcium, which is usually extremely low. The levels of vitamin D and its metabolites are reduced in the serum. Bone biopsy is a simple procedure that should be employed whenever the diagnosis is in question; the accuracy is improved by administration of tetracycline prior to biopsy, in order to label the mineralization front (Frame and Parfitt 1978).

The serum CPK activity is normal or, infrequently, slightly elevated (Dastur et al. 1975). The EMG shows myopathic abnormalities, without spontaneous activity (Skaria et al. 1975). Motor nerve conduction velocity was slightly reduced in the peroneal nerves in one study (Skaria et al. 1975) but not in another (Irani 1976). Muscle biopsy with routine histologic stains shows only scattered or diffuse muscle fiber atrophy, while histochemical muscle fiber typing may show type-2 fiber atrophy (Isenberg et al. 1982).

TREATMENT. The response to vitamin-D therapy is rather variable. All of the 14 patients treated with intramuscular vitamin D by Irani (1976) experienced a marked reduction of bone pain in 2 to 4 weeks, and most were completely relieved of pain in 8 to 10 weeks. The muscle weakness responded much more slowly, improvement beginning as late as 12 weeks after initiation of therapy. Of 14 patients treated by Skaria and associates (1975) for an average of 7 months, 12 were free of bone pain, 4 had recovered normal muscle power, and 6 showed improvement of strength. In another report four women with nutritional "pre-osteomalacia" and quadriceps weakness showed no improvement of muscle strength after 6 months of vitamin-D therapy, though serum levels of phosphorus, 25-hydroxyvitamin D, and parathormone returned to normal (Isenberg et al. 1982).

Other Types of Osteomalacia

Smith and Stern (1967) drew attention to the frequent occurrence of proximal muscle weakness in patients with osteomalacia, regardless of the etiology. They surveyed the hospital records of all patients with osteomalacia or hyperparathyroidism who had been studied at the Metabolic Unit of University College Hospital, London, during a period of 5 years. Proximal weakness was present in 20 (44 percent) of 45 patients with osteomalacia and was among the presenting symptoms in 15 patients. Muscle weakness occurred in each of nine etiologic categories, of which the most numerous was gluten-sensitive enteropathy. Fourteen of the 45 patients developed secondary or "tertiary" hyperparathyroidism (parathyroid hyperplasia or adenoma, respectively), and all 14 had proximal weakness. By contrast, weakness occurred in only six (6.6 percent) of 91 patients with primary hyperparathyroidism, and three of those had radiologic or bone-biopsy evidence of accompanying osteomalacia.

Because of the pitfalls of retrospective surveys, Smith and Stern (1969) carried out a prospective study of 11 patients with osteomalacia and 44 patients with hyperparathyroidism. Three of the 11 had so much bone pain that muscle strength could not be accurately assessed, but the other 8 patients with osteomalacia (73 percent) had clear-cut clinical evidence of myopathy, as did 2 of 3 patients with "tertiary" hyperparathyroidism; but only 1 of 41 patients with primary hyperparathyroidism had myopathy. The neuromuscular findings were identical to those of nutritional osteomalacia, except that muscular atrophy was not prominent. The EMG showed myopathic abnormalities in seven of the eight patients; CPK showed a borderline elevation in one patient and was normal in the remainder. Serum levels of vitamin D were below normal in most but not all of the patients with osteomalacic myopathy. Oral administration of vitamin D restored muscle power completely or nearly so, though at varying rates; one patient regained normal strength in 10 days, but others improved gradually over several months, and there was little correlation between the improvement of the metabolic bone disease and of the myopathy. One patient with renal tubular acidosis was treated only with sodium bicarbonate and also improved.

Many other publications confirm the association of a proximal myopathy, clinically identical to the myopathy of vitamin-D deficiency, with almost all varieties of osteomalacia except X-linked vitamin D-resistant hypophosphatemic rickets (Table 21). Myopathy and osteomalacia have also

TABLE 21. Myopathy in Vitamin D-Deficient Osteomalacia

Mechanism of Vitamin-D Deficiency	Reference
Nutritional	Irani (1976) Skaria et al. (1975) Smith & Stern (1967) Smith & Stern (1969) Isenberg et al. (1982)*
Malabsorption	
Gluten-sensitive enteropathy	Smith & Stern (1967, 1969) Banerji & Hurwitz (1971a) Mallette et al. (1975)*
Postgastrectomy	Morgan et al. (1970) Banerji & Hurwitz (1971b)
Jejunal bypass for obesity	Franck et al. (1979)
Pancreatic insufficiency	Smith & Stern (1969)
Laxative abuse	Mallette et al. (1975)*
Scleroderma	Mallette et al. (1975)*
Vitamin-D resistance	
Vitamin D-dependent rickets	Rasmussen & Anast (1978)
Renal tubular acidosis	Smith & Stern (1967) Mallette et al. (1975)*
Anticonvulsant therapy	Marsden et al. (1973) Mallette et al. (1975)*

*Type-2 muscle fiber atrophy demonstrated.

been associated with *chronic phosphate depletion* and with *chronic renal failure.* Since these disorders involve complex metabolic alterations, they will be discused in greater detail.

Myopathy and Chronic Renal Failure

The occurrence of proximal muscle weakness in uremic patients began to be reported in 1967, only a few years after the initial description of uremic polyneuropathy. By 1974, Floyd and coworkers (1974) in Newcastle were able to give a detailed description of 11 patients with "uremic myopathy." In 4 of these patients proximal weakness was the presenting problem and uremia was discovered during the initial workup, while in the other 7 patients a myopathy developed during maintenance hemodialysis—an incidence of 14 percent in the dialyzed population at that institution. The weakness came on gradually, affecting the pelvic girdle first, and in a few patients was associated with pain in the proximal lower extremities. On physical examination muscle atrophy was mild or absent; weakness was concentrated in the pelvic girdle and was also present in the shoulder girdle and neck; muscle stretch reflexes were often unusually brisk; and there was no abnormality of cranial nerves or sensation. Quantitative EMG in 10 patients showed a significant reduction of the mean motor unit potential duration and an increased percentage of polyphasic motor unit potentials in deltoid and quadriceps muscles. Motor nerve conduction velocities in upper and lower extremities were within the normal range. Quadriceps muscle biopsies in 10 patients showed atrophy of type-2 muscle fibers in every case, without other morphologic abnormalities, though evidence of muscle fiber degeneration was detected by electron microscopy in four cases.

Although the myopathy was clinically identical in the undialyzed and dialyzed patients, in the former group bone biopsies showed a combination of severe osteomalacia and osteitis fibrosa (the usual findings in renal osteodystrophy), while the dialyzed group had severe osteopenia (osteoporosis) with only mild osteomalacia and osteitis fibrosa. Furthermore, large doses of vitamin D improved muscle power and bone disease in the undialyzed patients but not in the dialyzed ones. Two dialyzed patients subsequently received renal allografts, and afterward their muscle power improved dramatically.

These observations suggested that relative deficiency of vitamin D might be an important cause of myopathy in the undialyzed patients, but that a different mechanism might be operating in the dialyzed patients. It soon became apparent that dialysis centers located in Newcastle and in several other cities around the world had an unusually high frequency of severe metabolic bone disease characterized by bone pain, fractures, myopathy, and resistance to vitamin-D therapy (Alvarez-Ude et al. 1978). Physicians in the same centers were also beginning to see patients with a newly recognized neurologic syndrome, progressive dialysis encephalopathy. In those units the water used for dialysis contained a high concentration of aluminum, and when deionized water was substituted the incidences of metabolic bone disease, myopathy, and dialysis encephalopathy fell sharply (Ward et al. 1978; Pierides 1978). Bone aluminum is extremely high in patients with dialysis osteodystrophy, and bone histology shows severe osteomalacia and osteopenia with little or no evidence of secondary hyperparathyroidism (osteitis fibrosa) (Hodsman et al. 1981). Unfortunately for our purposes, these articles provide few diagnostic details concerning the myopathy, but it seems likely that the well-documented myopathy described a few years earlier by Floyd and colleagues (1974) in dialyzed patients was of this type. Whether aluminum is the true culprit is still uncertain, but the dialysis fluid was certainly implicated in some cases. Aluminum toxicity has also been attributed to the chronic ingestion of aluminum-containing antacids.

Uremic bone disease (renal osteodystrophy) represents the interaction of several processes, including osteomalacia and osteitis fibrosa owing to secondary hyperparathyroidism. It is an old observation that renal osteodystrophy may respond to treatment with vitamin D, but that very large doses are needed in many cases. The conversion of vitamin D to 25-hydroxyvitamin D takes place in the liver, while the conversion of 25-hydroxyvitamin D to 1,25-dihydroxyvitamin D takes place in the renal cortex. Most investigators in this field now consider 1,25-dihydroxyvitamin D to be the principal biologically active form of vitamin D, although there is conflicting evidence for an additional role for 25-hydroxyvitamin D or 24,25-dihydroxyvitamin D. Blood levels of 25-hydroxyvitamin D are normal in patients with advanced renal failure, while levels of 1,25-dihydroxyvitamin D are low or undetectable, and treatment with small doses of 1,25-dihydroxyvitamin D reduces or eliminates bone pain and muscle weakness in some patients (Henderson et al. 1974). Goldstein and associates (1979) observed that muscle strength increased after 2 to 5 weeks of therapy with 1,25-dihydroxyvitamin D, while bone pain did not improve before 6 to 27 weeks of therapy.

An absolute or relative deficiency of 1,25-dihydroxyvitamin D may be an important cause of secondary hyperparathyroidism, by reducing intestinal absorption of calcium and by inducing skeletal resistance to parathyroid hormone. In patients with moderate renal insufficiency Massry and colleagues (Massry 1980) rectified serum levels of parathyroid hormone and reversed osteodystrophy by giving small doses of 1,25-dihydroxyvitamin D without restricting dietary phosphate intake. Thus, uremic osteodystrophy (and presumably uremic myopathy) may be partly due to abnormal vitamin-D metabolism, and the reason that such large doses of vitamin D are required in treatment may be the fact that very little of the administered dose is converted to the active metabolite.

Other investigators have had less success with 1,25-dihydroxyvitamin-D therapy, and it appears that nonresponders tend to have predominant osteomalacia on bone biopsy, with little or no osteitis fibrosa (Velentzas et al. 1981). Among a group of 19 hemodialysis patients with pure osteomalacic bone disease, there were 14 patients with severe myopathy, 7 showed improvement of muscle strength during treatment with 1,25-dihydroxyvitamin D, though bone histology did not improve in any patient. These puzzling observations suggest that some factor other than 1,25-dihydroxyvitamin-D deficiency can produce both osteomalacia and myopathy; this could be aluminum, the concentration of which was greatly increased in bone biopsies from patients with uremic osteomalacia (Hodsman et al. 1981).

Pathophysiology of Myopathy in Vitamin-D Deficiency. There is conflicting evidence about the biologic functions of various vitamin-D metabolites. If 1,25-dihydroxyvitamin D is the active form in all tissues, why are the biochemical features of dietary vitamin-D deficiency so different from those of the osteomalacia caused by mesenchymal tumors that induce a selective deficiency of 1,25-dihydroxyvitamin D? In fact, 1,25-dihydroxyvitamin-D levels were normal in three patients with nutritional osteomalacia, while levels of 25-hydroxyvitamin D and 24,25-dihydroxyvitamin D were quite low (Eastwood et al. 1979). Some investigators maintain that deficiency of 1,25-dihydroxyvitamin D is mainly responsible for uremic osteomalacia and anticonvulsant osteomalacia (Eastwood et al. 1976), and others have suggested that 24,25-dihydroxyvitamin D may be the preferred metabolite for bone mineralization (Hodsman et al. 1981).

At a cellular level, vitamin D acts on the nucleus to induce synthesis of specific messenger ribonucleic acid (RNA), which stimulates the production of cytoplasmic calcium-binding protein or proteins that are responsible for the translocation of extracellular calcium into the cell. These actions have been studied primarily in intestinal cells and kidney; little is known about the effects of vitamin D on muscle, where calcium influences the membrane permeability to monovalent cations and plays a central role in excitation-contraction coupling. Birge and Haddad (1975) observed that ATP content and protein synthesis were diminished in vitamin D-deficient rat muscle, and in tissue culture these abnormalities were corrected by 25-hydroxyvitamin D but not by 1,25-dihydroxyvitamin D. The influence of vitamin D on synthesis of other calcium-binding proteins of muscle—calmodulin, which regulates key glycolytic enzymes; the several calcium-binding proteins of sarcoplasmic reticulum; and troponin C, which mediates the calcium-sensitivity of the contractile proteins—has not been examined. (The amount of troponin C in muscle was reported to be reduced in vitamin D-deficient rabbits, but the data were unconvincing [Pointon et al. 1979]).

Experimental vitamin-D deficiency markedly slows the growth of young chicks, rabbits, and rats. In these rachitic animals, muscle mass is reduced to the same degree as body weight, and the animals often appear to be weak. In rats there is atrophy of type-2B (fast-glycolytic) muscle fibers more than of type-1 or type-2A fibers (Swash et al. 1979; Schimrigk et al. 1975). Vitamin D-deficient animals are much less active than normal, and their bones are more yielding, so that the atrophy may simply be due to reduced activity. Pleasure and coworkers (1979) did not find a reduction of muscle-fiber diameter in vitamin D-deficient chicks, a puzzling result since the muscle weights were reduced. No other notable pathologic observations emerged from these studies.

The rate of muscle relaxation was slow in vitamin D-deficient rats (Rodman and Baker 1978) and chicks (Pleasure et al. 1979), and maximum tetanic tension was reduced in chicks (Pleasure et al. 1979). These abnormalities were not present to the same degree in animals with hypocalcemic rickets induced by dietary deficiency of calcium. Calcium uptake by fragmented sarcoplasmic reticulum was reduced in vitamin D-deficient rabbits (Curry et al. 1974) and chicks (Pleasure et al. 1979). The calcium content of isolated mitochondria was reduced in chick muscle (Pleasure et al. 1979). Thus, it is possible that the contractile abnormality of vitamin D-deficient muscle results from various abnormalities of function of sarcoplasmic reticulum, including reduced calcium stores, diminished release of calcium during contraction, and slower uptake of calcium during relaxation.

However, these experiments do not really explain the clinical findings in patients with osteomalacic myopathy and do not account for the "myopathic" EMG abnormalities. All the foregoing experiments were performed on rapidly growing animals raised from birth in the dark on vitamin D-deficient diets. When animals are exposed to light, dietary deficiency of vitamin D does not produce rickets, and it is extremely difficult to induce vitamin-D deficiency in adult animals. A better animal model might be provided if inhibitors of the metabolic activation of vitamin D were available for laboratory experimentation.

Hypophosphatemic Osteomalacia

Acute hypophosphatemia causes various acute neuromuscular and cerebral symptoms, including acute generalized paralysis and rhabdomyolysis. These disorders are discussed in Chapter 2. *Chronic phosphorus depletion,* however, leads to slowly progressive proximal muscle weakness, bone pain, and osteomalacia, developing over a period of months or years. This syndrome may result from simple dietary deficiency of phosphorus or from intestinal malabsorption, but most of the reported cases are due to chronic ingestion of large amounts of antacids containing aluminum hydroxide, which binds dietary phosphate (Insogna et al. 1980; Ravid and Robson 1976; Goodman et al. 1978). The published reports do not include data on serum enzymes, EMG, or muscle biopsy, except that the serum activity of glutamic oxalacetic transaminase was normal in one case (Insogna et al. 1980). The biochemical findings are pathognomonic: normal serum calcium, low serum phosphorus, hypercalcuria, and absent urinary phosphorus. The patients recover within a few weeks after antacids are withdrawn and phosphate supplements are given.

Pathophysiology. The mechanisms of osteomalacia and of myopathy caused by dietary phosphorus depletion are not well understood. Severe cellular phosphorus deficiency is known to limit phosphorylation reactions and the synthesis of ATP, and Goodman and colleagues (1978) demonstrated a marked depression of ATP synthesis in platelets from a patient with chronic muscular weakness caused by antacid ingestion. Fuller and associates (1976) showed a 16-percent reduction of the muscle membrane resting potential in dogs depleted of phosphorus for 4 weeks. Some of the dogs appeared weak and lethargic and recovered promptly during phosphorus replacement. Muscle excitability, contractility, and resistance to fatigue have not been studied in chronic phosphorus depletion, but there is preliminary information that muscle ATP concentration may decline substantially (Fuller, cited by Knochel 1981). This subject is discussed in Chapter 2.

Urinary wastage of phosphate is the hallmark of *renal hypophosphatemic osteomalacia.* Adult patients present with debilitating bone pain and muscle weakness, and laboratory studies show normal serum calcium, hypophosphatemia, diminished renal tubular reabsorption of phosphate, low urinary calcium, and mild elevation of serum alkaline phosphatase activity. The syndrome is usually not familial in adults. In a subgroup of patients with glycinuria, a primary defect of renal tubular function is presumed to be present, but absorption of calcium and phosphorus from the intestine is also diminished, and successful treatment requires vitamin D as well as phosphate supplements (Dent and Stamp 1971). The myopathy appears to be clinically identical to that of vitamin-D deficiency, and muscle biopsy shows atrophy of type-2 muscle fiber (Schott and Wills 1975).

The same clinical and biochemical findings, with urinary wastage of phosphate, can be due to the presence of a *mesenchymal tumor,* removal of which cures both the myopathy and the osteomalacia (Pollack et al. 1973). About 25 such cases have been reported in adults and children; most of the patients had bone tumors variously described as fibromas, giant cell tumors, hemangiomas, or hemangiopericytomas; a few had soft tissue tumors described as sclerosing hemangiomas. Since many of the tumors were benign and were discovered only by accident, it remains uncertain what proportion of cases of hypophosphatemic osteomalacia is caused by such tumors. In several recent cases, serum levels of 1,25-dihydroxyvitamin D were depressed, while the levels of other vitamin-D metabolites were normal (Drezner and Feinglos 1977; Sweet et al. 1980; Parker et al. 1981; Fukomoto et al. 1979). In one case administration of small amounts of 1,25-dihydroxyvitamin D before surgery completely reversed the metabolic abnormalities (Drezner and Feinglos 1977). It seems that the tumors may secrete a substance that interferes with renal 1-hydroxylation of 25-hydroxyvitamin D.

Proximal Muscle Weakness in Hyperparathyroidism

Incidence and Clinical Features

Patients with primary hyperparathyroidism often complain of muscle weakness and fatigability, but overt signs of neuromuscular disease are infrequent. In Western countries the incidence of primary hyperparathyroidism is several times greater than that of osteomalacia, but reports of proximal weakness in hyperparathyroidism are much fewer than reports of myopathy in osteomalacia. Frame and colleagues (1968) described 3 patients with muscle weakness out of a total of 76 patients with hyperparathyroidism. The 3 patients had predominantly proximal weakness and muscle atrophy, no fasciculations or muscle tenderness, and normal reflexes. The serum enzymes were normal, EMG showed a high percentage of small, polyphasic motor unit potentials compatible with a myopathy, and a muscle biopsy showed scattered degeneration of muscle fibers. Henson (1966) found symptoms of muscular weakness in 11 (32 percent) of 34 patients with primary hyperparathyroidism (apparently by chart review) and stated that muscle weakness was "substantial" in 5 patients (15 percent). The clinical features were identical to those described by Vicale (1949): proximal muscle weakness and wasting, hypotonia, discomfort on movement, and exaggerated tendon reflexes. Again, EMG showed short-duration polyphasic potentials with no evidence of denervation, and muscle biopsy showed isolated muscle-fiber necrosis and proliferation of sarcolemmic nuclei, without denervation atrophy.

It was with this background that Smith and Stern inquired into the incidence of muscle weakness among patients with osteomalacia and hyperparathyroidism, first with a retrospective review of the medical records of 136 patients (Smith and Stern 1967) and then by personal examination of 55 patients admitted consecutively to the same metabolic unit within a period of 18 months (Smith and Stern 1969). With respect to primary hyperparathyroidism, they found proximal muscle weakness in 6 (6.6 percent) of 91 patients in the retrospective study, and in 1 (2.4 percent) of 41 patients in the prospective study. In contrast, among patients with osteomalacia, proximal weakness was reported in 44 percent in the first study and was observed in 8 (73 percent) of 11 patients in the second study, the other 3 having too much bone pain for accurate assessment. The clinical and EMG findings were apparently the same in the few hyperparathyroid patients with weakness as in the osteomalacic cases, and they conformed closely to those described by Vicale (1949), Henson (1966), and Frame and associates (1968).

In a recent retrospective series of 100 cases of primary hyperparathyroidism (Lafferty 1981), only 7 percent had signs or symptoms of muscle weakness (not specifically described), while 20 percent had "mental changes" and 47 percent were asymptomatic. The high proportion of asymptomatic cases reflects the recent trend toward early diagnosis of hyperparathyroidism by means of routine chemical testing.

Myopathic vs Neurogenic Muscle Weakness

In a frequently-cited pair of articles, W. K. Engel and his collaborators (Patten et al. 1974; Mallette et al. 1975) reported the presence of proximal muscle weakness in 14 of 16 patients with primary hyperparathyroidism and in each of 6 patients with osteomalacia; they concluded that the weakness had a neurogenic cause in every case. The uniquely high incidence of muscle weakness in the series of hyperparathyroid patients is puzzling, but more importantly, the neurogenic hypothesis is open to several criticisms.

1. Only 10 of the 16 hyperparathyroid patients had a verified parathyroid tumor; one of these clearly had amyotrophic lateral sclerosis and at least 3 of the 6 unverified cases were probably examples of osteomalacia with secondary hyperparathyroidism.

2. EMG showed typical myopathic abnormalities of motor unit potential in 5 cases, nonspecific minor changes in 3, no abnormality in 2, and neurogenic reinnervation potentials in 2, including the patient with amyotrophic lateral sclerosis. There were no fibrillations in any case. The authors argued that the myopathic EMG could, in theory, have resulted from nonfunction of some of the terminal nerve branches in each motor unit. That is certainly possible, but a purely myopathic EMG is rarely encountered in proven neurogenic diseases, and the latter usually cause fibrillations.

3. Muscle biopsies showed scattered, angulated, atrophic muscle fibers, which were predominantly or exclusively type 2. There were no signs of reinnervation (fiber type grouping). The authors argued that the presence of atrophy of muscle fiber was direct evidence of denervation, but in fact there is no proof that denervation is the only cause of angulated atrophy of muscle fibers. Similar atrophy occurs in other metabolic "myopathies" whose pathogenesis is still unsettled (hypothyroid, hyperthyroid, and steroid myopathies). It is equally plausible that atrophy results from inexcitability of muscle fibers (Gruener and Stern 1972b).

4. Muscle fasciculations were not described except in the patient with amyotrophic lateral sclerosis. Peculiar gross twitching or jerking of the tongue, which did not resemble ordinary fasciculations, was observed in almost all the patients with hyperparathyroidism and also in those with osteomalacia. This sign has not been mentioned in descriptions of the neuromuscular signs of hyperparathyroidism or osteomalacia by other neurologists, including some of considerable reputation (Vicale 1949; Henson 1966; Princas et al. 1965; Ekbom et al. 1964; Marsden et al. 1973; Floyd et al. 1974; Serratrice et al. 1978).

Role of Hypercalcemia

The relationship of hyperparathyroid weakness to hypercalcemia is difficult to unravel. It is often claimed that hypercalcemia itself produces neuromuscular symptoms; mild hypercalcemia causes apathy, depression, and fatigue, while calcium levels of 15 mg per dl or higher are said to cause generalized weakness, drowsiness, and confusion. The latter state has been referred to as calcium intoxication or hypercalcemic crisis, and it subsides rapidly following correction of the hypercalcemia (O'Dorisio 1978). However, there is no evidence that hypercalcemic weakness is due to a motor-unit disorder; the neuromuscular symptoms of hypercalcemia are probably central in origin (see Chapter 2).

Among the many accounts of hypercalcemic crisis in primary hyperparathyroidism (Lemann and Donatelli 1964), there is no case in which muscle paralysis was actually described, except for two patients with signs resembling a transverse myelopathy. One patient had been unable to walk for a month and had severe, generalized weakness, bilateral Babinski's signs, and loss of vibration sense at the ankles. His serum calcium level was 17 mg per dl. He began to improve 2 days after removal of a parathyroid adenoma, and his muscle strength was normal by the seventh day (Murphy et al. 1960). A second patient presented with severe, hypotonic weakness of all extremities, depressed sensorium, bilateral ankle clonus, Babinski's signs, a sensory level at C-2, and loss of bladder and bowel control. Serum calcium levels varied between 10 mg per dl and 14 mg per dl. Previous neck exploration having failed to reveal a tumor, the patient was treated with oral phosphates, and as her serum calcium level declined, the neurologic signs gradually subsided (Dyro 1977). These two cases are presumably *not* examples of the "generalized weakness" referred to in standard discussions of hypercalcemia.

From the information at hand, it is possible that subjective symptoms of weakness and easy fatigue in primary hyperparathyroidism may be related to hypercalcemia, since they subside quickly after removal of the parathyroid adenoma. Actual proximal weakness is uncommon, and is unlikely to be due to hypercalcemia, though in several cases the weakness resolved remarkably quickly following removal of a parathyroid adenoma. In the three cases reported by Frame and associates (1968) there was complete recovery of muscle power within a few days in one case and within 2 weeks in another. Patten and colleagues (1974) recorded the response to parathyroid surgery in six cases; improvement began within hours of surgery in some patients, and the four patients who improved after surgery recovered completely in 3 days to several weeks. This early and rapid recovery contrasts with the delayed and slow improvement of muscle strength that occurs during treatment of nutritional osteomalacia with vitamin D, and it suggests that muscle weakness in hyperparathyroidism may have a different pathogenesis from that of osteomalacic myopathy.

Relation to Vitamin-D Metabolism

The mechanism responsible for muscle weakness in hyperparathyroidism is completely unknown. Surprisingly, there is no experimental information about the effects of parathyroid hormone on motor function. Most patients do not become weak, and it is not rare for patients to have active hyperparathyroidism for several decades without neuromuscular impairment (Kosinski et al. 1976). To add to the confusion, patients with vitamin D-deficient osteomalacia generally develop secondary hyperparathyroidism, and occasionally the parathyroid hyperplasia gives rise to one or more adenomas, an outcome that has been dubbed "tertiary" hyperparathyroidism (Davies et al. 1968). Smith and Stern (1967, 1969) observed that proximal myopathy was an almost invariable finding in tertiary hyperparathyroidism. When primary hyperparathyroidism occurs in a patient with vitamin-D deficiency, serum calcium levels may be normal but become elevated during treatment with vitamin D. Some hypercalcemic patients with what appears to be primary hyperparathyroidism have coexistent osteomalacia on bone biopsy, and muscle weakness in such patients may resolve completely with vitamin-D treatment *before removal of the adenoma.* Chronic phosphate deficiency caused by hyperparathyroidism could explain the weakness in such cases (Woodhead et al. 1980), but Lumb and Stanbury (1974) have suggested that primary hyperparathyroidism itself may produce a relative deficiency of active vitamin-D metabolites in patients with low vitamin-D stores. The question arises, then, whether the infrequent occurrence of chronic myopathy in primary hyperparathyroidism is really a consequence of phosphate depletion or of vitamin-D deficiency, rather than of hyperparathyroidism.

Hypoparathyroidism and Pseudohypoparathyroidism

The principal neuromuscular symptom in these disorders is tetany, which is described in Chapter 2. The peripheral manifestations of tetany are much more common than the central ones. In a retrospective chart review of 34 patients with secondary hypoparathyroidism, Fonseca and Calverley (1967) found signs of peripheral tetany in 21 patients, but only 6 patients had seizures, 6 had psychiatric disturbances, and 1 had chorea.

There are several reports of elevated serum enzyme levels in patients with hypoparathyroidism and pseudohypoparathyroidism (Shane et al. 1980; Walters 1979; Kuhn et al. 1981; Piechowiak et al. 1981; Kruse et al. 1982). Only two patients had clear-cut clinical evidence of myopathy, but muscle-fiber degeneration was demonstrated histologically in several cases. The serum enzyme levels returned to normal in parallel with serum calcium levels.

Hypoparathyroidism has been observed in several cases of the Kearns-Sayre syndrome, a nonhereditary multisystem disease characterized by onset in childhood of progressive external ophthalmoplegia, short stature, pigmentary degeneration of the retina, neural deafness, cardiac conduction defects, myopathy with "ragged-red" muscle fibers, and polyneuropathy (Pellock et al. 1978).

PITUITARY DISEASES

Acromegaly

Myopathy

Pierre Marie, a French neurologist, recorded the presence of proximal muscle weakness and atrophy in the first two cases of acromegaly, a term that he coined (Marie 1886). He mentioned that some patients felt unusually strong in the early stages of the disease, an observation that calls to mind the acromegalic wrestler who fought under the name of the Angel several decades ago. The post mortem studies in the French literature that followed Marie's report suggested various neurogenic causes for the weakness, and it was not until 1970 that English (Mastaglia et al. 1970) and Swedish (Lundberg et al. 1970) neurologists published unequivocal clinical and EMG evidence of a mild, chronic myopathy in many cases of acromegaly.

In a series of 17 consecutive patients with acromegaly (Pickett et al. 1975), three fourths of the patients reported easy fatigability, and half had symptoms suggestive of proximal weakness. These complaints began 8 to 21 years after the onset of acral enlargement. Mild weakness and flabbiness of proximal limb muscles, without tenderness or irritability, were present on examination in 40 percent, similar to the incidence noted by others (Mastaglia et al. 1970; Lundberg et al. 1970). Using quantitative EMG, Mastaglia and colleagues (1970) showed a striking reduction of the mean duration of motor unit potentials in proximal muscles, and standard EMG showed myopathic abnormalities without fibrillations in half to three fourths of patients, including some without overt weakness (Lundberg et al. 1970; Pickett et al. 1975). The serum CPK level was slightly elevated in one fifth of the cases. Muscle biopsy samples often showed hypertrophy of type-1 fibers and atrophy or deficient numbers of type-2 fibers (Mastaglia 1973; Nagulesparen et al. 1976); muscle fiber necrosis was infrequent, internal nuclei were increased in number, and glycogen stores appeared increased (Mastaglia 1973).

Following pituitary surgery, improvement of strength was very slow and was still incomplete 12 to 21 months later; since levels of growth hormone did not return to normal in every case, it is hard to interpret this observation. There was no apparent correlation between the presence of myopathy and of any associated endocrine abnormalities such as diabetes or hypothyroidism (Pickett et al. 1975)

Pathophysiology. Little is known about the mechanism of muscle dysfunction in acromegaly. Perhaps this is not surprising, considering that years of exposure to excessive growth hormone precede the development of myopathy. Early animal studies showed that growth hormone produces considerable enlargement of muscles, especially proximal and axial ones, without a change in muscle force; in other words, strength is unchanged for the whole muscle but is reduced in terms of muscle weight (Bigland and Jehring 1952). Recently Prysor-Jones and Jenkins (1980) reported preliminary results with a new animal model of acromegaly induced by subcutaneous injection of a cultured rat pituitary tumor into mature rats. After 3 months body weight had doubled, there was widespread visceromegaly, and incorporation of thymidine into DNA was increased in skeletal muscle and heart. The size of type-1 muscle fibers was increased more than that of the other fiber types, reminiscent of the findings in human patients, but no atrophic fibers were seen. Perhaps this animal model will eventually clarify the pathogenesis of acromegalic myopathy.

Acromegalic muscle utilizes lipid fuels in preference to carbohydrates (Rabinowitz and Zierler 1963), perhaps as a consequence of the selective enlargement of muscle fibers high in oxidative enzymes. Similarly, in animals chronic administration of growth hormone depletes body fat stores and stimulates, albeit transiently, oxidation of fatty acids by muscle (Winckler et al. 1964). But there is no indication that these metabolic alterations are pertinent to the development of myopathy.

Peripheral Neuropathy

Symptoms of the disorder that we now recognize as the carpal tunnel syndrome were recorded in acromegaly as early as 1899 (Sternberg 1899). A recent survey showed that unilateral or bilateral median nerve compression at the wrist was present in about half of patients with long-standing acromegaly. The symptoms sometimes improved spontaneously, and in five out of six cases they resolved completely within 6 weeks after pituitary surgery, though neurologic and electrophysiologic deficits persisted. This rapid improvement may have resulted from a reduction in tissue water content after surgery. Only one of the patients relapsed after pituitary surgery, indicating that carpal tunnel surgery may not be needed in most patients who are going to have direct treatment of the endocrine disorder (Pickett et al. 1975).

Low and associates (1974) found clinical signs of a distal, symmetrical polyneuropathy of sensorimotor type in five of eleven patients, and eight patients had mild slowing of motor nerve conduction velocity and absent sural nerve sensory responses. Enlargement of ulnar or peroneal nerves was judged to be present in five cases. Sural nerve biopsies showed a slight reduction in the number of myelinated and unmyelinated fibers, and an increased amount of endoneurial and perineurial connective tissue. There was segmental demyelination and rare axonal degeneration, but 90 percent of the teased nerve fibers examined were normal. Others have found little clinical or electrophysiologic evidence of a diffuse polyneuropathy, and no enlargement of peripheral nerves, though compression neuropathies are fairly common (Pickett et al. 1975; Lundberg et al. 1970). Nerve roots may become compressed by hypertrophic soft tissue in the vertebral foramina, and rarely peripheral nerves may be enlarged by overgrowth of connective tissue (Stewart 1966).

Nelson Syndrome

In recent years, as a result of technical advances in pituitary surgery, there has been a return to Cushing's original view that the spontaneous occurrence of bilateral adrenal hyperplasia (Cushing's disease) is nearly always caused by a pituitary tumor, usually a chromophobe microadenoma, less often a basophilic or mixed-cell tumor. The preferred treatment of Cushing's disease is now trans-sphenoidal resection of the pituitary adenoma, which can be selectively removed in the majority of cases (Tyrell et al. 1978). For many years, however, total bilateral adrenalectomy was standard treatment, and there are a number of follow-up studies documenting the emergence of a symptomatic pituitary tumor some years later. Over half of adrenalectomized patients develop hyperpigmentation despite adequate steroid replacement therapy, and many of these patients eventually develop a frank pituitary tumor (Nelson's syndrome). Serum ACTH levels in such patients are extremely high.

Prineas and coworkers (1968) investigated 16 patients who had undergone bilateral total or subtotal adrenalectomy for Cushing's disease and no longer had active hyperadrenalism. Four of the five hyperpigmented patients complained of muscular weakness or excessive tiredness on effort, and on examination two of these had mild proximal weakness without other neuromuscular abnormalities. EMG was abnormal in all five pigmented patients, with increased insertional activity, pseudomyotonic discharges, fibrillations and positive waves, reduced mean duration of motor-unit potentials, and an increased percentage of polyphasic motor-unit potentials. No clinical or electromyographic abnormality was discovered in the nonpigmented patients. Serum CPK levels were normal. Muscle biopsy in four pigmented patients showed an accumulation of fat droplets beneath the sarcolemma in both type-1 and type-2 muscle fibers, without other histologic or ultrastructural abnormalities.

Although subsequent publications dealing with Nelson's syndrome do not mention neuromuscular symptoms (Hopwood and Kenny 1977; Cohen et al. 1978; Moore et al. 1976), the observations of Prineas and coworkers (1968) suggest that marked hypersecretion of ACTH may induce a lipid-storage myopathy with electrical hyperirritability. It is possible that these abnormalities are due to a direct action of ACTH, but nothing is known about the muscular effects of ACTH in the absence of hyperadrenalism.

DIABETES MELLITUS AND HYPERINSULINISM

Diabetic Neuropathies

Incidence

The motor manifestations of diabetic neuropathy fall into three categories: isolated nerve palsies, distal sensorimotor polyneuropathy, and diabetic amyotrophy. The incidence of these disorders is difficult to determine, because most of the published surveys do not distinguish between varieties of diabetic neuropathy. The main exception is Fry's survey (Fry et al. 1962) of 490 unselected patients from the Guy's Hospital Diabetes Clinic. Excluding patients whose only sign of neuropathy was loss of ankle jerks and vibration sense, there were 66 patients with neuropathy, an incidence of 13 percent. Of these, two thirds (44 patients) had symmetrical polyneuropathy; their ages ranged from 36 to 76 years. Eighteen patients had isolated neuropathies: twelve in the limbs (ages 19 to 65 years), three ocular (ages 54 to 80), and three facial (ages 40 to 61 years). Six patients had diabetic amyotrophy; their ages ranged from 47 to 59 years. (Two of the 66 patients had combined lesions.)

Indirect information gives some idea about the incidence of the different neuropathies. Fraser and colleagues (1979) encountered 51 cases of symptomatic mononeuropathy over a 3-year period at a large diabetic clinic in Edinburgh. Casey and Harrison (1972) found 12 cases of diabetic amyotrophy in 10 years at the National Hospital in London. Gibbels and Schliep (1970), reviewing 100 cases of diabetic neuropathy diagnosed in a university neurology clinic in Cologne during the 20-year period 1950 to 1969, classified 17 percent as amyotrophy, 32 percent as distal sensory polyneuropathy, and 52 percent as mixed forms.

Mononeuropathies

Motor nerve lesions with a *gradual* onset are usually due to compression or entrapment. In the 51 patients with diabetic mononeuropathy examined by Fraser and colleagues (1979), 30 had a gradual, progressive course; all of these were in the upper extremities, affecting the median nerve in 15 patients (13 of them female) and the ulnar nerve in 15 patients (10 of them male). In every case there was electrophysiologic evidence of conduction delay across the wrist or elbow, and the dominant arm was affected solely or predominantly, strongly suggesting that chronic trauma occurred during use of the limb. A distal, sensory or sensorimotor polyneuropathy was also present in 80 percent of the patients with ulnar neuropathy but in only 20 percent of those with carpal tunnel syndrome. Thus, diffuse diabetic abnormality of the peripheral nerves seemed to be an important factor in the development of ulnar neuropathy at the elbow.

The carpal tunnel syndrome developed in 12 percent of 995 diabetic patients over the age of 30 who were followed at the Mayo Clinic between 1945 and 1970 (Palumbo et al. 1978). In three series of cases of the carpal tunnel syndrome, diabetes was present in 7.5 to 11.5 percent of the patients (Czeuz et al 1966; Phalan 1966; Frymoyer and Bland 1973).

In contrast, the *acute* neuropathies in the study by Fraser and colleagues (1979) were confined to the lower extremities and cranial nerves and affected both sexes equally. Three involved the sciatic nerve, three the femoral nerve, eight the peroneal nerve, four the oculomotor or abducens nerve, and three the facial nerve. In the legs, motor conduction velocity was reduced in the affected nerve compared with the unaffected nerve on the opposite side. A polyneuropathy was present in 57 percent of the cases but was almost always mild in degree.

Acute neuropathies of large mixed nerves of the lower extremities are often accompanied by deep, aching pain in the affected muscles, which become wasted and may fasciculate. The corresponding muscle stretch reflexes are diminished or lost, but there is little sensory impairment. Recovery of muscle strength takes place over a period of months or years and is often incomplete in the distal muscles. Acute neuropathy of the oculomotor nerve causes orbital pain in about half of the cases. Pupillary function is spared in 80 percent of cases, a finding attributed to the fact that pupillomotor nerve fibers are carried in the periphery of the nerve, which tends to escape ischemic injury. Recovery of function is usually good but incomplete, and can be expected within 3 months.

There is fairly secure evidence that acute diabetic mononeuropathies are due to ischemic injury. Patchy ischemic degeneration of the oculomotor nerve has been documented in two postmortem studies (Dreyfus et al. 1957; Asbury et al. 1970), and there is one report of ischemic pathology in a case of multiple mononeuropathies in one leg (Raff et al. 1968). In the latter case, an elderly diabetic patient had suffered the apoplectic onset of multiple motor neuropathies in one leg, 6 weeks before death. Postmortem examination showed numerous small areas of patchy nerve degeneration scattered throughout the obturator, femoral, sciatic, and posterior tibial nerves on that side. Only one intraneural arterial occlusion was identified, and it was therefore presumed that atherosclerosis of small extraneural feeding arteries was responsible for the ischemic lesions.

Distal Sensorimotor Polyneuropathy

The *clinical features* of this very common type of diabetic neuropathy are familiar to most physicians. The earliest abnormalities usually consist of asymptomatic depression of the Achilles reflexes and reduced vibratory perception in the feet. Typically the onset is insidious, the distal sensory deficits increasing slowly over the course of many years, eventually being joined by distal muscle weakness and atrophy. The upper extremities are involved electrophysiologically, but clinically are much less affected than the lower extremities. In their study of 72 patients with muscle weakness caused by diabetic neuropathy, Gibbels and Schliep (1970) found symmetrical distal weakness in the legs in 28 percent and in the arms in 13 percent of their patients.

The onset of distal, symmetrical polyneuropathy is not always gradual; symptoms may appear subacutely or even explosively soon after the onset of diabetes, even in adolescents (Lawrence and Locke 1963). Symptoms of neuropathy sometimes begin soon after initiation of insulin treatments, a serious illness, or the stress of surgery (Thomas and Eliasson 1975). In the Guy's Hospital series, 9 percent of the cases of distal symmetrical polyneuropathy had an acute onset (Fry et al. 1962).

The prevalence of polyneuropathy increases steadily with increasing duration of the diabetes. Gamstorp and associates (1966) found minor clinical and nerve conduction abnormalities in 11 out of 107 diabetic children under the age of 17 years. The affected children had been diabetic for 4 years longer, on the average, than the children without neuropathy. In a prospective study of 4400 patients observed between 1947 and 1973, Pirart (1977) observed that the prevalence of clinical polyneuropathy increased linearly with increasing duration of diabetes, so that about 50 percent of patients had clinical signs after 25 years. (However, 94 percent of those patients had only asymptomatic loss of Achilles reflexes or reduction of vibration sense in the feet, so the prevalence of clinically important neuropathy was only 3 percent!) Motor nerve conduction velocity likewise tends to decrease with increasing duration of diabetes (Gregersen 1967).

Electrophysiologic studies frequently show mild abnormalities of motor and sensory nerve conduction in asymptomatic subjects without clinical signs of neuropathy, and the frequency of such findings increases with the duration of diabetes (Gregersen 1967). Lamontagne and Buchthal (1970) compared the electrophysiologic and clinical findings in 30 patients with diabetic neuropathy. Motor conduction velocity in the peroneal nerve was 18 to 50 m per second (mean 36 m per second) and was below the normal range in 80 percent of the patients; the degree of slowing correlated well with the clinical severity of the neuropathy. EMG showed fibrillations, loss of motor units, or reinnervation potentials in an even higher proportion of the patients; the abnormalities were more numerous in distal muscles, but their presence was not related to the clinical severity. Abnormalities of median nerve sensory conduction, the most frequent finding, were present in many patients with normal distal median motor nerve conduction and did match the sensory findings on clinical examination. In a later study, Behse and associates (1977) found pronounced EMG abnormalities (denervation, loss of motor units, and signs of reinnervation) in patients with sensorimotor polyneuropathy, while patients with mainly sensory polyneuropathy had little evidence of active denervation or of reinnervation. This latter group, however, still showed moderate to severe loss of motor units in nearly all muscles.

Kimura and colleagues (1979) used F-wave responses to study conduction throughout the length of the motor nerves of 102 otherwise healthy diabetic patients with "symmetric peripheral neuropathy," all of whom were ambulatory and without mononeuropathy, asymmetry, or predominantly proximal weakness. Motor conduction was mildly slowed in both proximal and distal nerve segments, being slightly worse in the distal segments and worse in the legs than in the arms.

All of these studies suggest that a diffuse abnormality of motor nerve function appears early in the course of diabetic polyneuropathy, affects the entire length of the nerve fibers, and is more severe in distal segments of the longest motor nerves (those in the lower extremities).

Our information about the *pathology* of diabetic polyneuropathy is derived almost entirely from biopsies of sensory (sural) nerves, but the foregoing discussion suggests that the same process probably affects motor and sensory nerves. Thomas and Lascelles (1966) demonstrated widespread segmental demyelination in teased nerve fiber preparations, and they considered this abnormality to be the primary pathologic process, axonal degeneration being a later development in severe, chronic cases. However, the recent study by Behse and associates (1977) showed loss of large and small myelinated and unmyelinated nerve fibers early in the disease; remyelination was also prominent, but active demyelination was infrequent. Axonal degeneration and Schwann cell damage seemed to proceed independently of each other. The conduction velocity in most of the sural nerves was 10 to 30 percent slower than would be expected from the normal linear relationship between the diameter of the largest myelinated fibers and the maximal conduction velocity. This discrepancy could reflect conduction slowing caused by remyelination, or it could be the result of a metabolic disturbance that does not produce morphologic changes.

In a recent postmortem study of lower extremity nerves in two patients with symmetric distal polyneuropathy, Sugimura and Dyck (1982) found a patchy loss of myelinated nerve fibers in the proximal and middle portions of the sciatic nerves. The focal distribution of the nerve fiber loss, which varied within fascicles and between adjacent fascicles, suggested an interstitial disease process rather than a metabolic cause.

The *spinal fluid protein* is increased (over 50 mg per dl) in two thirds of cases; in one series the mean value was 72 mg per dl and the highest value was 224 mg per dl. The spinal fluid protein is normal in diabetes in the absence of neuropathy or other causes of raised spinal fluid protein (Madonick and Margolis 1952). The high incidence of spinal fluid protein abnormalities in patients with polyneuropathy again suggests that the pathologic process is not restricted to the most distal portions of the motor nerves and involves the intraspinal nerve roots in most cases.

Diabetic Amyotrophy

The emergence of this syndrome as a distinct variety of diabetic neuropathy is a fascinating and perhaps unfinished chapter in recent neurologic history. Although Bruns described the syndrome in 1890, in modern times it was Garland and Taverner (1953) who first directed medical attention to this little-known motor complication of diabetes. The main features were deep pain, muscle weakness, atrophy, and areflexia, concentrated in the pelvic girdle and thighs, without loss of sensation. The symptoms and signs were unilateral or asymmetrical, progressed over a period of months or years, and showed a striking tendency to resolve slowly during treatment of the diabetes (which often was first diagnosed after the onset of neuromuscular symptoms). Because three of the original five patients had Babinski's signs, Garland and Taverner suggested that the seat of pathology was probably in the spinal cord—hence the name amyotrophy (Garland 1955), which implies anterior horn cell disease.

Around the same time, other neurologists were beginning to distinguish the acute diabetic mononeuropathies, largely motor and often painful, from the more familiar distal symmetrical polyneuropathy, which was mainly sensory. As we have seen, the former process usually involves recognizable mixed nerves of the lower extremities such as the femoral, sciatic, or peroneal nerves. Sullivan (1958) suggested that such neuropathies might be caused by occlusive vascular disease, and Gregersen (1969) argued that "amyotrophy" was merely a clustering of multiple mononeuropathies, which might be due to either vascular or metabolic causes. Moreover, an autopsy in a case of diabetic amyotrophy showed no spinal cord pathology except for chromatolysis of anterior horn cells, as occurs in peripheral nerve damage (Matthews 1958). Thus, when Raff and Asbury (1968) produced pathologic evidence of ischemic degeneration of multiple thigh nerves in an elderly diabetic man with unilateral lower-extremity weakness, they argued that diabetic amyotrophy was simply a proximal form of ischemic mononeuropathy multiplex. However, the patient studied by Raff and Asbury developed leg weakness over a period of only 12 to 24 hours and remained unchanged until his death 6 weeks later, whereas the proximal leg weakness of diabetic amyotrophy progresses for weeks or months. Furthermore, some patients with the clinical picture of amyotrophy also have proximal upper extremity involvement (Williams and Mayer 1976). Reviewing these conflicting facts, Asbury (1977) acknowledged that subacute proximal motor polyneuropathy seemed to be clinically distinct from the acute mononeuropathies, and that a metabolic rather than a vascular explanation seemed more plausible in the former group of cases.

CLINICAL FEATURES. Almost all the patients are over the age of 50, and the majority have become diabetic within a year before the onset of muscular symptoms. The neurologic symptoms often begin soon after a period of weight loss caused by a surgical operation, a serious illness, or deliberate weight reduction. Pain is often the initial symptom; it was present in 92 percent of 24 patients in three recent series (Casey and Harrison 1972; Chokroverty et al. 1977; Subramony and Wilbourn 1982). Very often the patients describe a deep ache in the lower back, hip, or thigh, initially unilateral and sometimes radiating down the leg. At this stage lumbar disc disease or arthritis of the hip is often suspected. A deep, burning sensation may be felt in the anterior thigh muscles, at times associated with unpleasant dysesthesias of the overlying skin. The pain persists and is sometimes so severe that narcotic analgesics are required for sleep. During this time wasting and weakness of the pelvifemoral muscles develop insidiously, and walking begins to be impaired. After weeks or months the pain and weakness may spread to the other leg, although both legs may be affected from the beginning. Not uncommonly the patient becomes unable to walk, is in constant pain, becomes depressed, and loses weight—a picture that Ellenberg (1974) termed "diabetic neuropathic cachexia."

Physical examination shows wasting and weakness of the pelvifemoral muscles in a pattern that does not conform to a nerve root or peripheral nerve distribution, since all the thigh muscles are involved to some degree, while the muscles below the knees are normal or much less involved. Usually the weakness is bilateral, but almost invariably it is worse in one leg. Straight-leg raising is not restricted or painful, and hip motion does not reproduce the pain. Fasciculations are rarely observed. Less severe muscle weakness and wasting are sometimes found in the lower legs, and very infrequently weakness is detected in the scapulohumeral muscles or lumbar spinal muscles (Williams and Mayer 1976; Casey and Harrison 1972; Garland 1961). The patellar reflexes are absent or reduced when the quadriceps muscles are involved; the Achilles reflexes may be depressed if the motor neuropathy involves the calf muscles, or if sensory polyneuropathy is also present. Cutaneous sensory loss in the femoral nerve distribution is usually absent or ill-defined. However, a few patients have large areas of thoracoabdominal sensory loss and dysesthesia, resulting from neuropathies of multiple thoracic spinal nerves (Sun and Streib 1981; Kikta et al. 1982), and the abdominal or lumbar muscles may be weak in such cases. Unilateral or bilateral extensor plantar responses were present in half of the 27 cases followed by Garland (1962), in 2 of the 12 cases of Casey and Harrison (1972), and in 1 of the 12 cases of Chokroverty and colleagues (1977), but were not found in other surveys (Subramony and Wilbourn 1982; Bastron and Thomas 1981).

LABORATORY FINDINGS. Serum CPK activity is normal. The spinal fluid protein is increased in the large majority of cases. In the active stage of the disease, electromyography of the affected muscles shows fibrillations, reduced numbers of motor units, a mixture of normal and long-duration motor units, and an excess of polyphasic potentials. In a high proportion of cases, increased insertional activity, fibrillations, and positive waves are found in the lumbar or thoracic paraspinal muscles of one or both sides, and spontaneous activity is also demonstrable in intercostal or abdominal muscles in patients with thoracoabdominal symptoms (Bastron and Thomas 1981; Sun and Streib 1981; Kikta et al. 1982). Motor nerve conduction is often slowed in the femoral nerve and may be slowed to different degrees in nerve branches supplying different portions of the quadriceps muscles (Chokroverty et al. 1977; Subramony and Wilbourn 1982). Conduction in the peroneal nerve proximal to the knee is slowed to a greater extent than in the segment of nerve distal to the knee (Chokroverty 1982). Muscle biopsy shows small or large groups of atrophic, angular fibers belonging to either type 1 or type 2, compatible with chronic and recent denervation. Electron microscopy shows degenerative changes of intramuscular nerve terminals and motor endplates in weak quadriceps muscles (Chokroverty 1982).

Prognosis and Treatment

There is no specific treatment for any type of diabetic neuropathy, and there is disagreement as to whether one can prevent or ameliorate these complications by controlling hyperglycemia. There is some evidence that good metabolic control is useful in the prevention and management of diabetic neuropathies, but the evidence is still fragmentary.

Many clinicians have maintained a skeptical, fatalistic attitude toward the need for strict control of diabetes in patients with neuropathy, in part because severe neuropathy may occur in patients with rather mild diabetes, and in part because the available statistics do not stand up well to critical analysis. However, several studies suggest that diabetic neuropathy occurs much more often in patients with poorly controlled than in those with well controlled diabetes. In the prospective Mayo Clinic study, symmetrical polyneuropathy and asymmetrical mononeuropathy developed 2.4 times as often in poorly controlled as in well-controlled diabetics (Palumbo et al. 1978). Among 4400 diabetics observed by Pirart (1977), the prevalence of neuropathy in poorly controlled patients increased linearly with the duration of diabetes, reaching 65 percent after 25 years. In contrast, in well-controlled patients the prevalence of neuropathy varied between 10 and 15 percent regardless of the duration of diabetes. The results were similar for retinopathy and nephropathy. The prevalance of coronary artery disease and peripheral vascular disease, however, did not vary with respect to metabolic control.

Thus, sustained hyperglycemia over a long period of time appears to be an important determinant of distal sensorimotor polyneuropathy (which accounted for most of the cases in the two studies cited). No such information is available concerning mononeuropathy and amyotrophy. Compression neuropathies might theoretically be preventable by reducing the "background damage" caused by diffuse polyneuropathy. Among the patients with mononeuropathy studied by Fraser and colleagues (1979) there was a high incidence of retinopathy and nephropathy in those with ulnar compression neuropathy but not in those with acute lower-limb or cranial neuropathies; this could imply that acute ischemic neuropathies are less likely to be preventable by good metabolic control.

Once neuropathy has begun, does it help to tighten metabolic control? A randomized, controlled study would be necessary to answer this question convincingly. The preliminary results of a randomized, controlled trial of strict diabetic treatment seem to indicate that eye and kidney lesions improve in patients treated by continuous subcutaneous insulin infusion (administered by a portable infusion pump), while these complications deteriorate in patients treated by conventional therapy (Steno Study Group 1982). With respect to neuropathy, the available information is only suggestive. Follow-up of 43 patients with symptomatic polyneuropathy at Guy's Hospital (Fry et al. 1962) showed good or fair recovery of function in 16 of the 28 patients who maintained good metabolic control after the onset of neuropathy, while recovery was poor in all 15 patients whose diabetes was poorly controlled. Motor nerve conduction velocities increased within 3 months when a group of patients with adult-onset diabetes were started on diabetic therapy; the degree of improvement was roughly proportional to the amount of reduction of fasting blood glucose concentrations (Porte et al. 1981).

Other follow-up studies show a striking tendency for improvement or recovery in patients with amyotrophy and thoracoabdominal neuropathy, but do not provide information about the value of metabolic control (Garland 1961; Casey and Harrison 1972; Sun and Streib 1981; Bastron and Thomas 1981). Garland believed that complete control of diabetes was essential for recovery from amyotrophy, but he acknowledged that some patients continued to deteriorate for several months after good control was achieved. Paradoxically, some patients suffer an acute exacerbation of neuropathy following institution of insulin treatment (Ellenberg 1974). Other patients improve rapidly following imposition of good diabetic treatment, as if a reversible "metabolic" nerve lesion were present (White et al. 1981). Most patients with diabetic amyotrophy, however, improve slowly over the course of several years, perhaps as a result of nerve regeneration. In acute ischemic mononeuropathies, recovery may be partly rapid (reflecting reversible ischemic injury) and partly slow (reflecting nerve degeneration and regeneration).

In summary, there is circumstantial evidence that good metabolic control may prevent the development and retard the progression of distal polyneuropathy. Acute mononeuropathies and diabetic amyotrophy show a striking tendency toward spontaneous recovery, which is often delayed; there is not much evidence that good control promotes this recovery, but there is no evidence to the contrary. At this stage of our knowledge, a prudent conclusion seems to favor vigorous control of diabetes.

When pain dominates the picture of diabetic neuropathy, phenytoin and carbamazepine are occasionally helpful, but a combination of amitriptyline and fluphenazine is more often effective (Gade et al. 1980). In elderly patients, these drugs should be used with great caution, starting at a low dosage and increasing it slowly. The entire dose of amitriptyline can be given at bedtime, to take advantage of its sedative property, for the pain is often most severe at night.

Pathophysiology. Theories about the mechanism of diabetic neuropathies cover a wide range of possibilities; vascular disease, metabolic Schwann-cell disease, and metabolic neuraxonal disease. Evidence can be marshalled for and against all theories, but direct proof is lacking for any of them.

The *acute mononeuropathies* are perhaps the best understood, for an ischemic pathology has been shown convincingly in several cases. However, the nature of the underlying vascular disease is still uncertain, because no vascular occlusions were found to account for the nerve infarctions. Raff and coworkers (1968) concluded that diabetic microangiopathy was not the cause; they suspected that small extraneural arteries might be involved, though this has not been proven. Atherosclerotic peripheral vascular disease without diabetes rarely causes acute mononeuropathies, and in diabetes there is no correlation between the occurrence of atherosclerotic symptoms (intermittent claudication) and of acute mononeuropathies (Fraser et al. 1979).

The pathology of *symmetrical polyneuropathy* is still controversial. Thomas and Lascelles (1966) described segmental demyelination in sural nerve biopsy specimens and suggested that Schwann-cell disease might be the primary process. More recent pathologic studies, however, show both axonal degeneration and segmental demyelination and remyelination, which seem to occur independently of each other and to affect all sizes of nerve fibers equally (Behse et al. 1977; Dyck et al. 1980). The early microangiopathic explanation has been discounted by recent workers who did not find occlusive disease of the vasa nervorum (Thomas and Lascelles 1966). Dissenting opinions continue to be heard, however. Williams and associates (1980) examined the ultrastructure of the vasa nervorum in sural nerve biopsies from 11 patients with diabetic neuropathy. Thrombus and endothelial-cell degeneration were present in at least one vessel in six biopsies, four of which were from patients who had recently recovered from severe ketoacidosis. In seven cases there was endothelial-cell hyperplasia of sufficient degree to occlude the lumen completely; these included patients with severe sensory polyneuropathy, severe generalized motor neuropathy, and recent ketoacidosis. It may be premature to discard microangiopathy as an explanation for diabetic polyneuropathy, especially since Pirart's (1977) data show that control of diabetes has a very similar effect on the prevalence of polyneuropathy, retinopathy, and nephropathy. The postmortem study of Sugimura and Dyck (1982) likewise suggested that an interstitial, proximal, patchy process was responsible for nerve degeneration, a process that could be ischemia or altered capillary permeability.

Diabetic amyotrophy and thoracoabdominal neuropathy raise even more puzzling questions. How is one to account for the peculiar restriction of amyotrophy to pelvic and thigh muscles, first in one leg and then in the other? Or the large swatches of cutaneous sensory disturbance that extend for many segments on either side of the torso? Even the location of the disease process along the nerve fiber is still uncertain. Bastron and Thomas (1981) and other authors have asserted that the EMG finding of denervation in the paraspinal muscles means that the nerve lesions are located in the spinal roots, proximal to the emergence of the posterior primary rami that supply those muscles. That argument, however, is only valid when one is trying to determine whether a *focal* lesion is in the nerve root or in a more distal site such as the plexus; it does not apply to a *diffuse* neuropathy. It is quite possible, for instance, that the nerve lesions are located in the distal segments of the motor nerves that supply both paraspinal and proximal limb muscles. This explanation fits with the observation that motor nerve conduction is slowed to different degrees in various nerve branches within the same muscle (Chokroverty et al. 1977). On clinical grounds it is difficult to accept the concept of a polyradiculopathy that causes severe proximal amyotrophy, while sparing the distal limb muscles supplied by the same nerve roots.

The selective involvement of proximal lower-extremity muscles in diabetic amyotrophy is analogous to the curious predilection of brachial neuritis for the proximal upper-extremity muscles. (In brachial neuritis, moreover, both clinical and electroneurographic findings indicate that the disease process is usually located distal to the brachial plexus.) At present, no hypothesis exists to account for the proximal localization in either disorder. In diabetic amyotrophy, the main clues to pathogenesis are the fact that most of the patients are middle-aged or elderly persons, many of whom have mild diabetes without microvascular or macrovascular complications; and the fact that active progression tends to run its course in a few months, as if the factors responsible were present for only a limited period of time.

In experimental rat diabetes produced by streptozotocin (Jakobsen 1979), as well as in the mutant diabetic mouse (Robertson and Sima 1980), there is an early and progressive reduction of motor nerve conduction velocity without any degenerative changes of axons or myelin. Later there is a concomitant reduction of axonal diameter ("axonal dwindling") of both myelinated and unmyelinated nerve fibers. Both the morphologic and physiologic changes can be prevented if insulin treatment begins early in the disease, but not if treatment is delayed. In rats given streptozotocin the volume of motor and sensory nerve cell bodies is reduced (Sidenius and Jakobsen 1980), and the rate of axonal transport of structural proteins is reduced (Jakobsen and Sidenius 1980). These observations suggest that slowing of motor nerve conduction is "metabolically" determined and reversible until structural changes appear. Whether these animal experiments are pertinent to human diabetic neuropathy remains to be established, since the characteristic pathology of the human disease has not been duplicated in the animal models (Brown et al. 1982; Sugimura and Dyck 1981).

Diabetic Infarction of Thigh Muscles

Spontaneous infarction of muscle is an extremely unusual occurrence that has been reported in four diabetic patients who were in the third to sixth decades of life (Banker and Chester 1973). In each case there was a sudden onset of pain, swelling, and tenderness in one thigh, with a palpable mass in the muscle. The process resolved over the course of several weeks, but a few months later the same thing happened in the other thigh.

Pathologic examination showed infarction of muscle fibers and small nerves, accompanied by occlusion of arterioles and of small and medium-sized arteries, caused by a combination of diabetic microangiopathy, atherosclerosis, and medial sclerosis. There appears to be some unusual deficiency of thigh-muscle circulation in diabetics that has not been defined. Banker and Chester (1973) emphasized that regeneration of muscle is ineffective in large infarctions, so that repair depends mainly on connective tissue proliferation.

The proper treatment appears to be bed rest and immobilization of the limb. Premature resumption of activity can lead to hemorrhage into the damaged muscle. Surgical exploration and arteriography could aggravate the problem and should be avoided.

Hypoglycemic Amyotrophy

There are about 30 published cases of distal muscle wasting and weakness in patients with severe spontaneous hypoglycemia (Jaspan et al. 1982). In almost every case the neuromuscular symptoms appeared after the patient had suffered episodes of hypoglycemic confusion or coma; in some patients the neuromuscular symptoms were gradually progressive, in others the symptoms came on abruptly after a severe hypoglycemic episode. The muscle weakness and atrophy were almost invariably distal in distribution and usually symmetrical; they were often worse in the upper extremities than in the lower. In a few cases proximal muscles were also affected. Fasciculations were sometimes prominent but were present in only one fourth of the cases. About one third of the patients had purely motor symptoms and signs; the others had distal numbness and paresthesias, but some of those had no sensory signs. Muscle stretch reflexes were sometimes depressed in muscles that were not weak, which suggests sensory involvement.

An insulinoma of the pancreas was identified in all but two early cases, in which no etiology was found. Following surgical removal of the tumor, sensory symptoms usually improved more than motor symptoms, so that most patients were left with some degree of distal amyotrophy.

Electromyography in the initial stages showed fibrillations and a reduced number of motor unit potentials; during recovery there was evidence of reinnervation by distal sprouting, in the form of large-amplitude motor unit potentials (Harrison 1976). Motor nerve conduction velocity was normal at all stages of the disorder, except in severely depleted motor units. Sensory nerve conduction was normal in one case (Harrison 1976), but sensory responses were nearly all absent in another case (Jaspan et al. 1982). Spinal fluid protein was normal.

There has been some controversy over whether the site of abnormality is the peripheral nerves or the anterior horn cells, but the weight of evidence favors a motor neuron disorder, with lesser involvement of the sensory ganglia. In two autopsied cases (Moersch and Kernohan 1938; Tom and Richardson 1951) there was neuronophagia in the ventral horns, and experimental hypoglycemia has produced anterior horn cell degeneration in cats (Winkelman and Moore 1940). Several clinical features also favor a neuronal pathology: the predilection for the upper limbs and for motor nerves, the normal conduction velocities, the permanence of the deficits, and EMG evidence of reinnervation by distal sprouting.

REFERENCES

Abbas, DH, Schlagenhauff, RE and Strong, HE: *Polyradiculoneuropathy in Addison's disease.* Neurology 27:494–495, 1977.

Adams, RD, Denny-Brown, D and Pearson, CM: *Diseases of Muscle: A Study in Pathology,* ed 2. Harper & Row, New York, 1962.

Afifi, AK, Bergman, RA, and Harvey, JC: *Steroid myopathy. Clinical, histologic and cytologic observations.* Johns Hopkins Med J 123:158–174, 1968.

Afifi, A, Najjar, SS, Mire-Salman J, et al: *The myopathy of the Kocher-Debre-Semelaigne syndrome.* J Neurol Sci 22:445–470, 1974.

Alvarez-Ude, F, Feest, TG, Ward, MK, et al: *Hemodialysis bone disease: Correlation between clinical, histologic, and other findings.* Kidney Int 14:68–73, 1978.

Amino, N, Yuasa, T, Yabu, Y, et al: *Exophthalmos in autoimmune thyroid disease.* J Clin Endocrinol Metab 51:1232–1234, 1980.

Arnett, FC and Michels, RG: *Inflammatory ocular myopathy in systemic sclerosis (scleroderma). A case report and review of the literature.* Arch Intern Med 132:740–743, 1973.

Asbury, AK: *Proximal diabetic neuropathy.* Ann Neurol 2:179–180, 1977.

Asbury, AK, Aldredge, H, Hershberg, R, et al: *Oculomotor palsy in diabetes mellitus: A clinicopathological study.* Brain 93:555–566, 1970.

Askari, A, Vignos, PJ and Moskowitz, RW: *Steroid myopathy in connective tissue disease.* Am J Med 61:485–492, 1976.

Aubertin, E and Bergouignan, M: *Syndrome de contracture musculaire au cours de la maladie d'Addison; action bien-faisante de la cortisone.* Ann Endrocrinol (Paris) 12:888–890, 1951.

Baldwin, KM, Ernst, SB, Herrick, RE, et al: *Exercise capacity and cardiac function in trained and untrained thyroid-deficient rats.* J Appl Physiol 49:1022–1026, 1980a.

Baldwin, KM, Hooker, AM, Herrick, RE, et al: *Respiratory capacity and glycogen depletion in thyroid-deficient muscle.* J Appl Physiol 49:102–106, 1980b.

Ballantyne, JP and Hansen, S: *A new method for the estimation of the number of motor units in a muscle. 1. Control subjects and patients with myasthenia gravis.* J Neurol Neurosurg Psychiatry 37:907–915, 1974a.

Ballantyne, JP and Hansen, S: *A new method for the estimation of the number of motor units in a muscle. 2. Duchenne, limb-girdle and facioscapulohumeral, and myotonic muscular dystrophies.* J Neurol Neurosurg Psychiatry 37:1195–1201, 1974b.

Banerji, NK and Hurwitz, LJ: *Neurological manifestations in adult steatorrhoea (probable gluten enteropathy).* J Neurol Sci 14:125–141, 1971a.

Banerji, NK and Hurwitz, LJ. *Nervous system manifestations after gastric surgery.* Acta Neurol Scand 47:485–513, 1971b.

Banker, BQ and Chester, CS: *Infarction of thigh muscle in the diabetic patient.* Neurology 23:667–677, 1973.

Bastron, JA and Thomas, JE: *Diabetic polyradiculopathy. Clinical and electromyographic findings in 105 patients.* Mayo Clin Proc 56:725–732, 1981.

Behan, PO: *Immune disease and HLA associations with myasthenia gravis.* J Neurol Neurosurg Psychiatry 43:611–621, 1980.

Behse, F, Buchthal, F and Carlsen, F: *Nerve biopsy and conduction studies in diabetic neuropathy.* J Neurol Neurosurg Psychiatry 40:1072–1082, 1977.

Bergouignan, M, Vital, C and Bataille, JM: *Les myopathies hypothyroidiennes. Aspects cliniques et histopathologiques.* Presse Medicale 75:1551–1556, 1967.

Bernard, JD, Larson, JA and Norris, FH: *Thyrotoxic periodic paralysis in Californians of Mexican and Filipino ancestry.* Calif Med 116:70–74, 1972.

Bigland, B and Jehring, B: *Muscle performance in rats, normal and treated with growth hormone.* J Physiol 116:129–136, 1952.

Birge, SJ and Haddad, JG: *25-Hydroxycholecalciferol stimulation of muscle metabolism.* J Clin Invest 56:1100–1107, 1977.

Birket-Smith, E and Olivarius, BF: *Polyradiculo-myopathia in transient thyrotoxicosis.* Dan Med Bull 4:217–219, 1957.

Blodi, FC and Gass, JDM: *Inflammatory pseudotumour of the orbit.* Br J Ophthal 52:79–93, 1968.

Braund, KG, Dillon, AR and Mikeal, RL: *Experimental investigation of glucocorticoid-induced myopathy in the dog.* Exp Neurol 68:50–71, 1980.

Bronsky, D, Kaganiec, GI and Waldstein, SS: *An association between the Guillain-Barré syndrome and hyperthyroidism.* Am J Med Sci 247:196–200, 1964.

BROWN, MR, DYCK, PJ, MCCLEARN, GE, ET AL: *Central and peripheral nervous system complications.* Diabetes 31 (Suppl 1): 65–70, 1982.

BRUCE, DS AND NICOL, CJM: *Contractile and fibre population changes induced by hyperthyroidism in rat skeletal muscle.* J Physiol (Lond) 310: 57P–58P, 1981.

BULL, GM, CARTER, AB AND LOWE, KG: *Hyperpotassaemic paralysis.* Lancet ii:60–63, 1953.

BURROWS, AW AND BARNETT, D: *Diagnostic problems in unilateral proptosis.* Lancet i:495, 1981.

BUTCHER, DL AND SAHN, SA: *Epidural lipomatosis: A complication of steroid therapy.* Ann Intern Med 90:60, 1979.

CAMBIER, J, MASSON, M AND DELAPORTE, P: *Le syndrome de contracture abdomino-crurale au cours de la maladie d'Addison.* Presse Medicale 78:2281–2282, 1970.

CASEY, EB AND HARRISON, MJG: *Diabetic amyotrophy: A follow-up study.* Br Med J 1:656–659, 1972.

CASSAN, SM, DIVERTIE, MB, HOLLENHORST, RW, ET AL: *Pseudotumor of the orbit and limited Wegener's granulomatosis.* Ann Intern Med 72:687–693, 1970.

CASTAIGNE, P, BUGE, A, LAPLANE, D, ET AL: *Insuffisance surrenale lente revelee par des crampes musculaires des membres inferieurs subintrantes et d'une rare violence.* Bull Soc Med Hop Paris 75:262–268, 1959.

CASTAIGNE, P, LAPLANE, P, MAUVAIS-JARVIS, P, ET AL: *Contractures des membres inferieurs au cours d'un panhypopituitarisme.* Ann Med Interne (Paris) 126:591–594, 1974.

CHARCOT, JM: *Lecons du Mardi a la Salpetriere.* Policlinique 1888–1889. Paris, 1889, pp 231–242.

CHOKROVERTY, S: *Proximal nerve dysfunction in diabetic proximal amyotrophy. Electrophysiology and electron microscopy.* Arch Neurol 39:403–407, 1982.

CHOKROVERTY, S, REYES, MG, RUBINO, FA, ET AL: *The syndrome of diabetic amyotrophy.* Ann Neurol 2:181–194, 1977.

CHOLLET, P, RIGAL, J-P AND PIGNIDE, L: *Une complication méconnue de l'hyperthyroidie: La neuropathie périphérique.* Presse Medicale 79:145, 1971.

CLAUSEN, T AND FLATMAN, JA: *The effect of catecholamines on Na-K transport and membrane potential in rat soleus muscle.* J Physiol 270:383–414, 1977.

CLEMENS, TL, HENDERSON, SL, ADAMS, JS, ET AL: *Increased skin pigment reduces the capacity of skin to synthesize vitamin D_3.* Lancet i:174–176, 1982.

COHEN, KL, NOTH, RH AND PECHINSKI, T: *Incidence of pituitary tumors following adrenalectomy. A long-term follow-up study of patients treated for Cushing's disease.* Arch Intern Med 138:575–579, 1978.

COLLINS, JA, ZIMMER, FE, JOHNSON, WJ, ET AL: *The many faces of hypothyroidism.* Postgrad Med 36:371–384, 1964.

COMINGS, DE, SKUBI, KB, VAN EYES, J, ET AL: *Familial multifocal fibrosclerosis: Findings suggesting that retroperitoneal fibrosis, mediastinal fibrosis, sclerosing cholangitis, Reidel's thyroiditis, and pseudotumor of the orbit may be different manifestations of a single disease.* Ann Intern Med 66:884–892, 1967.

CONN, JW: *Aldosteronism in man. Some clinical and climatological aspects.* Part II. JAMA 183:871–878, 1963.

CONWAY, MJ, SEIBEL, JA AND EATON, RP: *Thyrotoxicosis and periodic paralysis: Improvement with beta blockade.* Ann Intern Med 81:331–336, 1974.

CURRY, OB, BASTEN, JF, FRANCIS, MJO, ET AL: *Calcium uptake by sarcoplasmic reticulum of muscle from vitamin D-deficient rabbits.* Nature 249:83–84, 1974.

CZEUZ, KA, THOMAS, JE, LAMBERT, EH, ET AL: *Long-term results of operation for carpal tunnel syndrome.* Mayo Clin Proc 41:232–241, 1966.

DASTUR, DK, GAGRAT, BM, WADIA, NH, ET AL: *Nature of muscular change in osteomalacia: Light- and electron-microscope observations.* J Pathol 117:211–228, 1975.

DAVIES, DR, DENT, CE AND WATSON, L: *Tertiary hyperparathyroidism.* Br Med J 3:395–399, 1968.

DENNY-BROWN, D AND PENNYBACKER, JB: *Fibrillation and fasciculation in voluntary muscle.* Brain 61:311–332, 1938.

DENT, CE AND SMITH, R: *Nutritional osteomalacia.* Q J Med 38:195–209, 1969.

DENT, CE AND STAMP, TCB: *Hypophosphataemic osteomalacia presenting in adults.* Q J Med 40:303–329, 1971.

DREYFUS, PM, HAKIM, S AND ADAMS, RD: *Diabetic ophthalmoplegia: Report of a case with posmortem study and comments on vascular supply of human oculomotor nerve.* Arch Neurol Psychiatry 77:337–349, 1957.

DREZNER, MK AND FEINGLOS, MN: *Osteomalacia due to 1,25-dihydroxycholecalciferol deficiency. Association with a giant cell tumor of bone.* J Clin Invest 60:1046–1053, 1977.

Du Bois, DC and Almon, RR: *Disuse atrophy of skeletal muscle is associated with an increase in number of glucocorticoid receptors.* Endocrinology 107:1649–1651, 1980.

Dyck, PJ and Lambert, EH: *Polyneuropathy associated with hypothyroidism.* J Neuropath Exp Neurol 29:631–658, 1970.

Dyck, PJ, Sherman, WR, Hallcher, LM, et al: *Human diabetic endoneurial sorbitol, fructose, and myo-inositol related to sural nerve morphometry.* Ann Neurol 8:590–596, 1980.

Dyro, FM: *Quadriparesis as an unusual manifestation of hypercalcemia.* J Maine Med Assoc 68:370–371, 1977.

Eastwood, JB, Gray, RW, de Wardener, HE, et al: *Normal plasma 1,25-$(OH)_2$-vitamin-D concentrations in nutritional osteomalacia.* Lancet i:1377–1378, 1979.

Eastwood, JB, Stamp, TCB, Harris, E, et al: *Vitamin-D deficiency in the osteomalacia of chronic renal failure.* Lancet ii:1209–1212, 1976.

Ekbom, K, Kirstein, L and Astrom, KE: *Weakness of proximal limb muscles, probably due to myopathy after partial gastrectomy.* Acta Med Scand 176:493–496, 1964.

Ellenberg, M: *Diabetic neuropathic cachexia.* Diabetes 23:418–423, 1974.

Engel, AG: *Electron microscopic observations in thyrotoxic and corticosteroid-induced myopathies.* Mayo Clin Proc 41:785–796, 1966.

Enzmann, DR, Donaldson, SS and Kriss, JP: *Appearance of Graves' disease on orbital computed tomography.* J Comput Assist Tomogr 3:815–819, 1979.

Enzmann, D, Donaldson, SS, Marshall, WH, et al: *Computed tomography in orbital pseudotumor (idiopathic orbital inflammation).* Radiology 120:597–601, 1976.

Everts, ME, van Hardeveld, C, Ter Keurs, HEDJ, et al: *Force development and metabolism in skeletal muscle of euthyroid and hypothyroid rats.* Acta Endrocrinol 97:221–225, 1981.

Fanburg, BL: *Calcium transport by skeletal muscle sarcoplasmic reticulum in the hypothyroid rat.* J Clin Invest 47:2499–2506, 1968.

Farid, NR, Stone, E and Johnson, G: *Graves' disease and HLA: Clinical and epidemiological associations.* Clin Endocrinol 13:535–544, 1980.

Feibel, JH and Campa, JF: *Thyrotoxic neuropathy (Basedow's paraplegia).* J Neurol Neurosurg Psychiatry 39:491–497, 1976.

Fincham, RW and Cape, CA: *Neuropathy in myxedema. A study of sensory nerve conduction in the upper extremities.* Arch Neurol 19:464–466, 1968.

Fitts, RH, Winder, WW, Brooke, MH, et al: *Contractile, biochemical and histochemical properties of thyrotoxic rat soleus muscle.* Am J Physiol 238:C15-C20, 1980.

Floyd, M, Ayyar, DR, Barwick, DD, et al: *Myopathy in chronic renal failure.* Q J Med 53:509–524, 1974.

Fonseca, OA and Calverley, JR: *Neurological manifestations of hypoparathyroidism.* Arch Intern Med 120:202–206, 1967.

Forsham, PH: Personal communication, 1981.

Frame, B, Heinze, EG, Block, MA, et al: *Myopathy in primary hyperparathyroidism. Observations in three patients.* Ann Int Med 68:1022–1027, 1968.

Frame, B and Parfitt, M: *Osteomalacia: current concepts.* Ann Intern Med 89:966–982, 1978.

Franck, WA, Hoffman, GS, Davis, JS, et al: *Osteomalacia and weakness complicating jejunal bypass.* J Rheumatol 6:51–56, 1979.

Fraser, DM, Campbell, IW, Ewing, DJ, et al: *Mononeuropathy in diabetes mellitus.* Diabetes 28:96–101, 1979.

Fry, IK, Hardwicke, C and Scott, GW: *Diabetic neuropathy: A survey and follow-up of 66 cases.* Guy's Hosp Rep 111:113–129, 1962.

Frymoyer, JW and Bland, J: *Carpal-tunnel syndrome in patients with myxedematous arthropathy.* J Bone Joint Surg 55A:78–82, 1973.

Fukomoto, Y, Tarui, S, Tusukiyama, K, et al: *Tumor-induced vitamin D-resistant hypophosphatemic osteomalacia associated with proximal renal tubular dysfunction and 1,25-dihydroxyvitamin D deficiency.* J Clin Endocrinol Metab 49: 873–879, 1979.

Fuller, TJ, Carter, NW, Barcenas, C, et al: *Reversible changes of the muscle cell in experimental phosphorus deficiency.* J Clin Invest 57:1019–1024, 1976.

Gaan, D: *Chronic thyrotoxic myopathy with involvement of respiratory and bulbar muscles.* Br Med J 3:415–416, 1967.

Gade, GN, Hofeldt, FD and Treece, GL: *Diabetic neuropathic cachexia. Beneficial response to combination therapy with amitryptiline and fluphenazine.* JAMA 243:1160–1161, 1980.

Gamstorp, I, Shelburne, SA, Engleson, G, et al: *Peripheral neuropathy in juvenile diabetes.* Diabetes 15:411–418, 1966.

GARCIA, CA AND FLEMING, H: *Reversible corticospinal tract disease due to hyperthyroidism.* Arch Neurol 34:647–648, 1977.

GARDINER, PF, BOTTERMAN, BR, ELDRED, E, ET AL: *Metabolic and contractile changes in fast and slow muscles of the cat after glucocorticoid-induced atrophy.* Exp Neurol 62:241–255, 1978.

GARDINER, PF AND EDGERTON, VR: *Contractile responses of rat fast and slow muscles to glucocorticoid treatment.* Muscle Nerve 2:274–281, 1979.

GARDINER, PF, HIBL, B, SIMPSON, DR, ET AL: *Effects of a mild weight-lifting program on the progress of glucocorticoid-induced atrophy in rat hindlimb muscles.* Pflugers Arch 385:147–153, 1980a.

GARDINER, PF, MONTANARO, G, SIMPSON, DR, ET AL: *Effects of glucocorticoid treatment and food restriction on rat hindlimb muscles.* Am J Physiol 238:E124–E130, 1980b.

GARLAND, H: *Diabetic amyotrophy.* Br Med J 2:1287–1290, 1955.

GARLAND, H: *Diabetic amyotrophy.* Br J Clin Pract 15:9–13, 1961.

GARLAND, H AND TAVERNER, D: *Diabetic myelopathy.* Br Med J 1:1405–1408, 1953.

GELBERMAN, RH, ARONSON, D AND WEISNER, MH: *Carpal-tunnel syndrome. Results of a prospective trial of steroid injection and splinting.* J Bone Joint Surg 62A:1181–1184, 1980.

GIBBELS, E AND SCHLIEP, G: *Diabetische Polyneuropathie: Probleme der diagnostik und Nosologie. Dargestellt auf Grund des neuern Schrifttums und einer Analyse von 100 eigenen Fallen.* Fortschr Neurol Psychiat 38:369–436, 1970.

GOLD, EM: *The Cushing syndromes: Changing views of diagnosis and treatment.* Ann Int Med 90: 829–844, 1979.

GOLD, HK, SPANN, JF, JR AND BRAUNWALD, E: *Effect of alterations in the thyroid state on the intrinsic contractile properties of isolated rat skeletal muscle.* J Clin Invest 49:849–854, 1970.

GOLDBERG, AL AND GOODMAN, HM: *Relationship between cortisone and muscle work in determining muscle size.* J Physiol 200:667–675, 1969.

GOLDING, DN: *Hypothyroidism presenting with musculoskeletal symptoms.* Ann Rheum Dis 29:10–14, 1970.

GOLDSTEIN, DA, MALLUCHE, HH AND MASSRY SG: *Management of renal osteodystrophy with 1,25(OH)$_2$D3. I. Effects on clinical radiographic and biochemical parameters.* Min Elect Metabol 2:35–47, 1979.

GOODMAN, M, SOLOMONS, CC AND MILLER, PD: *Distinction between the common symptoms of the phosphate-depletion syndrome and glucocorticoid-induced disease.* Am J Med 65:868–872, 1978.

GRAIG, FA AND SMITH, JC: *Serum creatine phosphokinase activity in altered thyroid states.* J Clin Endocrinol 25:723–731, 1965.

GREGERSEN, G: *Diabetic neuropathy: Influence of age, sex, metabolic control, and duration of diabetes on motor conduction velocity.* Neurology 17:972–980, 1967.

GREGERSEN, G: *Diabetic amyotrophy—a well-defined syndrome?* Acta Med Scand 185:303–310, 1969.

GRIFFITHS, PD: *Serum enzymes in diseases of the thyroid gland.* J Clin Path 18:660–663, 1965.

GROSSIE, J AND ALBUQUERQUE, EX: *Extensor muscle response to triamcinoline.* Exp Neurol 58: 435–445, 1978.

GRUENER, R AND STERN, LZ: *Corticosteroids. Effects on muscle membrane excitability.* Arch Neurol 26:181–185, 1972a.

GRUENER, RP AND STERN, LZ: *Diphenylhydantoin reverses membrane effects in steroid myopathy.* Nature New Biology 235:54–55, 1972b.

HALL, R, KIRKHAM, K, DONIACH D, ET AL: *Ophthalmic Graves disease. Diagnosis and pathogenesis.* Lancet i:375–378, 1970.

HALPERN, AA, HOROWITZ, BG AND NAGEL, DA: *Tendon ruptures associated with corticosteroid therapy.* West J Med 127:378–382, 1977.

HALVERSON, PB, KOZIN, F, RYAN, LM, ET AL: *Rhabdomyolysis and renal failure in hypothyroidism.* Ann Int Med 91:57–58, 1979.

HARMAN, JB AND RICHARDSON, AT: *Generalized myokymia in thyrotoxicosis. Report of a case.* Lancet i:473–474, 1954.

HARRISON, MJG: *Muscle wasting after prolonged hypoglycemic coma: Case report with electrophysiological data.* J Neurol Neurosurg Psychiatry 39:465–470, 1976.

HAVARD, CWH: *Progress in endocrine exophthalmos.* Br Med J 1:1001–1004, 1979.

HENDERSON, RG RUSSELL, RGG, LEDINGHAM, JGG, ET AL: *Effects of 1,25-dihydroxycholecalciferol on calcium absorption, muscle weakness, and bone disease in chronic renal failure.* Lancet i:379–384, 1974.

Henson, RA: *The neurological aspects of hypercalcemia: With special reference to primary hyperparathyroidism.* JR Coll Physicians Lond 1:41–50, 1966.

Hodes, BL, Frazee, L and Szmyd, S: *Thyroid orbitopathy: An update.* Ophthalmic Surg 10:25–33, 1979.

Hodsman, AB, Sherrard, DJ, Wong, EGC, et al: *Vitamin D-resistant osteomalacia in hemodialysis patients lacking secondary hyperparathyroidism.* Ann Intern Med 94:629–637, 1981.

Hofmann, WW and Denys, EH: *Effects of thyroid hormone at the neuromuscular junction.* Am J Physiol 223:283–287, 1972.

Hofmann, WW and Smith, RA: *Hypokalemic periodic paralysis studied in vitro.* Brain 93:445–474, 1970

Hopwood, NJ and Kenny, FM: *Incidence of Nelson's syndrome after adrenalectomy for Cushing's disease in children.* Am J Dis Child 131:1353–1356, 1977.

Hurwitz, LJ, Mc Cormick, D and Allen, IV: *Reduced muscle α-glucosidase (acid-maltase) activity in hypothyroid myopathy.* Lancet i:67–69, 1970.

Ianuzzo, D, Patel, P, Chen, V, et al: *Thyroidal trophic influence on skeletal muscle myosin.* Nature 270:74–76, 1977.

Insogna, KL, Bordley, DR, Caro, JF, et al: *Osteomalacia and weakness from excessive antacid ingestion.* JAMA 244:2544–2546, 1980.

Irani, PF: *Electromyography in nutritional osteomalacic myopathy.* J Neurol Neurosurg Psychiatry 39:686–693, 1976.

Isenberg, DA, Newham, D, Edwards, RHT, et al: *Muscle strength and pre-osteomalacia in vegetarian Asian women.* Lancet i:55, 1982.

Jakobsen, J: *Early and preventable changes of peripheral nerve structure and function in insulin-deficient diabetic rats.* J Neurol Neurosurg Psychiatry 42:509–518, 1979.

Jakobsen, J and Sidenius, P: *Decreased axonal transport of structural proteins in streptozotocin diabetic rats.* J Clin Invest 66:292–297, 1980.

Janssen, JW, van Hardeveld, C and Kassenaar, AAH: *Evidence for a different response of red and white skeletal muscle of the rat in different thyroid states.* Acta Endocrinol 87:768–775, 1978.

Jaspan, JB, Wollman, RL, Bernstein, L, et al: *Hypoglycemic peripheral neuropathy in association with insulinoma: Implication of glucopenia rather than hyperinsulinism. Case report and literature review.* Medicine 61:33–44, 1982.

Jellinek, EH: *The orbital pseudotumour syndrome and its differentiation from endocrine exophthalmos.* Brain 92:35–58, 1969.

Joasoo, A, Murray, IPC and Steinbeck, AW: *Involvement of bulbar muscles in thyrotoxic myopathy.* Aust Ann Med 4:338–340, 1970.

Johnson, MA, Mastaglia, FL, Montgomery, AG, et al: *Changes in myosin light chains in the rat soleus after thyroidectomy.* FEBS Lett 110:230–235, 1980.

Kammer, GM and Hamilton, CR: *Acute bulbar muscle dysfunction and hyperthyroidism. A study of four cases and review of the literature.* Am J Med 56:464–470, 1974.

Kanayama, Y, Shiota, K, Horiguchi, T, et al: *Correlation between steroid myopathy and serum lactic dehydrogenase in systemic lupus erythematosus.* Arch Intern Med 141:1176–1179, 1981.

Karlsberg, RP and Roberts, R: *Effect of altered thyroid function on plasma creatine kinase clearance in the dog.* Am J Physiol 235:E614–E618, 1978.

Katz, AL and Pate, D: *Floppy head syndrome.* Arthritis Rheum 23:131–132, 1980.

Keane, JR: *Alternating proptosis. A case report of acute orbital myositis defined by the computerized tomographic scan.* Arch Neurol 34:642–643, 1977.

Kikta, DG, Breuer, AC and Wilbourn, AJ: *Thoracic root pain in diabetes: The spectrum of clinical and electromyographic findings.* Ann Neurol 11:80–85, 1982.

Kimura, J, Yamada, T and Stevland, NP: *Distal slowing of motor nerve conduction velocity in diabetic polyneuropathy.* J Neurol Sci 42:291–302, 1979.

Klein, I, Mantell, P, Parker, M, et al: *Resolution of abnormal muscle enzyme studies in hypoparathyroidism.* Am J Med Sci 279:159–162, 1980.

Knochel, JP: *Hypophosphatemia (Nutrition in Medicine).* West J Med 134:15–26, 1981.

Kosinski, K, Roth, SI and Chapman, EH: *Primary hyperparathyroidism with 31 years of hypercalcemia.* JAMA 236:590–591, 1976.

Kruse, K, Scheunemann, W, Baier, W, et al: *Hypocalcemic myopathy in idiopathic hypoparathyroidism.* Eur J Pediatr 138:280–282, 1982.

Kuhn, E, Eberwein, P, Fiehn, W, et al: *Gibt es eine Myopathie bei Unterfunktion der Parathyreoidea?* Akt Neurol 8:127–129, 1981.

LAFFERTY, FW: *Primary hyperparathyroidism. Changing clinical spectrum, prevalence of hypertension, and discriminant analysis of laboratory tests.* Arch Intern Med 141:1761–1766, 1981.

LAMBERT, EH, UNDERDAHL, LO, BECKETT, S, ET AL: *A study of the ankle jerk in myxedema.* J Clin Endocrinol 11:1186–1205, 1951.

LAMONTAGNE, A AND BUCHTHAL, F: *Electrophysiological study in diabetic neuropathy.* J Neurol Neurosurg Psychiatry 33:442–452, 1970.

LAWRENCE, DG AND LOCKE, S: *Neuropathy in children with diabetes mellitus.* Br Med J 1:784–785, 1963.

LAWSON, JD: *The free Achilles reflex in hypothyroidism and hyperthyroidism.* N Engl J Med 259:761–764, 1958.

LAYZER, RB: *Motor unit hyperactivity states.* In VINKEN, PJ AND BRUYN, GW (EDS): *Handbook of Clinical Neurology, Vol 41.* American Elsevier Publishing, New York, 1979, pp 295–316.

LAYZER, RB: *Medical progress: Periodic paralysis and the Na-K pump.* Ann Neurol 6:547–552, 1982.

LAYZER, RB AND GOLDFIELD E: *Periodic paralysis caused by abuse of thyroid hormone.* Neurology 24:949–952, 1974.

LEMANN, J AND DONATELLI, AA: *Calcium intoxication due to primary hyperparathyroidism. A medical and surgical emergency.* Ann Intern Med 60:447–459, 1964.

LEVY, IS, WRIGHT, JE AND LLOYD, GAS: *Orbital and retro-orbital pseudo-tumours.* Mod Probl Ophthalmol 14:364–367, 1975.

LEYS, D, DESTEE, A AND WAROT, P: *Contrature abdominocrurale en flexion revelatrice d'une insuffisance surrenalienne.* Nouv Presse Med 11:604, 1982.

LI, JB AND GOLDBERG, AL: *Effects of food deprivation on protein synthesis and degradation in rat skeletal muscles.* Am J Physiol 231:441–448, 1976.

LIPSON, SJ, NAHEEDY, MH, KAPLAN, MM, ET AL: *Spinal stenosis caused by epidural lipomatosis in Cushing's syndrome.* N Engl J Med 302:36, 1980.

LOW, PA, MC LEOD, JG, TURTLE, JR, ET AL: *Peripheral neuropathy in acromegaly.* Brain 97: 139–152, 1974.

LUDIN, HP, SPIESS, H AND KOENIG, MP: *Neuromuscular dysfunction associated with thyrotoxicosis.* Eur Neurol 2:269–278, 1969.

LUMB, GA AND STANBURY, SW: *Parathyroid function in human vitamin D deficiency and vitamin D deficiency in primary hyperparathyroidism.* Am J Med 56:833–839, 1974.

LUNDBERG, PO, OSTERMAN, PO AND STALBERG, E: *Neuromuscular signs and symptoms in acromegaly.* In WALTON JN, CANAL N, SCARLATA G, ET AL (EDS): *International Congress on Muscle Diseases, Milan, 1969.* Excerpta Medica, Amsterdam, 1970, pp 531–534.

MADONICK, MJ AND MARGOLIS, J: *Protein content of spinal fluid in diabetes mellitus.* Arch Neurol Psychiatry 68:641–644, 1952.

MALLETTE, LE, PATTEN, BM AND ENGEL, WK: *Neuromuscular disease in secondary hyperparathyroidism.* Ann Intern Med 82:474–483, 1975.

MARIE, P: *Sur deux cas d'acromegalie; hypertrophie singuliere, non congenitale, des extremites superieures, inferieures et cephalique.* Rev de Med (Paris) 6:297-333, 1886.

MARSDEN, CD, REYNOLDS, EH, PARSONS, V, ET AL: *Myopathy associated with anticonvulsant osteomalacia.* Br Med J 2:526–527, 1973.

MASSRY, SG: *Requirements of vitamin D metabolites in patients with renal disease.* Am J Clin Nutr 33:1530–1535, 1980.

MASTAGLIA, FL: *Pathological changes in skeletal muscle in acromegaly.* Acta Neuropathol 24:273–286, 1973.

MASTAGLIA, FL, BARWICK, DD AND HALL, R: *Myopathy in acromegaly.* Lancet ii:907–909, 1970.

MATTHEWS, WB: *Discussion on some clinical, genetic and biochemical aspects of metabolic disorders of the nervous system.* Proc R Soc Med Lond 51:859–963, 1958.

MCCOMAS, AJ, SICA, REP, MC NABB, AR, ET AL: *Evidence for reversible motor neuron dysfunction in thyrotoxicosis.* J Neurol Neurosurg Psychiatry 37: 548–558, 1974.

MCDANIEL, HG, PITTMAN, CS, OH, SJ, ET AL: *Carbohydrate metabolism in hypothyroid myopathy.* Metabolism 26:867–873, 1977.

MCEACHERN, D AND ROSS, WD: *Chronic thyrotoxic myopathy. A report of three cases with a review of previously reported cases.* Brain 65:181–192, 1942.

MCFADZEAN, AJS AND YEUNG, R: *Periodic paralysis complicating thyrotoxicosis in Chinese.* Br Med J 1:451–455, 1967.

MCKERAN, RO, SLAVIN, G, ANDREWS, TM, ET AL: *Muscle fibre type changes in hypothyroid myopathy.* J Clin Path 18:659–663, 1975.

McKeran, RO, Ward, P, Slavin, G, et al: *Central nuclear counts in muscle fibers before and during treatment in hypothyroid myopathy.* J Clin Path 32:229–233, 1979.

Meier, C and Bischoff, A: *Polyneuropathy in hypothyroidism. Clinical and nerve biopsy study of 4 cases.* J Neurol 215:103–114, 1977.

Mizusawa, H, Takagi, A, Sugita, H, et al: *Mounding phenomenon: An experimental study in vitro.* Neurology 33:90–93, 1983.

Moersch, FP and Kernohan, JW: *Hypoglycemia: Neurologic and neuropathologic studies.* Arch Neurol Psychiatry 39:242–257, 1938.

Moore, TJ, Dluhy, RG, Williams, GH, et al: *Nelson's syndrome: Frequency, prognosis, and effect of prior pituitary irradiation.* Ann Intern Med 85:731–734, 1976.

Morgan, DB, Hunt, G and Paterson, CR: *The osteomalacia syndrome after stomach operations.* Q J Med 39:395–410, 1970.

Morkin, E: *Stimulation of cardiac myosin adenosine triphosphatase in thyrotoxicosis.* Circ Res 44:1–7, 1979.

Murphy, TR, Remine, WH and Burbank, MK: *Hyperparathyroidism: Report of a case in which parathyroid adenoma presented primarily with profound muscular weakness.* Proc Mayo Clin 35:629–640, 1960.

Murray, IPC and Simpson, JA: *Acroparaesthesia in myxoedema. A clinical and electromyographic study.* Lancet i:1360–1363, 1958.

Nagulesparen, M, Trickey, R, Davies, MJ, et al: *Muscle changes in acromegaly.* Br Med J 2:914–915, 1976.

Najjar, SS: *Muscular hypertrophy in hypothyroid children: The Kocher-Debré-Sémélaigne syndrome.* J Pediatr 85:236–239, 1974.

Nerup, J: *Addison's disease—clinical studies. A report of 108 cases.* Acta Endocrinol 76:127–141, 1974.

Nickel, SN, Frame, B, Bebin, J, et al: *Myxedema neuropathy and myopathy. A clinical and pathologic study.* Neurology 11:125–137, 1961.

Nikoskelainen, E, Enzmann, DR, Sogg, RL, et al: *Computerized tomography of the orbits. A report of 196 patients.* Acta Ophthalmol 55:885–900, 1977.

Norris, FH Jr: *Neuromuscular transmission in thyroid disease.* Ann Intern Med 64:81–86, 1966.

Norris, FH Jr: *Use of acetazolamide in thyrotoxic periodic paralysis.* N Engl J Med 286:893, 1972.

Norris, FH and Panner, BJ: *Hypothyroid myopathy. Clinical, electromyographic and ultrastructural observations.* Arch Neurol 14:574–589, 1966.

Nugent, RA, Rootman, J, Robertson, WD, et al: *Acute orbital pseudotumors—classification and CT features.* Amer J Roentgenol 137:957–962, 1981.

Nwoye, L, Mommaerts, WFHM, Simpson, DR, et al: *Evidence for a direct action of thyroid hormone in specifying muscle properties.* Am J Physiol 242:R401–R408, 1982.

O'Dorisio, TM: *Hypercalcemic crisis.* Heart Lung 7:425–435, 1978.

Okihiro, MM and Nordyke, RA: *Hypokalemic periodic paralysis. Experimental precipitation with sodium liothyronine.* JAMA 198:949–951, 1966.

Okinaka, S, Shizume, K, Iino, S, et al: *The association of periodic paralysis and hyperthyroidism in Japan.* J Clin Endocrinol 17:1454–1459, 1957.

Palumbo, PJ, Elveback, LR and Whisnant, JP: *Neurologic complications of diabetes mellitus: Transient ischemic attack, stroke, and peripheral neuropathy.* Adv Neurol 19:593–601, 1978.

Parker, MS, Klein, I, Haussler, MR, et al: *Tumor-induced osteomalacia. Evidence of a surgically correctible alteration of vitamin D metabolism.* JAMA 245:492–493, 1981.

Patten, BM, Bilezikian, JP, Malette, LE, et al: *Neuromuscular disease in primary hyperparathyroidism.* Ann Intern Med 80:182–193, 1974.

Payne, MW, Watters, LC, Bailey, CE, et al: *Periodic paralysis with thyrotoxicosis—treatment with propranolol.* J Med Assoc Ga 68:701–703, 1979.

Pellock JM, Behrens, M, Lewis, L, et al: *Kearns-Sayre syndrome and hypoparathyroidism.* Ann Neurol 3:455–458, 1978.

Perez, G, Siegel, L and Schreiner, GE: *Selective hypoaldosteronism with hyperkalemia.* Ann Int Med 76:757–763, 1972.

Phalen, GS: *The carpal-tunnel syndrome. Seventeen years' experience in diagnosis and treatment of 654 hands.* J Bone Joint Surg 48A:211–228, 1966.

Pickett, JBE, Layzer, RB, Levin, SR, et al: *Neuromuscular complications of acromegaly.* Neurology 25:638–645, 1975.

Piechowiak, H, Grobner, W, Kremer, H, et al: *Pseudohypoparathyroidism and hypocalcemic "myopathy." A case report.* Klin Wochenschr 59:1195–1199, 1981.

Pierides, AM: *Dialysis dementia, osteomalacic fractures and myopathy: A syndrome due to chronic aluminum intoxication.* Int J Artif Organs 1:208–211, 1978.

Pimstone, N, Marine, N and Pimstone, B: *Beta-adrenergic blockade in thyrotoxic myopathy.* Lancet ii:1219–1220, 1968.

Pirart, J: *Diabete et complications degeneratives. Presentation d'une etude prospective portant sur 4400 cas observes entre 1947 et 1973.* Diabete Metab 3:97–107;173–182; 245–256, 1977.

Pleasure, DE, Walsh, GO and Engel, WK: *Atrophy of skeletal muscle in patients with Cushing's syndrome.* Arch Neurol 22:118–125, 1970.

Pleasure, D, Wyszynski, B, Sumner, A, et al: *Skeletal muscle calcium metabolism and contractile force in vitamin D-deficient chicks.* J Clin Invest 64:1157–1167, 1979.

Pointon, JJ, Francis, MJO and Smith, R: *Effect of vitamin D deficiency on sarcoplasmic reticulum and troponin C concentration of rabbit skeletal muscle.* Clin Sci 57:257–263, 1979.

Pollack, JA, Schiller, AL and Crawford, JD: *Rickets and myopathy cured by removal of nonossifying fibroma of bone.* Pediatrics 52:364–371, 1973.

Pollard, JD, Mc Leod, JG, Angel Honnibal, TG, et al: *Hypothyroid polyneuropathy. Clinical, electrophysiological and nerve biopsy findings in two cases.* J Neurol Sci 53:461–471, 1982.

Porte, D jr, Graf, RJ, Halter, JB, et al: *Diabetic neuropathy and plasma glucose control.* Am J Med 70:195–200, 1981.

Posner, JB and Jacobs, DR: *Isolated analdosteronism. I. Clinical entity, with manifestations of persistent hyperkalemia, periodic paralysis, salt-losing tendency, and acidosis.* Metabolism 13:513–521, 1964.

Preece, MA, Tomlinson, S, Ribot, CA, et al: *Studies of vitamin D deficiency in man.* Q J Med 44:575–589, 1975.

Prineas, J, Hall, R, Barwick, DD, et al: *Myopathy associated with pigmentation following adrenalectomy for Cushing's syndrome.* Q J Med 37:63–77, 1968.

Prineas, JW, Mason, SA and Henson, RA: *Myopathy in metabolic bone disease.* Br Med J 1:1034–1036, 1965.

Prysor-Jones, RA and Jenkins, JS: *Effect of excessive secretion of growth hormone on tissues of the rat, with particular reference to the heart and skeletal muscle.* J Endocrinol 85:75–82, 1980.

Purcell, JJ, jr and Taulbee, WA: *Orbital myositis after upper respiratory tract infection.* Arch Ophthalmol 99:437–438, 1981.

Purnell, DC, Daly, DD and Lipscomb, PR: *Carpal-tunnel syndrome associated with myxedema.* Arch Intern Med 108:751– 756, 1961.

Puvanendran, K, Cheah, JS, Naganathan, N, et al: *Thyrotoxic myopathy. A clinical and quantitative analytic electromyographic study.* J Neurol Sci 42:441–451, 1979a.

Puvanendran, K, Cheah, JS, Naganathan, N, et al: *Neuromuscular transmission in thyrotoxicosis.* J Neurol Sci 43:47–57, 1979b.

Puvanendran, K, Cheah, JS and Wong, PK: *Electromyography (EMG) study in thyrotoxic periodic paralysis.* Aust N Z J Med 7:507–510, 1977.

Rabinowitz, D and Zierler, KL: *Differentiation of active from inactive acromegaly by studies of forearm metabolism and response to intra-arterial insulin.* Bull J Hopkins Hosp 113:211–224, 1963.

Rado, JP, Marosi, J, Tako, J, et al: *Hyperkalemic intermittent paralysis associated with spironolactone in a patient with cardiac cirrhosis.* Am Heart J 76:393–398, 1968.

Raff, MC and Asbury, AK: *Ischemic mononeuropathy and mononeuropathy multiplex in diabetes mellitus.* N Engl J Med 279: 17–22, 1968.

Raff, MC, Sangalang, V and Asbury, AK: *Ischemic mononeuropathy multiplex associated with diabetes mellitus.* Arch Neurol 18:487–499, 1968.

Ramsay, ID: *Thyrotoxic myopathy—electromyography.* Q J Med 34:255–267, 1965.

Ramsay, ID: *Muscle dysfunction in hyperthyroidism.* Lancet ii:931–934, 1966.

Ramsay, ID:*Thyroid Disease and Muscle Dysfunction.* Year Book Medical Publishers, Chicago, 1974.

Rao, SN, Katiyar, BC, Nair, KRP, et al: *Neuromuscular status in hypothyroidism.* Acta Neurol Scand 61: 167–177, 1980.

Rasmussen, H and Anast, C: *Familial hypophosphatemic (vitamin D-resistant) rickets and vitamin D-dependent rickets.* In Stanbury, JB, Wyngaarden, JG and Frederickson, DS (eds): *The Metabolic Basis of Inherited Disease.* McGraw-Hill, New York, 1978, pp 1537–1562.

Ravid, M and Robson, M: *Proximal myopathy caused by iatrogenic phosphate depletion.* JAMA 236:1380–1381, 1976.

RESNICK, JS, DORMAN, JD AND ENGEL, WK: Thyrotoxic periodic paralysis. Am J Med 47:831–836, 1969.

RIVES, KL, FURTH, ED AND BECKER, DV: *Limitations of the ankle jerk test. Intercomparison with other tests of thyroid function.* Ann Int Med 62:1139–1146, 1965.

ROBERTSON, DM AND SIMA, AAF: *Diabetic neuropathy in the mutant diabetic mouse [C57BL/ks(db/db)]. A morphometric study.* Diabetes 29:60–67, 1980.

RODMAN, JS AND BAKER, T: *Changes in the kinetics of muscle contraction in vitamin D-depleted rats.* Kidney Int 13:189–193, 1978.

ROSENFELD, M: *Akute aufsteigende Lahmung bei Morbus Basedow.* Berl Klin Wochenschr 39:538–540, 1902.

ROSS, EJ AND LINCH, DC: *Cushing's syndrome-killing disease: Discriminatory value of signs and symptoms aiding early diagnosis.* Lancet ii:646–649, 1982.

ROSS, EJ, MARSHALL-JONES, P AND FRIEDMAN, M: *Cushing's syndrome: Diagnostic criteria.* Q J Med 35:149–192, 1966.

ROWNTREE, LG AND SNELL, AM: *A Clinical Study of Addison's Disease.* WB Saunders, Philadelphia, 1931.

RUFF, RL, STÜHMER, W AND ALMERS, W: *Effect of glucocorticoid treatment on the excitability of rat skeletal muscle.* Pflugers Arch 395:132–137, 1982.

SALICK, AI, COLACHIS, SC AND PEARSON, CM: *Myxedema myopathy: Clinical, electrodiagnostic, and pathological findings in advanced cases.* Arch Phys Med Rehabil 49: 230–237, 1968.

SALICK, AI AND PEARSON, CM: *Electrical silence of myoedema.* Neurology 17:899–901, 1967.

SATOYOSHI, E, MURAKAMI, K, KOWA, H, ET AL: *Periodic paralysis in hyperthyroidism.* Neurology 13: 746–752, 1963.

SCARPALEZOS, S, LYGIDAKIS, C, PAPAGEORGIOU, C, ET AL: *Neural and muscular manifestations of hypothyroidism.* Arch Neurol 29:140–144, 1973.

SCHAMBELAN, M AND SEBASTIAN, A: *Hyporeninemic hypoaldosteronism.* Adv Intern Med 24:385–405, 1979.

SCHIMRIGK, K, LASSMANN, R AND STRODER, J: *Morphological and morphometric studies of the skeletal muscles of rachitic rats.* Z Kinderheilk 119:235–243, 1975.

SCHOTT, GD AND WILLS, MR: *Myopathy in hypophosphataemic osteomalacia presenting in adult life.* J Neurol Neurosurg Psychiatry 38:297–304, 1975.

SCHOTT, GD AND WILLS, MR: *Muscle weakness in osteomalacia.* Lancet i:626–629, 1976.

SERGOTT, RC, GLASER, JS AND CHARYULU, K: *Radiotherapy for idiopathic inflammatory orbital pseudotumor. Indications and results.* Arch Ophthalmol 99:853–856, 1981.

SERRATRICE, G, PELLISSIER, JF AND CROS, D: *Les atteintes musculaires des osteomalacies. Etude clinique, histoenzymologique et ultrastructurale de 10 cas.* Rev Rhum Mal Osteoartic 45:621–630, 1978.

SHAMMAS, HJF, MINCKLER, DS AND OGDEN, C: *Ultrasound in early thyroid orbitopathy.* Arch Ophthalmol 98:277–279, 1979.

SHANE, E, MCCLANE, KA, OLARTE, MR, ET AL: *Hypoparathyroidism and elevated serum enzymes.* Neurology 30:192–195, 1980.

SHERMAN, L, GOLDBERG, M AND LARSON, FC: *The Achilles reflex. A diagnostic test of thyroid function.* Lancet i:243–245, 1963.

SHIRABE, T, TAWARA, S, TERAO, A, ET AL: *Myxoedematous polyneuropathy: A light and electron microscopic study of the peripheral nerve and muscle.* J Neurol Neurosurg Psychiatry 38:241–247, 1975.

SHISHIBA, Y, SHIMIZU, T, SAITO, T, ET AL: *Elevated immunoreactive insulin concentration during spontaneous attacks in thyrotoxic periodic paralysis.* Metabolism 21:285–290, 1972.

SHIZUME, K, SHISHIBA, Y, SAKUMA, M, ET AL: *Studies on electrolyte metabolism in idiopathic and thyrotoxic periodic paralysis. I. Arteriovenous differences of electrolytes during induced paralysis.* Metabolism 15:138–144, 1966.

SHOJI, S, TAKAGI, A, SUGITA, H, ET AL: *Muscle glycogen metabolism in steroid-induced myopathy of rabbits.* Exp Neurol 45:1–7, 1974.

SIDENIUS, P AND JAKOBSEN, J: *Reduced perikaryal volume in lower motor and primary sensory neurons in early experimental diabetes.* Diabetes 29:182–187, 1980.

SIMPSON, JA: *Myasthenia gravis: A new hypothesis.* Scot Med J 5: 419–436, 1960.

SKARIA, J, KATIYAR, BC, SRIVASTAVA, TP, ET AL: *Myopathy and neuropathy associated with osteomalacia.* Acta Neurol Scand 51:37–58, 1975.

SLAVIN, ML AND GLASER, JS: *Idiopathic orbital myositis. Report of six cases.* Arch Ophthalmol 100:1261–1265, 1982.

SMITH, R AND STERN, G: *Myopathy, osteomalacia and hyperparathyroidism.* Brain 90:593–602, 1967.

SMITH, R AND STERN, G: *Muscular weakness in osteomalacia and hypoparathyroidism.* J Neurol Sci 8:511–520, 1969.

STENO STUDY GROUP: *Effect of 6 months of strict metabolic control on eye and kidney function in insulin-dependent diabetics with background retinopathy.* Lancet i:121–124, 1982.

STERNBERG, M: *Acromegaly.* New Sydenham Society, London, 1899.

STEWART, BM: *The hypertrophic neuropathy of acromegaly.* Arch Neurol 14:107–110, 1966.

SUBRAMONY, SH AND WILBOURN, AJ: *Diabetic proximal neuropathy. Clinical and electromyographic studies.* J Neurol Sci 53:293–304, 1982.

SUGIMURA, K AND DYCK, PJ: *Sural nerve myelin thickness and axis cylinder caliber in human diabetes.* Neurology 31:1087–1091, 1981.

SUGIMURA, K AND DYCK, PJ: *Multifocal fiber loss in proximal sciatic nerve in symmetric distal diabetic neuropathy.* J Neurol Sci 53:501–509, 1982.

SULLIVAN, JF: *The neuropathies of diabetes.* Neurology 8:243–249, 1958.

SUN, SF AND STREIB, EW: *Diabetic thoracoabdominal neuropathy: Clinical and electrodiagnostic features.* Ann Neurol 9:75–79, 1981.

SUSAC, JO, GARCIA-MULLIN, R AND GLASER, JS: *Ophthalmoplegia in dermatomyositis.* Neurology 23:305–309, 1973.

SWASH, M, SCHWARTZ, MS AND SARGEANT, MK: *Osteomalacic myopathy: An experimental approach.* Neuropathol Appl Neurobiol 5:295–302, 1979.

SWEET, R, MALES, JL, HAMSTRA, AJ, ET AL: *Vitamin D metabolite levels in oncogenic osteomalacia.* Ann Intern Med 93:279–280, 1980.

TAKAMORI, M, GUTMANN, L, CROSBY, TW, ET AL: *Myasthenic syndromes in hypothyroidism. Electrophysiological study of neuromuscular transmission and muscle contraction in two patients.* Arch Neurol 26:326–335, 1972.

TAKAMORI, M, GUTMANN, L AND SHANE, SR: *Contractile properties of human skeletal muscle. Normal and thyroid disease.* Arch Neurol 25:535–546, 1971.

TAMAI, H, NAKAGAWA, T, OHSAKO, N, ET AL: *Changes in thyroid functions in patients with euthyroid Graves' disease.* J Clin Endocrinol Metab 50:108–112, 1980.

THOMAS, PK AND ELIASSON, SG: *Diabetic neuropathy.* In DYCK, PJ, THOMAS, PK AND LAMBERT, EH (EDS): *Peripheral Neuropathy.* WB Saunders, Philadelphia, 1975, pp 956–981.

THOMAS, PK AND LASCELLES, RG: *The pathology of diabetic neuropathy.* Q J Med 35:489–509, 1966.

THOMSEN, M, PLATZ, P, ANDERSEN, OO, ET AL: *MLC typing in juvenile diabetes mellitus and idiopathic Addison's disease.* Transplant Rev 22:125–147, 1975.

THORN, GW, FORSHAM, PH AND EMERSON, K JR: *The Diagnosis and Treatment of Adrenal Insufficiency,* ed 2. Charles C Thomas, Springfield, Illinois, 1951.

TOM, MI AND RICHARDSON, JC: *Hypoglycemia from islet cell tumor of pancreas with amyotrophy and cerebrospinal nerve cell changes.* J Neuropath Exp Neurology 10:57–66, 1951.

TOYO-OKA, T AND ROSS, J: *Influence of hyperthyroidism on the superprecipitation response and Ca^{2+}-sensitivity of natural actomyosin in cardiac and skeletal muscle.* Biochim Biophys Acta 590:407–410, 1980.

TROKEL, SL AND HILAL, SK: *Recognition and differential diagnosis of enlarged extraocular muscles in computed tomography.* Am J Opthalmol 87:503–512, 1979.

TSE, J, WRENN, RW AND KUO, JF: *Thyroxine-induced changes in characteristics and activities of β-adrenergic receptors and adenosine 3', 5' -monophosphate and guanosine 3', 5' -monophosphate systems in the heart may be related to reputed catecholamine supersensitivity in hyperthyroidism.* Endocrinology 107:6–16, 1980.

TSENG, CS, CROMBIE, AL, HALL R, ET AL: *An evaluation of supervoltage orbital irradiation for Graves' ophthalmopathy.* Clin Endocrinol 13:545–551, 1980.

TYRELL, JB, BROOKS, RM, FITZGERALD, PA, ET AL: *Cushing's disease: Selective trans-sphenoidal resection of pituitary microadenomas.* N Engl J Med 298:753–758, 1978.

URBANIC, RC AND GEORGE, JM: *Cushing's disease—18 years' experience.* Medicine 60:14–24, 1981.

VAN DELLEN, RG AND PURNELL, DC: *Hyperkalemic paralysis in Addison's disease.* Mayo Clin Proc 44:904–914, 1969.

VAN MARLE, W AND WOODS, KL: *Acute hydrocortisone myopathy.* Br Med J 281:271–272, 1980.

VAUGHN, NJA, SLATER, JDH, LIGHTMAN, SL, et al: *The diagnosis of primary hyperaldosteronism.* Lancet i:120–125, 1981.

VELENTZAS, C, OREOPOULOS, DG, PIERRATOS, A, ET AL: *Treatment of renal osteodystrophy with 1,25-dihydroxycholecalciferol.* Can Med Assoc J 124:577–583, 1981.

VENABLES, GS, BATES, D AND SHAW, DA: *Hypothyroidism with true myotonia.* J Neurol Neurosurg Psychiatry 41:1013–1015, 1978.

VICALE, CT: *The diagnostic features of a muscular syndrome resulting from hyperparathyroidism, osteomalacia owing to renal tubular acidosis, and perhaps to related disorders of calcium metabolism.* Trans Am Neurol Assoc 74:143–147, 1949.

VILCHEZ, JJ, CABELLO, A, BENEDITO, J, ET AL: *Hyperkalemic paralysis, neuropathy and persistent motor neuron discharges at rest in Addison's disease.* J Neurol Neurosurg Psychiatry 43:818–822, 1980.

WAAL-MANNING, HJ: *Effect of propranolol on the duration of the Achilles reflex.* Clin Pharmacol Ther 10:199–206, 1969.

WALTERS, RO: *Idiopathic hypoparathyroidism with extrapyramidal and myopathic features.* Arch Dis Child 54:236–238, 1979.

WARD, MK, ELLIS, HA, FEEST, TG, ET AL: *Osteomalacic dialysis osteodystrophy: Evidence for a water-borne aetiological agent, probably aluminium.* Lancet i:841–845, 1978.

WARON, M, ALKAN, WJ AND MERA, A: *Hyperkalemic quadriplegia in Addison's disease without hyperpigmentation.* Isr J Med Sci 6:650–654, 1970.

WEINSTEIN, R, SCHWARTZMAN, R AND LEVEY, GS: *Propranolol reversal of bulbar dysfunction and proximal myopathy in hyperthyroidism.* Ann Intern Med 82:540–541, 1975.

WHITE, EA, SCHAMBELAN, M, ROST, CR, ET AL: *Use of computed tomography in diagnosing the cause of primary aldosteronism.* N Engl J Med 303:1503–1507, 1980.

WHITE, NH, WALTMAN, SR, KRUPIN, T, ET AL: *Reversal of neuropathic and gastrointestinal complications related to diabetes mellitus in adolescents with improved metabolic control.* J Pediat 99:41–45, 1981.

WILES, CM, YOUNG, A, JONES, DA, ET AL: *Muscle relaxation rate, fibre-type composition and energy turnover in hyper- and hypo thyroid patients.* Clin Sci 57:375–384, 1979.

WILLIAMS, E, TIMPERLEY, WR, WARD, JD, ET AL: *Electron microscopical studies of vessels in diabetic peripheral neuropathy.* J Clin Pathol 33:462–470, 1980.

WILLIAMS, JR AND MAYER, RF: *Subacute proximal diabetic neuropathy.* Neurology 26:108–116, 1976.

WILSON, J AND WALTON, JN: *Some muscular manifestations of hypothyroidism.* J Neurol Neurosurg Psychiatry 22:320–324, 1959.

WINCKLER, B, STEELE, R, ALTSZULLER, N, ET AL: *Effect of growth hormone on free fatty acid metabolism.* Am J Physiol 206:174–178, 1964.

WINDER, WW AND HOLLOSZY, JO: *Response of mitochondria of different types of skeletal muscle to thyrotoxicosis.* Am J Physiol 232:C180–C184, 1977.

WINKELMAN, NW AND MOORE, MT: *Neurohistopathologic changes with metrazol and insulin shock therapy. An experimental study on the cat.* Arch Neurol Psychiatry 43:1108–1137, 1940.

WOODHEAD, JS, GHOSE, RR AND GUPTA, SK: *Severe hypophosphatemic osteomalacia with primary hyperparathyroidism.* Br Med J 281:647–648, 1980.

YEUNG, RTT AND TSE, TF: *Thyrotoxic periodic paralysis. Effect of propranolol.* Am J Med 57:584–590, 1974.

Chapter 4

INFECTION

BACTERIAL INFECTIONS

Bacterial Myositis

Primary Suppurative Myositis

Spontaneous infection of muscle by pyogenic bacteria, commonly referred to as "tropical pyomyositis," is a rare disease in temperate climates, but it accounts for about 3 percent of surgical admissions to hospitals in tropical Africa. In developed countries the diagnosis is often delayed because physicians are unfamiliar with this entity and because presenting signs and symptoms often do not suggest an infection.

The clinical picture can be divided into two syndromes: a subacute disorder, caused mainly by staphylococcal infection, with a benign outcome; and a hyperacute infection by beta-hemolytic streptococci, with severe toxemia and often a fatal outcome.

In *subacute pyomyositis*, the infection may lodge in almost any muscle mass of the limbs or trunk (Chiedozi 1979). Several muscles are infected in about one third of the cases. The initial symptoms are pain, tenderness, swelling, and induration localized to one or more muscles. There is a low-grade fever, but external signs of inflammation are slight. The muscle feels hard or rubbery rather than fluctuant, pain is not severe, and the patient does not appear very ill. At this stage there is little or no pus, and needle aspiration may be diagnostically unrewarding. After a week or two the mass becomes fluctuant, the patient becomes more febrile and toxic, and the regional lymph nodes enlarge.

Routine laboratory tests reveal a moderate leukocytosis, with a shift to the left, and elevation of the erythrocyte sedimentation rate. (Eosinophilia is usually present in tropical cases, but this finding is probably unrelated.) Contrary to expectation, the CPK is usually normal (Levin et al. 1971; Swarts et al. 1981), although myoglobinuria occurred in one case (Armstrong 1978). The causative organism is Staphylococcus aureus in 94 percent of cases, S albus in 3.5 percent, Escherichia coli in 1 percent and streptococcus in 1 percent (Chiedozi 1979). Gonococcal pyomyositis has also been reported (Swarts et al. 1981). Blood cultures are negative in over 95 percent of cases. The bacteriologic diagnosis can be made by aspiration of pus from a fluctuant abscess. Computed tomography can help to define the initial muscle enlargement and the later low-density central zone (Fig. 14) (Schlech et al. 1981) and to guide needle aspiration (Ralls et al. 1980). Radionuclide gallium scanning is especially useful in locating multiple abscesses (Hirano et al. 1980).

Recently, a more serious picture of tropical pyomyositis was described in Nigerian children (Aderele and Osinusi 1980). Blood cultures were positive in 60 percent of the patients, and 25 percent developed osteomyelitis. Late referral to hospital and coexisting malnutrition may account for the dissemination of infection in those patients; in another series of cases from Nigeria (Chiedozi 1979), only 5 percent of patients presented with such advanced disease.

At an early stage, staphylococcal pyomyositis usually responds to antibiotic treatment alone, but if pus is present, incision and drainage are necessary. When multiple muscles are involved the fever and toxic symptoms usually persist until the last abscess has been located and drained (Levin et al. 1971; Goldberg et al. 1979).

The pathogenesis of staphylococcal pyomyositis is rather mysterious. Skeletal muscle is remarkably resistant to pyogenic infection, and muscle abscesses are rarely encountered in staphylococcal septicemia. By the same token, bacteremia is rarely documented in pyomyositis except at an advanced stage, and although muscle infections are often multiple, other organs are not usually involved. Most of the reported cases in the United States have been in boys (Altrocchi 1971; Levin et al. 1971; Goldberg et al. 1979; Sirinavin and McCracken 1979; Sty et al. 1980), but in Nigeria two thirds of the patients are adults, the incidence being lowest between the ages of 10 and 25 years (Chiedozi 1979). Closed trauma and skin furuncles may be predisposing factors, but in most cases no underlying cause is discovered.

Hyperacute streptococcal myositis is a rare condition that has been reported mainly from developed countries with temperate climates (Barrett

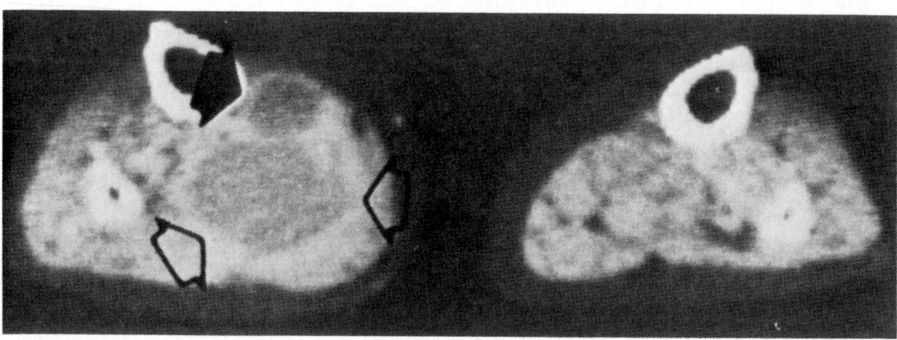

FIGURE 14. CT radiographs of the lower legs in a case of pyomyositis. The open arrows point to a large hypodense abscess in the medial head of the gastrocnemius muscle. A smaller, satellite abscess in the subcutaneous tissue is indicated by the solid arrow. (From Schlech et al., 1981, with permission.)

and Greshom 1958; Svane 1971). The disease begins abruptly with severe pain, swelling, and tenderness in one muscle, usually without external signs of inflammation. Over the next 2 or 3 days toxemia develops rapidly, leading to shock, acute renal failure, and cardiac arrhythmia. Most of the patients have died despite incision and drainage of the muscle abscess and administration of large amounts of penicillin. In a recent case (Svane 1971), there was autopsy evidence of disseminated intravascular coagulation, and this process may have contributed to the fulminating course in other fatal cases. Although all of the reported cases of hyperacute pyogenic myositis were caused by beta-hemolytic streptococcus, this organism can cause a less fulminating, subacute myositis similar to staphylococcal pyomyositis. In a recent case of streptococcal psoas myositis, which was detected by CT scan before an abscess had formed, the infection resolved completely with penicillin therapy (McLaughlin 1980).

The source of streptococcal myositis is usually not evident. However, Porter and associates (1981) reported two patients with simultaneous streptococcal and picornavirus infections of muscle, presenting as an acute, generalized, necrotizing myopathy with myoglobinuria. In these cases, a viral myositis may have provided an entry for the streptococcal infection.

Clostridial Myonecrosis (Gas Gangrene)

Localized infection of skeletal muscle with gas-forming, histotoxic clostridial organisms constitutes a life-threatening surgical emergency that is easier to prevent than to treat. In civilian practice most cases result from compound fractures, contaminated wounds, ischemic ulcers, and amputations for peripheral vascular disease. It is generally agreed that clostridial wound infection is largely preventable by avoiding primary closure of a contaminated wound, performing early and adequate debridement and cleansing of the wound, and administering prophylactic penicillin. However, amputation for peripheral vascular insufficiency carries an unavoidable risk of leaving behind nonviable tissue that can act as a seat of infection (Cameron and Ford 1978). There are rare examples of clostridial myositis occurring after intramuscular injections; from reactivation of spores in an old, healed wound; by distant seeding from a bowel lesion, especially a colon carcinoma; or as a spontaneous infection in patients with leukemia (Jendrzejewski et al. 1978).

Because the local and systemic toxicity of clostridial myonecrosis accelerates so rapidly, it is important to recognize the early signs and to act promptly and decisively. The presenting symptom is *the rapid onset of severe pain in the affected part*, worse than would be expected from the external appearance, which is often tense and shiny but not inflamed. Soon afterward, the onset of systemic toxicity is manifest by tachycardia and a feeling of great apprehension, with clear sensorium. The site of infection is extremely tender, and if a wound is present it often exudes a watery discharge that may have a sweet odor. The overlying skin soon takes on a red or coppery hue, the edema becomes brawny, and blisters may appear. Crepitus may be present but is not as prominent as it is in clostridial cellulitis, a less malignant process. Increasing systemic toxicity brings on hypotension, hemolytic jaundice, and renal failure, and death may occur in 24 to 36 hours.

Although gas gangrene is traditionally associated with clostridial infections, many cases involve mixed infections that include other fecal organisms, and muscle infections with gas-forming anaerobic streptococci or E coli carry at least as high a mortality as clostridial infections (Darke et al. 1977). In order to determine the appropriate treatment, it is important to seek a preliminary bacteriologic diagnosis by Gram stain of the wound exudate or of necrotic tissue obtained at the time of debridement. Clostridial organisms are recognized as large, Gram-positive rods. In gas gangrene, the necrotic muscle appears dark red or black and does not contract on mechanical stimulation. The presence of gas in the tissue is often demonstrable by radiography even if it is not detected clinically.

The two mainstays of treatment are hyperbaric oxygen therapy (if available) and extensive debridement, with amputation if necessary. Clinical experience suggests that hyperbaric oxygen is most effective in pure clostridial infection, is less effective in mixed infections, and is ineffective in infections with anaerobic streptococci or E coli. Some authors recommend treating clostridial infection initially by a limited surgical procedure—opening the wound and draining any abscesses that are present and then administering hyperbaric oxygen. If the first hyperbaric oxygen treatment produces prompt improvement in the toxemic manifestations, extensive debridement can be postponed, thus lowering the risk of anesthetic death during the toxemic state. In these favorable cases, further debridement can be carried out when the borders of nonviable tissue become better demarcated, and the limb can often be saved. In nonclostridial infections, and in cases in which the response to hyperbaric oxygen is inadequate, early extensive debridement is required. Gangrene following amputations for peripheral vascular disease usually require a higher amputation (Darke et al. 1977; Henderson et al. 1978; Cameron and Ford 1978). Aqueous penicillin is given intravenously in a dosage of 20 million units per day: cephalosporin or chloramphenicol can be substituted if the patient is allergic to penicillin. Hypotension and fluid losses are treated with intravenous fluids, plasma, volume expanders, and blood transfusions.

Disorders Caused by Bacterial Toxins

Botulism

Botulism is a form of rapidly developing paralysis caused by the exotoxin of Clostridium botulinum, an anaerobic soil bacillus. Botulinum toxin blocks the release of acetylcholine from peripheral cholinergic nerve terminals, but does not affect central nervous system synapses. The resulting symptoms can all be attributed either to paralysis of skeletal muscle or to parasympathetic blockade.

Until recently botulism was regarded mainly as a form of food poisoning, though a few cases were known to be caused by wound infection. Recently, however, Pickett and colleagues (1976) discovered that botulism can occur spontaneously in infants as a result of colonization of the colon by C botulinum. The incidence of infant botulism has, in fact, proven to be greater than that of food-borne botulism, and spontaneous botulism is now recognized as the commonest cause of rapidly progressive weakness in the first 6 months of life (Arnon 1980).

Among the eight toxigenic strains of C botulinum, types A, B, E, and F are known to cause human illness, with the first three types accounting for almost all cases. In the United States type-A organisms predominate in soils west of the Mississippi River and type-B organisms predominate in the East; food-borne intoxications tend to follow the same pattern. Type-A infection has been prevalant in wound botulism (Merson and Dowell 1973).

Until recently only type-A and type-B organisms had been isolated from the feces of babies with infant botulism. Type-E toxin is mainly associated with botulism caused by seafood. There may be differences in the severity or pattern of toxicity among the different strains, but these have only minor clinical importance.

CLINICAL FEATURES. About 23 cases of *food-borne botulism* are reported yearly in the United States (Merson et al. 1974). Symptoms usually begin 12 to 72 hours after ingestion of the tainted food, but the latency can be as short as 6 hours in severe cases. About half of the patients experience nausea, vomiting, abdominal pain, or diarrhea, usually before or coincident with the onset of paralytic symptoms. Invariably the cranial muscles are involved first, causing dysphagia, dysphonia, ptosis, diplopia, lingual dysarthria, and weakness of the facial and chewing muscles. Dry mouth, dizziness, and inability to focus vision on near objects are the common symptoms of parasympathetic insufficiency. The pupillary reactions are impaired in about half of the cases. Constipation is often present but bladder paralysis is infrequent. Weakness of the neck, trunk, thoracic, and diaphragmatic muscles soon joins the cranial muscle symptoms, and limb weakness appears soon afterward. The muscle stretch reflexes are preserved until the limb weakness is fairly severe. Weakness advances relentlessly; in the worst cases ventilatory failure occurs less than 23 hours after the onset of symptoms, while in milder cases weakness progresses for as long as a week and then reaches a plateau. Improvement begins after 1 or 2 weeks in mild cases, after several weeks in severe cases. Complete recovery can be expected within 2 months in mild cases and within 1 year in severe cases (Ryan and Cherington 1971; Hughes et al. 1981).

Wound botulism produces an identical clinical picture except that the preliminary gastrointestinal disturbances are lacking. Among eight cases reviewed by Merson and Dowell (1973), the wound appeared clean when reopened in four cases and appeared infected in four cases, two of which had gas formation. The syndrome is rare; in the United States, only six cases were reported to the National Communicable Disease Center in the 4-year period 1970 to 1973 (Merson et al. 1974).

Infant botulism occurs mainly between the ages of 1 and 6 months. It has been estimated that 500 cases occur annually in the United States; half of these children die at home with sudden infant death syndrome (Arnon 1980). Hospitalized babies usually present with poor sucking and feeding, a weak cry, ptosis, loss of head control, and generalized, flaccid weakness. Constipation is commonly reported. These manifestations usually stabilize after a week or two and then improve. However, about 30 percent of infants with botulism admitted to a hospital have subsequently suffered respiratory arrest (Arnon 1980).

Recently a type-G strain of C botulinum was isolated at necropsy from four adults and one 4-month old infant, all of whom died suddenly and unexpectedly at home (Sonnabend et al. 1981). Three of the adults had had preceding symptoms compatible with early botulism. Type-G toxin was present in the serum in three cases, and two patients had concomitant type-A botulism. In addition, type-D organisms and toxin and type-A toxin were detected in five other infants and adults who died suddenly and unexpectedly. In all there were 10 identifications of botulism among 40 infants and 55 adults with sudden death unexplained at autopsy. These cases were part of a series of over 600 autopsies in which complete bacteriologic studies were done; botulinal organisms or toxin were never identified in cases in which the cause of death was apparent at autopsy (Sonnabend et al 1981). If these results are correct, as many as 10 percent of pathologically unexplained sudden deaths may be due to botulism.

DIAGNOSIS. The clinical picture of botulism is so distinctive that there is little likelihood of confusion with other causes of acute generalized paralysis (see Chapter 1). Myasthenia gravis never causes such rapidly progressive paralysis in so short a time without any prior history of neuromuscular symptoms. At an early stage of botulism there is often a positive response to anticholinesterase drugs, but this response wanes as the paralysis deepens (Ryan and Cherington 1971). Routine laboratory tests and spinal fluid examination give normal results.

Rapid (but not specific) confirmation of the diagnosis can be obtained through *electrophysiologic tests.* EMG often shows low-amplitude, short-duration motor unit potentials in weak muscles; the number of motor unit potentials activated by maximal voluntary effort is reduced if the muscle is severely weak. Motor nerve conduction velocity is normal. In mildly weak muscles, the amplitude of the response to nerve stimulation is normal or mildly reduced, and modest facilitation may occur during rapid repetitive stimulation. In severely weak muscles, the amplitude of the evoked response is low and may decline during stimulation at 3 Hz, but there is usually no facilitation at rapid rates of stimulation (Oh 1977). Posttetanic facilitation, if present, tends to persist as long as 10 or 15 minutes after activation (Gutmann and Pratt 1976), much longer than in myasthenia gravis or the Lambert-Eaton syndrome. The amplitude of evoked muscle responses can often be increased by the administration of calcium gluconate or guanidine (Oh 1977; Messina et al. 1979). After about 2 weeks, EMG often reveals fibrillations at rest, a consequence of the denervation produced by the severe presynaptic block of neuromuscular transmission. The fibrillations disappear by the time the patient has recovered completely.

Specific confirmation of botulism requires identification of the toxin or the organism in the patient or in a food source. In infant botulism C botulinum and botulinal toxin can invariably be isolated from the feces but are virtually never found in the serum (Arnon 1980). In nine cases of wound botulism, toxin was identified in the serum in three of the six patients tested, and wound culture was positive in four of eight patients (Merson and Dowell 1973). When food-borne botulism is suspected, both serum and stool samples should be tested for toxin and the stool should be cultured for C botulinum. Of 48 patients with clinical botulism, 73 percent were positive by at least one of these three tests, but only 35 percent had toxin in the serum. If the search is enlarged to include examination of foods and testing of other symptomatic persons in outbreaks, a positive diagnosis can be made in 88 percent of cases (Dowell et al. 1977).

PATHOPHYSIOLOGY. Botulinum toxin is a protein weighing about 150,000 daltons. The various toxin types have the same mode of action despite their antigenic differences. This consists of selective interference with the release of quanta or packets of acetylcholine from synaptic vesicles within cholinergic nerve terminals. Electrical transmission along the nerve terminals is not impaired (Harris and Miledi 1971).

The normal mechanism for release of acetylcholine by a nerve impulse is mediated by a rise in intracellular calcium concentration, caused by an influx of calcium during the action potential (Fig. 15) (Katz and Miledi 1968). Botulinum toxin probably makes the transmitter release mechanism relatively insensitive to calcium, since the effect of the toxin can be overcome by increasing the calcium concentration in the nerve terminals (Cull-Candy et al. 1977). Repetitive stimulation of the nerve

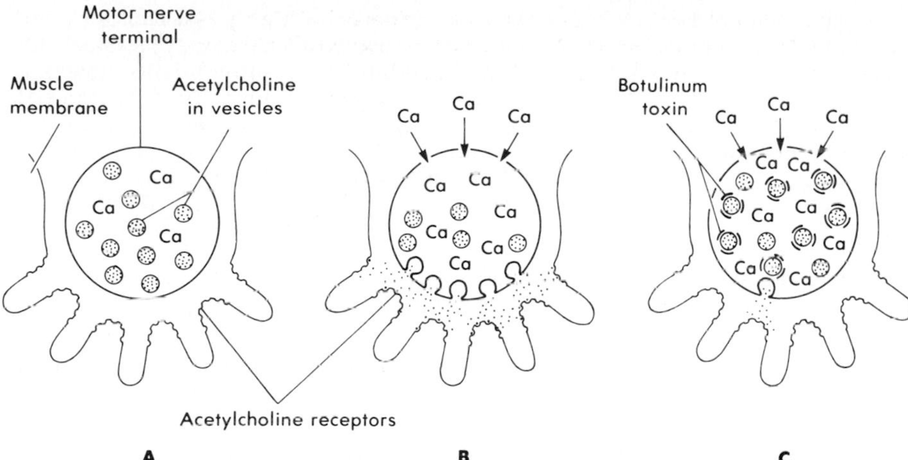

FIGURE 15. Pathophysiology of botulism. At a normal neuromuscular junction, the resting nerve terminals (*A*) contain synaptic vesicles filled with acetylcholine. The arrival of an action potential (*B*) promotes an influx of calcium, which triggers the release of acetylcholine into the synaptic cleft. Botulinum toxin (*C*) probably interacts with the membrane of the synaptic vesicles, inhibiting the releasing action of calcium.

at fast rates likewise facilitates transmitter release by increasing the intracellular calcium concentration, a fact that explains the clinical improvement in neuromuscular transmission produced by tetanic stimulation. Cull-Candy and associates (1977) found that transmitter release in botulinum-poisoned muscle was considerably enhanced by the presence of tetraethyl ammonium (TEA). This substance prolongs the duration of the nerve terminal action potential by blocking the transient increase of potassium conductance that follows the transient increase in sodium conductance; prolonged depolarization permits more calcium to enter the nerve terminals, thereby enhancing transmitter release. Guanidine also facilitates the calcium-mediated release of acetylcholine, but the mechanism of action of this drug is less well understood. In experiments with rats, both TEA and guanidine restored normal neuromuscular transmission in vitro when the extracellular calcium concentration was elevated (Lundh et al. 1977).

During prolonged botulinal poisoning, muscle fibers atrophy and fibrillate as if the motor nerves had been cut. After the first week of paralysis the intramuscular nerves and nerve terminals begin to sprout, and several weeks later they begin to establish new neuromuscular junctions. After some months these new synapses mature and the extraneous nerve sprouts regress (Duchen and Strich 1968). Thus, in severe cases of botulinal poisoning, recovery of neuromuscular function results from the formation of a new synapse for each denervated muscle fiber, a fact that accounts for the long duration of convalescence.

Bacteriology. Food-borne botulism occurs when the heat-resistant spores of C botulinum germinate in foodstuffs that provide a relatively anaerobic environment. Toxin production is reduced at low pH, so that low-acid foods such as vegetables, meat, and fish are especially dangerous for preservation or canning. The toxin itself, however, is readily inactivated by heat (80°C for 30 minutes or 100°C for 10 minutes); this is why most cases of botulinal poisoning are caused by preserved foods that received little or no cooking before being eaten.

Unlike other clostridial organisms, C botulinum is rarely found as an incidental contaminant in wounds. Presumably the factors favoring wound infection by C botulinum are similar to those responsible for gas gangrene. Considering the rarity of wound botulism compared with tetanus and gas gangrene, however, it seems likely that C botulinum spores do not readily germinate in animal tissues, but there is little direct information on this subject (Merson and Dowell 1973).

The colon of normal adult animals and humans is highly resistant to colonization by C botulinum, but infant animals are susceptible (Arnon 1980). Stool cultures are almost invariably negative for C botulinum in healthy infants; however, affected infants may be susceptible because of a different enteric flora. Wilcke and colleagues (1980) found that the feces of infants with botulism contained one tenth of the number of organisms present in the stools of normal infants, with a higher proportion of facultative anaerobes. Honey has been incriminated as a possible source of the organism in some patients (Arnon 1980).

TREATMENT. If the diagnosis of food-borne botulism is suspected, the physician should collect 10 ml of serum, obtain a stool specimen, and contact the state Health Department to arrange for prompt testing of the specimens and to obtain antitoxin. Since mouse toxicity tests take at least 24 hours, initial treatment must proceed without a definitive diagnosis. Trivalent (ABE) antiserum, in doses recommended by the Health Department, is administered intravenously after subcutaneous tests for hypersensitivity to horse serum. If the diagnosis is delayed more than a few days, it may be too late for antitoxin to be of much value, and there is a 10-percent risk of inducing anaphylaxis or serum sickness by giving antitoxin (Merson et al. 1974). Thus, antitoxin can reasonably be omitted in late cases. A human preparation of botulinal antitoxin is being developed.

Aside from these measures, treatment consists of assuring an open airway and administering mechanical ventilation if necessary. The controversial role of guanidine is discussed below. Low-dose heparin therapy would probably reduce the incidence of thrombophlebitis during the prolonged convalescence.

When wound botulism is suspected, the possibility of food-borne botulism should not be forgotten; a patient in a San Francisco hospital developed botulism while recovering from a surgical operation, but the cause was found to be home-canned food brought in by the patient's wife! Serum and stool specimens should be collected as above, and the wound should be explored, cultured, and thoroughly debrided and irrigated. Antitoxin therapy is useful here because the toxin is still being produced in the wound. It is standard practice to give penicillin, but whether this is useful is not known.

In cases of infant botulism, the stool is sent to be cultured and assayed for toxin. For reasons not yet understood, the infants recover spontaneously without specific treatment to eradicate the organism, and indeed the organism persists in the colon during recovery. Neither antitoxin nor antibiotic treatment is recommended (Arnon 1980).

Guanidine has been convincingly shown to improve muscle strength and neuromuscular transmission in some patients (Cherington and Ryan 1968, 1970) but it has not been as useful as originally hoped (Puggiari and Cherington 1978). In particular, the drug seems to have little effect on severely weak muscles, so that it does not often rescue patients from mechanical ventilation. A double-blind trial showed no clinical benefit from guanidine in 12 patients, but there were no objective measurements of muscle strength or vital capacity (Kaplan et al. 1979). Nevertheless, it is clear that a better drug is needed.

Lundh and coworkers (1977) showed that 4-aminopyridine, which acts similarly to tetraethyl ammonium (TEA), could reverse botulinal paralysis in rats. Ball and associates (1979) gave 4-aminopyridine to four patients with severe botulism. There was marked improvement in limb strength and ocular movements but little effect on ventilation; moreover, two patients developed generalized convulsions after 4 hours of intravenous drug therapy. It is possible that a lower dose of 4-aminopyridine could be combined with guanidine for greater safety, but a better approach would be to find a similar agent that does not enter the central nervous system (Ball et al. 1979). Meanwhile, the usefulness of guanidine should still be assessed case by case.

OUTCOME. Excluding infant botulism, the fatality rate for botulism is about 23 percent (Merson et al. 1974). The main reason for this high mortality is failure of physicians to recognize the seriousness of the disease or to be prepared for the rapid worsening of paralysis. In the patients who survive, recovery of muscle function is essentially complete. For that reason, it is important to avoid hypoxic brain damage by *anticipating* the need for mechanical ventilation rather than waiting until emergency tracheal intubation is required. In modern intensive care units the fatality rate for botulism should probably not be more than 5 percent.

Tetanus

While botulism kills by paralysis, tetanus incites the neuromuscular system to lethal overactivity. Both disorders are caused by a clostridial exotoxin that blocks synaptic transmission, peripherally in the former disorder and centrally in the latter. Wound botulism is rare, but tetanus is invariably caused by a wound infection. C tetani organisms are ubiquitous in the soil, and though they are more numerous in hot, moist climates, tetanus is still common in tropical regions mainly because of poor hygiene and low levels of immunization. It is estimated that there are 350,000 cases of tetanus in the world every year (Trujillo et al. 1980). Most of the enormous amount of medical skill and money expended on caring for these patients, not to mention the 160,000 fatalities, could be spared by putting into effect simple, inexpensive prophylactic measures that have been available for decades. In the United States and Britain, where the annual incidence of tetanus is 0.3 to 0.9 cases per million, almost all cases occur in nonimmunized persons, and the remaining patients did not obtain a booster dose of tetanus toxoid at the time of injury (Edmondson and Flowers 1979; Blake et al. 1976). In Munich, between 9 and 12 percent of young persons aged 18 to 22 years have no detectable tetanus antibodies (Pilars de Pilar and Spiess 1981), and in an Alabama family practice 26 percent of the populace were unprotected (Pieroni et al. 1980). Truly, tetanus is "the inexcusable disease."

CLINICAL FEATURES. The infection responsible for tetanus may reside in a wound or skin ulcer, in the female genital tract following childbirth or septic abortion, or in the umbilical stump of newborn infants. Puerperal and neonatal tetanus are rare in developed countries. In Britain, no source of infection was identified in fully 25 percent of the cases; 65 percent were due to wounds; 8 percent to infection of a chronic skin ulcer; and 2 percent to elective surgical operations. Because most of the wounds were minor, nearly half of the patients did not seek medical attention (Edmondson and Flowers 1979). In New York during the past few decades narcotic addiction has been the most frequent cause, mainly in those who inject drugs subcutaneously (Brust and Richter 1974). The incubation period varies from 4 to 20 days. The main symptoms are *muscle rigidity and spasms.* Trismus (persistent spasm of jaw closure) and dysphagia are the presenting symptoms in most patients. Others complain initially of muscle stiffness in the neck, back, abdomen, or one limb, and a few patients with wounds of the head or neck present with unilateral facial weakness or ocular muscle palsies (cephalic tetanus), but trismus appears soon afterward. Except in the few patients whose symptoms remain localized to one limb ("local tetanus"), muscle rigidity soon becomes generalized and affects the face, larynx, throat, spine, and limbs. Reflex spasms develop within a few days in most cases but may not appear for up to 12 days after the onset of rigidity. An early onset of spasms is more typical of severe cases, but a delayed onset does not insure a benign course (Edmondson and Flowers 1979).

The spasms consist of a sudden, localized or generalized contraction of opposing muscles, lasting for a few seconds but occurring repeatedly for several minutes. Tetanic spasms are extremely painful; they cause respiratory embarrassment, injure the muscles, and sometimes even fracture the spine or long bones. The spasms tend to be triggered by sensory stimulation, emotion, or movement, but they may occur for no apparent reason.

The standard neurologic examination is difficult to perform without eliciting spasms, but aside from muscle rigidity, hyperactive stretch reflexes, and cranial nerve palsies (in cephalic tetanus), there are no abnormal signs.

Severely affected patients have sustained hypertension and persistent tachycardia with a heart rate of 140 to 180. Fever and sweating occur even without muscular overactivity, and the metabolic rate is so high that the caloric intake must be increased to prevent exhaustion. These manifestations have been attributed to direct involvement of the sympathetic nervous system (Kerr et al. 1968). Occasionally there are wide swings of blood pressure, possibly resulting from alternating stimulation of alpha-adrenergic and beta-adrenergic receptors (Kanarek et al. 1973).

LABORATORY FINDINGS. The diagnosis is based entirely on the characteristic clinical picture. Routine laboratory tests are unrevealing, and the cerebrospinal fluid (CSF) is normal. The serum CPK level is moderately or markedly elevated as a result of the forceful, isometric muscle contractions, and myoglobinuria sometimes develops. EMG recordings from muscles involved by rigidity or spasms show a continuous discharge of normal motor unit potentials, resembling voluntary muscle contraction. An important EMG finding is the abolition or curtailment of the normal silent period during reflex contraction of muscles. This can almost always be demonstrated in the masseter muscles, as described below.

C tetani can be cultured from a wound in about one fourth of the cases. In partly immunized patients known not to have received tetanus toxoid in the past 10 years, an elevated serum titer of tetanus antitoxin is evidence for an amnestic immune response caused by a recent infection with C tetani (Risk et al. 1981).

DIFFERENTIAL DIAGNOSIS. Few conditions mimic the clinical picture of tetanus. Strychnine poisoning produces a very similar syndrome, but the symptoms begin abruptly an hour or two after ingestion of the poison, and reflex spasms tend to be more prominent than rigidity. Acute dystonic reactions to phenothiazine drugs and related neuroleptics have been confused with tetanus, and vice versa. Trismus owing to oral pathology occasionally suggests tetanus but is not associated with rigidity elsewhere in the body.

TREATMENT. All patients should be admitted to an intensive care unit, because even those with mild symptoms can develop laryngospasm very suddenly, necessitating the use of intravenous succinylcholine in order to intubate the trachea. If the airway is even slightly compromised the patient should be intubated at once; a tracheostomy can be performed electively if it appears that prolonged mechanical ventilation will be needed. Centrally acting sedative-relaxant drugs are given to reduce rigidity and control spasms, usually diazepam (10 to 20 mg IV or IM every 4 to 6 hours) and chlorpromazine (25 to 50 mg IV or IM every 6 hours). In severe cases (about 90 percent of the patients in two recent series) the spasms are not adequately controlled by sedation, and the current approach in most centers is to administer a neuromuscular blocking drug like curare or pancuronium and to provide mechanical ventilation (Edmondson and Flowers 1979; Trujillo et al. 1980). Additional standard treatment includes intramuscular administration of antitoxin (preferably human type, 500 to 4000 units); penicillin 1 million units IM every 6 hours for 1 week; debridement and cleansing of the wound; and careful attention to fluid, electrolyte, and blood replacement. Initially intravenous alimentation is given; when the respiratory status is stable, nasogastric tube feeding can be used in some patients, but since gastrointestinal stasis is commonly present, intravenous hyperalimentation may be necessary. Low-dose heparin therapy is probably indicated in paralyzed patients. Every patient should be started on a course of active immunization with toxoid, because natural tetanus does not confer active immunity.

The value of intrathecal antitoxin therapy has been controversial. Recently a controlled trial of human tetanus immunoglobulin in 97 patients with early tetanus (before the onset of spasms) showed a death rate of 2 percent in patients given 250 units of antitoxin by the intrathecal route, compared with a 21 percent death rate among patients given 1000 units intramuscularly. Only 6 percent of the former group progressed to a moderate or severe grade of tetanus, while 31 percent of the latter did so (Gupta et al. 1980). Unfortunately, intrathecal human tetanus immunoglobulin was not beneficial in patients with more advanced tetanus (Vakil and Armitage 1979) or in neonatal tetanus (Sedaghatian 1979), though intrathecal therapy with equine antitoxin has been reported to be effective in such cases (Sanders et al. 1977). Since there have been no adverse reactions to the intrathecal therapy, it seems reasonable to administer 250 units of human tetanus immunoglobulin as soon as possible after admission, in addition to the standard intramuscular dose.

There is considerable uncertainty about how to manage the sympathetic instability. Some authors have had good results with small doses of propranolol (Trujillo et al. 1980) or propranolol and bethanidine (Prys-Roberts et al. 1969, Kanarek et al. 1973), but Edmondson and Flowers (1979) attributed two episodes of cardiac arrest during tracheal suction to the use of propranolol, perhaps because of unopposed vagal reflexes. Until more is known about these risks, sympathetic blocking agents should be used with great caution, if at all.

COURSE AND OUTCOME. The active phase of the illness generally lasts about 4 weeks regardless of the severity of the symptoms (Edmondson and Flowers 1979). In the Leeds series of 100 patients, the average duration of mechanical ventilation with pharmacologic paralysis was 21 days (Edmondson and Flowers 1979), and for 233 patients in Caracas the average stay in the intensive care unit was 22 days (Trujillo et al. 1980). It is clear that the use of curarization and artificial ventilation has eliminated uncontrolled spasms as a cause of death, but patients still die from unexpected cardiac arrest, shock, renal failure, and sepsis. The mechanism of cardiac arrest is not always apparent; cardiac standstill may occur without any apparent metabolic disturbance, even when a functioning cardiac pacemaker is in place (Brust and Richter 1974). Renal failure is probably not due to myoglobinuria when the spasms have been well controlled; in a recent series it was thought that treatment of hypotension with sympathomimetic agents might have been responsible (Seedat et al. 1981).

In two recent series of patients treated with total curarization, the fatality rate was about 10 percent; this figure may be close to the lowest obtainable for severe tetanus (Trujillo et al. 1980; Edmondson and Flowers 1979), but the promising results with intrathecal human tetanus immunoglobulin suggest that the fatality rate can be reduced to around 2 percent in patients treated before the onset of spasms. In undeveloped countries the fatality rate is 15 to 28 percent in large referral centers that use tracheotomy without curarization (Vakil and Armitage 1979; Gupta et al. 1980; Garnier 1975; Sanders et al. 1977). In the United States, however, the fatality rate was 62 percent for the period 1965 to 1971 (Blake 1976)! This sobering statistic demonstrates that most American physicians do not understand the basic principles of tetanus therapy. In Britain, where the fatality rate is only 10 percent, although the incidence of tetanus is even lower than in the United States, a system of regional referral centers probably helps to standardize therapy and to maintain a core of experienced medical personnel.

After recovery, only 4 percent of patients have any significant residual disability (Flowers and Edmondson 1980). Mild rigidity and reflex myoclonus occasionally continue, with diminishing intensity, for a few months, in rare cases persisting for nearly 2 years (Illis and Taylor 1971; Risk et al. 1981). Depression, disorientation, and emotional lability are common during convalescence, in part, perhaps, owing to withdrawal from diazepam. In one series these symptoms subsided in a few weeks (Flowers and Edmondson 1980), but in another series sleep disturbance, irritability, or impairment of memory sometimes persisted for a year or more (Illis and Taylor 1971). Shahani and associates (1979) reported mononeuropathies of the median, ulnar, peroneal, and other nerves in 80 percent of 34 cases of severe tetanus; they attributed the neuropathies to a direct effect of tetanus toxin, but mechanical trauma is a more plausible mechanism. The neuropathies recovered in most cases. One infant who survived neonatal tetanus had a permanent, flaccid quadriplegia of undetermined cause (Gadoth et al. 1981).

Pathophysiology. Tetanus toxin, a protein of 150,000 daltons, passes from the site of its production in a peripheral wound into skeletal muscle, where it is taken up by motor nerve terminals, moving from there by retrograde transport within motor axons to the central nervous system (Price et al. 1975). In generalized tetanus, it is presumed that the toxin enters the blood stream and is widely distributed to the skeletal muscles, where it gains access to the motor nerves. In local tetanus the symptoms are confined to the part of the body with the wound, suggesting that in such cases the toxin does not enter the blood stream. It appears that, in the central nervous system, the toxin crosses the motor nerve cell plasma membrane to enter the presynaptic nerve terminals of inhibitory interneurons, because the main action of the toxin is to block the release of the inhibitory transmitters glycine and gamma-aminobutyric acid (GABA) (Fig. 16) (Mellanby and Green 1981). The physiologic consequence of this presynaptic block of inhibitory synapses is a release of spinal and brainstem motor neurons from normal polysynaptic inhibitory controls (Brooks et al. 1957). Excitatory stimulation produces exaggerated motor responses because the usual dampening mechanisms are in abeyance. There are short and long excitatory

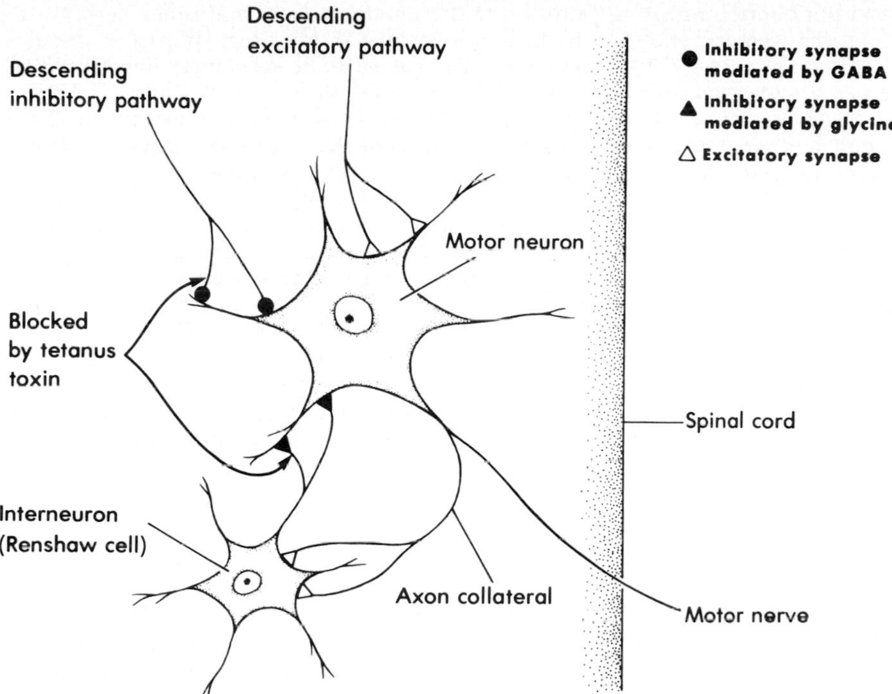

FIGURE 16. Pathophysiology of tetanus. Tetanus toxin selectively blocks inhibitory synapses in the brainstem and spinal cord, by preventing the release of inhibitory neurotransmitters. One type of inhibitory reflex is the recurrent inhibition of Renshaw, which is partly responsible for the silent period that occurs during the normal muscle stretch reflex (see Fig. 17).

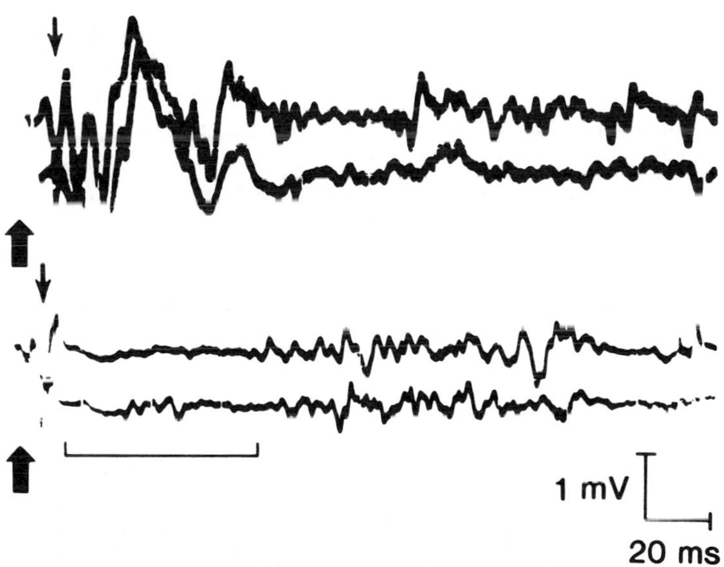

FIGURE 17. Loss of silent period of stretch reflex in tetanus. These are surface EMG recordings from both masseter muscles of a patient with tetanus *(upper two tracings)* and from a normal control *(lower two tracings)*. The sweep is triggered by a jaw tap *(bottom arrows)*, which elicits the masseter reflex *(top arrows)*. The upper tracings from the patient show an exaggerated reflex response with no silent period. The lower tracings show a normal silent period of 60 msec following the reflex response. (From Risk et al., 1981, with permission.)

and inhibitory connecting pathways in the spinal cord and brainstem, permitting a localized sensory stimulus to have a widespread excitatory impact in tetanus. Reflexes with long polysynaptic pathways appear to be selectively impaired (Bratzlavsky and Vander Eecken 1980). Likewise, excitatory and inhibitory influences descend from the brain to the lower centers, explaining the adverse effect of light, noise, and emotional arousal. Animal experiments have also demonstrated disinhibition of spinal sympathetic neurons (Habermann and Welhöner 1974).

The deficiency of reflex inhibition can be demonstrated in patients by studying the "silent period" that occurs during the normal muscle stretch reflex. This is a brief cessation of motor nerve activity that lasts 50 to 100 msec and is due mainly to recurrent (Renshaw) inhibition of motor neuron excitability. In tetanus, the inhibitory synapse is blocked, so that the silent period is abolished or reduced in duration in muscles that exhibit continuous spontaneous activity (Fig. 17). Thus, abbreviation of the silent period is regularly found in the masseter muscles of patients with trismus, but in localized tetanus is found only in the affected limb muscles (Struppler et al. 1963; Ricker et al 1971; Bratzlavsky and Vander Eecken 1980). Interestingly, the silent period is normal in the stiff-man syndrome, a useful feature for distinguishing that disorder from tetanus (Risk et al. 1981).

Diphtheria

Infection by one of the toxin-producing strains of Corynebacterium diphtheriae produces a demyelinative multiple neuropathy in about 20 percent of the cases, depending on the severity of the infection and the immune status of the patient. The neuropathy is delayed in onset and may run a long course but it does not, as a rule, leave permanent sequelae. Myocardial toxicity, however, occurs in two thirds of the patients and is largely responsible for the 10 percent death rate for diphtheria in the United States (Weinstein 1977a).

The primary infection is usually located in the upper respiratory tract, especially in the pharynx; nasal, laryngeal, or tracheal infections occur infrequently. Toxin-producing diphtheritic infections can also occur in the middle ear, conjunctiva, esophagus, intestine, umbilical stump of newborn infants, genitalia, wounds, and skin. In developed countries, improved hygiene and routine immunization of infants against diphtheria toxin have made diphtheria a rare disease, and consequently most physicians are now unfamiliar with the neuromuscular complications. In other areas of the world, diphtheria is still endemic (Kazemi et al. 1973; Khuri-Bulos 1980), and even in the United Stated the incidence has been rising in recent years (Brooks et al. 1974). An interesting recent development has been the rising number of cases of cutaneous diphtheria in the northwestern United States and Canada (Pedersen et al. 1977).

CLINICAL FEATURES. There are two types of neuropathic complication: mononeuropathies, which affect the motor cranial nerves predominantly, and a generalized sensorimotor polyneuropathy. A curious feature of both neuropathies is their delayed onset and their tendency to appear in stepwise fashion over a long period of time, so that some symptoms are improving at the same time that new symptoms appear.

In pharyngeal diphtheria, the earliest and commonest neuropathic symptoms are dysphonia and nasal regurgitation of fluids caused by palatal paralysis, which occurs in about 15 percent of patients. Palatal weakness usually appears in the second week but can begin at any time between the first and seventh weeks after the first symptoms of infection. When it occurs in the first 2 weeks it is clearly related to the local effects of the toxin, since palatal paralysis is ipsilateral in one-sided faucial infections (Scheid 1952) and rarely occurs in cutaneous diphtheria (Gaskell and Korb 1946). Other mononeuropathies tend to occur 4 to 7 weeks after the throat symptoms; paralysis of accommodation (nearly always sparing pupillary reactions) occurs in 10 percent of patients, extraocular muscle palsies occur in 3 percent, and paralysis of facial, laryngeal, masticatory, tongue, diaphragm, or other muscles occurs in fewer than 1 percent. Occasionally there is numbness of the pharynx or tongue or loss of taste. The mononeuropathies may be bilateral or unilateral, and they usually resolve within 6 weeks.

Polyneuropathy usually appears between the sixth and twelfth weeks of the illness; this complication develops in nearly half of the patients with palatal paralysis but in only 5 percent of patients without palatal weakness. The onset is gradual, with disappearance of the muscle stretch reflexes followed by distal numbness and tingling in the extremities; diffuse weakness of the limbs, trunk, and neck; and sensory ataxia of the trunk and limbs. The weakness may be asymmetrical, is usually more proximal than distal (Kurdi and Abdul-Kader 1979; Scheid 1952), and is often greater in the legs than in the arms. In severe cases, which are uncommon, there may be respiratory paralysis, loss of sphincter control, and distal muscle wasting. Recovery usually occurs in 6 to 12 weeks but takes longer in severe cases.

In a study of cutaneous diphtheria among American soldiers in Burma during the Second World War, Gaskell and Korb (1946) found that neuropathies occurred in one third of the patients, beginning 23 to 158 days after the estimated onset of the infection. In two thirds of the patients polyneuropathy occurred without cranial neuropathies; in the remainder, cranial neuropathies (mainly loss of accommodation) occurred first and the generalized polyneuropathy that followed tended to be more severe than in patients without cranial nerve involvement.

LABORATORY FINDINGS. In patients with polyneuropathy, the CSF protein is usually increased and may exceed 300 mg per dl (Gaskell and Korb 1946). Slight or moderate CSF pleocytosis occurs in 14 percent of the cases (Scheid 1952). Motor nerve conduction velocities and distal motor latencies tend to be normal or mildly abnormal in the first 2 weeks of the generalized polyneuropathy, even when limb weakness is marked. After that time, conduction velocities decline, even as muscle strength begins to improve, and they reach the lowest values of 15 to 35 m per second (about 45 percent of the mean normal value) after 5 to 10 weeks and gradually return to normal by 35 weeks. Prolongation of the distal motor latencies follows the same time course (Kurdi and Abdul-Kader 1979).

RELATION OF THE NEUROPATHY TO THE IMMUNE STATUS. In pharyngeal diphtheria the incidence of neurologic complications parallels the severity of the local manifestations. Thus, Scheid (1952) recorded a frequency of neuropathy ranging from 2 percent in mild cases to 77 percent in severe cases of pharyngeal infection. Full immunization against diphtheria toxin lowers the attack rate and lessens the severity of the infections that do occur (Brooks et al. 1974), thus reducing the incidence and severity of neurologic complications. Although most cases of diphtheria in the United States now occur in persons from low socio-economic groups, especially American Indians and blacks, population surveys suggest that the level of immunization in the general population is probably low enough to permit more widespread epidemics at any time (Pilars de Pilar and Spiess 1981).

TREATMENT. Early administration of equine diphtheria antitoxin affords considerable protection against the development of neuropathy. For example, Paley and Truelove (1948) recorded neuropathy in 17 percent of patients who received antitoxin after the first 2 days of pharynegeal infection, compared with 6 percent of patients who received antitoxin within the first 2 days. The case fatality rate is reduced even when antitoxin is given as late as the fourth day, but at that time it is 40 times higher than when antitoxin is given on the first day (Hodes 1979). In cutaneous diphtheria, antitoxin may be protective after a much longer delay; Gaskell and Korb (1946) found that the incidence of neuropathy was 14 percent when antitoxin was given before the 32nd day of the infection, 31 percent after the 32nd day, and 61 percent in untreated cases. For maximal protection it is the usual practice to give antitoxin before the diagnosis of diphtheria is confirmed by bacterial culture, after first testing the patient for hypersensitivity to horse serum. Recommended doses vary; one regimen is to give 40,000 units IV in early cases and 80,000 to 120,000 units in late or severe cases (Hodes 1979). A 10-day course of penicillin or erythromycin will usually eradicate the infection, but antibiotic treatment does not appreciably alter the incidence of serious complications. The paralytic complications are treated by the usual supportive measures.

PATHOPHYSIOLOGY. Diphtheria toxin produces paranodal and segmental demyelination of peripheral nerves in man and in experimental animals (Mc Donald and Kocen 1975). This is a direct effect of the toxin, not a hypersensitivity reaction, but its precise mechanism is not known. The toxin is a single polypeptide chain of 62,000 daltons, one portion of which serves to bind to cell surface receptors while the other portion enters the cell. Inside the cytoplasm the toxin inhibits protein synthesis by inactivating the enzyme translocase (elongation factor 2), which regulates the addition of amino acids to growing peptide chains (Pappenheimer and Gill 1973). Diphtheria toxin has been shown to inhibit the synthesis of several constituents of myelin (Pleasure et al. 1973), but whether this action accounts for the demyelination is not known, because the time course of the biochemical changes has not been correlated with the onset of pathologic or physiologic changes.

The clinical features of human diphtheritic neuropathy are fairly well reproduced in guinea pigs by subcutaneous injection of toxin. Muscle weakness appears 16 to 41 days later and reaches a peak in the second week of illness; improvement begins 4 to 10 days after a plateau is reached, and recovery is complete by 27 days after the onset of neuropathic signs (Morgan-Hughes 1968). The weakness is most marked in axial and proximal muscles and affects chewing and swallowing in severe cases. The conduction velocity of the motor nerves remains normal during the latent period, declines abruptly at or shortly after the onset of weakness, and does not return to normal until 10 to 19 weeks after the injection of toxin, although clinical recovery is complete well before that time. During the period of severe weakness, compound muscle action potentials in response to nerve stimulation are markedly reduced in amplitude and dispersed in time. During recovery the amplitude of the muscle responses increases strikingly, but temporal dispersion persists, reflecting different degrees of slowing of conduction in various nerves (Morgan-Hughes 1968). Thus it appears that block of electrical conduction at multiple sites in many nerves is responsible for weakness in the early phase of the illness; at this stage conduction velocity may be normal or reduced in the few nerve fibers that still conduct impulses between the point of stimulation and the muscle. During recovery, conduction block is gradually relieved in various demyelinated nerve segments; conduction velocity is slow in these nerves, though the summated muscle response improves as more nerves regain function. At the peak of weakness, microscopic examination of teased nerve fibers shows complete destruction of segments of myelin between nodes of Ranvier; during recovery there is remyelination and a gradual increase in myelin thickness as conduction velocities return toward normal (Morgan-Hughes 1968).

In human diphtheria, severe neuropathy may be accompanied by distal muscle wasting, and in such cases recovery may take many months, a finding that suggests that some nerves have suffered axonal degeneration. Likewise, in experimental diphtheritic neuropathy a variable degree of axonal degeneration has been observed in severely affected animals. It is not known whether diphtheria toxin affects motor axons directly, independently of demyelination. However, there is experimental evidence that demyelination itself can alter axonal function. Injection of diphtheria toxin beneath the perineurium of chicken sciatic nerve causes focal demyelination and electrical conduction block; in addition, fast axonal transport of proteins down the axons is blocked at the site of demyelination, and the muscle fibers supplied by those nerves undergo atrophy (Kidman et al. 1978a, 1978b). Slow axonal transport, however, is not blocked (Kidman et al. 1979).

Necrotizing Myopathy and Myoglobinuria

Some bacterial infections cause myalgia, muscle tenderness, and elevated serum CPK levels. Bacterial toxins, rather than direct infection of the muscles, are suspected to be responsible for these manifestations.

In *Weil's disease,* the severe form of leptospirosis, about 70 percent of patients complain of myalgia, and myoglobinuria occurs in a few of them. Ho and Scully (1980) suggested that unnoticed myoglobinuria might explain the occurrence of acute renal failure in Weil's disease. *Typhoid fever* has been reported to cause myoglobinuria or elevated CPK levels in the absence of bacteremia (David and Tolaymat 1978). Isolated cases of myoglobinuria have occurred in patients with septicemia caused by mixed enteric organisms (Kalish et al. 1982), Staphylococcus epidermidis, Legionella pneumophila, and aspergillus (El Nahas et al. 1983).

Myalgia is a prominent feature of the *toxic shock syndrome,* an acute multisystem illness caused by a staphylococcal exotoxin. Originally described in children, the disease appeared in epidemic form in connection with the use of tampons during menstruation (Tanner et al. 1981; Tofte and Williams 1981; Fisher et al. 1981), and it has also been reported in patients with skin infections, surgical and nonsurgical wounds, and postpartum sepsis (Reingold et al. 1982). The major manifestations include fever, hypotension, scarlatiniform rash, vomiting or diarrhea, and myalgia. The serum CPK activity is increased in about 70 percent of the cases, sometimes reaching levels above 10,000 IU per liter. The clinical features of the muscular disorder have not yet been adequately described; during convalescence the patients are said to experience prolonged fatigue and weakness for as long as several months (Chesney et al. 1981, 1982).

An acute febrile illness of infants, known as Kawasaki's disease or mucocutaneous lymph node syndrome, has been reported to produce muscle tenderness, weakness, and EMG abnormality (Koutras 1982). Some adult patients with similar manifestations have shown high serum CPK levels (Hicks et al. 1982), but the classification of these cases is in doubt because of their close resemblance to cases of the toxic shock syndrome (Chesney et al. 1981).

Syphilitic Amyotrophy

Early in this century, when syphilis was still a common disease, some cases of lower motor neuron disease were attributed to neurosyphilis under the rubric of syphilitic amyotrophy. Even then the diagnosis was a subject of controversy; now there are few neurologists who have seen even a single example of the syndrome, and several authorities doubt that it exists.

Nevertheless, cases of "syphilitic amyotrophy" continue to be published (Heathfield and Turner 1951; Schwob 1952; Datta et al. 1966; Hewitt 1967; Luxon et al. 1979), and hence it is appropriate to reassess the clinical data that gave rise to this diagnosis.

There is no disagreement about the occurrence of amyotrophy in the well-established forms of spinal syphilis. Focal amyotrophy can result from ischemic myelomalacia or from inflammation of the spinal nerve roots in patients with meningovascular syphilis, and in the rare syndrome of syphilitic pachymeningitis. In such cases there are sensory and long-tract signs of a myeloradiculitis. Syphilitic amyotrophy, however, is said to cause widespread lower motor neuron degeneration, often in the absence of other signs of myelopathy.

We owe most of the early accounts of this syndrome to French neurologists writing at the turn of the century, especially Leri, who considered syphilitic amyotrophy to be the most frequent cause of amyotrophy in his clinical practice (Martin 1925). Similar views have been expressed by Martin (1925), Winkelman (1932), Mackay and Hall (1933), and Wechsler and colleagues (1944).

According to Martin (1925), muscular weakness and atrophy usually begin in the small muscles of one or both hands, are often accompanied by pain in the shoulder or neck, and progress slowly up the arms over a period of months or years. The extensor muscles of the fingers and wrists may be the first muscles to be affected, producing "syphilitic wrist-drop" (Heathfield and Turner 1951). In 20 percent of the cases amyotrophy starts in the shoulder girdle muscles, while in 10 percent of the cases the anterolateral muscles of the lower legs are affected first, followed by the calf and thigh muscles. Wasting may spread to the muscles of the neck, back, or chest and may skip from lumbar to cervical segments or vice versa. The process may become arrested but more often progresses to complete, flaccid paralysis of one or more limbs, sometimes causing death from respiratory failure. Fasciculations are usually present and the reflexes are lost. Sensory disturbance may be seen in the form of impaired vibration sense in the legs or vague patches of numbness over the extremities. Pyramidal tract signs are present in some cases, even within spinal segments manifesting amyotrophy (Heathfield and Turner 1951; Datta et al. 1966), a feature usually considered typical of amyotrophic lateral sclerosis. In some cases the spastic features predominate and amyotrophy is slight. Urinary sphincter disturbances of the upper motor neuron type are said to be fairly common. Cases of progressive bulbar palsy (Cook 1953) and acute anterior poliomyelitis (Barker 1943), have also been attributed to neurosyphilis.

In Martin's review (1925) the blood Wassermann's reaction was negative in 25 percent of cases, but the CSF reaction was positive in untreated cases. In other reports, the CSF displayed a modest lymphocytic pleocytosis of up to 100 cells per cu mm, and the concentration of protein and gamma globulin were usually increased.

I have reviewed most of the case reports of syphilitic amyotrophy published in English since 1925, together with a sampling of French articles of the same period, amounting to 20 cases in all. The reports are not very convincing. In 13 cases there was no postmortem examination and no documented response to treatment (Luxon et al. 1979; Heathfield and Turner 1951; Mackay and Hall 1933; Schwob 1952; Wechsler and colleagues 1944; Martin 1925). In 4 cases (including three patients with Argyll Robertson's pupils) there was no autopsy, but there was a suggestive response to treatment (Martin 1925; Mackay and Hall 1933; Datta et al. 1966). In the 3 remaining cases autopsy showed changes consistent with meningovascular syphilis and myelitis, but there was no response to treatment (Martin 1925; Winkelman 1932; Lhermitte et al. 1945).

It is difficult to avoid the suspicion that most of these cases were instances of amyotrophic lateral sclerosis (ALS), coincidentally associated with meningovascular syphilis or tabes dorsalis. The case of Lhermitte and associates (1945) showed pathologic changes typical of ALS in addition to those of meningovascular syphilis, but the authors attributed all the abnormalities to syphilis. Alajouanine and coworkers (1950) have documented the coincidental occurrence of typical ALS late in the course of tabes dorsalis. A case of "acute syphilitic poliomyelitis" reported by Barker (1943) is more reasonably interpreted as an example of poliomyelitis in a patient with asymptomatic neurosyphilis, while a carefully detailed account of a patient with "progressive bulbar palsy due to syphilis" appears to be a description of meningovascular and tabetic neurosyphilis with prominent involvement of the lower cranial nerves and spinal cord (Cook 1953).

To summarize, in the English and French literature of the past half century there are no pathologically proven examples of syphilitic amyotrophy that responded convincingly to therapy. No doubt focal amyotrophy can occur in the course of neurosyphilis as a result of tabetic neuropathies, of radicular involvement by leptomeningitis or pachymeningitis, or of focal myelomalacia caused by meningomyelitis. It is very doubtful, however, that patchy, widespread, lower motor neuron signs, with or without pyramidal tract signs (the typical picture of ALS), can be attributed to syphilis.

VIRAL INFECTIONS

Myopathy in Viral Infections

Myalgia and Fatigue

Myalgia is a prominent symptom in many acute infectious diseases caused by viruses, bacteria, and protozoa. The generalized muscle aching usually occurs at the beginning of the illness; there is little or no muscle tenderness, and movement does not increase the discomfort. The cause of this myalgia is not known. There is no indication of actual muscle infection, and muscle histology in a few biopsies has been unremarkable. In a group of adult patients with influenza A2, serum CPK levels rose slightly in the acute phase and returned to normal during convalescence, but the CPK changes did not correlate with the presence or severity of myalgia (Friman 1976).

Similarly, subjective muscle weakness and fatigue are common complaints during the acute and convalescent phases of influenza and other viral illnesses, but objective muscle weakness is rarely encountered. Friman and associates (1977) performed single-fiber EMG in a group of 14 patients with influenza or echovirus infections, all of whom complained of myalgia, and in a group of 9 patients with mumps who did not complain of myalgia. EMG "jitter," a nonspecific indication of delayed neuromuscular transmission, was observed in 5 to 6 percent of muscle action-potential pairs in both groups of patients, compared with the reported normal value of 1 percent; but the observations were not controlled, and the clinical significance of these minor findings is doubtful. Friman (1977) also reported a slight reduction (5 to 15 percent) of isometric muscle strength in 39 patients who were tested just after the febrile period of various acute infections, mainly of viral or mycoplasmal origin; but since these measurements require full voluntary effort, the finding could be due to simple lassitude rather than to motor unit dysfunction.

In the case of *pleurodynia* (epidemic myalgia, Bornholm's disease, devil's grip), myalgia is the main clinical feature. An acute vital illness characterized by fever and severe pain in the chest, pleurodynia occurs primarily in children and young adults. The chest pain may be unilateral, bilateral, or substernal, and like pluerisy it is accentuated by movements of the chest wall. (Genuine pleuritis does in fact occur in a few cases.) Headache and abdominal muscle pain are commonly present, and pain may spread to the neck, upper back, and shoulder-girdle muscles. Occasionally there is localized swelling of intercostal or other muscles. The symptoms last between 2 days and 2 weeks. The majority of cases are caused by one of the group-B Coxsackie viruses, but a similar syndrome occurs in patients infected with group-A Coxsackie viruses and echo viruses. Other manifestations of Coxsackie-B infection, such as meningitis, myocarditis, or hepatitis, may accompany pleurodynia (Lerner 1977; Dallsdorf and Melnick 1965).

Pathophysiology. The cause of myalgia in pleurodynia is not known, but the clinical signs suggest that a restricted myopathy of some sort is present. Serum enzyme levels do not seem to have been reported. Coxsackie viruses have a special affinity for skeletal muscle, at least in some animal species. Suckling mice infected with group-A Coxsackie viruses develop generalized muscle necrosis without significant lesions in other tissues, while group-B infections cause encephalomyelitis, myocarditis, and restricted muscle necrosis (Dallsdorf and Melnick 1965; Ray et al. 1979).

Viruses are present in abundance in these lesions. Cell-mediated host immunity may contribute to the pathogenesis of heart muscle damage in experimental Coxsackie virus-B infections, since immune lymphocytes from infected mice have a cytolytic effect on myocardial cells in tissue culture (Huber et al. 1980).

Benign Influenza Myopathy

A transient, painful myopathy of the lower extremities may occur during convalescence from influenza (Middleton et al. 1970; Dietzman et al. 1976; Farrell et al. 1980). Most of the affected persons are children between 6 and 12 years of age, and about two thirds of the patients are boys, though the syndrome occurs occasionally in older children and rarely in adults. The muscle symptoms begin 2 to 7 days after the onset of the influenza symptoms, usually when the fever and respiratory symptoms are improving. Pain appears abruptly in the calf muscles and sometimes in other leg and thigh muscles; the pain is so severe that the child may refuse to walk, preferring to crawl along the floor, or he may walk with a bizarre, antalgic gait. The affected muscles may be swollen and tender, so that it is difficult for the examiner to estimate muscle strength in the legs; weakness is probably not a prominent feature, however, and the remainder of the neurologic examination is normal. Recovery is very rapid; the symptoms and signs usually resolve in 1 to 5 days, and the patients walk normally within a week.

During the symptomatic phase, serum CPK activity is almost always increased, averaging 10 times the upper limit of normal and ranging up to 60 times normal. In two cases, EMG showed myopathic motor unit potentials in affected muscles (Ruff and Secrist 1982). Muscle biopsies were abnormal in three fourths of cases in one series, showing scattered necrosis of long segments of muscle fibers with little or no evidence of primary inflammation, although necrotic fibers were often invaded by neutrophils, other inflammatory cells, and mononuclear phagocytes (Farrell et al. 1980).

Most of the cases are caused by influenza-B infection, but influenza A, adenovirus type 2, and parainfluenza virus 4A have also been implicated (McKinlay and Mitchell 1976). Specimens from muscle biopsy in 12 cases with influenza-B infection did not contain detectable antibody, immune complexes, or viral particles, and the virus was successfully cultured from only one specimen (Farrell et al. 1980). Thus, benign influenza myopathy appears to be a restricted form of rhabdomyolysis, without clear evidence of either an inflammatory process or a direct infection of muscle. The mechanism of the muscle necrosis remains unknown.

Myoglobinuria

In contrast to the restricted muscle necrosis typical of benign influenza myopathy, generalized rhabdomyolysis and myoglobinuria may develop in the course of influenza and other viral infections. In adult patients this appears to be a fairly benign illness. Josselson and associates (1980) reviewed 15 cases in patients over the age of 12; 7 were associated with influenza-A infection, and the others occurred in patients with Coxsackie, herpes simplex, Epstein-Barr, echo, and parainfluenza infections. One case has been reported with serologic evidence of adenovirus infection (Meshkinpour and Vaziri 1981). In some patients rhabdomyolysis occurs at the beginning of the febrile illness; in others myalgia, muscle weakness, and dark urine begin during the convalescent stage. Although transient renal insufficiency occurred in half of the patients, all made a good recovery. There was no previous or family history of similar episodes except in two patients: a 27-year-old man who had had several similar episodes in childhood in association with respiratory infections (Simon et al. 1970), and a 22-year-old man who had had repeated episodes of myoglobinuria in association with febrile respiratory infections and during febrile reactions following immunizations, routine surgery, and experimental administration of typhoid vaccine (Berg and Frenkel 1958). Thus, a few individuals may be unusually susceptible to muscle injury during viral infections or fever, but this is probably not true of most adult patients who develop myoglobinuria during a viral illness.

The childhood cases of viral myoglobinuria present a more serious picture; the course of the illness is often fulminating, with a fatal outcome in about 35 percent of cases. Savage and associates (1971), reviewing 23 published cases of children with nonexertional idiopathic rhabdomyolysis, noted a history of a similar illness among siblings in 9 patients, while 10 patients had experienced two or more episodes of myoglobinuria. Furthermore, 7 children died during the first and only episode, so that 63 percent of those who survived the first attack had multiple episodes. These data suggest that the majority of children with viral myoglobinuria have some sort of inherent muscle defect. So far, no biochemical abnormality has been discovered in this syndrome.

Muscle pathology in both children and adults with viral myoglobinuria consists merely of muscle fiber necrosis with a secondary inflammatory and phagocytic reaction; there is little convincing evidence of a primary inflammatory process (Ghatak et al. 1973; Fukuyamata et al. 1977; Greco et al. 1977). Electron microscopy in one case was thought to show particles resembling myxovirus (Greco et al. 1977) and picornavirus in another case (Fukuyamata et al. 1977), but viral cultures of muscle have been negative except in one recent case in which influenza-B virus was isolated (Gamboa et al. 1979). As in the syndrome of benign influenza myopathy, we do not know whether the muscle necrosis is related to a viral infection of muscle, to an immune reaction, or to some other unidentified toxic mechanism.

Viral Myositis

Virus-like particles have been detected in electron-microscopic studies of muscle from patients with polymyositis and dermatomyositis. (For a review, see Gamboa et al. 1979.) In these cases the ultrastructural identification of viruses was not confirmed by culture, immunofluorescence, or serologic tests. There is thus no convincing evidence for a persistent viral infection in ordinary polymyositis or dermatomyositis. Recently, however, adenovirus type 2 was isolated from skeletal muscle of a patient with chronic inclusion-body myositis, an atypical form of polymyositis long suspected to have a viral origin (see Chapter 5). The patient's serum had a high titer of neutralizing antibodies to the same virus (Mikol et al. 1982).

Several patients with X-linked agammaglobulinemia have developed persistent echovirus infection of the central nervous system, skeletal muscles, skin, and subcutaneous tissues, a syndrome somewhat resembling dermatomyositis (Bardelas et al. 1977; Mease et al. 1981). In these patients the serum enzymes were markedly elevated, EMG showed myopathic abnormalities, and muscle biopsies showed perivascular lymphocytic inflammation and scattered muscle fiber degeneration. One patient was successfully treated with type-specific human immune globulin (Mease et al. 1981).

The question of a viral etiology of polymyositis and dermatomyositis is also discussed in Chapter 5.

Acute Anterior Poliomyelitis

In addition to the three strains of poliovirus, several viruses are capable of causing fairly selective infection of the motor nerve cells of the spinal cord and lower brainstem. Now that poliovirus infections have become rare in many countries, these viral diseases must be considered in the differential diagnosis of acute anterior poliomyelitis. Viral infections that cause acute anterior poliomyelitis include the following:

Poliovirus
Coxsackie viruses
Echoviruses
Enterovirus 71
Enterovirus 70
Mumps
Herpes simplex
Adenovirus 7
Arboviruses

Poliovirus Infection

The clinical and pathologic features of paralytic poliomyelitis have been extensively reviewed (Weinstein 1977b; Price and Plum 1978). The following brief summary is intended for comparison of poliovirus with other viral infections that have a similar clinical picture.

CLINICAL FEATURES. Paralysis usually begins in a setting of aseptic meningitis, with fever, headache, stiff neck, and vomiting. In children there may have been a transient upper respiratory infection or gastroenteritis a week earlier. At first the involved muscles tend to ache, become tight, or twitch, but these symptoms of motor nerve hyperactivity are soon replaced by flaccid paralysis. The patchy weakness can affect any muscles of the limbs, trunk, and lower four cranial nerves; it is often concentrated in one limb, but it does not follow strict radicular patterns. Respiratory weakness, brainstem disturbances of respiratory control, autonomic disorders, and bladder paralysis occur in a minority of patients. The paralysis spreads and intensifies, then levels off in 3 to 5 days.

Severe pain may continue for several weeks in severely paralyzed muscles. Paresthesias and dysesthesias are common during the acute illness, but outright sensory loss is extremely rare, though in two cases proven by viral culture and serologies there was a flaccid paraplegia with a sensory level in the lumbar region (Plum 1956; Seggey et al. 1976). Even so, pathologic studies indicate that neuronal degeneration is not confined strictly to the motor neurons of the spinal cord and brainstem but may involve neurons of the sensory ganglia, posterior and intermediolateral horns of the spinal cord, brainstem reticular formation, cerebellum, hypothalamus, thalamus, and precentral gyrus.

LABORATORY FINDINGS. During the preparalytic phase the CSF white blood cell count averages 185 cells per cu mm, after which it declines gradually although it remains abnormal during the first week after the onset of paralysis. At first there is often a predominance of neutrophils, but lymphocytes quickly take their place. The protein concentration is usually normal during the first week of paralysis and rarely exceeds 100 mg per dl; afterward it tends to increase, reaching an average level of 164 mg per dl 3 to 4 weeks after onset, before returning gradually to normal. The immunoglobulin concentration may be increased (Fishman 1980).

EMG during the acute phase of paralysis shows none of the classic signs of denervation except for a reduction of the number of motor unit potentials that can be activated voluntarily. After about 1 month the EMG shows increased insertional activity, fibrillations, positive waves, and fasciculations. Somewhat later the motor unit potential changes of reinnervation appear: prolonged, polyphasic action potentials of large amplitude (Aminoff 1978). Eventually the fibrillations disappear or become much less numerous, but fasciculations may persist indefinitely. If patients are tested many years later, muscles that appear normal clinically sometimes show a reduced number of motor unit potentials under voluntary control, with many large reinnervation potentials, indicating that some of the motor neurons supplying these muscles had been involved by polio and that function was restored by distal sprouting of surviving nerve fibers (Hayward and Seaton 1979; Lutschg and Ludin 1981).

Motor nerve conduction tests during the first few weeks show neither slowing of velocity nor reduction in amplitude of the compound muscle action potential. Later, after a significant proportion of the motor axons have degenerated, motor nerve conduction velocity is still normal or is slightly reduced, but the compound muscle action potential is smaller because of the loss of excitable nerve fibers. Still later the reinnervation of denervated muscle fibers by surviving motor nerves permits the size of the compound muscle action potential to increase toward normal.

Other Enterovirus Infections

Coxsackie virus A-7 has been isolated from cases of paralytic poliomyelitis during epidemics in Russia since 1952; two of the thirteen reported patients died. A single case has been reported from the United States (Ranzenhofer et al. 1958), and in an outbreak in Scotland in 1959 there were six cases closely resembling poliomyelitis among thirty-three cases of aseptic meningitis caused by this organism. All the paralyzed patients were boys under 6 years of age; one died of fulminating paralytic illness, and two had residual weakness 8 or 9 months later (Combined Scottish Study 1961).

Other Coxsackie viruses accounted for 25 cases of polio-like illness in California from 1955 to 1957 and represented 5 percent of all cases reported as "poliomyelitis." The viruses isolated were type A-9 (three cases), B-2 (six cases), B-3 (one case), B-4 (eight cases), B-5 (six cases), and both B-4 and B-5 (one case). A rise in serum antibody titers to the same virus type was documented in 14 of 15 cases. All but 3 of the patients were below the age of 12, and the weakness was of mild or moderate severity, except in one patient with severe weakness. No follow-up information was obtained (Magoffin et al 1961b).

During an epidemic of echovirus-6 infection in 1955, mild muscle weakness was found in 39 percent of 130 patients with acute aseptic meningitis, most of whom were between 4 and 15 years of age. Of the 42 cases only 6 had limb weakness; the others had weakness of the anterior neck, trunk, and abdomen. The motor signs were considered questionable in many cases, and at follow-up 3 years later there was no residual weakness or amyotrophy (Karzon et al. 1962; King and Karzon 1962). In an epidemic of echovirus "Frater" there was one case of flaccid arm paralysis among 63 patients with meningitis; no follow-up was obtained (Combined Scottish Study 1961). Echovirus was also listed as a cause of mild polio-like illness in a large California survey by Magoffin and colleagues (1961a).

An epidemic of enterovirus-71 infection in Bulgaria in 1975 caused about 700 cases of aseptic meningitis, among which there were 52 cases of "poliomyelitis-like disease" and 68 cases of bulbar encephalomyelitis (Shindarov et al. 1979). The Bulgarian strain of enterovirus 71 regularly produced polio-like disease when inoculated into monkeys (Chumakov et al. 1979). Two outbreaks of enterovirus-71 infection in Japan, in 1973 and in 1978, were characterized by hand, foot, and mouth disease (a syndrome usually linked to Coxsackie A-16 infections), with meningoencephalitis in 8 to 24 percent of the cases; in addition, a flaccid, hyporeflexic paralysis of one leg occurred in 2.5 percent of cases (Ishimaru et al. 1980). A small outbreak of 12 cases in New York State in 1977 included 2 cases with paralytic polio-like illness as well as cases of aseptic meningitis, meningoencephalitis, respiratory disease, gastroenteritis, and hand-foot-mouth disease (Chonmaitree et al. 1981).

Enterovirus 70 is one of the agents responsible for acute hemorrhagic conjunctivitis (AHC), a new, pandemic form of conjunctivitis that originated in Ghana in 1969 and swept across North Africa, Malaysia, Indonesia, India, Southeast Asia, Japan, and Taiwan (Hung and Kono 1979). (Epidemics of AHC have also been caused by Coxsackie virus A-24 infection, but no paralytic sequelae were observed in those cases [John et al. 1981]). The first report of a severe polio-like illness complicating AHC came from India (Wadia et al. 1973), and by 1976 there were 76 published cases (Hung et al. 1976). This is a very small proportion of the millions of patients who have had AHC, but milder forms of paralytic illness may have gone unrecognized. Recently, enterovirus 70 has been isolated from patients with AHC in Florida, suggesting that this new paralytic disease may soon appear in Western countries (Hatch et al. 1981).

The neurologic illness, which comes on 1 to 5 weeks after the conjunctivitis, consists of an aseptic meningitis, lancinating and paresthetic pains in the legs, and rapidly progressive lower motor neuron weakness involving the legs to a greater extent than the arms. The bulbar muscles may be affected (Thakur 1981; Katiyar et al. 1981), but respiratory weakness is mild and infrequent. The muscle involvement is asymmetrical and predominantly proximal in the extremities; as in true poliomyelitis, the reflexes are depressed or lost in weak muscles, muscle wasting appears quickly, and prolonged or permanent disability is common. (Nearly two thirds of the Indian patients with paralytic symptoms remained handicapped 10 years later [Wadia et al. 1981].) A few patients have regional sensory deficits, sphincter disturbances, or extensor plantar responses, but these manifestations are transient. EMG has confirmed the presence of acute denervation, with fibrillations and diminished recruitment of motor units, but no fasciculations have been seen. Velocity of motor nerve conduction has been normal in almost all cases. These clinical and electrophysiologic findings are compatible with a myelitis predominantly affecting the ventral gray matter. Because of the sensory symptoms some authors have suggested that a radiculitis might also be present, but no autopsy studies have been reported.

Other Infections

A mild paralytic illness has been described in a few cases of meningitis caused by mumps (Lennette et al. 1960), adenovirus 7 (Combined Scottish Study 1961), and herpes simplex (Magoffin et al. 1961b). A case attributed to infectious mononucleosis was probably an example of brachial neuritis (Mukherjee 1965). Focal flaccid paralysis is also a recognized complication of several arbovirus infections including St. Louis encephalitis, California encephalitis, and tick-borne Central European and Russian spring-summer encephalitides (Holmgren et al. 1959). In these cases the paralysis is usually transient, and cerebral symptoms are much more prominent.

Recently there have been several reports of a "poliomyelitis-like illness" in children during an acute exacerbation of bronchial asthma. No infectious agent has been incriminated, and the clinical and electrophysiologic findings are more compatible with a radiculoplexitis than a poliomyelitis. This syndrome is discussed in Chapter 5.

Late Progression of Muscle Weakness Following Poliomyelitis

For more than a century it has been recognized that some persons with old polio develop progressive muscular weakness and atrophy many years after the original acute illness. The syndrome is not rare, though only a small proportion of patients with old polio appear to be affected. These cases have given rise to considerable speculation. Some authors regard the association as coincidental and attribute the late motor neuron disease to amyotrophic lateral sclerosis (ALS); for others, the disorder is a special form of motor neuron disease with a more benign prognosis than ALS (Campbell et al. 1969; Mulder et al. 1972). Still other authors attribute the progressive weakness to the effects of aging on surviving motor neurons (Hayward and Seaton 1979; Wiechers and Hubbell 1981), or of prolonged stress on weakened muscles (Drachman et al. 1967) and unstable joints (Anderson et al. 1972). Each of these explanations may be correct in some cases, but the preponderance of evidence suggests that the major cause of late progression of weakness in old polio is a motor neuron degeneration that differs in several respects from typical ALS.

Campbell and colleagues (1969) reviewed 83 published cases of this syndrome and presented 6 cases of their own, while Mulder and associates (1972) reported 34 patients examined personally at the Mayo Clinic between 1942 and 1970. From these accounts, a fairly consistent picture emerges. The majority of the patients (74 to 92 percent) are men. The original attack of acute poliomyelitis usually takes place in early childhood, and the time elapsed before the onset of new weakness averages 37 years (a range of 8 to 65 years). The new weakness appears insidiously in one of several muscles, accompanied by muscle atrophy and fasciculations, often in limbs or muscles not previously impaired by the old polio. EMG shows signs of recent denervation (fibrillations) in the newly affected muscles. About one fifth of the patients have Babinski's signs, but there is usually no spasticity or heightening of reflexes, and sensation is normal. The course is generally much more gradual than in typical ALS, in which the median length of survival is less than 3 years; in the Mayo Clinic series the patients were followed for an average of 12 years after the onset of weakness, yet only one patient died from neuromuscular causes.

A few patients do have a rapidly fatal course. Some of those patients could have coincidental ALS (as illustrated by a recent autopsied case [Roos et al. 1980]), but the patient reported on by Steegman (1937) probably did not have ALS. She was 20 years old at the onset of progressive muscular atrophy, 17 years after having acute poliomyelitis, yet she died from respiratory paralysis 2 years later. At autopsy there were no inflammatory changes in the spinal cord; the anterior horns showed widespread degeneration of motor nerve cells and pronounced gliosis, but the corticospinal tracts were normal.

The cause of late motor neuron degeneration after old polio is completely unknown. There is no pathologic evidence of an active viral infection, and CSF antibodies to poliovirus and other viruses are not increased (Kurent et al. 1979). One theory attributes the syndrome to a "normal" dropout of motor neurons with advancing age, producing an exaggerated effect in patients with old polio because even their strong muscles are supplied by a depleted pool of motor neurons (Hayward and Seaton 1979). Furthermore, the surviving motor neurons, which have enlarged their terminal ramifications by sprouting to reinnervate denervated muscle fibers, carry an extra metabolic burden in maintaining this enlarged motor unit territory. In support of this hypothesis, Wiechers and Hubbell (1981) found increased jitter in single-fiber EMG recordings from persons with old polio, the abnormalities being greater the longer the time since the attack of polio. There are several clinical observations, however, that weigh against this explanation: the random involvement of muscles, often attacking strong muscles rather than weak ones, although the former are supplied by many fewer motor neurons; the fact that many patients are under 40 and some are under 30 years of age when late amyotrophy begins; the relentless progression of weakness once it begins; and the presence of Babinski's signs in some patients. Furthermore, EMG in patients with severe but stable residual weakness does not show active denervation (fibrillations) as late as 50 years after the original acute illness (Hayward and Seaton 1979; Lutschg and Ludin 1981). Mulder and associates (1972) pointed out that the syndrome resembles ALS in most respects except for the better prognosis and the relative paucity of pyramidal tract signs in the former disease, and they suggested that ALS itself could be the result of an acute viral infection early in life. This may be true, but so far there is no compelling evidence for a persistent viral infection in either disease (Rowland 1982).

Herpes Zoster

Primarily an infection of sensory nerves and skin, herpes zoster produces focal muscle weakness in about 5 percent of cases (Thomas and Howard 1972). Paralysis of cranial motor nerves accounts for nearly half of this group, and most of the other cases of weakness are in one arm or leg; thoracoabdominal weakness is either rare or (more likely) difficult to detect (Kendall 1957; Gupta et al. 1969). Thus, weakness is found in 12 to 22 percent of patients with zoster involving dermatomes C5 to T1 or L2 to S1, but in only 0.3 percent of cases with zoster of T2 to L1 (Thomas and Howard 1972).

CLINICAL FEATURES. The skin eruption either precedes the onset of weakness or appears concurrently; the interval can be less than 1 day or as long as 3 months, but is generally less than a month. In the limbs and trunk the rash and the weakness are always on the same side, and there is a fairly close correspondence between the cutaneous segments and the myotomes involved, though occasionally there is a discrepancy of several spinal segments. The motor deficit is usually in the distribution of one or two adjacent nerve roots and rarely may involve the entire nerve supply of one limb. A patchy diminution and distortion of sensation is often present in the affected dermatomes, and the corresponding reflexes are depressed or absent.

Once detected, weakness reaches a maximum within a few days. The severity of weakness is usually not uniform in the muscles supplied by the involved spinal segments. Recovery begins some weeks later and is generally very slow, so that it may take more than a year before the extent of the permanent deficits can be assessed. Follow-up studies show that complete recovery of muscle power occurs in 50 to 70 percent of patients; about 15 percent of patients do not improve (Gupta et al. 1969; Thomas and Howard 1972; Molloy and Goodwill 1979; Gardner-Thorpe et al. 1976).

CRANIAL MOTOR NEUROPATHIES. Isolated facial nerve paralysis is the most common motor complication of herpes zoster. Zoster, in turn, is present in 5 to 10 percent of patients with Bell's palsy (Mair and Flugsrud 1976). About half of these patients have otic zoster, with vesicles on the tympanum, the external ear canal, the outer surface of the ear, the anterior pillar of the fauces, or the junctional zone between the ear and the mastoid bone. These areas represent the cutaneous sensory territory of the facial nerve. In the remaining patients the rash lies either in the two upper cervical dermatomes or on the face. Taste is often impaired over the anterior tongue owing to involvement of the chorda tympani nerve, and there are sometimes auditory or vestibular symptoms caused by eighth nerve involvement. Paralysis of one or more of the oculomotor nerves occurs in about 4 percent of patients with opthalmic-division zoster, sometimes in company with facial paralysis. Paralysis of bulbar cranial nerves, an even more uncommon complication, occurs in association with facial zoster (Thomas and Howard 1972).

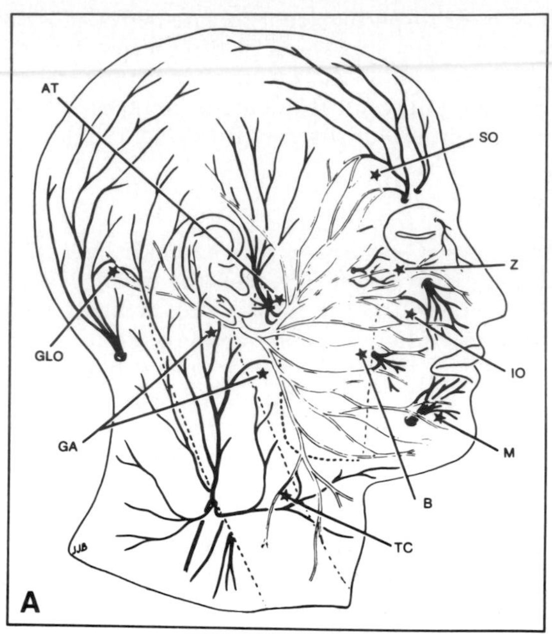

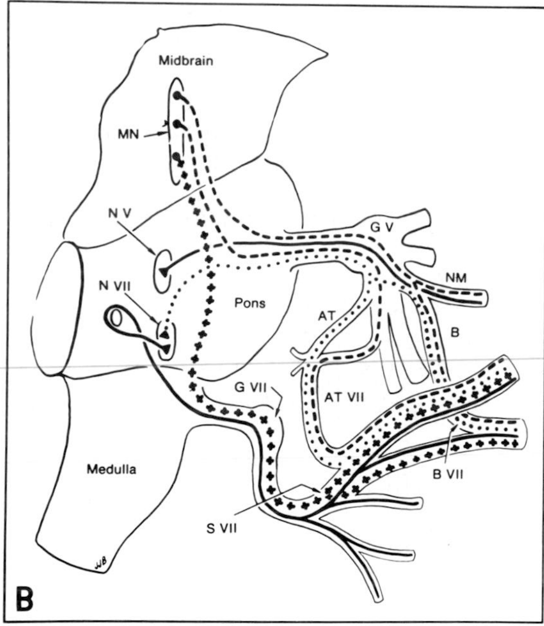

FIGURE 18. Communications of facial nerve with trigeminal and cervical nerves. (*A*) The superficial communications of the facial nerve (white outline) and the trigeminal and cervical nerves (solid black) are depicted. The communicating sensory nerves are denoted by the following abbreviations: AT, auriculotemporal; B, buccal; GA, greater auricular; GLO, greater and lesser occipital; IO, infraorbital; M, mental; SO, supraorbital; TC, transverse cervical; Z, zygomatic.

(*B*) The deep communications of the motor fibers of the seventh and fifth cranial nerves (solid and dotted lines) and the afferent fibers for proprioception and deep sensibility (dashed and crossed lines) are depicted. AT, auriculotemporal nerve. B, buccal nerve. AT VII, communicating ramus of auriculotemporal with facial nerve. B VII, communicating ramus of buccal with facial nerve. GV, trigeminal ganglion. G VII, geniculate ganglion. NM, nerves to muscles of mastication. MN, mesencephalic (sensory) nucleus of trigeminal nerve. NV, motor nucleus of trigeminal nerve. N VII, motor nucleus of facial nerve. S VII, superior division of facial nerve. (From Baumel, 1974, with permission.)

PATHOLOGY. Herpes zoster is thought to be a reactivation of a latent infection of the dorsal root ganglia with varicella-zoster virus, but the anatomic pathways by which motor nerves become involved is still unclear. Based on a few autopsy studies, it is thought that the inflammatory process extends from the dorsal root ganglion into the posterior horn of the spinal cord, causing a unilateral, segmental, posterior and anterior poliomyelitis and leptomeningitis. In addition, inflammatory cell infiltration may involve the ventral (motor) root, probably by contiguous spread from the adjacent dorsal root ganglion, and patchy inflammation may extend throughout the length of the peripheral nerve (Denny-Brown et al. 1944). Thus, the lower motor neuron may be damaged at any place along its length, from the spinal cord to the muscle. The occasional lack of correspondence between the dermatomal distribution of the rash and the involved motor segments could be a result of longitudinal spread of the infection within the ventral gray matter.

The anatomic basis of cranial motor neuropathies is harder to account for. An important clinical clue is the fact that oculomotor nerve paralyses are associated only with zoster of the ophthalmic division of the trigeminal nerve, while facial palsy occurs with skin eruptions in the sensory territory of either the seventh nerve, the trigeminal nerve, or the upper two cervical nerves. As Gupta and associates (1969) suggested, the anatomic link between the sensory and motor nerve fibers in these cases could be proprioceptive or other sensory fibers supplying the muscles. The sensory fibers of the ocular muscles are derived from the ophthalmic division of the trigeminal nerve; infection of the sensory ganglion could spread down these sensory nerve fibers into the adjacent third, fourth, or sixth motor nerves. Similarly, some of the sensory nerve fibers that supply the facial muscles are derived from the trigeminal nerve (and presumably from the upper cervical nerves in the case of the platysma muscle); these sensory nerve fibers communicate with the facial nerve via auriculotemprol, buccal, and other extracranial connections (Fig. 18) (Baumel 1974). Thus, varicella-zoster infection of the trigeminal or cervical ganglia could spread distally along sensory nerve fibers to contact the adjacent motor branches of the facial nerve, and involvement of the chorda tympani and eighth cranial nerves could be due to contiguous spread from the adjacent facial nerve.

TREATMENT. A 3-week course of corticosteroid therapy, given soon after onset of the rash, reduces the duration of postherpetic neuralgia in patients aged 60 years or more (Eaglestein et al. 1970) and does not appear to spread or disseminate the infection. There is no information about the effect of steroid therapy on the incidence or severity of motor complications. Steroid therapy is commonly used in idiopathic Bell's palsy, where there is evidence that treatment within 72 hours reduces the incidence of permanent motor sequelae. Facial paralysis owing to zoster is generally treated the same way, although there is no published evidence that it is effective. The hypothetical rationale for early steroid therapy in Bell's palsy is to prevent nerve compression by inflammatory edema in the facial canal. There is no clear rationale for using steroids to prevent postherpetic neuralgia, but the fact that it seems to work suggests that the inflammatory component of zoster may have deleterious effects. Thus, an argument could be made for undertaking a controlled trial of steroid therapy in patients with paralytic zoster, but until this is done steroid therapy cannot be recommended solely for the prevention of motor sequelae.

Rabies

It is not widely realized that about 20 percent of patients with rabies do not exhibit the classic signs of "furious" rabies, which are encephalitic manifestations, but present with a rapidly spreading paralysis very similar to the Guillain-Barré syndrome. The epithets of "dumb rabies" and "paralytic rabies" have been applied to this syndrome. Actually, even in furious rabies limb paralysis of lower motor neuron origin develops eventually in many patients (Warrell 1976). Although rabies is now rare in most developed countries, it is important for physicians to be aware of the existence of paralytic rabies, because medical personnel who handle these patients may need to be given immunoprophylaxis (Lamas et al. 1980).

CLINICAL FEATURES. In paralytic rabies, the incubation period can range from 7 to 90 days following an animal bite, but there is no history of a bite in about 20 percent of cases. Pain and paresthesias at the site of the animal bite are soon followed by weakness of the same limb, and then by rapid spread of weakness to other limbs; in some patients, however, weakness affects all four limbs simultaneously. There may be fever and headache, but meningeal signs are usually slight. Fasciculations may be seen, the muscle stretch reflexes disappear, and extensor plantar responses are sometimes found, but sensation is usually preserved. As the flaccid paralysis ascends, respiratory and bulbar paralysis develops. In most cases the mental state remains clear until late in the course, but anxiety, shivering, or excitement may be seen, and tachycardia is frequently present. Without mechanical ventilation, patients die in 7 to 11 days; with support they may live a few weeks longer, but the outcome is the same as in the encephalitic form of rabies. Only two patients are alleged to have survived rabies encephalomyelitis (Hattwick et al. 1972; Porras et al. 1976); in those cases the diagnosis was unproven, and the clinical course was more suggestive of allergic encephalomyelitis.

LABORATORY FINDINGS. In a recent series the CSF was examined in 10 patients: 2 had normal results and the others showed pleocytosis, raised protein, or both abnormalities (Chopra et al. 1980). A lymphocytic pleocytosis of up to 950 cells and protein increases up to 350 mg per dl have been reported in ordinary rabies. The glucose content of CSF remains normal (Warrell 1976). In two unvaccinated patients with rabies accompanied by limb paralysis, EMG on day 11 and day 14 showed no voluntary or spontaneous electrical activity in the paralyzed muscles, and peripheral nerve excitability was greatly reduced. A week later there were fibrillations on EMG, and all nerves were inexcitable in both patients (Prier et al. 1979). These results suggested that the peripheral nerves were directly involved, since pure anterior horn cell disease does not usually alter peripheral nerve excitability in such a short time. These are the only electrophysiologic studies that have been reported in paralytic rabies.

PATHOPHYSIOLOGY. Recently Chopra and colleagues (1980) undertook a thorough pathologic study of the central and peripheral nervous system in 11 patients with paralytic rabies. The findings in the central nervous system were the same as those in the encephalitic form of rabies, except that in the paralytic cases the inflammatory changes and neuronal degeneration were concentrated in the spinal cord, especially the lumbar and lower dorsal segments, and were most severe in the ventral horns. Less severe inflammatory and neuronal changes were present in the dorsal root ganglia and medulla, and mild, focal changes were sometimes found elsewhere in the brain. In classical rabies the inflammatory process is most prominent in the thalamus, hypothalamus, cerebellum, limbic system, cerebral cortex, and brainstem, although the spinal cord is also affected.

These findings were the same as others have described, but of greater interest were the changes in the peripheral nervous system. The spinal nerve roots all showed some degree of wallerian degeneration, but the peripheral nerves showed axonal degeneration in only four of the eleven cases, suggesting that wallerian degeneration in the nerve roots was due to anterior horn cell destruction but had not yet extended beyond the roots in most cases (the patients having survived only 7 to 11 days). In every case, however, examination of teased fibers from the peripheral nerves showed segmental demyelination and remyelination, and in half of the nerves this was the major abnormality. Inflammation was observed in one nerve root but not in the peripheral nerves. These findings prompted Chopra and colleagues to suggest that the peripheral nerve lesions reflected a primary demyelinative neuropathy caused by an autoimmune reaction akin to the Guillain-Barré syndrome.

Until now it has been assumed that paralytic rabies is due to viral anterior poliomyelitis (Lancet editorial 1978). However, the electrophysiologic abnormalities reported by Prier and associates (1979) raise the possibility of a widespread peripheral neuropathy; those authors interpreted their findings as evidence of an axonal process, but an acute demyelinative polyneuropathy, if sufficiently severe, would give the same results. It is interesting that rabies immunization may predispose to the development of the paralytic rather than the encephalitic form of the disease (Warrell 1976; Chopra et al. 1980). Rabies-specific antibody has also been shown to cause a paradoxical shortening of the incubation period in human patients (Chopra et al. 1980) and in experimental animals (Prabhakar and Nathanson 1981). Whether the polyneuropathy of paralytic rabies is caused by spread of the viral infection throughout the peripheral nervous system or by an autoimmune process cannot be determined without further viral and immunologic studies.

DIFFERENTIAL DIAGNOSIS. Paralytic rabies may initially be difficult to distinguish from an allergic polyneuritis caused by prophylactic immunization. The incidence of paralytic reactions is about 1:32,000 for duck embryo vaccine; only one case has been reported so far following vaccination with the new human diploid cell rabies vaccine (Bøe and Nyland 1980). Postimmunization polyneuritis usually begins within 3 weeks of the first dose of vaccine (Adaros and Held 1971), while the incubation period for rabies is ordinarily longer, but two of the patients reported by Chopra and colleagues (1980) became ill 7 and 12 days after exposure to rabies; both had received rabies vaccine but had rabies at autopsy. A rapid fluorescent technique for measuring serum antibodies against rabies is now available, but this test does not unequivocally distinguish rabies from a reaction to immunization. It is sometimes possible to identify rabies antigen by immunofluorescence studies of corneal smears taken from patients during life (Miller and Nathanson 1977)

TREATMENT. The treatment of persons exposed to known rabies consists of passive immunization with rabies immune globulin and active immunization with some type of rabies vaccine. Until recently the decision whether to give immune prophylaxis to persons exposed to possible rabies was weighed very carefully, because of the high incidence of allergic reactions to antirabies horse serum and to the duck embryo vaccine (Corey and Hattwick 1975). However, the introduction of human rabies immune globulin and of a highly effective rabies vaccine prepared in human diploid cell cultures (Anderson et al. 1980) has virtually eliminated such risks, leaving only questions of expense and inconvenience. Widespread availability of the new preparations should lessen the public fear of rabies prophylaxis and encourage victims of animal bites to seek medical attention sooner.

PROTOZOAN INFECTIONS

Toxoplasmosis

In recent years there has been considerable interest in the role played by toxoplasmosis in the pathogenesis of inflammatory muscle disease. Toxoplasmosis is a worldwide infection of man and many other mammals and birds. The intracellular protozoan parasite Toxoplasma gondii remains alive in animal tissues for long periods of time, especially in skeletal muscle, so that human infection can occur from eating undercooked meat. Other sources of primary infection in healthy persons (other than congenital infection) are uncertain, but may include oocysts shed into the soil in cat feces (Frenkel and Ruiz 1981). Cases of disseminated toxoplasmosis, with symptoms primarily affecting the central nervous system, are being seen increasingly in immunologically compromised patients (Gleason and Hamlin 1974; Townsend and Wolinsky 1975).

Acute Toxoplasma Myositis

While there is a high prevalence of inapparent infection in many human populations, cases of acute, noncongenital toxoplasmosis are documented infrequently. The clinical picture consists of fever, lymphadenopathy, and myalgia, sometimes with sore throat, a maculopapular skin rash, hepatosplenomegaly, and meningoencephalitis. In a few patients the clinical picture includes generalized muscle pain and weakness resembling polymyositis. Of the four cases of this type that have been reported (Rowland and Greer 1961; Chandar et al. 1968; McNicholl and Underhill 1970; Pollock 1979), three involved boys 7 to 12 years old and the fourth a 33-year-old man. Over a period of several weeks the patients experienced fever, malaise, myalgia, lymphadenopathy, sore throat, and generalized weakness. Two patients had a transient skin rash on the trunk, and one presented with skin changes on the face, elbows, and knees as well as Gottron's papules on the knuckles, a picture reminiscent of dermatomyositis (Pollock 1979). There was diffuse muscle weakness of the trunk and limbs, greater in the proximal than the distal muscles. The muscles were diffusely tender, and in two patients some muscles were swollen. The muscle stretch reflexes were depressed but sensation was normal. One patient had a mild meningoencephalitis and hepatosplenomegaly. The serum activity of muscle enzymes was markedly elevated in two patients, moderately elevated in another, and normal in one patient who was improving. EMG, performed in two patients, showed myopathic abnormalities, with fibrillations in one case. A muscle biopsy was obtained in three patients; light microscopic examination showed no abnormality in two of these, and in another patient there were mild abnormalities consisting of focal areas of muscle fiber degeneration, round cell infiltration, and fibroblastic activity. In all the patients there were high and changing titers of toxoplasma antibodies, and specific IgM antibody was demonstrated in the most recent case, but no organisms were identified in the muscle. All the patients recovered completely: two patients recovered in 4 to 6 months without treatment, one recovered in 6 months after a 4-week course of pyrimethamine and sulfadimidine, and one recovered soon after a brief course of sulfadiazine and pyrimethamine that had to be stopped because of a drug reaction.

Toxoplasmosis in Patients with Polymyositis

In several other cases toxoplasmosis was associated with myositis but the relationship was less clear-cut. Hendrickx and coworkers (1979) described an 8-year-old boy with classic dermatomyositis of 9 months' duration, well documented by EMG and muscle biopsy although the serum CPK activity was only slightly elevated. Toxoplasma antibody titers were high, but specific IgM antibody was not found. No organisms were detected by light microscopy of routinely stained muscle sections, but a fluorescent antibody technique showed free toxoplasma organisms. Under treatment with prednisone, methotrexate, pyrimethamine, and sulfadiazine the patient improved slowly, eventually developing subcutaneous calcification. In this case it is difficult to be confident that active toxoplasmosis was present or, if present, that it was the cause of the dermatomyositis. Similarly, a 49-year-old woman reported by Samuels and Rietschel (1976) seems to have had classic polymyositis, with Raynaud's phenomenon and absent peristalsis of the lower esophagus. After 6 months of steroid therapy, she became ill, and toxoplasma antibody titers, obtained for the first time, were found to be high. The titers eventually came down during treatment with sulfadiazine and pyrimethamine, but the muscle weakness persisted. In this case it can be argued that toxoplasmosis did not begin until after 6 months of steroid treatment, which had made the patient susceptible to a new or reactivated toxoplasma infection. In another case (Karasawa et al. 1981), toxoplasma myositis was identified at autopsy in a patient with angioimmunoblastic lymphadenopathy, but serologic evidence indicated that infection occurred secondarily, during immunosuppressive therapy.

The case of a 44-year-old woman described by Topi and colleagues (1979) is even harder to classify. She had an indolent, 3-year illness with a skin rash said to resemble that of dermatomyositis, myalgia, arthralgia, and muscle wasting; her muscle strength was not described. Laboratory abnormalities included eosinophilia, a high sedimentation rate, increased IgG in the serum, a positive rheumatoid factor, high toxoplasma antibody titers, and normal serum levels of CPK. EMG suggested the presence of a myopathy, and muscle biopsy showed myositis as well as numerous free and encysted toxoplasma organisms, confirmed both by immunofluorescence and by inoculation into mice. Treatment with pyrimethamine and sulfadiazine led to resolution of the clinical and laboratory abnormalities. This patient undoubtedly had toxoplasmosis, but was the 3-year illness caused by toxoplasmosis, or did she have an unrelated collagen-vascular disease complicated by toxoplasmosis?

Finally, Greenlee and associates (1975) described the remarkable case of a 60-year-old man with a gradual onset of fever, muscle "cramps," incoordination, and confusion. He showed ataxia of station and gait, ataxic limb movements, widespread fasciculations, Babinski's sign, diminished reflexes, and diminished vibration sense in the legs. There was eosinophilia and a very high sedimentation rate, and the EEG was diffusely slow. Although there was no muscle weakness or tenderness, the serum CPK activity was markedly increased; muscle biopsy showed areas of muscle cell necrosis and inflammation with scattered muscle fiber atrophy and target fibers suggesting denervation, and EMG showed a diffuse neurogenic disorder with evidence of a motor and sensory polyneuropathy. Toxoplasma antibody titers were elevated in the serum and CSF; the CSF was acellular but the protein was 77 mg per dl with 27 percent gamma globulin. Toxoplasma cysts were demonstrated in the muscle biopsy (Fig. 19). Treatment with sulfadiazine and pyrimethamine for 3 months was followed by a steady improvement of the clinical and laboratory abnormalities, but subsequently there was a protracted, relapsing course requiring more antitoxoplasma drug treatment, to which the clinical response was less clear-cut. In this patient, proven toxoplasmosis was associated with a diffuse disorder of the central and peripheral nervous systems and with an inflammatory, necrotizing myopathy. The apparent response to treatment suggests that all of these abnormalities may have been due to toxoplasmosis, but it is difficult to believe that direct infection was responsible for the polyneuropathy, which has not been reported to occur in toxoplasmosis. An alternative explanation is that the neurologic disorders were caused by an autoimmune reaction triggered by toxoplasmosis.

Autoimmune mechanisms have not been discussed in previous accounts of toxoplasmosis. However, in five of the eight cases cited above there were skin changes or other features reminiscent of a collagen-vascular disease, and in four cases toxoplasmosis occurred without preceding steroid therapy. An autoimmune mechanism could explain why toxoplasma organisms have rarely been identified in muscle biopsies from patients with polymyositis complicating toxoplasmosis. In this regard it is interesting that toxoplasma organisms were found postmortem in skeletal muscle in only one of five patients dying with disseminated toxoplasmosis, though organisms were numerous in brain, heart, and lungs (Gleason and Hamlin 1974).

What is the role of toxoplasmosis in ordinary cases of idiopathic inflammatory myopathy? Kagen and coworkers (Kagen et al. 1974; Phillips et al. 1979) examined the prevalence of serum antibodies to toxoplasma in

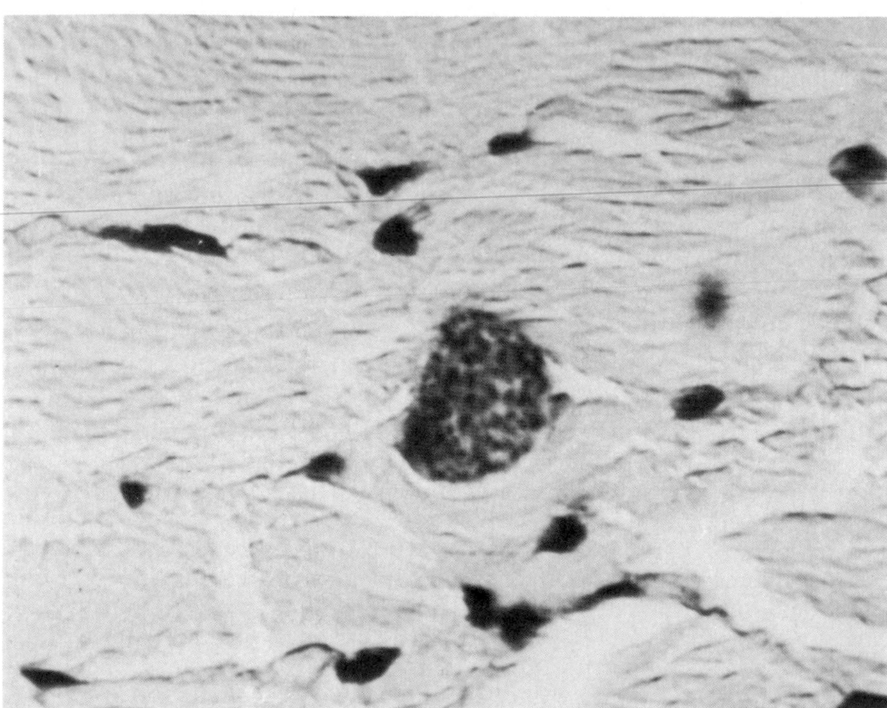

FIGURE 19. Toxoplasma myositis. Encysted Toxoplasma gondii organisms are seen in an area of intact muscle fibers (hematoxylin and eosin). (From Greenlee et al., 1975, with permission.)

patients with polymyositis, dermatomyositis, or myositis complicating connective tissues disease, compared with a matched group of patients with unrelated diseases. Of 20 patients with polymyositis, 35 percent had complement-fixing antibodies, compared to 4 percent of controls, and the mean titer of complement-fixing antibodies was increased in the myositis patients. Although Sabin-Feldman (SF) dye-test antibodies were prevalent in all groups, 30 percent of polymyositis patients had titers of 10 to 16 dilutions while only 3 percent of controls had titers as high as 10 dilutions. High SF antibody titers were also found in 3 of 24 patients with dermatomyositis and in one of 25 patients with connective tissue disease. None of the 10 children under age 16 (including seven patients with dermatomyositis) had increased SF antibody titers; if the children are excluded from the analysis, high SF titers were present in 32 percent of adults with polymyositis, in 18 percent of adults with dermatomyositis, and in 3 percent of adult controls. There was no indication of a nonspecific increase of antibodies in these patients, since the titers of viral antibodies were not increased. These results suggest that a significant proportion of adult patients with idiopathic inflammatory myopathy have had a recent toxoplasma infection. However, it is still not clear whether toxoplasmosis is a cause or a result of the disease, or a result of the treatment. Until this question is settled, serologic tests for toxoplasmosis should probably be performed in the initial workup of all patients with idiopathic inflammatory myopathy, and the serologies should be repeated periodically during immunosuppressive therapy. A trial of specific treatment for toxoplasmosis should be considered in patients who have serologic or pathologic evidence of toxoplasmosis.

HELMINTHIC INFECTIONS

Trichinosis

Trichinosis (or trichinellosis) is a subacute myositis resulting from infection with larvae of the nematode Trichinella spiralis, which enter the body through ingestion of infected meat or meat products. The disease is widely distributed throughout the world, but is most prevalent in North America, Central Europe, and the Arctic (Gould 1970). The most frequent source of infection is raw or undercooked pork, but lately there have been several cases caused by consumption of wild animal meat such as bear, walrus, and wild boar, and two large outbreaks have been traced to infected horse meat (Bellani et al. 1978; Bourée et al. 1979).

The parasites are ingested in the form of encysted larvae in meat; free larvae are released, by the action of digestive enzymes, into the lumen of the small intestine, where they reach sexual maturity and copulate. The resulting second generation of motile larvae is responsible for the major manifestations of the disease. Invading the lymphatic system of the intestine, larvae are disseminated through the blood stream, infecting the skeletal muscles and, to a much smaller extent, the myocardium, brain, skin, and retina. They do not survive long except in skeletal muscle, where they become intracellular parasites within muscle fibers and develop a protective cyst wall. The cysts start to calcify after a number of months, but the larvae may survive for years (Gould 1970).

CLINICAL FEATURES. The symptoms of trichinosis are traditionally divided into intestinal, invasive, and convalescent stages. The *intestinal stage,* when the first generation of female larvae penetrate the intestinal mucosa and reproduce, occupies the first week after infection; during this period gastrointestinal symptoms, malaise, and mild fever occur in a minor proportion of patients, ranging from 37 percent in severe cases to 7 percent in mild cases (Kassur et al. 1978).

The stage of *muscle invasion* by the second generation of larvae begins about 5 days after infection and may continue for several weeks as successive crops of larvae are hatched in the intestinal lumen. At 1 to 3 weeks after ingestion of the contaminated food, the major symptoms of the illness appear, many of which are due primarily to inflammatory and allergic reactions to the presence of larvae in the tissues. The most frequent manifestations are fever, myalgia, edema of the eyelids and face, headache, malaise, anorexia, arthralgia, chemosis of the bulbar conjunctivae, splinter hemorrhages in the nailbeds, itching, and a generalized macular or petechial skin rash. Muscle pain and tenderness, which may affect all of the voluntary musculature including the extraocular muscles, are sometimes accompanied by muscle swelling, induration, and weakness. There may be oculomotor weakness, and trismus from involvement of the chewing muscles is not infrequent. In severe cases there may be myocarditis, allergic pneumonitis, impairment of ventilation owing to involvement of the diaphragm and intercostal muscles, and rarely central nervous system manifestations such as confusion, stupor, focal cerebral signs, or seizures. A necrotizing arteritis resembling polyarteritis nodosa, with mononeuritis multiplex, has been reported in two patients with trichinosis who were negative for hepatitis B surface antigen but had extremely high levels of serum IgE (Frayha 1981).

During the second or third month the symptoms begin to subside, and *convalescence* continues for another 1 to 3 months, with complete recovery in the great majority of patients. Muscle contractures may require physical therapy, and a few patients complain of fatigue and rheumatic pains for years afterwards.

LABORATORY FINDINGS. Eosinophilia occurs in close to 100 percent of cases, generally appearing about 10 days after infection, reaching its highest point during the third or fourth week, and subsiding gradually over a period of months. The peak eosinophil count is generally 15 to 50 percent of the leukocyte count and may be even higher. Leukocytosis occurs in about two thirds of the cases, sometimes reaching counts of 20,000 to 50,000 per mm^3, so that the absolute eosinophil count can be very high indeed. The sedimentation rate is normal or only moderately increased. Serum IgM and IgE levels tend to increase transiently after the third week, while IgA and IgG levels are depressed (Rosenberg et al. 1974). Transient hypocalcemia occurs in 91 percent of cases (Bourée et al. 1979). The serum CPK activity is increased in 75 to 90 percent of patients, reaching a peak in the fourth to fifth week of infection with values 10 to 20 times the normal upper limit, and returning to normal during the next several months (Bourée et al. 1979: Kassur et al. 1978). Electromyography in severe cases reveals increased insertional activity, profuse fibrillations and positive waves, and myopathic changes in the recruitment pattern and in the individual motor unit potentials (Gross and Ochoa 1979). However, in a recent outbreak of mild to moderate severity, EMG showed myopathic abnormalities in only 4 of 52 patients (Bourée et al. 1979).

PATHOLOGY. Muscle biopsy shows clusters of neutrophils, plasma cells, lymphocytes, histiocytes, and eosinophils between muscle fibers and around small blood vessels. Necrotic muscle fibers tend to be located in the vicinity of an inflammatory focus and may be seen to be undergoing phagocytosis. Regenerating muscle fibers and an increase of interstitial connective tissue are seen in later stages (Drachman and Tunchay 1965). Trichinella larvae, either free or encysted depending on the duration of the infection, can sometimes be seen within muscle fibers, but larvae were detected in only 9 percent of biopsies taken from 32 patients with mild to moderate illness (Bourée et al. 1979). Gross and Ochoa (1979) observed that live larvae reacted with histochemical stains for NADH-tetrazolium reductase and myofibrillar ATPase.

DIAGNOSIS. The specific diagnostic tests consist of (1) microscopic examination of fresh or digested tissue, and (2) various serologic assays. Although larvae begin to invade muscle on the fifth day and continue to arrive for several weeks, only in very heavy infestations are larvae numerous enough to be detected in a muscle biopsy before the third or fourth week of infection. The simplest method for direct demonstration of larvae is by compression. A weighed sample of muscle (preferably taken near a tendinous insertion, where larvae are more numerous) is placed in normal saline at 5°C until used. Portions of the muscle are teased out, compressed between glass slides, and examined with a low-power microscope, so that the total number of larvae per gram of muscle can be estimated. This method is several times more sensitive than light microscopy of fixed tissue sections and gives more accurate information about the severity of the infestation.

Serologic tests begin to be positive in the third or fourth week of illness; they can remain positive for several years afterward, so that conversion from a negative to a positive reaction, or a rising titer, is more useful than one positive or negative reaction. (The trichinella intradermal skin test suffers from a high incidence of false negative and positive results and its use is not currently recommended.) Several serologic tests are in use; each of them is sometimes negative in proven cases, and many cross-react with other helminths or with Salmonella typhi and paratyphi. The indirect fluorescent antibody test detects IgM antibodies, while the complement fixation, bentonite flocculation, and latex agglutination tests detect IgG antibodies (Gould 1970).

TREATMENT. Despite the sometimes alarming manifestations of trichinosis, the overall mortality rate is low. In the United States during the decade 1947 to 1956 there were 3576 cases of trichinosis with a case fatality ratio of 2.3 percent, while in the decade 1966 to 1975 there were 1327 cases and the case fatality ratio was 1.0 percent (Juranek and Schultz 1978). In the USSR there were no deaths among 45 patients with severe trichinosis treated with corticosteroids (Klein 1978). However, severe infection can confine a patient to bed with unremitting pain for as long as 6 weeks, and the aftereffects may be noticeable for 6 months or longer. Fortunately, drugs are now available that reduce the incidence and ameliorate the symptoms of severe trichinosis.

Corticosteroid therapy suppresses many of the symptoms and signs of the invasive stage, which are probably due in large part to hyperimmunity. An initial daily dose of 40 to 60 mg prednisone generally brings rapid resolution or improvement of fever, myalgia, headache, facial edema, splinter hemorrhages, skin rash, pneumonitis, myocarditis, and cerebral symptoms. There has been some concern over the results of animal experiments showing that early steroid therapy increases the severity of the muscle infestation, by preventing the normal immunologic "rejection" of parasites during the intestinal stage of the disease. Human cases, however, usually present at a later stage, when the intestinal stage is ending (Gould 1970; Klein 1978). At any rate, the infection itself can now be controlled by one of the benzimidazole drugs, which are larvicidal both in the intestinal and invasive stages. Treatment of infected mice with thiabendazole for 2 weeks, beginning on day 21, reduced the number of larvae recovered from muscle by 62 to 96 percent, depending on the dose, and concomitant steroid treatment did not affect this result (Campbell and Blair 1978). In another study, mebendazole (Vermox, Ortho Pharmaceuticals) was given to infected mice in an oral dose of 3 mg per kg twice a day for 3 days, either 14 days or 28 days after infection. The number of larvae recovered from muscle was reduced by 75 and 86 percent, respectively, and all of the larvae that were recovered appeared to be dead (McCracken and Taylor 1980). This dosage schedule is essentially the same as that currently used for treating children and adults for pinworms, ascaris, and other intestinal nematode infestations, and it is very well tolerated.

While treatment with a larvicidal agent alone may aggravate the hyperimmune manifestations of trichinosis, the combination of steroids and a benzimidazole drug appears to be safe and efficacious. The benzimidazole drugs themselves have a mild anti-inflammatory effect in illness of mild to moderate severity, even without steroid therapy (Bourée et al. 1979).

Cysticercosis

A peculiar enlargement of the skeletal muscles has been reported in a total of 16 patients with generalized cysticercosis (Pallis and Lewis 1981). This complication is a minor and unusual feature of the disorder, compared with the well-known cerebral manifestations, which are an important cause of neurologic disability in Mexico, Africa, Asia, and Eastern Europe.

Cysticercosis occurs when man becomes an *intermediate* host in the life cycle of the pork tapeworm, Taenia solium. Ordinarily man functions as the *primary* host, becoming infected by eating undercooked pork containing live, encysted larvae (cysticerci). The larvae mature to become hermaphroditic adults, which survive for up to 5 years in the lumen of the jejunum, periodically releasing eggs or gravid proglottids that may contain many thousands of eggs. In the normal cycle the eggs are discharged with the feces into the soil, where they are ingested by pigs; the eggs hatch in the pig's intestine, releasing embryo larvae that penetrate the intestinal wall and are disseminated via the blood stream to the skeletal muscles and other body tissues. In the pig's tissues the larvae encyst and eventually die, unless ingested by a human host, whereupon the cycle resumes. Man becomes an intermediate host *when he ingests the eggs produced by his own tapeworm.* As in the pig, the eggs release embryo larvae that invade the intestinal wall and are carried via the blood stream to various body tissues including brain and muscle. Separate crops of larvae are frequently present in the tissues as a result of repeated episodes of egg ingestion.

When encysted larvae die in body tissues, between 1 and 10 years after infection, a violent inflammatory response may ensue, with fever, myalgia, subjective weakness, and eosinophilia. These symptoms can be controlled with a course of steroid therapy, which is especially valuable for suppressing the periodic relapses of cysticercal meningoencephalitis. After death of the larvae the cysts gradually calcify and can then be detected by roentgenography, especially in the subcutaneous tissues.

Although some cysticerci are deposited in muscle, in man as in swine, the number of larvae is rarely large enough to cause muscle symptoms. Patients with diffuse muscle enlargement caused by cysticercosis have an extraordinarily dense infestation of the skeletal muscles (Fig. 20), so that at biopsy numerous distended cysts can be seen to bulge out of the incised muscle (Fig. 21). Surprisingly, there is little or no histologic evidence of inflammation in the adjacent muscle, and this finding is in keeping with the paucity of muscular symptoms. The typical history is a rather rapid enlargement of the skeletal muscles, starting locally and becoming generalized over a period of a few months, usually without muscle pain, tenderness, or weakness, and without fever or other systemic symptoms. Nodules are usually not palpable in the muscles but can be identified in the subcutaneous tissues (14 of 16 cases) or in the tongue (10 of 16 cases). The muscle cysts are not calcified at the time of presentation, but are easily found by biopsy of an enlarged muscle. Fourteen of the patients had epilepsy or other signs of cerebral involvement.

Despite the lack of tissue reaction to the muscle cysticerci, it has been suggested that muscle enlargement occurs not at the time of the original massive infestation but some years later, when the larvae begin to die and the cysts become intensely swollen (Jolly and Pallis 1971). The cuticle of parasitic helminth larvae is poorly antigenic, a property that helps to prolong the viability of larvae in the tissue phase so that the life cycle of the

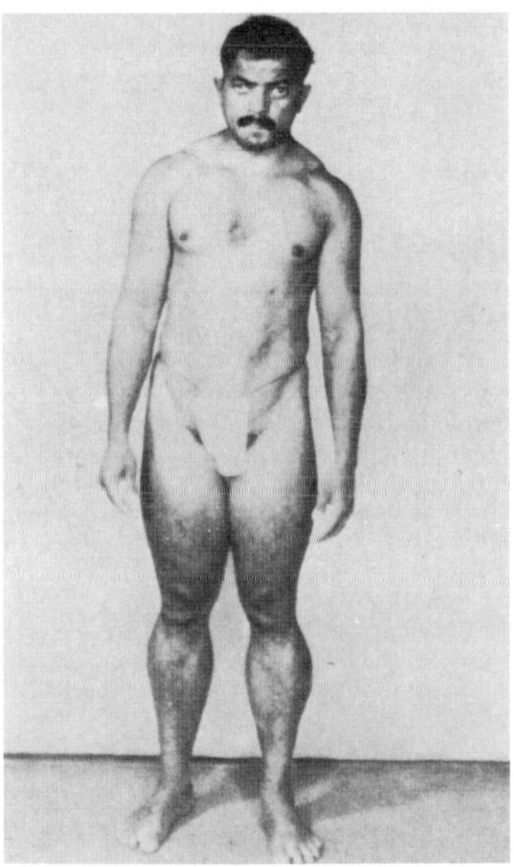

FIGURE 20. A patient with massive enlargement of muscles caused by cysticercosis. (From Jacob and Mathew, 1968, with permission.)

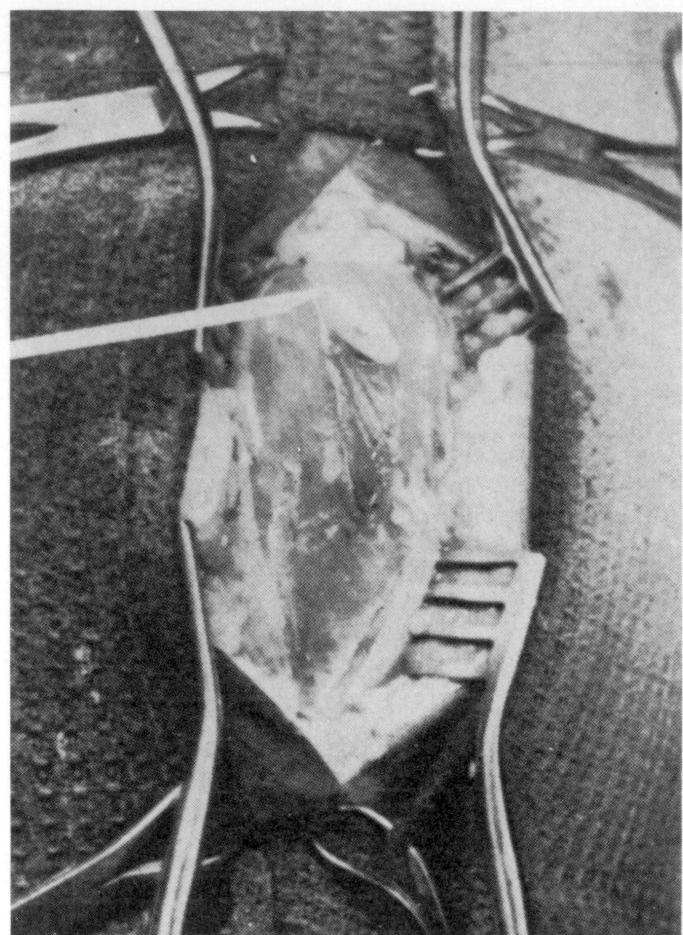

FIGURE 21. Muscle biopsy in a patient with cysticercosis. The pointer indicates a cyst lying free between muscle fibers. (From Jacob and Mathew, 1968, with permission.)

worm can continue. However, it is hard to explain why there should be so little local or systemic reaction to dying larvae in muscle, whereas patients without muscle enlargement commonly experience episodes of fever, myalgia, muscle tenderness, and eosinophilia in association with larval death. The viability of larvae recovered from muscle biopsies has not usually been examined, but viable larvae were mentioned in one case (McGill 1948), and in another case the anatomic details of the larval scolex were well preserved under microscopic examination (Jacob and Mathew 1968).

The prognosis of massive cysticercosis of muscle is not mentioned in the published reports. At the time of the initial studies, muscle enlargement had been present for up to 2 years, but none of the patients was followed beyond that time.

Muscle Masses Caused by Tapeworm Larvae

Hydatid cysts sometimes present as a slowly enlarging, tumor-like, deep muscle mass. In areas of the world where echinococcosis is endemic, these larval cysts may be the commonest cause of a benign muscle tumor. The mass is painless unless secondarily infected (Pallis and Lewis 1981). In the US there have been about 50 cases of *sparganosis* characterized by a solitary subcutaneous or superficial muscle cyst containing a tapeworm larva of the genus Spirometra. The resulting mass, which is a few centimeters in size, is sometimes tender and occasionally migrates slowly downward (Ali-Khan et al. 1973; Cho and Patel 1978).

BENIGN MYALGIC ENCEPHALOMYELITIS (EPIDEMIC NEUROMYASTHENIA)

The controversy over the existence or nonexistence of the disease variously termed benign myalgic encephalomyelitis, epidemic neuromyasthenia, and Iceland disease, has at times assumed the character of a religious war. While many physicians ardently espouse a concept of the disease as an infection involving the central nervous system and the muscles (Lyle and Chamberlain 1978), others attribute most of the manifestations to psychologic elaboration and hysterical contagion, unwittingly encouraged by medical personnel (McEvedy and Beard 1970b; May et al. 1980).

CLINICAL FEATURES. The clinical syndrome has been reviewed thoroughly in a recent symposium (Lyle and Chamberlain 1978). After a few days of symptoms resembling a viral upper respiratory or gastrointestinal infection, there are complaints of headache, muscle pain and tenderness, lethargy, subjective weakness, and fatigue. The fatigue is especially characteristic; a patient may start the day feeling fairly well, but after minor exertion feels exhausted and has to rest. Vertigo, tinnitus, diplopia, and photophobia are sometimes mentioned. Mental symptoms are almost invariably present, especially depression, irritability, weeping spells, mood swings, impaired concentration, and frequent nightmares.

On the initial physical examination there may be minor signs of a viral illness such as red throat, adenopathy, or conjunctival infection. Mild fever is present in a few patients, but meningeal signs have not been found. Muscle weakness of some kind is commonly described; often it is hemiplegic, monoplegic, or paraplegic, and sometimes it is generalized. Muscle atrophy is rarely mentioned. Coarse muscle twitches are seen but not true fasciculations. "Myoclonus" has been frequent in some epidemics. Muscle stretch reflexes are rarely altered even when profound weakness persists for months, and Babinski's signs have been reported in very few cases. Sensory complaints consist mostly of vague areas of dysesthesia and hyperesthesia, but on examination many patients demonstrate cutaneous sensory deficits in a stocking and glove pattern. Cranial nerve signs are uncommon, but ptosis, nystagmus, and facial weakness have been described. Retention of urine may occur, but confusion, dementia, and seizures have not been reported.

Laboratory abnormalities have been few and inconsistent. The CSF is almost always normal. Viral cultures have been negative except in a few instances, and positive isolations have not been confirmed by serologic tests. Routine hematology, blood chemistry, urinalysis, ECG, and radiography have been unrevealing. Minor EEG abnormalities were frequent in the Royal Free Hospital epidemic. EMG has been reported to show peculiar abnormalities of motor unit firing that experienced readers interpret as variations in voluntary effort, though these findings were claimed to be objective evidence of muscle disease (Lyle and Chamberlain 1978). Other EMG abnormalities, such as fibrillations or abnormal configuration of motor unit potentials, have rarely been seen. Motor nerve conduction velocity is normal. In a recent epidemic, 12 of 14 acute-phase sera were anticomplementary, suggesting the possible presence of circulating immune complexes (Dillon et al. 1974).

The most remarkable and controversial feature of the illness is the protracted convalescence. Many patients do not recover for several months, and a variable proportion run a relapsing course, suffering recurrent or heightened symptoms when they attempt normal activities. A few patients continue to be disabled for many years, although objective signs of neurologic disability remain absent.

About 30 epidemics of this type of illness have been reported since 1934, many of them involving nurses and other hospital personnel. In several instances there was a peculiar restriction of symptoms to a single group within an institution, sparing other persons who were also exposed to contagion. For example, during an epidemic at an Air Force hospital there were many cases among medical personnel but almost none among the hospital patients or among the nonmedical residents of the base barracks, where many of the affected medical personnel lived (Graybill et al. 1972). There is a preponderance of female cases, which is not surprising since several epidemics were confined to nurses' residences. Very young children have not been affected.

There is another peculiar characteristic of these epidemics: hardly any of the articles describing them were written by neurologists, and few of the neuromuscular evaluations were conducted by physicians experienced in neuromuscular diagnosis. This is true of recent as well as of older publications, and it is especially puzzling since the possibility that the neurologic findings might be spurious has been frequently discussed in the medical literature for over 20 years.

Comparison with Established Infectious Diseases

Myalgia is, as discussed earlier in this chapter, a frequent symptom in many viral infections, and it is especially severe in pleurodynia (epidemic myalgia), which may have a protracted, relapsing course. The enteroviruses that cause pleurodynia are also frequently responsible for aseptic meningitis and occasionally cause meningoencephalitis or polio-like illness. Epidemic vertigo has been reported in the setting of viral-like illness, with inflammatory changes in the CSF (Pedersen 1959). Postviral fatigue and depression are well known, especially following influenza, infectious hepatitis, and infectious mononucleosis. Thus, there is no difficulty in accepting the validity of the *symptoms* of myalgia, dizziness, fatigue, and postviral depression. The real stumbling blocks in these articles are (1) the peculiar lack of laboratory abnormalities, and (2) the reports of neurologic signs that evoke skeptical reactions among many neurologists.

Validity of Neurologic and Muscular Signs

The reported incidence of muscle weakness on examination varies widely in the different articles; it is present in the majority of cases in some epidemics and completely absent in others. In most reports there is a paucity of clinical detail regarding muscle tone, reflex changes, and tests for functional weakness, but in some reports it was noted that hemiplegia or paraplegia was almost never accompanied by the usual reflex changes expected in upper motor neuron lesions. Spurious muscle weakness is one of the most common hysterical manifestations, and muscle or joint pain may simulate weakness. There are well-known methods for attempting to distinguish genuine from spurious weakness, and the fact that most of the articles did not address this problem suggests that the examiners either did not consider the possibility that the weakness was spurious or did not know how to evaluate this possibility. In one outbreak the neurologic manifestations were regarded as hysterical, but the hysterical reaction was thought to be a physical effect of encephalitis. (Pool et al. 1961). In most cases in which EMG, nerve conduction velocities, and repetitive stimulation tests were done, the results were normal; but in the Royal Free Hospital epidemic an EMG pattern of intermittent volitional effort was misinterpreted as proof of an "organic" disorder, and this egregious error is still being offered in evidence 20 years later (Lyle and Chamberlain 1978). Recently, Ramsay and Rundle (1979) made much of the finding of elevated serum myoglobin levels, with normal CPK levels, in eight patients with chronic muscle fatigue of up to 35 years' duration, which the authors attributed to benign myalgic encephalomyelitis. Myoglobinemia without CPK elevation is a finding so improbable as to make laboratory error a much more likely explanation. All of these errors and omissions point to one conclusion: the authors of most of these reports were extremely naive with respect to neurologic and neuromuscular diagnosis.

Among the remaining neurologic abnormalities reported there is a preponderance of "soft" signs and a paucity of unambiguous ones. Nystagmus, deafness, hyperacusis, facial weakness, and ptosis were cited but not described, and there was no mention of solid findings such as oculomotor paralysis, unilateral facial paralysis, or other common manifestations of brain stem encephalitis or postinfectious demyelination. Electronystagmography was not performed, so the "nystagmus" could have been normal end-point nystagmus, and the "hyperacusis" was not documented by audiometric testing. Ptosis is a common hysterical manifestation, notorious for eliciting mistaken diagnoses of myasthenia gravis. Urinary retention was not documented by cystometry; it is another common hysterical symptom.

In summary, virtually all of the neurologic signs can be classified as either the kind that are frequently observed in hysteria, or the sort of normal finding that is frequently misinterpreted as abnormal by naive observers. Unambiguous clinical signs and confirmatory laboratory abnormalities, which are usually plentiful in cases of infectious or postinfectious encephalomyelitis, are conspicuously lacking. Under these circumstances it is not surprising that many physicians who have never seen patients with this syndrome are inclined to believe the views of McEvedy and Beard (1970a, 1970b) and May and associates (1980) that most of the epidemics were compounded of varying proportions of patient elaboration, medical self-deception, and invalid case ascertainment.

Does Benign Myalgic Encephalomyelitis Exist?

There is, however, a core of *symptoms* that is not so easy to dismiss. In the thoughtful account of the Great Ormond Street epidemic by Dillon and colleagues (1974), hardly any patients were considered to have objective neurologic signs, though the array of symptoms was much the same as in the other epidemics. The patients were seen early and repeatedly by one physician, who noted nonspecific signs of upper respiratory tract infection in many patients, but few other abnormalities. Although the physician made a deliberate attempt to reassure the patients, there was a protracted, relapsing course in about one fifth of the patients, lasting up to 1 year. I see no reason to doubt the validity of this epidemic, even though no infectious agent was isolated.

Schwartz and coworkers (1978) have recently described six patients with complaints of myalgia and excessive muscular fatigue lasting 1 or 2 years after a febrile, influenza-like illness. Neurologic examination was normal, with no weakness being found in any patient; the serum CPK levels were normal, while EMG and muscle biopsy showed minor, nonspecific abnormalities. The patients eventually recovered completely. The authors distinguished these cases from benign myalgic encephalomyelitis by the lack of central nervous system or psychiatric involvement and suggested that they had a benign form of polymyositis; but the clinical picture was much closer to the former syndrome.

Chronic, relapsing symptoms of fatigue, myalgia, fasciculation, and depression have been reported in a few patients following proven coxsackie virus infection (Innes 1970). Recently, seven patients with prolonged, relapsing symptoms resembling those of myalgic encephalomyelitis were found to have persistent elevation of serum IgM antibodies to the viral capsid antigen of Epstein-Barr virus (Tobi et al. 1982). They had vague symptoms of low-grade fever, malaise, emotional distress, gastrointestinal discomfort, myalgia, and weakness; some had lymphadenopathy, hepatomegaly, or mild splenomegaly, but liver function tests and other laboratory investigations gave normal results. The Paul-Bunnell test for infectious mononucleosis was negative in every case. The authors postulated that their patients had a persistent Epstein-Barr virus infection. This has not been proven, but persistent infection is a characteristic feature of the herpes family of viruses.

Thus, the clinical syndrome of benign myalgic encephalomyelitis seems to occur occasionally on a sporadic basis in several different viral infections, but whether there is a single epidemic illness of this type remains in dispute. If another epidemic surfaces, it would be desirable to have the patients evaluated by experts in the clinical and laboratory diagnosis of neuromuscular disease, in addition to the usual specialists in infectious disease, epidemiology, and psychiatry.

REFERENCES

Adaros, HL and Held, JR: *Guillain-Barré syndrome associated with immunization against rabies: Epidemiological aspects.* Proc Assoc Res Nerv Ment Dis 49:178–185, 1971.

Aderele, WI and Osinusi, K: *Pyomyositis in childhood.* J Trop Med Hyg 83:99–104, 1980.

Alajouanine, T, Thurel, R, Castaigne, P, et al: *Deux cas de sclerose laterale amyotrophique associee au tabes.* Rev Neurol 83:291–294, 1950.

Ali-Khan, Z, Irving, RT, Wignall N and Bowmer, EJ: *Imported sparganosis in Canada.* Can Med Assoc J 108:590–593, 1973.

Altrocchi, PH: *Spontaneous bacterial myositis.* JAMA 217:819–820, 1971.

Aminoff, MJ: *Electromyography in Clinical Practice.* Addison-Wesley Publishing, Menlo Park, California, 1978, pp 95–96.

Anderson, AD, Levine SA and Gellert, H: *Loss of ambulatory ability in patients with old anterior poliomyelitis.* Lancet ii:1061–1063, 1972.

Anderson, LJ, Winkler, WG, Hafkin, B, et al: *Clinical experience with a human diploid cell rabies vaccine.* JAMA 244:781–784, 1980.

Armstrong, JH: *Tropical pyomyositis and myoglobinuria.* Arch Intern Med 138: 1145–1146, 1978.

Arnon, SS: *Infant botulism.* Ann Rev Med 31:541–560, 1980.

Atrachki, SA and Wilson, DH: *Who is likely to get tetanus?* Br Med J 1:179, 1977.

BALL, AP, HOPKINSON, RB, FARRELL, ID, ET AL: *Human botulism caused by* Clostridium botulinum *type E: The Birmingham outbreak.* Q J Med 48:473–491, 1979.

BARDELAS, JA, WINKELSTEIN, JA, SETO, DSY, ET AL: *Fatal ECHO 24 infection in a patient with hypogammaglobulinemia: Relationship to dermatomyositis-like syndrome.* J Pediat 90:396–399, 1977.

BARKER, LF: *Acute syphilitic anterior poliomyelopathic syndrome: Report of a case.* Arch Neurol Psychiat 49:118–119, 1943.

BARRETT, AM AND GRESHOM, GA: *Acute streptococcal myositis.* Lancet i:347–351, 1958.

BAUMEL, JJ: *Trigeminal-facial nerve communications.* Arch Otolaryngol 99:34–44, 1974.

BELLANI, L, MANTOVANI, A, PAMPIGLIONE, S, ET AL: *Observations on an outbreak of human trichinellosis in northern Italy.* In KIM, CW AND PAWLOWSKI, ZS (EDS): *Proceedings of the Fourth International Conference on Trichinellosis, August 26–28, 1976.* University Press of New England, 1978, pp 535–539.

BERG, P AND FRENKEL, EP: *Myoglobinuria after spontaneous and induced fever: Report of a case.* Ann Intern Med 48:380–389, 1958.

BØE, E AND NYLAND, H: *Gullain-Barré syndrome after vaccination with human diploid cell rabies vaccine.* Scand J Infect Dis 12:231–232, 1980.

BLAKE, PA, FELDMAN RA, BUCHANAN, TM, et al: *Serologic therapy of tetanus in the United States, 1965–1971.* JAMA 238: 42–44, 1976.

BOURÉE , P, BOUVIER, JB, PASSERON, J, ET AL: *Outbreak of trichinosis near Paris.* Br Med J 1:1047–1049, 1979.

BRATZLAVSKY, M AND VANDER EECKEN, H: *La physiopathologie de l'hypertonie musculaire du tétanos.* Rev Neurol 12:815–823, 1980.

BROOKS, GF, BENNETT, JV and FELDMAN, RA: *Diptheria in the United States, 1959 1970.* J Infect Dis 129:172–178, 1974.

BROOKS, VB, CURTIS, DR AND ECCLES, JC: *The action of tetanus on the inhibition of motor neurons.* J Physiol 135:655–672, 1957.

BRUST, JCM AND RICHTER, RW: *Tetanus in the inner city.* NY State J Med 74:1735–1742, 1974.

CAMERON, HU AND FORD, M: *Gas gangrene—need it occur?* Can Med Assoc J 119:1207–1209, 1978.

CAMPBELL, AMG, WILLIAMS, ER AND PEARCE, J: *Late motor neuron degeneration following poliomyelitis.* Neurology 19:1101–1116, 1969.

CAMPBELL, WC AND BLAIR, LS: *Combined anthelminthic and corticosteroid therapy of trichinellosis in mice.* In KIM, CW AND PAWLOWSKI, ZS (EDS): *Proceedings of the Fourth International Conference on Trichinellosis, August 26–28, 1976.* University Press of New England, 1978, pp 409–417.

CHANDAR, K, MAIR, H AND MAIR, NS: *Case of toxoplasma myositis.* Br Med J 1:158–159, 1968.

CHERINGTON, M AND RYAN, DW: *Botulism and guanidine.* N Eng J Med 278:931–933, 1968.

CHERINGTON, M AND RYAN, DW: *Treatment of botulism with guanidine. Early neurophysiologic studies.* N Eng J Med 282:195–197, 1970.

CHESNEY, PJ, CRASS, BA, POLYAK, MB, ET AL: *Toxic shock syndrome: Management and long-term sequelae.* Ann Intern Med 96 (part 2):847–851, 1982.

CHESNEY, PJ, DAVIS, JP, PURDY, WK, WAND, PJ AND CHESNEY, RW: *Clinical manifestations of toxic-shock syndrome.* JAMA 246:741–748, 1981.

CHIEDOZI, LC: *Pyomyositis. Review of 205 cases in 112 patients.* Am J Surg 137:255–259, 1979.

CHO, C AND PATEL, SP: *Human sparganosis in northern United States.* NY State J Med 78:1456–1458, 1978.

CHONMAITREE, T, MENGUS, MA, SCHERVISH-SWIERKOSZ, EM, ET AL: *Enterovirus 71 infection: Report of an outbreak with two cases of paralysis and a review of the literature.* Pediatrics 67:489–493, 1981.

CHOPRA, JS, BANERJEE, AK, MURTHY, JMK, ET AL: *Paralytic rabies. A clinico-pathological study.* Brain 103:789–802, 1980.

CHUMAKOV, M, VOROSHILOVA, M, SHINDAROV, L, ET AL: *Enterovirus 71 isolated from cases of epidemic poliomyelitis-like disease in Bulgaria.* Arch Virol 60:329–340, 1979.

COMBINED SCOTTISH STUDY: Poliomyelitis-like disease in 1959. Br Med J 2:597–605, 1961.

COOK, RE: *Progressive bulbar palsy due to syphilis.* Am J Syph 37:161–164, 1953.

COREY, L AND HATTWICK, M: *Treatment of persons exposed to rabies.* JAMA 232:272–276, 1975.

CULL-CANDY, SG, LUNDH, H AND THESLEFF, S: *Effects of botulinum toxin on neuromuscular transmission in the rat.* J Physiol 260:177–203, 1977.

DALLSDORF, G AND MELNICK, JL: *Coxsackie viruses.* In HORSFALL, FL, JR AND TAMM, I (EDS): *Viral and Rickettsial Infections of Man*, ed 4. JB Lippincott, Philadelphia, 1965, pp 474–512.

DARKE, SG, KING, AM AND SLACK, WK: *Gas gangrene and related infection: Classification, clinical features and aetiology, management and mortality. A report of 88 cases.* Br J Surg 64:104–112, 1977.

DATTA, A, DASADHIKARY, C AND GHOSH, S: *Syphilitic amyotrophy.* J Indian Med Assoc 47:287–300, 1966.

DAVID, CB AND TOLAYMAT, A: *Typhoid fever: Unusual presentation.* J Pediatr 93:533, 1978.

DENNY-BROWN, D, ADAMS, RD AND FITZGERALD, PJ: *Pathologic features of herpes zoster.* Arch Neurol Psychiatry 51:216–231, 1944.

DIETZMAN, DE, SCHALLER, JG, RAY G, ET AL: *Acute myositis associated with influenza B infection.* Pediatrics 57:255–258, 1976.

DILLON, MJ, MARSHALL, WC, DUDGEON, JA, ET AL: *Epidemic neuromyasthenia: Outbreak among nurses at a children's hospital.* Br Med J 1:301–305, 1974.

DOWELL, VR, MCCROSKEY, LM, HATHEWAY, CL, ET AL: *Coproexamination for botulinal toxin and* Clostridium botulinum. *A new procedure for laboratory diagnosis of botulism.* JAMA 238:1829–1832, 1977.

DRACHMAN, DA AND TUNCHAY, TO: *The remote myopathy of trichinosis.* Neurology 15:1127–1135, 1965.

DRACHMAN, DB, MURPHY, SR, NIGAM, MP, ET AL: *"Myopathic" changes in chronically denervated muscle.* Arch Neurol 16:14–24, 1967.

DUCHEN, LW AND STRICH, SJ: *The effects of botulinum toxin on the pattern of innervation of skeletal muscle in the mouse.* Q J Exp Physiol 53:84–89, 1968.

EAGLESTEIN, WH, KATZ, R AND BROWN, JA: *The effects of early corticosteroid therapy on the skin eruption and pain of herpes zoster.* JAMA 211:1681–1683, 1970.

EDMONDSON, RS AND FLOWERS, MW: *Intensive care in tetanus: Management, complications, and mortality in 100 cases.* Br Med J 1:1401–1404, 1979.

EL NAHAS, AM, FARRINGTON, K, QUYYUMI, S, ET AL: *Rhabdomyolysis and systemic infection.* Br Med J 286:349–350, 1983.

FARRELL, MK, PARTIN, JC AND BOVE, KE: *Epidemic influenza myopathy in Cincinnati in 1977.* J Pediatr 96:545–551, 1980.

FISHER, RF, GOODPASTURE, HC, PETERIE, JD AND VOTH, DW: *Toxic shock in menstruating women.* Ann Intern Med 94:156–163, 1981.

FISHMAN, RA: *Cerebrospinal Fluid in Diseases of the Nervous System.* WB Saunders, Philadelphia, 1980, pp 273–274.

FLOWERS, MW AND EDMONDSON, RS: *Long-term recovery from tetanus: A study of 50 survivors.* Br Med J 280:303–305, 1980.

FRAYHA, RA: *Trichinosis-related polyarteritis nodosa.* Am J Med 71:307–312, 1981.

FRENKEL, JK AND RUIZ, A: *Endemicity of toxoplasmosis in Costa Rica. Transmission between cats, soil, intermediate hosts and humans.* Am J Epidemiol 113:254–269, 1981.

FRIMAN, G: *Serum creatine phosphokinase in epidemic influenza.* Scand J Infect Dis 8:13–20, 1976.

FRIMAN, G: *Effect of acute infectious disease on isometric muscle strength.* Scand J Lab Clin Invest 37:303–308, 1977.

FRIMAN, G, SCHILLER, HH AND SCHWARTZ, MS: *Disturbed neuromuscular transmission in viral infections.* Scand J Infect Dis 9:99–103, 1977.

FUKUYAMATA, Y, ANDO, T AND YOKOTA, J: *Acute fulminant myoglobinuric polymyositis with picornavirus-like crystals.* J Neurol Neurosurg Psychiatry 40:775–781, 1977.

GADOTH, N, DAGAN, R, SANDBANK, U, LEVY, D AND MOSES, SW: *Permanent tetraplegia as a consequence of tetanus neonatorum. Evidence for widespread lower motor neuron damage.* J Neurol Sci 51:273–278, 1981.

GAMBOA, ET, EASTWOOD, AB, HAYS, AP, ET AL: *Isolation of influenza virus from muscle in myoglobinuric polymyositis.* Neurology 29:1323–1335, 1979.

GARDNER-THORPE, C, FOSTER, JB AND BARWICK, DD: *Unusual manifestations of herpes zoster. A clinical and electrophysiological study.* J Neurol Sci 28:427–447, 1976.

GARNIER, MJ: *Tetanus in patients 3 years of age and up. A personal series of 230 consecutive patients.* Am J Surg 129:459–463, 1975.

GASKELL, HS AND KORB, M: *Occurrence of multiple neuritis in cases of cutaneous diphtheria.* Arch Neurol Psychiatry 55:559–572, 1946.

Ghatak, NR, Erenberg, G, Hirano, A, et al: *Idiopathic rhabdomyolysis in children.* J Neurol Sci 20:253–268, 1973.

Gleason, TH and Hamlin, WB: *Disseminated toxoplasmosis in the compromised host.* Arch Intern Med 134:1059–1062, 1974.

Goldberg, JS, London, WL and Nagel, DM: *Tropical pyomyositis: A case report and review.* Pediatrics 63:298–300, 1979.

Gould, SE (ed): *Trichinosis in Man and Animals.* Charles C Thomas, Springfield, 1970.

Graybill, JR, Silva, J, Jr, O'Brien, MS, et al: *Epidemic neuromyasthenia. A syndrome or disease?* JAMA 219:1440–1443, 1972.

Greco, TP, Askenase, PW and Kashgarian, M: *Post-viral myositis: Myxovirus-like structures in affected muscle.* Ann Intern Med 86:193–194, 1977.

Greenlee, JE, Johnson, WD, Campa, JF, et al: *Adult toxoplasmosis presenting as polymyositis and cerebellar ataxia.* Ann Intern Med 82:367–371, 1975.

Gross, B and Ochoa, J: *Trichinosis: Clinical report and histochemistry of muscle.* Muscle Nerve 2:394–398, 1979.

Gupta, PS, Goyal, S, Kapoor, R, et al: *Intrathecal human tetanus immunoglobulin in early tetanus.* Lancet ii:439–440, 1980.

Gupta, SK, Helal, BH and Kiely, P: *The prognosis in zoster paralysis.* J Bone Joint Surg 51B:593–603, 1969.

Gutmann, L and Pratt, L: *Pathophysiologic aspects of human botulism.* Arch Neurol 33:175–179, 1976.

Habermann, E and Welhöner, HH: *Advances in tetanus research.* Klin Wochenschr 52:255–265, 1974.

Harris, AJ and Miledi, R: *The effect of type D botulinum toxin on frog neuromuscular junctions.* J Physiol 217:497–515, 1971.

Hatch, MH, Malison, MD and Palmer, EL: *Isolation of enterovirus 70 from patients with acute hemorrhagic conjunctivitis in Key West, Florida.* N Engl J Med 305:1648–1649, 1981.

Hattwick, MAW, Weiss, TT, Stechschulte, CJ, et al: *Recovery from rabies: A case report.* Ann Intern Med 76:931–942, 1972.

Hayward, M and Seaton, D: *Late sequelae of paralytic poliomyelitis: A clinical and electromyographic study.*J Neurol Neurosurg Psychiatry 42:117–122, 1979.

Heathfield, KWG and Turner, JWA: *Syphilitic wrist-drop.* Lancet ii:566–569, 1951.

Henderson, DK, Tillman, DB, Webb, HH, et al: *Infectious disease emergencies: The clostridial syndromes—Teaching Conference, University of California, Los Angeles, and Harbor General Hospital, Torrance (Specialty Conference).* West J Med 129:101–120, 1978.

Hendrickx, GFM, Verhage, J, Jennekens, FGI, et al: *Dermatomyositis and toxoplasmosis.* Ann Neurol 5:393–395, 1979.

Hewitt, AB: *Syphilitic amyotrophy.* Br J Vener Dis 43:272–274, 1967.

Hicks, JT, Korenyi-Both, A, Utsinger, PD, et al: *Neuromuscular and immunochemical abnormalities in an adult man with Kawasaki disease.* Ann Intern Med 96:607–610, 1982.

Hirano, T, Srinivasan, G, Janakiraman, N, et al: *Gallium 67 citrate scintigraphy in pyomyositis.* J Pediatrics 97:596–598, 1980.

Ho, KJ and Scully, KT: *Acute rhabdomyolysis and renal failure in Weil's disease.* Ala J Med Sci 17:133–137, 1980.

Hodes, HL: *Diphtheria.* Pediatr Clin North Am 26:445–459, 1979.

Holmgren, B, Lindahl, J, von Zeipel, G, et al: *Tick-borne meningoencephalomyelitis in Sweden.* Acta Med Scand 164:507–522, 1959.

Huber, SA, Job, LP, and Woodruff, JF: *Lysis of infected myofibers by Coxsackievirus B-3-immune lymphocytes.* Am J Pathol 98:681–694, 1980.

Hughes, JM, Blumenthal, JR, Merson, MH, Lombard, GL, Dowell, VR, Jr and Gangarosa, EJ: *Clinical features of types A and B food-borne botulism.* Ann Intern Med 95:442–445, 1981.

Hung, TP, Jung, SM, Liang, HC, et al: *Radiculomyelitis following acute haemorrhagic conjunctivitis.* Brain 99:771–790, 1976.

Hung, TP and Kono, R: *Neurologic complications of acute haemorrhagic conjunctivitis (a polio-like syndrome in adults).* In Vinken, PJ and Bruyn, GW (eds): *Handbook of Clinical Neurology, Vol. 38.* North-Holland, Amsterdam, 1979, pp 595–623.

Illis, LS and Taylor, FM: *Neurological and electroencephalographic sequelae of tetanus.* Lancet i:826–830, 1971.

Innes, SGB: *Encephalomyelitis resembling benign myalgic encephalomyelitis.* Lancet i:969–971, 1970.

Ishimaru, Y, Nakano, S, Yamaoka, K, et al: *Outbreaks of hand, foot, and mouth disease by enterovirus 71. High incidence of complication disorders of central nervous system.* Arch Dis Child 55:583–588, 1980.

Jacob, JC and Mathew, NT: *Pseudohypertrophic myopathy in cysticercosis.* Neurology 18:767–771, 1968.

Jendrzejewski, JW, Jones, SR, Newcombe, RL, et al: *Nontraumatic clostridial myonecrosis.* Am J Med 65:542–546, 1978.

John, TJ, Christopher, S and Abraham, J: *Neurological manifestation of acute haemorrhagic conjunctivitis due to enterovirus 70.* Lancet ii:1283–1284, 1981.

Jolly, SS and Pallis, C: *Muscular pseudohypertrophy due to cysticercosis.* J Neurol Sci 12:155–162, 1971.

Josselson, J, Pula, T and Sadler, JH: *Acute rhabdomyolysis associated with an echovirus 9 infection.* Arch Intern Med 140:1671–1672, 1980.

Juranek, DD and Schultz, MG: *Trichinellosis in humans in the United States: Epidemiologic trends.* In Kim, CW and Pawlowski, ZS (eds): *Proceedings of the Fourth International Conference on Trichinellosis, August 26–28, 1976.* University Press of New England, 1978, pp 523–528.

Kagen, LJ, Kimball, AC and Christian, CL: *Serologic evidence of toxoplasmosis among patients with polymyositis.* Am J Med 56:186–191, 1974.

Kalish, SB, Tallman, MS, Cook, FV and Blumen, EA: *Polymicrobial septicemia associated with rhabdomyolysis, myoglobinuria, and acute renal failure.* Arch Intern Med 142:133–134, 1982.

Kanarek, DJ, Kaufman, B and Zwi, S: *Severe sympathetic hyperactivity associated with tetanus.* Arch Intern Med 132:602–604, 1973.

Kaplan, JE, Davis, LE, Narayan, V, et al: *Botulism, type A, and treatment with guanidine.* Ann Neurol 6:69–71, 1979.

Karasawa, T, Takizawa, I, Morita, K, Ishibashi, H, Kanayama, S and Shikata, T: *Polymyositis and toxoplasmosis.* Acta Pathol Jpn 31:675–680, 1981.

Karzon, DT, Hayner, NS, Winkelstein, W, Jr, et al: *An epidemic of aseptic meningitis syndrome due to echo virus type 6. II. A clinical study of echo 6 infection.* Pediatrics 29:418–431, 1962.

Kassur, B, Januszkiewicz, J and Poznavska, H: *Clinic of trichinellosis.* In Kim, CW and Pawlowski, ZS (eds): *Proceedings of the Fourth International Conference on Trichinellosis, August 26–28, 1976.* University Press of New England, 1978, pp 27–44.

Katiyar, BC, Misra, S, Singh, RB and Singh, AK: *Neurological syndromes after acute epidemic conjunctivitis.* Lancet ii:866–867, 1981.

Katz, B and Miledi, R: *The role of calcium in neuromuscular facilitation.* J Physiol 195:481–492, 1968.

Kazemi, B, Tahernia, C and Zandian, K: *Motor nerve conduction in diphtheria and diphtheritic myocarditis.* Arch Neurol 29:104–106, 1973.

Kendall, D: *Motor complications of herpes zoster.* Br Med J 2:616–618, 1957.

Kerr, JH, Corbett, JL, Prys-Roberts, C, et al: *Involvement of the sympathetic nervous system in tetanus. Studies on 82 cases.* Lancet ii:236–241, 1968.

Khuri-Bulos, N: *Diphtheria in Jordan: A diminishing yet important paediatric disease.* J Trop Med Hyg 83:79–83, 1980.

Kidman, AD, Baker, W de C and Sippe, HJ: *Effect of diphtheritic demyelination on axonal transport in the sciatic nerve and subsequent muscle changes in the chicken.* Adv Exp Biol Med 100:439–452, 1978a.

Kidman, AD, Dolan, L and Sippe, HJ: *Blockade of fast axonal transport by diphtheritic demyelination in the chicken sciatic nerve.* J Neurochem 30:57–61, 1978b.

Kidman, AD, Hanwell, M and Cooper, N: *Failure of diphtheritic demyelination to block slow axonal transport in the chicken sciatic nerve.* J Neurochem 33:357–359, 1979.

King, DL and Karzon, DT: *An epidemic of aseptic meningitis syndrome due to echovirus type 6. III. Sequelae three years after infection.* Pediatrics 29:432–437, 1962.

Klein, JS: *Treatment of severe trichinellosis.* In Kim, CW and Pawlowski, ZS (eds): *Proceedings of the Fourth International Conference on Trichinellosis, August 26–28, 1976.* University Press of New England, 1978, pp 535–539.

Koutras, A: *Myositis with Kawasaki's disease.* Am J Dis Child 136:78–79, 1982.

Kurdi, A and Abdul-Kader, M: *Clinical and electrophysiological studies of diphtheritic neuritis in Jordan.* J Neurol Sci 42:243–250, 1979.

Kurent, JE, Brooks, BR, Madden, DL, et al: *CSF viral antibodies. Evaluation in amyotrophic lateral sclerosis and late-onset postpoliomyelitis progressive muscular atrophy.* Arch Neurol 36:269–273, 1979.

LAMAS, CC, MARTINEZ, AJ, BARAFF, R, ET AL: *Rabies encephaloradiculomyelitis. Case report.* Acta Neuropathol 51:245–247, 1980.

LANCET: *Dumb rabies* (editorial). Lancet ii:1031–1032, 1978.

LAYZER, RB: *Motor unit hyperactivity states.* In VINKEN, PJ AND BRUYN, GW (EDS): *Handbook of Clinical Neurology, Vol 41.* North-Holland, Amsterdam, 1979, pp 295–316.

LENNETTE, EH, CAPLAN, GE AND MAGOFFIN, RL: *Mumps virus infection simulating paralytic poliomyelitis.* Pediatrics 25:788–797, 1960.

LERNER, AM: *Enteric viruses: Coxsackie viruses, echo viruses, reoviruses.* In THORN, GW, ADAMS, RD, BRAUNWALD, E, ET AL (EDS): *Harrison's Principles of Internal Medicine,* ed 8. McGraw-Hill, New York, 1977, pp 981–987.

LEVIN, MJ, GARDNER, P AND WALDVOGEL, FA: *"Tropical" pyomyositis. An unusual infection due to staphylococcus aureus.* N Engl J Med 284:196–198, 1971.

LHERMITTE, J, FAURE-BEAULIEU, VOGT-POPP MLLE, ET AL: *Sclerose laterale amyotrophique de Charcot et syphilis. Une observation anatomo-clinique.* Rev Neurol 77:131–133, 1945.

LUNDH, H, LEANDER, S AND THESLEFF, S: *Antagonism of the paralysis produced by botulinum toxin in the rat. The effects of tetraethylammonium, guanidine and 4-aminopyridine.* J Neurol Sci 32:29–43, 1977.

LUTSCHG, J AND LUDIN, H-P: *Electromyographic findings in patients after recovery from peripheral nerve lesions and poliomyelitis.* J Neurol 225:25–32, 1981.

LUXON, L, LEES, AJ AND GREENWOOD, RJ: *Neurosyphilis today.* Lancet i:90–93, 1979.

LYLE, WH AND CHAMBERLAIN, RN (EDS): *"Epidemic neuromyasthenia" 1934–1977: Current approaches.* Postgrad Med J 54:705–774, 1978.

MACKAY, RP AND HALL, GW: *Syphilitic amyotrophy.* Arch Neurol Psychiatry 29:241–254, 1933.

MAGOFFIN, RL, LENNETTE, EH, HOLLISTER, AC JR, ET AL: *An etiologic study of clinical paralytic poliomyelitis.* JAMA 175:269–278, 1961a.

MAGOFFIN, RL, LENNETTE, EH AND SCHMIDT, NJ: *Association of coxsackie viruses with illnesses resembling mild paralytic poliomyelitis.* Pediatrics 28:602–613, 1961b.

MAIR, IWS AND FLUGSRUD, LB: *Peripheral facial palsy and herpes zoster infection.* J Laryngol Otol 90:373–379, 1976.

MARTIN, JP: *Amyotrophic meningo-myelitis (spinal progressive muscular atrophy of syphilitic origin).* Brain 48: 153–182, 1925.

MAY, PGR, ASHTON, JR, DONNAN, SPB, ET AL: *Personality and medical perception in benign myalgic encephalomyelitis.* Lancet ii:1122–1124, 1980.

MCCRACKEN, RO AND TAYLOR, DD: *Mebendazole therapy of parenteral trichinellosis.* Science 207:1220–1222, 1980.

MCDONALD, WI AND KOCEN, RS: *Diphtheritic neuropathy.* In DYCK, PJ, THOMAS, PK AND LAMBERT, EH (EDS): *Peripheral Neuropathy.* WB Saunders, Philadelphia, 1975, pp 1281–1300.

MCEVEDY, CP AND BEARD, AW: *Royal Free epidemic of 1955: A reconsideration.* Br Med J 1: 7–11, 1970a.

MCEVEDY, CP AND BEARD, AW: *Concept of benign myalgic encephalomyelitis.* Br Med J 1:11–15, 1970b.

MCGILL, RJ: *Cysticercosis resembling myopathy.* Lancet ii:728–730, 1948.

MCKINLAY, IA AND MITCHELL, J: *Transient myositis in childhood.* Arch Dis Child 51:135–137, 1976.

MCLAUGHLIN, MJ: *CT and percutaneous fine-needle aspiration biopsy in tropical myositis.* AJR 134:167-168, 1980.

MCNICHOLL, B AND UNDERHILL, D: *Toxoplasmic polymyositis.* Ir J Med Sci 3:525–527, 1970.

MEASE, PJ, OCHS, HD AND WEDGWOOD, RJ: *Successful treatment of echovirus meningoencephalitis and myositis-fasciitis with intravenous immune globulin therapy in a patient with x-linked agammaglobulinemia.* N Engl J Med 304:1278–1281, 1981.

MELLANBY, J AND GREEN, J: *How does tetanus toxin act?* Neuroscience 6:281–300, 1981.

MERSON, MH AND DOWELL, VR, JR: *Epidemiologic, clinical and laboratory aspects of wound botulism.* N Engl J Med 289:1005–1010, 1973.

MERSON, MH, HUGHES, JM, DOWELL, VR, ET AL: *Current trends in botulism in the United States.* JAMA 229:1305–1308, 1974.

MESHKINPOUR, H AND VAZIRI, ND: *Acute rhabdomyolysis associated with adenovirus infection.* J Infect Dis 148:133, 1981.

Messina, C, Dattola, R and Ginlanda, P: *Effect of guanidine on the neuromuscular block of botulism. An electrophysiological study.* Acta Neurol Napoli 34:459–462, 1979.

Middleton, PJ, Alexander, RM and Szymanski, MT: *Severe myositis during recovery from influenza.* Lancet ii:533–535, 1970.

Mikol, J, Felton -Papaiconomou, A, Ferchal, F, Perol, Y, Gautier, B, Haguenau, M and Pepin, B: *Inclusion-body myositis: Clinicopathological studies and isolation of an adenovirus type 2 from muscle biopsy specimen.* Ann Neurol 11:576–581, 1982.

Miller, A and Nathanson, N: *Rabies: Recent advances in pathogenesis and control.* Ann Neurol 2:511–519, 1977.

Molloy, MG, and Goodwill, CJ: *Herpes zoster and lower motor neurone paresis.* Rheumatol Rehabil 18:170–173, 1979.

Morgan-Hughes, JA: *Experimental diphtheritic neuropathy. A pathological and electrophysiological study.* J Neurol Sci 7:157–175, 1968.

Mukherjee, SK: *Involvement of anterior horn of spinal cord in infectious mononucleosis.* Br Med J 1:1112, 1965.

Mulder, DW, Rosenbaum, RA and Layton, DD, Jr: *Late progression of poliomyelitis or forme fruste amyotrophic lateral sclerosis?* Mayo Clinic Proc 47:756–761, 1972.

Oh, SJ: *Botulism: Electrophysiological studies.* Ann Neurol 1:481–485, 1977.

Paley, RG and Truelove, SC: *Diphtheria in the Army in the United Kingdom: Study of its Complications.* J R Army Med Corps 90:109–116, 1948.

Pallis, CA and Lewis, PD: *Involvement of human muscle by parasites.* In Walton, JN (ed): *Disorders of Voluntary Muscle,* ed. 4. Churchill-Livingstone, London, 1981, pp 569–584.

Pappenheimer, AM, Jr and Gill, DM: *Diphtheria. Recent studies have clarified the molecular mechanisms involved in its pathogenesis.* Science 182:353–358, 1973.

Pedersen, AHB, Spearman, J, Tronca, E, et al: *Diphtheria on Skid Road, Seattle, Wash., 1972–75.* Public Health Rep 92:336–342, 1977.

Pedersen, E: *Epidemic vertigo. Clinical picture, epidemiology and relation to encephalitis.* Brain 82:566–580, 1959.

Phillips, PE, Kassan, SS and Kagen, LJ: *Increased toxoplasma antibodies in idiopathic inflammatory muscle disease. A case-controlled study.* Arthritis Rheum 22:209–214, 1979.

Pickett, J, Berg, B, Chaplin, E, et al: *Syndrome of botulism in infancy: Clinical and electrophysiologic study.* N Engl J Med 295:770–772, 1976.

Pierone, RE, Coplin, TW and Leeper, JD: *Tetanus and diphtheria immune status of patients in a family practice.* J Fam Pract 11:403–406, 1980.

Pilars de Pilar, CE and Spiess, H: *Diphtherie-und Tetanusantikorper bei Kindern und jungen Erwachseuen.* Dtsch Med Wochenschr 106:1341–1345, 1981.

Pleasure, DE, Feldmann, B and Prockop, DJ: *Diphtheria toxin inhibits the synthesis of myelin proteolipid and basic protein by peripheral nerve* in vitro. J Neurochem 20:81–90, 1973.

Plum, F: *Sensory loss with poliomyelitis.* Neurology 6:166–172, 1956.

Pollock, JL: *Toxoplasmosis appearing to be dermatomyositis.* Arch Dermatol 115:736–737, 1979.

Pool, JH, Walton, JN, Brewis, EG, et al: *Benign myalgic encephalomyelitis in Newcastle upon Tyne.* Lancet i:733–737, 1961.

Porras, C, Barboza, JJ and Fuenzalida, E: *Recovery from rabies in man.* Ann Intern Med 85:44–48, 1976.

Porter, CB, Hinthorn, DR, Couchonnal, G, et al: *Simultaneous streptococcus and picornavirus infection. Muscle involvement in acute rhabdomyolysis.* JAMA 245:1545–1547, 1981.

Prabhakar, BS and Nathanson, N: *Acute rabies death mediated by antibody.* Nature 290:590–591, 1981.

Price, DL, Griffin, J, Young, A, et al: *Tetanus toxin: Direct evidence for retrograde transport.* Science 188:945–947, 1975.

Price, RW and Plum, F: *Poliomyelitis.* In Vinken, PJ, Bruyn, GW and Klawans (eds): *Handbook of Clinical Neurology, Vol 34.* North-Holland, Amsterdam, 1978, pp 93–132.

Prier, S, Gibert, C, Bodros, A, et al: *Neurophysiological changes in non-vaccinated rabies patients.* Lancet i:620, 1979.

Prys-Roberts, C, Kerr, JH, Corbett, JL, et al: *Treatment of sympathetic overactivity in tetanus.* Lancet i:542–546, 1969.

Puggiari, M and Cherington, M: *Botulism and guanidine. Ten years later.* JAMA 240:2276–2277, 1978.

Ralls, RW, Boswell, W, Henderson, R, et al: *CT of inflammatory disease of the psoas muscle.* AJR 134:767–770, 1980.

RAMSAY, AM AND RUNDLE, A: *Clinical and biochemical findings in ten patients with benign myalgic encephalomyelitis.* Postgrad Med J 55:856–857, 1979.

RANZENHOFER, ER, DIZON, FC, LIPTON, MM, ET AL: *Clinical paralytic poliomyelitis due to Coxsackie virus group A, type 7.* New Engl J Med 259:182, 1958.

RAY, GC, MENNICH, LL AND JOHNSON, PC: *Selective polymyositis induced by coxsackievirus B1 in mice.* J Infect Dis 140:239–243, 1979.

REINGOLD, AL, SHANDS, KN, DAN, BB AND BROOME, CV: *Toxic-shock syndrome not associated with menstruation. A review of 54 cases.* Lancet i:1–4, 1982.

RICKER, K, EYRICH, K AND ZWIRNER, R: *Seltenere Formen von Tetanuserkrankung. Klinische und elektromyographische Untersuchung.* Arch Psychiatr Nervenkr 215:75–91, 1971.

RISK, WS, BOSCH, EP, KIMURA, J, ET AL: *Chronic tetanus: Clinical report and histochemistry of muscle.* Muscle Nerve 4:363–366, 1981.

ROOS, RP, VIOLA, MV, WALLMANN, R, ET AL: *Amyotrophic lateral sclerosis with antecedent poliomyelitis.* Arch Neurol 37:312–313, 1980.

ROSENBERG, EG, WHALEN, GE AND POLMAR, SH: *Elevated IgE levels in trichinellosis.* In KIM, CW: *Proceedings of the Third International Conference on Trichinellosis, 1972.* Intext Educational Publishers, New York, 1974, pp 399–406.

ROWLAND, LP (ED): *Human Motor Neuron Diseases.* Raven Press, New York, 1982.

ROWLAND, LP AND GREER, M: *Toxoplasmic polymyositis.* Neurology 11:367–370, 1961.

RUFF, RL AND SECRIST, D: *Viral studies in benign acute childhood myositis.* Arch Neurol 39:261–263, 1982.

RYAN, DW AND CHERINGTON, M: *Human type A botulism.* JAMA 216:513–514, 1971.

SAMUELS, BS AND RIETSCHEL, RL: *Polymyositis and toxoplasmosis.* JAMA 235:60–61, 1976.

SANDERS, RKM, MARTYN, B, JOSEPH, R, ET AL: *Intrathecal antitetanus serum (horse) in the treatment of tetanus.* Lancet i:974–977, 1977.

SAVAGE, DCL, FORBES, M AND PEARCE, GW: *Idiopathic rhabdomyolysis.* Arch Dis Child 46:594–607, 1971.

SCHEID, W: *Diphtherial paralysis. An analysis of 2,292 cases of diphtheria in adults, which included 174 cases of polyneuritis.* J Nerv Ment Dis 116:1095–1101, 1952.

SCHLECH, WF III, MOULTON, P AND KAISER AB: *Pyomyositis: Tropical disease in a temperate climate.* Am J Med 71:900–902, 1981.

SCHWARTZ, MS, SWASH, M AND GROSS, M: *Benign postinfection polymyositis.* Br Med J 2:1256–1257, 1978.

SCHWOB, RA, FOUCQUIER, E AND FRANÇON, J: *Amyotrophie syphilitique et sclerose laterale amyotrophique.* Rev Neurol 86:334–337, 1952.

SEDAGHATIAN, MR: *Intrathecal serotherapy in neonatal tetanus: A controlled trial.* Arch Dis Child 54:623–625, 1979.

SEEDAT, YK, OMAR, MAK, SEEDAT, MA, ET AL: *Renal failure in tetanus.* Br Med J 282:360–361, 1981.

SEGGEY, J, OHRY, A, ROZIN, R, ET AL: *Sensory losses in poliomyelitis.* Arch Neurol 33:664, 1976.

SHAHANI, M, DASTUR, FD, DASTOOR, DH, ET AL: *Neuropathy in tetanus.* J Neurol Sci 41:173–182, 1979.

SHINDAROV, LM, CHUMAKOV, MP, VOROSHILOVA, MK, ET AL: *Epidemiological, clinical and pathomorphological characteristics of epidemic poliomyelitis-like disease caused by enterovirus 71.* J Hyg Epidemiol Microbiol Immunol 23:284–295, 1979.

SIMON, NM, ROVNER, RN AND BERLIN, BS: *Acute myoglobinuria associated with type A2 (Hong Kong) influenza.* JAMA 212:1704–1705, 1970.

SIRINAVIN, S AND MCCRACKEN, GH, JR: *Primary suppurative myositis in children.* Am J Dis Child 133:263–265, 1979.

SONNABEND, O, SONNABEND, W, HEINZLE, R, ET AL: *Isolation of* Clostridum botulinum *type G and identification of type G botulinal toxin in humans: Report of five sudden unexpected deaths.* J Infect Dis 148:22–27, 1981.

STEEGMAN, AT: *Poliomyelitis (poliomyelopathia) chronica: Report of a case.* Arch Neurol Psychiatry 38:537–549, 1937.

STRUPPLER, A, STRUPPLER, E AND ADAMS, RD: *Local tetanus in man. Its clinical and neurophysiological characteristics.* Arch Neurol 8:62–78, 1963.

STY, JR, BABBITT, DP, BOEDECKER, RA, ET AL: *"Tropical pyomyositis."* Wisc Med J 79:38–39, 1980.

SVANE, S: *Peracute spontaneous streptococcal myositis. A report on 2 fatal cases with review of literature.* Acta Chir Scand 137:155–163, 1971.

SWARTS, RL, MARTINEZ, LA AND ROBSON, HG: *Gonococcal pyomyositis.* JAMA 246:246, 1981.

TANNER, MH, PIERCE, BJ AND HALE, DC: *Toxic shock syndrome.* West J Med 134:477–484, 1981.

THAKUR, LC: *Cranial nerve paralysis associated with acute haemorrhagic conjunctivitis.* Lancet ii:584, 1981.

THOMAS, JE AND HOWARD, FM, JR: *Segmental zoster paresis—a disease profile.* Neurology 22:459–466, 1972.

TOBI, M, RAVID, Z, FELDMAN-WEISS, V, BEN-CHETRIT, E, MORAG, A, CHOWERS, I, MICHAELI, Y, SHALIT, M AND KNOBLER, H: *Prolonged atypical illness associated with serological evidence of persistent Epstein-Barr virus infection.* Lancet i:61–64, 1982.

TOFTE, RW AND WILLIAMS, DN: *Toxic shock syndrome: Clinical and laboratory features in 15 patients.* Ann Intern Med 94:149–156, 1981.

TOPI, GC, D'ALLESSANDRO, L, CATRICALA, C, ET AL: *Dermatomyositis-like syndrome due to toxoplasma.*Br J Dermatol 101:589–591, 1979.

TOWNSEND, JJ AND WOLINSKY, JS: *Acquired toxoplasmosis: A neglected cause of treatable nervous system disease.* Arch Neurol 32:335–343, 1975.

TRUJILLO, MJ, CASTILLO, A, ESPANA, JV, ET AL: *Tetanus in the adult: Intensive care and management experience with 233 cases.* Crit Care Med 8:419–423, 1980.

VAKIL, BJ AND ARMITAGE, P: *Therapeutic trial of intracisternal human tetanus immunoglobulin in clinical tetanus.* Trans R Soc Trop Med Hyg 73:579–583, 1979.

WADIA, NH, IRANI, PF AND KATRAK, SM: *Lumbosacral radioculomyelitis associated with pandemic acute hemorrhagic conjunctivitis.* Lancet i:350, 1973.

WADIA, NH, WADIA, PN, KATRAK, SM AND MISRA, VP: *Neurological manifestations of acute haemorrhagic conjunctivitis.* Lancet ii:528–529, 1981.

WARRELL, DA: *The clinical picture of rabies in man.* Trans R Soc Trop Med Hyg 70:188–195, 1976.

WECHSLER, IS, SAPIRSTEIN, MR AND STEIN, A: *Primary and symptomatic amyotrophic lateral sclerosis.* Am J Med Sci 208:70–81, 1944.

WEINSTEIN, L: *Diphtheria.* In THORN, GW, ADAMS, RD, BRAUNWALD, E, ISSELBACHER, KJ AND PETERSDORF, RG (EDS): *Harrison's Principles of Internal Medicine,* ed 8. McGraw-Hill, New York, 1977a, pp 877–881.

WEINSTEIN, L: *Poliomyelitis.* In THORN, GW, ADAMS, RD, BRAUNWALD, E, ISSELBACHER, KJ AND PETERSDORF, RG (EDS): *Harrison's Principles of Internal Medicine,* ed 8. McGraw-Hill, New York, 1977b, pp 999–1005.

WIECHERS, DO AND HUBBELL, SL: *Late changes in the motor unit after acute poliomyelitis.* Muscle Nerve 4: 524–528, 1981.

WILCKE, BW, JR, MIDURA, TF AND ARNON, SS: *Quantitative evidence of intestinal colonization by* clostridium botulinum *in four cases of infant botulism.* J Infect Dis 141:419–423, 1980.

WILSON, SAK: *Neurology.* Edward Arnold & Co, London, 1940, pp 475–480.

WINKELMAN, NW: *Chronic syphilitic poliomyelitis.* Arch Neurol Psychiatry 28:151–159, 1932.

Chapter 5

INFLAMMATORY AND IMMUNE DISORDERS

REACTIONS TO INFECTION AND IMMUNIZATION

Postinfectious and Allergic Neuropathies

Acute Brachial Neuritis

This disorder is a painful multiple neuropathy affecting the muscles of the shoulder girdle and arm. The syndrome goes under many other names, including neuralgic amyotrophy (Parsonage and Turner 1948) and brachial plexus neuritis, but the former term gives no hint of the anatomic location, while the latter term has misled a generation of neurology residents, since the brachial nerves are usually involved distal to the plexus. A rare but similar multiple neuritis occurs in the lower extremities (Sander and Sharp 1981); for the sake of consistency this should be called crural neuritis instead of lumbosacral plexus neuritis.

CLINICAL FEATURES. The clinical picture is rather stereotyped. Over a period of several hours the patient develops pain in the shoulder, scapula, and upper arm, sometimes extending into the neck and down the arm to the elbow or even to the hand. The pain is severe, often interfering with sleep and requiring treatment with narcotic analgesics, and it has a constant, deep, aching character made worse by movement of the arm but not by coughing, sneezing, or movement of the neck. The pain may last a day or two or may persist for several weeks; it may improve and then return, perhaps shifting to the other shoulder.

Weakness is noticed within a few days, usually after the pain improves; patients may not know whether weakness was present earlier, because the pain made them reluctant to use the arm, but once noticed the weakness usually does not get any worse. Partial or complete paralysis of individual muscles is found in a patchy distribution, usually concentrated in the muscles supplied by the C-5 and C-6 nerve roots. Sensory loss is absent or slight; if the deltoid muscle is affected there may be a patch of numbness on the overlying skin, corresponding to the sensory territory of the axillary nerve. Fasciculation is uncommon, and muscle stretch reflexes are impaired only in weak muscles. In about one third of the cases there is asymmetric involvement of both arms. Atrophy of the affected muscles begins in 2 to 3 weeks and becomes quite severe.

Careful examination shows that the muscle weakness is in a peripheral nerve distribution in almost every case. This fact was emphasized in the early descriptions of serum sickness neuritis (Wilson and Hadden 1932; Doyle 1933); Parsonage and Turner (1948) also recognized this anatomic pattern in many of their cases, but they thought that the findings in other cases indicated a plexus or even a spinal cord lesion, hence their term "neuralgic amyotrophy." Ironically, one example that they gave of paralysis that was "only explicable by an anterior-horn cell lesion" was the presence in several patients of selective weakness of distal flexion of the thumb and index finger: a pattern that we now recognize as characteristic of an anterior interosseous nerve palsy.

The axillary, suprascapular and long thoracic nerves are most often involved, causing deltoid, supraspinatus, infraspinatus, and serratus anterior muscle paralysis (Fig. 22). Separate motor nerve branches may be affected to a different degree; thus, the anterior part of the deltoid may be weaker than the posterior part, and the supraspinatus muscle may be spared while the infraspinatus is paralyzed. Among 136 cases reported by Parsonage and Turner (1948) there was isolated paralysis of the long thoracic nerve in 32 cases, bilateral in 2 cases, and in another 11 cases an isolated paralysis of this nerve on one side was accompanied by paralysis of other muscles on the other side. Other commonly affected nerves include the radial, musculocutaneous, phrenic, spinal accessory, and anterior interosseous branch of the median nerve.

LABORATORY FINDINGS. In the first week, EMG shows only a reduced number of motor unit potentials under voluntary control; afterward, fibril-

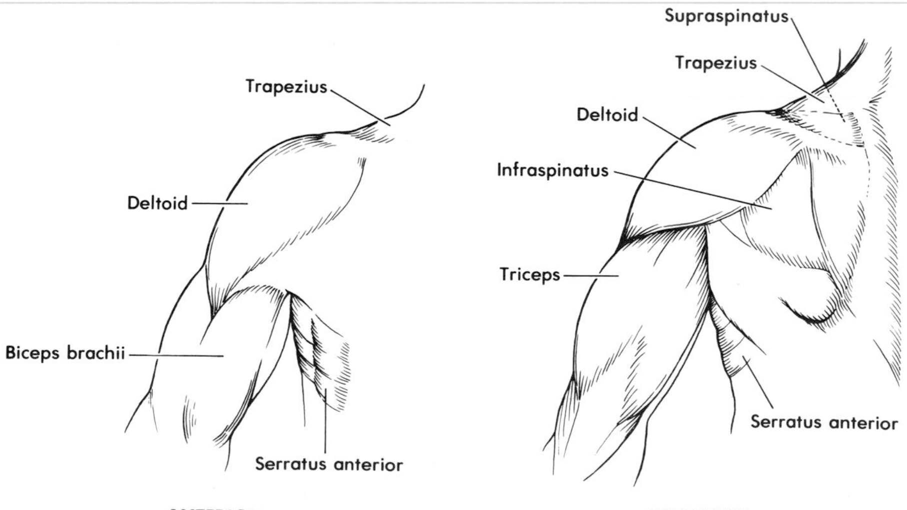

FIGURE 22. The muscles most frequently paralyzed in acute brachial neuritis.

lations become more numerous in the affected muscles but are not found in the paraspinal muscles. Motor nerve conduction is normal by routine techniques, but Martin and Kraft (1974) showed prolongation of the conduction time (up to 8 times normal) to affected muscles when motor nerves were stimulated above the clavicle. When the radial or median nerves were involved, conduction velocities were normal through the plexus but distal latencies were prolonged. CSF examination is normal in most cases, but in rare instances there is an increase in the number of lymphocytes, the protein level, or the gamma globulin concentration. These clinical, CSF, and electrophysiologic findings suggest that brachial neuritis is, in most cases, an affection of distal portions of motor branches of the brachial plexus and nerves.

ANTECEDENT EVENTS. In the wartime series of Parsonage and Turner (1948), half of the patients had an antecedent infection such as malaria, typhus, typhoid, pyogenic infections, or "minor fevers," while in 16 percent of the cases there was antecedent trauma or surgery. In a series of 99 patients at the Mayo Clinic (Tsairis et al. 1972), brachial neuritis was preceded by some type of infection (usually viral-like) in 35 patients, by immunization in 13 patients, and by a surgical operation in 2 patients, but half of the patients had no obvious predisposing cause. The viral infections are usually of the upper respiratory or "flu" variety; specific viruses have rarely been implicated, although a few cases have been related to cytomegalovirus or EB-virus infections (Duchowney et al. 1979; Tsairis et al. 1972). There is a report of an "epidemic" of brachial plexus neuritis among mill workers in Czechoslovakia, possibly caused by coxsackie A2 infection (Bardos and Somodska 1961). The most common types of preceding immunization are injections of tetanus toxoid or influenza vaccine. Serum sickness is now an unusual cause but many cases were reported in the first half of this century (Wilson and Hadden 1932; Doyle 1933); only a small fraction of patients treated with horse serum developed neurologic complications, however. In serum sickness, systemic symptoms of urticaria, fever, or arthritis nearly always precede the neurologic symptoms by a day or two. Brachial neuritis and mononeuritis account for 75 percent of the neurologic complications of serum sickness, 15 percent take the form of a generalized polyneuritis, and 10 percent present as encephalomyelitis. In a recent study, the frequency of neuropathy following tetanus toxoid administration was 0.4 cases per million vaccine doses distributed (Quast et al. 1979).

COURSE AND PROGNOSIS. In the mildest cases there is no nerve degeneration, and complete recovery occurs within a few weeks. In most cases, however, there is a mixture of reversible and irreversible nerve damage, so that full recovery requires a lengthy period of nerve regeneration. Despite this fact the long-term prognosis is very good. While only a third of patients show complete return of power at the end of 1 year, 75 percent have recovered completely after 2 years, and 80 to 90 percent are normal at the end of 3 years (Tsairis et al. 1972). In patients with full clinical recovery the EMG is generally normal (Devathasan and Tong 1980). There is little evidence that early steroid treatment affects the outcome, though it may hasten the subsidence of pain. Recurrence of brachial neuritis has been recorded in 5 to 10 percent of cases, but some of these patients have the rare hereditary form of recurrent brachial (and crural) neuritis (Taylor 1960).

Amyotrophy in Severe Asthma

Recently a number of children have been observed to develop severe paralysis of one limb during convalescence from an acute asthmatic attack. Hopkins (1974) first drew attention to this syndrome when he described a "poliomyelitis-like illness" following severe asthma in 10 children. An equal number of cases has been reported subsequently (Danta 1975; Ilett et al. 1977; Shapiro et al. 1979; Blonquist and Bjorksten 1980; Wheeler and Ochoa 1980; Manson and Thong 1980; Liebeschuetz 1981). The reported children, mostly boys, range in age from 1 to 11 years and usually have a history of chronic allergic asthma. Four to eleven days after onset of an acute asthmatic attack the patient suddenly develops severe, flaccid weakness in one limb, accompanied in some cases by pain and paresthesias. The arm is affected more often than the leg. Initially weakness may be more widespread, but residual weakness and atrophy are usually confined to one limb. There is no objective sensory loss, and fasciculations have not been seen. Recovery may begin as late as 9 months afterward, but the degree of recovery is poor; there is always some permanent weakness and atrophy, and some patients have been left with complete and permanent paralysis of one limb. CSF lymphocytic pleocytosis is present in almost every case, and the CSF protein is elevated in half of the patients.

Several authors have assumed that the paralysis is due to an anterior horn cell disease; in most of the cases, however, there were no meningeal signs or fever. Poliomyelitis infection was definitely excluded, and no consistent viral identification has been made. Furthermore, some of the electrophysiologic findings suggested a more distal nerve involvement. In one case, Danta (1975) performed EMG and motor nerve stimulation at 5 weeks, 11 months, and 19 months; initially there was no response to stimulation of nerves supplying completely paralyzed muscles, but in later tests a response was obtained with normal conduction velocity, indicating either recovery from nerve conduction block or late nerve regeneration. Wheeler and Ochoa (1980) found no motor response to median nerve stimulation 5 days after onset of paralysis, before fibrillations had appeared; this is too early for peripheral nerves to show Wallerian degeneration in anterior horn cell disease. Two-and-a-half years later there was evidence of misdirected reinnervation in the form of bursts of motor unit potentials in the biceps muscle, occurring synchronously with deep inspirations. The authors attributed this synkinesis to regenerative sprouting within the spinal cord, but it is much more likely that motor fibers of the phrenic nerve (C-3, C-4, C-5), damaged at the level of the nerve roots or upper trunk of the brachial plexus, regenerated and found their way into the musculocutaneous nerve (C-5, C-6). Respiratory-arm muscle synkinesis has been reported several times as a late consequence of upper cervical root or trunk lesions and, indeed, "provides objective evidence of antecedent nerve root or brachial plexus injury" (Swift et al. 1980).

Acute Motor Mononeuropathies

Isolated motor nerve palsies occur in serum sickness (Doyle 1933), and Parsonage and Turner (1948) included such neuropathies in the category of "neuralgic amyotrophy" when there was a history of preceding shoulder-girdle pain. Among the *spinal mononeuropathies*, the long thoracic, radial, axillary, and suprascapular nerves are most often affected, and the musculocutaneous, femoral, sciatic, anterior interosseous, intercostal, and phrenic nerves are occasionally involved.

Acute *phrenic nerve paralysis* deserves additional comment because of its pulmonary consequences. Tsairis and colleagues (1972) found six cases of diaphragmatic paralysis, including one case with bilateral involvement, in a retrospective chart review of 99 cases of brachial plexus neuritis at the Mayo Clinic. Since the presence of partial diaphragmatic paralysis can be difficult to document, even with fluoroscopy, and unilateral paralysis is often asymptomatic, it is possible that phrenic nerve involvement occurs in more than 6 percent of patients with brachial plexus neuritis. Yet there are only a few reports documenting the simultaneous occurrence of acute brachial plexus neuritis and phrenic nerve paralysis (Aleksic et al. 1973). There are, however, many reports in the non-neurologic literature of "idiopathic phrenic nerve paralysis." In these cases there is sometimes an antecedent febrile illness, and shoulder or chest pain may precede the paralysis. Simultaneous bilateral paralysis occurs in a small percentage of cases, and some patients suffer paralysis of the other hemidiaphragm long after the first attack. Spontaneous recovery occurs within 3 years in the majority of patients. It seems very likely, as Aleksic and associates (1973) suggested, that many cases of idiopathic diaphragmatic paralysis are due to postinfectious mononeuritis, and careful neuromuscular examination would probably reveal signs of brachial neuritis in many such patients.

Unilateral phrenic nerve paralysis is usually asymptomatic, but it may cause dypsnea in recumbency or reduced exercise tolerance. Bilateral phrenic nerve paralysis produces a much more dramatic impairment of pulmonary mechanics, of which the most distinctive feature is severe dyspnea in recumbency. In the standing position the vital capacity is 40 to 60 percent of normal; this value may fall slightly in the sitting position, but a profound reduction to 10 to 20 percent of normal occurs in recumbency, especially in the supine position. This is because the weight of the abdominal organs helps to expand the intrathoracic volume in the upright position but compresses it in recumbency (Comroe et al. 1951; Newsom-Davis 1976; Kreitzer 1978). Tachypnea is also noticeable on exertion because of the reduced vital capacity. Paradoxical inward movement of the abdomen on inspiration is a characteristic sign, best observed when the patient is supine. In some cases mechanical assistance to ventilation, such as a rocking bed, must be used at night, but many patients are able to sleep in a chair or with the upper body partly elevated. Improvement often does not begin for 6 months, yet complete recovery occurs within 2 to 3 years in most patients; nerve regeneration is the mechanism that best explains this delayed and protracted recovery, and it also explains why such patients rarely benefit from diaphragmatic pacing by phrenic nerve electrostimulation.

Cranial Motor Mononeuropathies

ABDUCENS PARALYSIS. Of the three ocular motor nerves, the abducens nerve is most subject to transient paralysis of unidentified cause. Sometimes the paralysis occurs suddenly, following a minor viral illness, and clears within a few months, suggesting a postinfectious inflammatory mechanism. Such cases have been reported in children (Knox et al. 1967) and are not uncommon in adults, although little has been written about them.

VAGUS NERVE PARALYSIS. Idiopathic vocal cord paralysis constitutes 10 to 30 percent of all cases of vocal cord paralysis (Clerf 1953; Williams 1959; Kearsley 1981). Clerf (1953) obtained a history of recent viral-like illness in over half of 85 idiopathic cases seen in a 10-year period. The left vocal cord was involved in three fourths of the viral cases, and the majority were young persons under 35 years of age. Using laryngeal EMG, Berry and Blair (1980) found involvement of only the recurrent laryngeal nerve in 14 unilateral cases, while in 8 cases both the superior and recurrent laryngeal branches were involved, probably indicating that the vagus nerve was involved proximal to the emergence of the superior laryngeal nerve. Palatal weakness is rare, however, suggesting that the vagus nerve is nearly always affected distal to the pharyngeal branches. Occasionally both vocal cords become paralyzed simultaneously, producing acute airway obstruction that may require tracheal intubation and tracheotomy. Spontaneous recovery may occur in 1 month but usually takes 5 or 6 months, and in a few cases recovery does not occur until 3 or 4 years after onset (Williams 1959). Although no prospective study exists, the recovery rate, partial or complete, has been reported to be between 50 and 90 percent (Williams 1959; Blau and Kapadia 1972; Berry and Blair 1980). Recurrent ipsilateral or contralateral vocal cord paralysis has been reported (Berry and Blair 1980).

FACIAL NERVE PARALYSIS. The annual incidence of Bell's palsy is about 23 cases per 100,000 population (Karnes 1975). The clinical picture is very well known. After a brief prodrome of pain in the mastoid region in about 60 percent of patients, there is a rapid development of unilateral facial weakness, which reaches a plateau within 4 days in almost all cases. In different series the proportion of patients with complete paralysis has ranged from 30 to 75 percent; the remaining patients have clinical and electrophysiologic evidence of different degrees of paralysis in various branches of the facial nerve (Boongird and Vejjajiva 1978). At the time of presentation patients occasionally describe a vague sensation of numbness or heaviness in the affected side of the face, but careful examination rarely shows any disturbance of sensation. There is ipsilateral impairment of taste on the anterior two thirds of the tongue (supplied by the chorda tympani branch of the facial nerve) in 50 to 60 percent of patients, and ipsilateral reduction of lacrimation occurs in 6 to 15 percent, but signs of involvement of the other cranial nerves are rarely detected in a standard clinical examination.

Examination of the CSF shows a mild lymphocytic pleocytosis in 12 percent of cases and a mild elevation of the protein level in 30 percent (Karnes 1975). Electrophysiologic studies sometimes show conduction block in the facial nerve proximal to the stylomastoid foramen (that is, within the skull) without damage to axons. This conclusion is based on two observations. First, in such cases EMG does not show muscle denervation (fibrillations), which usually are found after 2 weeks in cases in which nerve degeneration has occurred. Second, electrical stimulation of the nerve produces muscle potentials of normal amplitude in the upper, middle, and lower portions of the face, indicating that the nerves are normally excitable distal to the stylomastoid foramen. In other patients, some or all of the axons are irreversibly damaged inside the skull; the axons then undergo Wallerian degeneration, so that excitability of the extracranial portion of the facial nerve is reduced or absent by 6 days after the onset of paralysis, and muscle fibrillations appear in the EMG by 10 to 14 days after onset (Boongird and Vejjajiva 1978; Karnes 1975).

This conception of the pathophysiology was confirmed in one case by an autopsy performed 10 days after the onset of complete facial paralysis. There was degeneration and phagocytosis of myelin throughout the course of the facial nerve within the bony canal, while the axons were swollen but intact. There was diffuse lymphocytic infiltration of the entire nerve, including the chorda tympani, with proliferation of Schwann cells and fibroblasts. No vascular occlusions were identified in the vasa nervorum, though the vascular channels were compressed by edema of the nerve trunk (Proctor et al. 1976).

The timing and degree of functional recovery are determined by the underlying pathology. Where there is little or no axonal degeneration, recovery begins about 10 days after onset and is clinically complete in 2 to 6 weeks. If the entire nerve degenerates, recovery occurs by means of regeneration; EMG signs of recovery can be detected in the third or fourth month, but clinical signs of recovery appear somewhat later and continue until 8 to 12 months after the onset of paralysis. In the latter cases recovery is always incomplete (although not necessarily disfiguring), facial contracture develops, and synkinesis* can be demonstrated. When there is a mixture of conduction block in some axons and Wallerian degeneration in others, partial recovery occurs in 2 to 6 weeks followed by slow, delayed recovery in 4 to 12 months, and there may be late sequelae of contracture and synkinesis. Recurrent facial paralysis occurs in about 10 percent of patients; it is ipsilateral in two thirds of those cases (Mamoli et al. 1977).

Lately, several authors have reported abnormalities of other cranial nerves in patients with Bell's palsy. Safman (1971) found electrophysiologic abnormalities in the opposite facial nerve in 14 of 18 patients, though weakness was not clinically apparent; no controls were studied, however, and no quantitative data were reported. Djupesland and coworkers (1977) and Adour and colleagues (1978) described transient hypesthesia on the same side of the face and on the oropharyngeal mucous membranes in over 60 percent of their patients, but these authors did not describe their method of sensory examination. These claims are not in accord with the experience of most neurologists. Patients with facial paralysis commonly report a vague facial numbness initially, but this appears to be an entirely subjective sensation, perhaps related to the altered muscle tone, because sensory thresholds, the subjective perception of light touch and pain, the consensual corneal reflex, and the sternutatory reflex are very rarely altered. Spector and Schwartzman (1975) described two patients with Bell's palsy who had clear-cut deficits of all modalities of sensation in the trigeminal territory, with a diminished corneal reflex, but the purpose of their paper was to show that this combination of signs, rare as it is, does not necessarily mean that a mass lesion is present. Djupesland and coworkers (1977) reported transitory ipsilateral hearing deficits in 6 of 16 patients (2 with herpes zoster), but Adour and Doty (1973) found no audiometric abnormality in 48 consecutive patients. Phillipszoon (1962), Adour and Doty (1973), and Djupesland and coworkers (1977) found impaired caloric vestibular responses and positional nystagmus in many cases, and Djupesland and coworkers (1977) described difficulties with equilibrium and posture, impaired coordination of fine movements, and spontaneous nystagmus in 7 of 16 patients. In their examination of 70 patients with acute facial palsy (including four with auricular zoster), Tovi and associates (1980) detected involvement of the trigeminal nerve in 37 patients, of vestibular-cochlear function in 4 patients, and of the recurrent laryngeal, glossopharyngeal, hypoglossal, and spinal accessory nerves in 2 patients each. All these observations are so alien to

*Synkinesis is a simultaneous contraction of one part of the face during activation of another part, caused by misdirected regeneration of axons. Thus, an eye blink may cause an ipsilateral twitch near the mouth or in the platysma, and pursing the lips may cause the eye to close.

the experience of most neurologists that they are difficult to accept without more objective evidence.

Viral studies have likewise given confusing and conflicting results. In a retrospective chart review, only 28 percent of patients with idiopathic Bell's palsy recalled a preceding infectious illness (Kennedy et al. 1978). While overt herpes zoster infection has been found in 5 to 10 percent of patients with typical Bell's palsy, Djupesland and coworkers (1976) found a fourfold or greater change in the serum complement-fixing antibody titer to varicella-zoster virus in 7 of 49 patients with idopathic Bell's palsy, and changing antibody titers to several other viruses in five additional patients, so that 24 percent of the patients had signifcant changes in serum antibody titers. Adour and colleagues (1975), however, found no change in any viral antibody titers in 41 patients. Tovi and associates (1980) observed herpes simplex vesicles, fever, and cervical adenopathy in 24 percent of 70 patients, a much higher incidence than others have reported. Although the serum titer of antibodies to herpes simplex virus rarely changes in Bell's palsy, Adour and colleagues (1975), Tovi and associates (1980), and others have suggested that many or most cases of idiopathic facial palsy are due to reactivation of a herpes simplex infection in the trigeminal ganglion, spreading to the facial nerve by the same communicating branches that have been invoked to explain facial palsy in trigeminal herpes zoster. The main objection to this hypothesis is the fact that facial paralysis very rarely occurs during eruptions of trigeminal herpes simplex, even in the extensive eruptions that follow trigeminal root section. Likewise, herpetic skin lesions are uncommon in Bell's palsy, though Tovi and associates (1980) have claimed otherwise.

The majority of patients have "a good result" when evaluated 9 months after the onset of facial paralysis, but the fact is not particularly consoling to the 10 or 15 percent of patients with obtrusive sequelae such as weakness, synkinesis, contracture, or crocodile tears. There is now reasonably firm evidence that a short course of high-dose prednisone, administered within a few days after the onset of paralysis, substantially reduces the incidence and consequences of axonal degeneration. Taverner and associates (1971) gave prednisolone, 80 mg per day (adult dose) for 5 days, tapering the dose rapidly during the following 4 days. In a controlled, sequential trial of patients with moderate or severe paralysis, a poor result (less than 50 percent recovery) occurred in 6 percent of patients treated with ACTH and in none of the patients treated with prednisolone. Synkinesis occurred in 34 percent of the ACTH-treated patients compared with 14 percent of those treated with prednisone. Similar results have been obtained in a nonrandomized trial (Adour et al. 1978) and in a randomized trial in which the difference did not reach significance, probably because only one third of the patients had severe weakness (Wolf et al. 1978).

One would like to avoid treating patients unnecessarily, but it is difficult to identify in advance patients who are likely to develop denervation. Electrodiagnostic testing cannot distinguish this group before the fifth or sixth day, too late for steroid therapy to be of much value. Although patients with mild weakness nearly all recover fully, these patients make up only 10 to 20 percent of the total number. In the remaining majority of patients, the completeness of paralysis is not a very reliable prognostic indicator. Measurement of the anodal galvanic taste threshold has been recommended as an accurate means of selecting patients for steroid therapy (Aminoff 1973). About 40 percent of patients with early Bell's palsy have a normal taste threshold as compared with the opposite side of the tongue, and 93 percent of these patients recover completely without treatment (Taverner et al. 1967). Unfortunately, subjective alterations of taste and the results of ordinary clinical taste testing do not correlate well with outcome, and the electrogustometer is not commercially available. For all of these reasons it seems prudent to recommend a course of prednisone provided that (1) treatment can be instituted within 4 days of onset, (2) there are no medical contraindications, and (3) the weakness is at least moderately severe, or there is a subjective or objective impairment of taste. The dose schedule should approximate that employed by Taverner and colleagues (1971): 80 mg of prednisone for 5 days, tapered rapidly over the next 4 days.

MIGRATORY RECURRENT CRANIAL NEURITIS. This rare syndrome has been reported most often from Southeast Asia (Tay et al. 1974; Steele and Vasuvat 1970), but it is not unknown in Europe (Hokkanen et al. 1978). During a period of many years the patients experience repeated episodes, at intervals of months or years, of single or multiple cranial nerve palsies that generally resolve within a few weeks. The same or different nerves are involved in each episode. The episodes may be preceded by a mild upper respiratory infection or by nonspecific stress, and they are usually accompanied by headache. The cranial nerves most frequently affected are the facial nerve, the ocular motor nerves, the optic nerve, and the trigeminal nerve. The erythrocyte sedimentation rate and the white blood cell count are often mildly elevated, and the CSF may show a mild mononuclear pleocytosis and an elevated protein level. Corticosteroid therapy appears to bring prompt resolution of the episode in most cases. This syndrome bears some resemblance to the disorder known as acute painful ophthalmoplegia, especially since ocular involvement may be accompanied by mild proptosis and chemosis in both syndromes (Tay et al. 1974). Painful ophthalmoplegia is discussed further in Chapter 3.

Acute Idiopathic Polyneuritis

The Guillain-Barré syndrome (GBS) is an acute or subacute inflammatory polyneuropathy characterized by generalized muscle weakness and areflexia, usually followed by complete recovery of function. This dramatic disorder has received much medical attention in recent decades, although the annual incidence is only 0.6 to 1.9 cases per 100,000 population (Kennedy et al. 1978; Shoenberger et al. 1981), amounting to somewhat over 2,000 cases a year in the United States. Recent progress in immunologic research has stimulated a re-examination of the pathogenesis of GBS. Even the clinical and electrodiagnostic features, ably reviewed in an authoritative chapter by Arnason (1975b), have become better defined as a result of several studies published in the last few years (McLeod et al. 1976; Löffel et al. 1977; Andersson and Sidén 1982), and considerable interest has been aroused by recent evaluations of the therapeutic value of corticosteroids and plasmapheresis.

CLINICAL FEATURES. GBS occurs at all ages, but the incidence increases steadily with age. Men are affected somewhat more often than women. In about half of the patients a viral upper respiratory infection or other infectious illness precedes the symptoms of polyneuritis by 2 to 3 weeks, but the infectious symptoms have usually subsided by the time the neuritic symptoms begin.

The neurologic illness consists of three stages: a progressive phase, a plateau, and a recovery phase. Contrary to a widespread impression, sensory disturbance, especially paresthesia, is the presenting symptom in half of the patients, and in other patients paresthesias and weakness appear together; only about one fourth of the patients experience muscle weakness first. Pain in the legs and back is another common early symptom. Even so, muscle weakness dominates the clinical picture, quickly spreading through the limbs and the axial muscles. The weakness may "ascend" from the legs to the arms but this sequence tends to be overemphasized in some textbooks; in fact, weakness is usually diffuse but spotty and often asymmetric at the outset, and terms like "proximal" and "distal" do not adequately convey the findings. The weakness continues to increase, reaching a plateau within 2 weeks in about half of the cases and within 4 weeks in almost all cases. During this progressive phase the muscle stretch reflexes become depressed and disappear, although they may be preserved in a few mild cases. The pulmonary vital capacity declines in half of the patients.

At the peak of their disability, about 60 percent of the patients are unable to walk and 20 percent need mechanical ventilation. The muscles are often painful and are sometimes tender; neuropathic pain may also be present. Distal impairment of sensation, especially for touch, vibration, and position sense, is present in 50 to 80 percent of patients. Cranial neuropathies, especially facial weakness (often bilateral) and weakness of the throat, tongue, and jaws, are usually slow to appear but eventually are found in half of the patients. Weakness of the ocular muscles is infrequent. Extensor plantar responses have been described but are hard to evaluate in the presence of lower motor neuron weakness. Impairment of bladder control is infrequent, but other autonomic disturbances are commonly present, including persistent sinus tachycardia, orthostatic hypotension, episodes of hypertension and hypotension, and impairment of sweating and thermal regulation. Occasionally there is inappropriate secretion of antidiuretic hormone.

A rare clinical variant, usually termed the Miller Fisher syndrome, is characterized by external ophthalmoplegia, areflexia, and loss of truncal equilibrium. Pupillary function is sometimes spared, muscle strength is usually normal, and sensation may be intact despite the ataxia. The clinical course and CSF findings resemble those of GBS, but the anatomic basis of the ophthalmoplegia and ataxia is still debated (Fisher 1956; Elizan et al. 1972); a brainstem disorder has been invoked in some cases (Becker et al. 1981).

The plateau period lasts anywhere from a few days to 6 weeks; a prolonged delay before improvement begins is associated with severe disease. As in Bell's palsy, recovery occurs in two stages: an early stage, usually completed within 6 weeks, and a delayed, protracted stage associated with nerve regeneration. In mild cases complete recovery occurs within a few weeks; in severe cases the full extent of recovery may not be apparent for more than a year. About 80 percent of patients recover completely or have minor residual signs, and about 5 percent of patients are left with an important handicap, mainly in the form of distal weakness and sensory loss in the legs and hands. Relapses during convalescence or recurrence months or years later have been recorded in fewer than 5 percent of patients. The case mortality ratio is less than 5 percent; deaths occur primarily in elderly persons or patients with serious associated illness.

LABORATORY FINDINGS. An elevated CSF protein level is an important diagnostic sign but is not always found. The protein level rises after the first week in most patients (McLeod et al. 1976). There is no published series in which lumbar punctures were performed repeatedly during the first several weeks of illness in a large group of patients; however, individual patients with otherwise typical GBS have had a persistently normal CSF. The CSF white cell count is increased in 12 to 20 percent of the cases, and in the series of McCleod and associates (1976), contrary to the usual dictum, all of the increases occurred after the first week, with values of 30 to 148 leukocytes per mm^3 in 10 percent of the cases. Indeed, considering the inflammatory changes in the nerve roots, it is not surprising that CSF pleocytosis is found occasionally. An increased CSF concentration of gamma globulin, with oligoclonal bands in CSF and serum, has been found in two thirds of the patients (Link 1973; Dalakas et al. 1980).

Electrodiagnostic studies (McLeod 1981) are valuable for diagnosis but initially provide little information about prognosis. At the peak of weakness, abnormalities of motor or sensory nerve conduction are found in 80 to 90 percent of patients, if several nerves are tested in each patient. The abnormalities include slow motor nerve conduction, prolonged distal motor latency, reduced motor amplitude, and reduced amplitude or prolonged latency of sensory nerve or mixed nerve action potentials (Eisen and Humphreys 1974; McLeod et al. 1976; McQuillen 1971). Slowing of motor nerve conduction velocity in the "demyelinative range" can be found in at least one nerve in about half of the patients. Motor conduction blocks and temporal dispersion of motor responses or of sensory and mixed action potentials are typical findings (Wexler 1980). However, normal motor nerve conduction velocity has been reported in 20 to 40 percent of patients in some series, especially early in the illness, and serial studies tend to show progressive slowing of conduction even when patients are improving, followed by a progressive return toward normal (Hausmanowa-Petrusewicz et al. 1979; Wexler 1980).

These findings are not unlike those encountered in diphtheritic polyneuropathy (Chapter 4), and the explanation may be similar. In GBS, both conduction slowing (Miyoshi and Oh 1977; Kimura 1978) and demyelinative lesions (Asbury et al. 1969) are scattered throughout the length of the peripheral nerves, including the nerve roots. If conduction is blocked in the proximal part of a nerve trunk, weakness may be severe even when conduction is normal distal to the block. Likewise, there may be distal conduction block or axonal degeneration in some of the nerves in a nerve trunk, but the unaffected motor nerves may conduct with normal velocity. When distal nerve lesions are repaired, the amplitude of the response will increase but conduction velocity may be slow in the remyelinated or regenerated nerves. Indeed, permanent slowing of nerve conduction is frequently present in patients who have made a good recovery (Hausmanowa-Petrusewicz et al. 1979).

During the first several weeks, EMG provides no useful information about the prognosis for recovery. After that time, EMG evidence of denervation (fibrillations) indicates that axonal degeneration has occurred and suggests that recovery will probably be slow. Complete absence of motor and sensory responses to distal nerve stimulation also suggests that severe Wallerian degeneration has probably taken place.

PATHOLOGY (Prineas 1981). The important autopsy studies carried out by Asbury and associates (1969) established the fact that GBS is primarily a demyelinative polyneuropathy of inflammatory origin, with secondary axonal degeneration in severely affected nerves. The inflammatory picture consists of multiple focal, perivascular infiltrations of lymphocytes and macrophages in the endoneurium and epineurium of somatic and sympathetic nerves, extending in a patchy distribution from the roots to the nerve terminals. A segmental demyelinative process is closely associated with the focal inflammatory infiltrates. These features can usually be detected in sural nerve biopsies, especially if teased nerve fibers are also examined (McLeod et al. 1976), but nerve biopsy is rarely needed for the diagnosis and provides no information about prognosis.

PRECIPITATING CAUSES. The role of antecedent illness is more apparent for GBS than for Bell's palsy. Occurrence of a viral-like illness 1 to 4 weeks previously has been noted in 50 to 70 percent of cases. A number of specific virus infections have been incriminated, including measles, influenza, varicella, herpes zoster, cytomegalovirus disease, infectious mononucleosis, infectious hepatitis (Berger et al. 1981), and infections caused by coxsackie viruses and echoviruses (Arnason 1975b). In addition, mycoplasma pneumoniae, chlamydial infections, gram-negative infections, and legionnaire's disease (Morgan and Gawler 1981) have been identified in some cases. GBS may occur 2 to 3 weeks after fever therapy, and between 5 and 10 percent of GBS cases follow a surgical operation. Vaccination against smallpox (Spillane and Wells 1964), rabies immunization (especially with suckling mouse brain vaccine [Adaros and Held 1971]), and vaccination against influenza (Marks and Halpin 1980) are rare causes of GBS except during mass immunization programs. There is an increased incidence of GBS in patients with Hodgkin's disease, angioimmunoblastic lymphadenopathy, and other types of lymphoma.

Recent serologic surveys indicate that cytomegalovirus infection may account for 11 to 26 percent of all GBS cases, depending on whether the diagnostic criterion is the presence of specific IgM antibodies or a fourfold change in the titer of complement-fixing antibodies (Dowling et al. 1977; Schmitz and Enders 1977; Dowling and Cook 1981). IgM antibodies to EB-virus are present in 8 percent (Dowling and Cook 1981), and high titers of mycoplasma antibodies are found in 5 percent of GBS patients (Goldschmidt et al. 1980). Thus, perhaps a third of GBS cases, especially those occurring in young patients, may be caused by cytomegalovirus, infectious mononucleosis, or mycoplasma pneumoniae infections. These infections tend to induce cold agglutinins, and Dowling and coworkers (1977) found increased titers of cold agglutinins in one third of GBS patients.

TREATMENT. Corticosteroid and ACTH therapy was widely used during the 2 decades 1957 to 1977, with conflicting reports of their efficacy (Goodall et al. 1974). Finally, in London a randomized, prospective study was carried out in which 21 patients treated early with prednisolone for 2 weeks* were compared with 19 untreated patients. Contrary to expectation, the steroid-treated patients showed *less* improvement at 3 months and at 1 year after onset; six steroid-treated patients (29 percent) had considerable disability at 1 year compared with only one untreated patient (5 percent). There were three relapses (14 percent) in the steroid-treated group and none in the control group (Hughes et al. 1978).

When these discouraging results were published, they were all the more surprising because the effectiveness of steroid therapy was just becoming apparent in a related disorder, subacute or chronic (relapsing) idio-

*The schedule was 60 mg daily for 1 week, 40 mg daily for 4 days, and 30 mg daily for 3 days.

pathic polyneuritis. Furthermore, there was no treatment to take the place of steroids, since cytotoxic immunosuppressive drugs did not seem to be effective (in fact, there was one report of GBS in a renal transplant patient already on immunosuppressive therapy [Drachman et al. 1970]). At this point, anecdotal reports began to appear describing good, even dramatic, results from plasma exchange therapy during the progressive stage of GBS (Brettle et al. 1978; Ropper et al. 1980; Mark et al. 1980; Cook et al. 1980; Rumpl et al. 1981). Because of the danger of misinterpreting spontaneous recovery for a therapeutic effect, so vividly illustrated by the 20-year experience with steroid therapy, a randomized prospective trial of plasmapheresis therapy in GBS was undertaken by 21 collaborating hospitals in North America, beginning in February 1981. The results of the trial will not be known for a year or two. If circulating antibodies or immune complexes are responsible for nerve damage in GBS, it may be that plasmapheresis would have to be performed early in order to prevent axonal degeneration, which is responsible for the protracted course and incomplete recovery in severe cases.

Pathophysiology of Postinfectious Neuropathies. There are reasons for thinking that different pathogenic mechanisms may underly acute mononeuritis and brachial plexus neuritis, on one hand, and acute idiopathic polyneuritis (GBS) on the other hand. The former neuropathies appear abruptly and evolve rapidly over a few days; the manifestations are localized, and axonal degeneration occurs frequently, so that muscle denervation and delayed recovery occur frequently. In GBS the neuropathies appear gradually over several weeks, the manifestations are diffuse, and the primary disease process consists of widespread, multifocal, segmental demyelination, with varying degrees of secondary axonal degeneration. In serum sickness, acute mononeuritis and plexus neuritis occur five times as often as GBS. If immune processes are involved in the pathogenesis of these neuropathies, as seems very likely, it is logical to suspect, as Arnason (1975a) has suggested, that acute plexus neuritis is an antibody-mediated disorder, while GBS is primarily mediated by lymphocytes.

Nevertheless, the two types of neuropathy share a variety of predisposing factors: viral infections, especially minor upper respiratory or gastrointestinal illnesses, immunizations, and surgical operations. Furthermore, both types usually occur in otherwise healthy individuals with no prior history of hypersensitivity disorders, are usually not accompanied by systemic manifestations of acute or delayed hypersensitivity, and affect motor nerves preferentially.

The clinical manifestations of serum sickness result from the deposition of immune complexes and complement in the walls of blood vessels, provoking an inflammatory response that damages the surrounding tissues. If this process occurs in acute plexus neuritis, it is hard to understand why multiple nerves in one limb are affected, why the arm is so much more susceptible than the leg, and why there are no systemic signs of immune complex disease in the vast majority of patients. Alternatively, there could be antibodies directed against nerve tissue or against an infectious agent which has invaded peripheral nerves, leading to localized antigen-antibody reactions and complement-mediated tissue injury.

Much more information is available about GBS (Iqbal et al. 1981a; Cook and Dowling 1981; Nyland et al. 1981). The pathologic findings of perivenular lymphocytic infiltrates containing transformed lymphocytes are reminiscent of a delayed hypersensitivity reaction (Asbury et al. 1969). Peripheral blood lymphocytes from patients with GBS produce demyelination in peripheral nerve cultures, and when exposed to peripheral nerve or myelin antigens in vitro they undergo transformation and inhibit monocyte migration (Arnason 1975b). An animal model, experimental allergic neuritis (EAN), has been produced in rodents by immunization with an extract of peripheral nerve (Waksman and Adams 1955) or with a basic protein constituent of peripheral nerve myelin (antigenically distinct from central myelin basic protein, which produces allergic encephalomyelitis) (Brostoff et al. 1972). The clinical and pathologic features of EAN are very similar to GBS, and the disease can be transferred by immunocompetent lymphocytes but not by serum, suggesting that delayed hypersensitivity is the principle disease mechanism (Åström and Waksman 1962).

There is also evidence of antibody production in patients with GBS: increased levels of immunoglobulin, with oligoclonal bands in CSF and serum (Link 1973), deposition of immunoglobulins in nerve (Luijten and Baart de la Faille-Kuyper 1972), and circulating antibodies reacting with crude peripheral nerve antigen (Nyland and Aarli 1978). There are reports that GBS serum can produce demyelination when injected directly into nerves (Feasby et al. 1982; Sumner et al. 1982; Saida et al. 1982), but some investigators were unable to confirm this (Low et al. 1982). Antibodies directed against the myelin basic protein of peripheral nerves have not been found in patients with GBS, although they are present in animals with EAN (Iqbal et al. 1981b). Immune complexes containing hepatitis B surface antigen were noted to appear in serum and CSF coincident with the onset of GBS in a patient recovering from type B hepatitis (Penner et al. 1982). Studies such as these form the rationale for current trials of plasmapheresis therapy in GBS.

Recently Phillips and colleagues (1981) reported that serum from patients who developed GBS after being vaccinated for swine influenza contained antibodies reacting with a peripheral nerve antigen that was also a constituent of the vaccine. Of the vaccinated GBS patients, 65 percent had such antibodies, compared with 10 percent of nonvaccinated GBS patients. In both groups, however, over half of the patients showed binding of serum IgG to peripheral nerve in vitro. These interesting findings suggest that GBS may be mediated by immune responses directed against several different antigens. Some cases may be initiated by an immune reaction directed against an antigenic constituent of the infectious agent that happens to be similar or identical to a constituent of peripheral nerves.

However, it seems unlikely that all of the different viral infections implicated in GBS contain human nerve antigens. How then do infections trigger GBS? Diffuse infection of the peripheral nervous system seems an unlikely explanation; as Arnason (1975b) has stated, "It is difficult to envisage any simple basis on which so many different viral agents, each with its unique clinical features, would produce an identical clinical syndrome and an identical pathological picture in nerve by any direct invasive mechanism." Arnason suggested that viruses might provoke autoimmunity by incorporating host membrane material and rendering it antigenic, and this mechanism has also been invoked in mycoplasma infections (Davis et al. 1981). Nevertheless, there is some indication that direct invasion of the peripheral nerves by an infectious agent could be responsible for some cases of GBS. In a recent case, Mycoplasma pneumoniae organisms were identified by special techniques in CSF and circulating leukocytes of a GBS patient who had recently recovered from a mycoplasmal illness (Bayer et al. 1981). In Marek's disease of domestic chickens, which is caused by a herpes virus related to Epstein-Barr (EB) virus and cytomegalovirus, a demyelinative polyneuropathy occurs in association with a latent infection of the Schwann cells and other supporting cells of the peripheral nerves. The affected birds exhibit cellular and humoral immune responses to both peripheral nerve and myelin (Stevens et al. 1981). This animal model of GBS is especially interesting because it combines the infectious and immune mechanisms of pathogenesis, and also because herpes viruses have been incriminated in the etiology of GBS. The monophasic, transient character of GBS also fits an infectious model. If the immunologic reaction were directed primarily against the infectious agent rather than against myelin, one would expect to see (as has been described) a transient polyclonal increase in IgG and the CSF, deposits of immune complexes in the supporting tissue of peripheral nerves, and an inflammatory response to the immune complexes, leading to the release of harmful chemical substances by damaged cells—in other words, a localized Arthus reaction. It is noteworthy that the agent of Marek's disease cannot be recovered from peripheral nerves by traditional culture techniques, and that other herpes viruses, as well as mycoplasma organisms, are prone to establish latent infections in humans. Thus, there is reason to suspect that those GBS cases that are associated with infections caused by EB virus, cytomegalovirus, and Mycoplasma pneumoniae (about one third of all cases) may be due to a latent infection of the peripheral nervous system and to the resulting immunologic reactions, which may be directed against the infectious agent or against host peripheral nerve constituents rendered antigenic by the infection (Pepose 1982).

Other Neuromuscular Disorders

Polymyositis and *dermatomyositis* occasionally begin after vaccination or other immunizations (Cotterill and Shapiro 1978; Kåss 1978; Ehrengut 1978). The number of reported cases is small, so that it is difficult to know whether the association is meaningful. *Myasthenia gravis,* too, may begin a few weeks after a viral illness (Lubetzki Korn and Abramsky 1981). Two patients with myasthenia gravis had transient exacerbation of weakness beginning about 10 days after vaccination against smallpox (Spillane and Wells 1964); this reaction could represent a nonspecific stimulation of the immune system, resulting in increased production of antibodies against the acetylcholine receptor, but adverse reactions to other types of immunization (against influenza, for instance) do not seem to be common in myasthenia. However, exacerbations following minor viral infections are a well-known feature of myasthenia gravis, and it would be interesting to know whether the serum titer of actetylcholine receptor antibodies rises during intercurrent infections.

CHRONIC IDIOPATHIC POLYNEURITIS

In the past 10 or 15 years this syndrome has become recognized as one of the principle subgroups of polyneuropathy of obscure etiology (Prineas 1970). Like GBS, subacute or chronic demyelinative polyneuropathy typically occurs in healthy persons of any age. According to some authors (Prineas and McLeod 1976; Oh 1978; Dyck et al, 1975), a history of preceding viral illness, immunization, or insect bite is commonly obtained, but Dalakas and Engel (1981a) were unable to incriminate any precipitating factors.

CLINICAL FEATURES. Clinically the syndrome resembles a slow form of GBS. Muscle weakness is usually the predominant symptom, but paresthesias and numbness also occur and occasionally are the predominant feature. Weakness of the limbs begins gradually, often in the legs, and spreads through the limbs with increasing severity at a pace measured in weeks and months rather than days. Weakness usually continues to increase for months or years until steroid treatment is started. Some patients have a stepwise rather than steady progression of symptoms, and others show a relapsing and remitting course.

The limb muscle weakness usually has a diffuse distribution, involving proximal muscles at least as much as distal ones. There is little or no muscular atrophy, because axonal degeneration is usually not a prominent feature, and fasciculations are infrequent. The trunk muscles may be affected, but respiratory weakness is rarely noticeable. The proximal distribution of weakness in some patients may suggest a myopathy, but the muscle stretch reflexes are always depressed and often there is complete areflexia even in fairly strong muscles, a hallmark of peripheral nerve disease. Sensation is sometimes completely normal; in other cases, deep and superficial sensation are impaired in the distal portions of the limbs. When sensory loss is severe there is a sensory ataxia of gait and a coarse, postural tremor of the limbs and trunk. Any of the cranial nerves from 3 to 12 may be affected, but such findings are infrequent except in the series of Prineas and McLeod (1976), who recorded cranial neuropathies in 10 out of 34 patients.

LABORATORY FINDINGS. In most cases motor nerve conduction velocities are diffusely and strikingly slow, in the range of 20 to 30 m per second, and distal motor latencies are similarly prolonged. The responses are temporally dispersed, and regions of conduction block may be identified. Sensory nerve conduction is often abnormal despite a lack of clinical sensory signs, showing reduced amplitudes and prolonged latencies of the sensory action potentials. The CSF protein is increased in 90 percent of cases, ranging as high as 600 to 700 mg per dl, and a mild lymphocytic pleocytosis is present in about 10 percent of cases. The CSF concentration of gamma globulin was increased in 14 percent of the patients reported on by Dyck and associates (1975), but since the IgG/albumin ratio was not stated, the increase could have been a nonspecific result of a leaky blood-CSF barrier. Dalakas and coworkers (1980) found normal in-situ synthesis rates of IgG in the CSF, but a dense, monoclonal band of IgG was present in 14 of 15 cases. This abnormality persisted for many months, despite clinical fluctuations and steroid treatment. The monoclonal IgG did not bind to sections of normal human nerve in vitro, so that its pathologic significance is unknown. General laboratory tests including the sedimentation rate, are usually normal except for an increased concentration of serum gamma globulin in about 10 percent of the patients (Dyck et al. 1975).

PATHOLOGY. The pathology of sural nerve biopsies has been extensively studied (Dyck et al. 1975; Oh 1978; Prineas and McLeod 1976), and there is general agreement that the main features consist of segmental demyelination and remyelination, infrequent axonal degeneration and regeneration, occasional onion-bulb hypertrophic changes, and in a few cases a reduced density of myelinated fibers. Mononuclear cell infiltrates were observed by some investigators (Dyck et al. 1975; Prineas and McLeod 1976) but not by others (Dalakas and Engel 1981a). Autopsy studies showed similar findings, but in addition there was a scattered infiltration of mononuclear inflammatory cells in the spinal cord and brain, and the peripheral nerve changes were more marked in the roots and proximal portions of nerves than in the distal portions (Dyck et al. 1975). The pathologic findings are quite similar to those of GBS (Prineas and McLleod 1976; Dyck et al. 1975).

Other evidence suggests that antibody-mediated immune mechanisms may be involved. Using immunofluorescence light microscopy, Dalakas and Engel (1980) demonstrated granular deposits of IgM and C3 component of complement in the walls of blood vessels of peripheral nerves, as well as linear deposits of IgM on Schwann cell plasma membranes of unmyelinated nerve fibers. They suggested that the IgM could be an antibody toxic to Schwann cells.

TREATMENT. The response to corticosteroid therapy is usually excellent (Dalakas and Engel 1981a). It is usual to begin treatment with daily, single-dose prednisone (40 to 80 mg in adults), changing to an alternate-day schedule in 1 to 3 months if a good clinical response has been obtained. Because axonal degeneration is rarely severe, improvement is often apparent within a few weeks, and complete recovery usually occurs in 6 to 12 months. Treatment should be continued for about 1 year, with slowly tapered dosage, because relapse is likely if the dose is reduced too rapidly, and relapses may be much more severe than the original illness.

Some patients who respond incompletely, either on the first occasion or during subsequent relapses, may have a better response to a combination of prednisone with azathioprine or cyclophosphamide. A number of case reports indicate that intermittent courses of plasmapheresis, in combination with prednisone and a cytotoxic immunosuppressive drug, are useful in some refractory patients (Server et al. 1979; Levy et al. 1979; Gross and Thomas 1981).

It is now common practice to offer a trial of steroid therapy to patients with subacute or chronic polyneuropathy of unknown cause, after a thorough search for a specific etiology has been fruitless.* Experience has shown that the patients who are likely to respond to steroid treatment are those with marked slowing of motor nerve conduction velocity and increased CSF protein. Absence of either feature reduces the response rate, and if both features are absent the patient will almost certainly not respond to steroids (and probably does not have chronic inflammatory polyneuropathy). A sural nerve biopsy should be performed before embarking on steroid treatment, to strengthen the diagnosis in the event that prolonged treatment becomes necessary; however, a negative result does not exclude this diagnosis.

Pathophysiology. The pathogenesis of chronic idiopathic polyneuritis is still uncertain. Despite the clinical, pathologic, and electrophysiologic resmblances, there are equally impressive differences between this disorder and GBS. Steroid treatment appears to be ineffective in GBS but is often strikingly effective in chronic inflammatory polyneuropathy. Axonal degeneration occurs less often in the chronic than in the acute disorder. Plasmapheresis appears to be effective in the former while its response in the latter, though still being evaluated, is inconsistent. These findings suggest that the two disorders may have different immunologic mechanisms; in particular, evidence for a pathogenetic role of circulating antibodies is stronger in the chronic disorder. Studies of leukocyte antigens also suggest different immunologic backgrounds. Chronic inflammatory polyneuritis is associated with HLA antigens AW-30, AW-31, and DW-3, while GBS shows no definite association with any phenotype (Stewart et al. 1978).

VARIANT SYNDROMES. A few patients with chronic inflammatory polyneuropathy have exhibited the syndrome of muscular overactivity known as neuromyotonia, consisting of myokymia and muscle stiffness. In some of these cases the involved muscles became noticeably enlarged (Valenstein et al. 1978).

Recently a number of patients have been seen with a chronic, relapsing neuropathy that takes the form of a mononeuropathy multiplex rather than a polyneuropathy. The most distinctive feature of these cases is the presence of a *persistent conduction block* at locations where nerves are not usually subject to entrapment, especially in the upper arms and thighs (Lewis et al. 1982). Peripheral mononeuropathies and occasionally cranial mononeuropathies develop gradually over a period of weeks, months, or years, and then become stable or subside spontaneously. The disorder is not painful and there is no evidence of systemic illness even after many years of neuropathic symptoms. The peripheral nerve lesions produce focal

*In particular, the possibility of a polyneuropathy related to a paraproteinemia should be carefully investigated, as described in the next section.

weakness and variable degrees of muscle atrophy; focal sensory loss may also occur, but the motor signs are usually more striking. Muscle stretch reflexes are preserved except in the affected muscles. The nerve trunks are not enlarged to palpation; in fact, in one of my patients a segment of ulnar nerve with chronic conduction block appeared quite atrophic when exposed at surgery. Motor nerve conduction velocity is often normal across the uninvolved distal nerve segments, but stimulation at proximal sites reveals multiple areas of conduction block. Presumably the sites of chronic conduction block represent focal demyelinated lesions of the nerve trunks. Preliminary experience indicates that steroid and cytotoxic drug therapy may be effective, but in most cases the symptoms are not severe enough to warrant such treatment.

Acute, subacute, and chronic relapsing polyradiculoneuropathies have been reported in seven patients with *angioimmunoblastic lymphadenopathy*, a rare form of lymphoma characterized by a rapid evolution, hypergammaglobulinemia, and involvement of lymph nodes, bone marrow, and lungs (Brunet et al. 1981). Several patients had intractable aching pain in the back and extremities. The peripheral nerve pathology was similar to that of idiopathic polyneuritis, with segmental demyelination and multifocal inflammatory infiltration, but leptomeningeal invasion occurred in some patients, producing an inflammatory CSF picture. Some of the patients responded to treatment with steroids or intrathecal methotrexate.

NEUROMUSCULAR DISORDERS ASSOCIATED WITH PARAPROTEINEMIA

The rare sensorimotor polyneuropathy associated with multiple myeloma has long intrigued clinical investigators, but lately it has been found that some patients with polyneuropathy have monoclonal immunoglobulin abnormalities without a frank plasma cell malignancy. Although much remains to be learned about these disorders, the outlines of several distinct syndromes are beginning to emerge (Table 22).

Plasma Cell Malignancies

Polyneuropathy is usually regarded as a rare complication of multiple myeloma, with an incidence of 0.4 to 3 percent in retrospective chart reviews. However, in a prospective series Walsh (1971) found clinical signs of polyneuropathy in 13 percent and electrophysiologic signs in 39 percent of mye-

TABLE 22. Polyneuropathies Associated with Paraproteinemia

Disorder	Type of Neuropathy
A. Plasma cell malignancies	
1. Lytic multiple myeloma	Distal, sensorimotor, axonal, with or without amyloid
2. Waldenström's macroglobulinemia	Distal, sensorimotor, axonal, with or without amyloid
3. Sclerotic myeloma (including solitary plasmacytoma)	Diffuse, motor or sensorimotor, demyelinative
B. Nonmalignant paraproteinemias	Diffuse, motor or sensorimotor, demyelinative Distal, sensorimotor, axonal Amyloid neuropathy

loma patients. Hesselvik (1969) found clinical signs of polyneuropathy in 12 percent of myeloma patients, while nerve biopsy abnormalities were present in 65 percent. The incidence of polyneuropathy in Waldenstrom's macroglobulinemia, a less common disorder, has not been formally studied but is probably not less than that in myeloma, since more than 20 cases of this association have been reported (McLeod and Walsh 1975).

In a review of 54 published cases of multiple myeloma with polyneuropathy (not including Walsh's series), Driedger and Pruzanski (1980) noted several distinctive clinical features. About 80 percent of the patients were men, half of them less than 51 years old. Neuropathy was the presenting symptom in 80 percent of the patients. A solitary plasmacytoma was present in 26 percent, and fewer than three lesions were seen on x-ray in 42 percent of the cases; osteosclerotic or mixed sclerotic and lytic lesions were present in more than half of the cases. The serum paraprotein was usually present in low concentration, especially in cases of solitary plasmacytoma, where the paraprotein was often not detectable by routine serum protein electrophoresis. The abnormal immunoglobulin was an IgG in 78 percent of the cases and an IgA in the remainder. In 10 cases in which the light chains were classified, all were of lambda type. Kelly and colleagues (1981) found kappa and lambda light chains with equal frequency in patients with lytic multiple myeloma, while five of nine patients with sclerotic myeloma had lambda light chains and four had no detectable light chains. In patients with ordinary multiple myeloma, kappa light chains are twice as frequent as lambda chains, the same as in healthy persons.

CLINICAL FEATURES. The clinical features of polyneuropathy appear to differ in the lytic and sclerotic types of myeloma (Kelly et al. 1981). In *lytic myeloma,* the patients have a median age of 63 years and usually exhibit the typical clinical and laboratory signs of multiple myeloma. They have a gradually progressive, symmetric, sensorimotor polyneuropathy that is confined to the extremities in a decidedly distal distribution. Sensory symptoms usually appear first and often dominate the clinical picture; burning pain and unpleasant dysesthesia and paresthesia are common, and all modalities of sensation are affected. The muscle weakness is associated with atrophy, but fasciculations are uncommon. The muscle stretch reflexes are reduced or absent, especially in the distal portions of the limbs. The CSF protein is normal or slightly increased; motor nerve conduction velocities are only mildly slowed, and sensory nerve responses are diminished in amplitude. These findings are consistent with an axonal type of polyneuropathy.

Some patients with lytic multiple myeloma develop amyloid polyneuropathy. In the past this was considered a rare complication, but at the Mayo Clinic amyloid was present in 4 of the 10 cases of polyneuropathy associated with lytic myeloma (Kelly et al. 1981), and Benson and colleagues (1975) found 3 patients with polyneuropathy among 14 cases of amyloidosis secondary to malignant B-cell dyscrasia. The clinical features of amyloid polyneuropathy in multiple myeloma are similar to those of primary amyloid polyneuropathy, which is described below.

Patients with *sclerotic myeloma* are generally younger (median age 49 years), have a normal sedimentation rate, do not have myeloma cells in a random bone marrow sample, and have a small paraprotein spike (0.7 to 1.7 g per dl). These patients may have a predominantly motor polyneuropathy or a mixed motor-sensory polyneuropathy, with little or no pain. Respiratory weakness occurs in some cases. The CSF protein is increased and may reach values over 500 mg per dl. Papilledema, a complication also encountered in idiopathic inflammatory polyneuritis, was present in 3 of 10 patients with sclerotic myeloma neuropathy at the Mayo Clinic (Kelly et al. 1981). Motor nerve conduction velocity is moderately or markedly slowed, in the demyelinative range, and responses may be unobtainable.

A peculiar assortment of associated findings has recently been described in some patients with the polyneuropathy of sclerotic myeloma. These include skin changes (hyperpigmentation, thickening, hirsutism, and hyperhidrosis), endocrinopathy (gonadal failure, gynecomastia, and insulin-sensitive diabetes mellitus), hepatosplenomegaly, lymphadenopathy, peripheral edema, ascites, pleural effusions, and fever. Among the published series of patients with osteosclerotic myeloma and polyneuropathy, one or more of these symptoms were mentioned in 13 to 33 percent of the cases (Iwashita et al. 1977). No serum paraprotein was detected in 40 percent of the cases; two thirds of the remainder had IgG paraproteins, and the others had IgA paraproteins. Most of the cases have been reported from Japan, but the syndrome is beginning to be recognized in Western countries (Bardwick et al. 1980; Delauche et al. 1981; Driedger and Pruzanski 1980). The clinical and laboratory features of the polyneuropathy are the same as those observed in other cases of sclerotic myeloma neuropathy. In two of these patients, Driedger and Pruzanski (1980) were unable to detect any serum antibodies reacting with neurons, glia, or various non-neural tissue antigens, so the basis of these extraordinarily diverse manifestations remains unexplained.

PATHOLOGY. Microscopic examination of peripheral nerves obtained by biopsy and autopsy has given conflicting findings. Axonal degeneration has been seen in most cases, but a mixture of segmental demyelination and axonal degeneration has also been described, and Hesselvik (1969) found demyelination to be the predominant lesion, though she did not use the more reliable teased-fiber technique. Kelly and colleagues (1981) reported a mixture of axonal degeneration and demyelination in sural nerve specimens from patients with either lytic or sclerotic myeloma; small infiltrates of mononuclear cells were also observed, reminiscent of chronic inflammatory polyneuropathy.

COURSE AND TREATMENT. In most patients with lytic multiple myeloma, the neuropathy advances relentlessly to death within a year or two, and the neuropathy generally responds poorly to treatment. By contrast, patients with a solitary, sclerotic plasmacytoma respond surprisingly well to treatment of the tumor with radiation, with or without chemotherapy. Progression of the neuropathy is often arrested and there may be some degree of recovery, though eventually the tumor recurs, and new lesions may appear in other parts of the skeleton (Read and Warlow 1978). Even patients with more extensive sclerotic myeloma may respond to radiation and chemotherapy (Driedger and Pruzanski 1980). In view of these gratifying results, a special effort should be made to search for a sclerotic myeloma in patients with polyneuropathy whose clinical features fit the general picture outlined above. The workup should include not only an ordinary serum protein electrophoresis but serum immunoelectrophoresis, tests for light chains in the urine, and a full skeletal radiographic survey (a more sensitive test for myeloma than the radionuclide bone scan). Some paraproteins precipitate at room temperature or in the cold, so if a paraprotein is not found, a blood sample should be collected and processed at 37°C (Sherman et al. 1982).

Nonmalignant Paraproteinemia

The distinction between malignant and benign monoclonal gammopathies is uncertain and tenuous. In normal persons the frequency of asymptomatic paraproteinemia increases with age; paraproteins have been found in 3 to 7 percent of persons over the age of 70 and in up to 19 percent of persons over the age of 90 (Kohn 1974). Nevertheless, "benign" paraproteinemia sometimes evolves into a malignant syndrome or is associated with symptomatic illness other than neoplasia. The two major syndromes that have been strongly linked with nonmalignant paraproteinemia are idiopathic primary amyloidosis, which may cause polyneuropathy and myopathy, and a nonamyloid type of chronic or relapsing polyneuropathy that resembles chronic idiopathic polyneuritis.

The incidence of these disorders is not known, but they appear to be uncommon. At the Mayo Clinic, Kelly and coworkers (1981b) found that 10 percent of patients with polyneuropathy of undetermined cause had a monoclonal gammopathy; among these 28 patients there were 3 with myeloma, 1 with Waldenstrom's macroglobulinemia, 1 with heavy-chain disease, 8 with primary amyloidosis, and 15 with "benign" monoclonal gammopathy. Kahn and colleagues (1980) performed routine protein electrophoresis on sera from 14,000 neurologic patients admitted to the National Hospital in London during a period of 3½ years. Among the 26 patients with paraproteinemia there were 10 cases of known myeloma or Waldenstrom's macroglobulinemia, 2 patients subsequently shown to have a solitary plasmacytoma, and 14 unexplained cases. This last group included 9 patients with polyneuropathy not otherwise explained, all of whom had very slow motor nerve conduction velocities.

Chronic Relapsing Polyneuropathy with Benign Monoclonal Gammopathy

The clinical features of nonamyloid polyneuropathy in patients with nonmalignant paraproteinemia are just beginning to be reported. Dalakas and Engel (1981b) outlined a homogenous clinical syndrome in 11 patients: a slowly progressive, sensorimotor polyneuropathy, sparing the cranial nerves and affecting mainly large nerve fibers, so that pain and temperature sensation and autonomic function were spared. The CSF protein level was increased, with a mean value of 110 mg per dl, and the CSF concentrations of IgA and IgG were increased. Monoclonal immunoglobulin bands were present in the CSF of five out of six patients tested. Motor nerve conduction velocities were quite slow, in the range of 30 to 60 percent of normal. Sural nerve biopies showed axonal and myelin loss in all cases, with focal mononuclear cell infiltration in two patients. The serum paraprotein was either IgG or IgM, and the same immunoglobulin was deposited, along with complement, in the endoneurium, perineurium, and interstitial blood vessels of sural nerves. Bone marrow examination consistently failed to show any increase in the number of plasma cells or lymphocytes.

Contamin and coworkers (1976) described a patient with similar clinical features, whose polyneuropathy took a relapsing course over a period of 19 years. The relapses followed intercurrent infections and tended to progress more rapidly than the initial illness. An IgG serum paraprotein was documented during the last 13 years of the illness, during which the amount increased from 0.5 to 1.3 g per dl. Read and associates (1978) described a similar polyneuropathy in three patients who became bedridden over the course of 9 to 18 months; one patient became totally paralyzed except for eye movements and lost all sensation. Treatment with steroids and azathioprine was ineffective, but eventually the patients recovered spontaneously. One of the patients relapsed 14 years later after a nonspecific febrile illness; as in the case of Contamin and coworkers (1976), the deterioration was rapid, with the patient becoming bedridden 3 days after onset of the recurrent symptoms, but recovering spontaneously over a period of several months. The paraprotein was an IgG, with kappa light chains in two patients and lambda light chains in the other. Another patient had a pure motor neuropathy with diffuse muscular atrophy in the limbs, accompanied by widespread fasciculations. The picture resembled motor neuron disease, although the cranial muscles were spared and pyramidal tract signs were absent. Nerve conduction was slow and the CSF protein was 132 to 265 mg per dl. Postmortem examination confirmed the presence of a radiculoneuropathy with only secondary chromatolytic changes in the anterior horn cells (Rowland et al. 1982).

In three other series of patients, the serum paraprotein was IgM-kappa in 16 cases, IgG-kappa in 7 cases, and IgG-lambda in 1 case (Chazot et al. 1976; Kahn et al. 1980; Latov et al. 1981). Thus there appears to be an unusual prevalence of M heavy chains and of kappa light chains in this syndrome. As is true of solitary myelomas, the paraprotein spike is often quite small and should be searched for by immunoelectrophoresis and by avoiding cryoprecipitation.

Pathophysiology. Whether the paraprotein is itself responsible for the polyneuropathy is still uncertain. The most direct evidence for a circulating neurotoxic substance in patients with paraproteinemic neuropathy comes from a recent experiment (Besinger et al. 1981) in which mice were injected for 8 to 10 weeks with purified monoclonal IgG from patients with polyneuropathy associated with either myeloma or benign gammopathy. The mice developed a demyelinating polyneuropathy with slowed nerve conduction velocities; control mice, injected with monoclonal IgG from myeloma patients without neuropathy, did not develop neuropathy. However, Bosch and associates (1982) were unable to demonstrate any acute effects of injecting paraproteinemic serum into rat sciatic nerve.

Latov and colleagues (1980) demonstrated myelin-binding activity in an IgM-kappa paraprotein from one patient, and subsequently Latov and others (1981) detected myelin-binding activity in sera from two patients with IgM-kappa paraproteins, a possible reaction with axon material in a third patient, and no antibody activity against peripheral nerve fractions in seven other patients with paraproteinemic neuropathies. In the two cases with antimyelin activity, teased nerve fiber preparations showed primary segmental demyelination, whereas two patients whose sera did not react with nerve components showed axonal degeneration with secondary segmental demyelination (Nemni et al. 1981). Read and associates (1978) were unable to detect antibody activity against peripheral nerve in three cases, but this may have been a technical problem, since Sewell and coworkers (1981) observed that an IgG paraprotein showed specific binding to formalin-fixed sections of peripheral nerve but not to fresh-frozen sections. Chazot and colleagues (1976) found deposits of immunoglobulin, of the same type as the serum paraprotein, in sural nerve samples from five patients with idiopathic paraproteinemic polyneuropathy. Thus, the varied immunologic and pathologic findings suggest that there may be several different disease mechanisms in this syndrome. Whether there are corresponding differences in clinical attributes is still unknown. A diagnostic question that remains to be investigated is the relationship between this syndrome and chronic idiopathic polyneuritis, in which a monoclonal band may be present in CSF but not in serum (Dalakas et al. 1980).

Treatment has not been very successful in the few reported cases. Dalakas and Engel (1981b) mentioned "minimal to mild benefit" from steroids and azathioprine in four cases, while Read and associates (1978) observed no response to these drugs in two cases. Latov and colleagues (1980) reported slow clinical recovery, and disappearance of the serum IgM spike, in a patient treated with plasmapheresis, prednisone, and chlorambucil; however, other patients have recovered without treatment, and the patient described by Contamin and coworkers (1976) showed no change in a serum IgG spike during remissions or relapses, although he responded well to steroids. No doubt the response to treatment will soon be better defined, now that this syndrome is being recognized more often.

Neuropathy in Primary Generalized Amyloidosis

Amyloid polyneuropathy has been recognized for many years in both hereditary and nonhereditary forms. Formerly, the nonhereditary amyloidoses were classified into two groups: cases occurring in patients with malignant paraproteinemia, and a more common syndrome referred to as primary, generalized amyloidosis (PGA). In both primary and myeloma-related amyloidosis, polyneuropathy occurs in only a small proportion of cases (Benson et al. 1975; Pruzanski and Katz 1976). Recently it has been shown that the amyloid material in both of these groups is composed of fragments of immunoglobulin light chains that are homogeneous in a given individual, and that patients with PGA have a serum or urine paraprotein and an increased number of plasma cells or lymphocytes in the bone marrow. Thus, both types of amyloidosis appear to result from overproduction of immunoglobulins or their light chains and are associated with proliferation of B-cells, so that the distinction between malignant and benign plasma-cell dyscrasias seems arbitrary in this syndrome.

The clinical features of amyloid polyneuropathy are distinctive in several respects. First, the disease has a predilection for small-diameter autonomic and sensory nerves. Second, the carpal tunnel syndrome occurs in some cases, because of amyloid infiltration of the flexor retinaculum. Third, cardiac involvement is frequently associated (Trotter et al. 1977; Cohen and Benson 1975). Most of the patients are men, and the onset of symptoms is usually in middle age or late life, with slow progression of disability over many years. Autonomic symptoms, which may be the presenting feature, include orthostatic hypotension, bowel dysfunction, impotence, and lack of sweating. Sensory symptoms usually precede motor dysfunction and consist of distal paresthesia, dysesthesia, burning or stabbing pains, and numbness; the legs are usually affected first, and pain and temperature sensation are often impaired to a greater extent than the large-fiber sensory functions of touch, vibration, and position sense. Muscle weakness and atrophy eventually appear in a distal distribution; many patients exhibit prominent fasciculations, and some complain of muscle cramps. Less common features include purpura, hoarseness, leg edema, and trophic skin ulcers.

The CSF protein is normal or mildly increased, though occasional values over 200 mg per dl have been reported. While conduction velocities are usually not much reduced, nerve degeneration is prominent, as indicated by loss of nerve excitability and EMG signs of muscle denervation. Muscle biopsy shows scattered muscle fiber atrophy without fiber-type grouping, indicating that nerve regeneration occurs sluggishly at best (Trotter et al. 1977). Bone marrow examination disclosed an increase in the number of

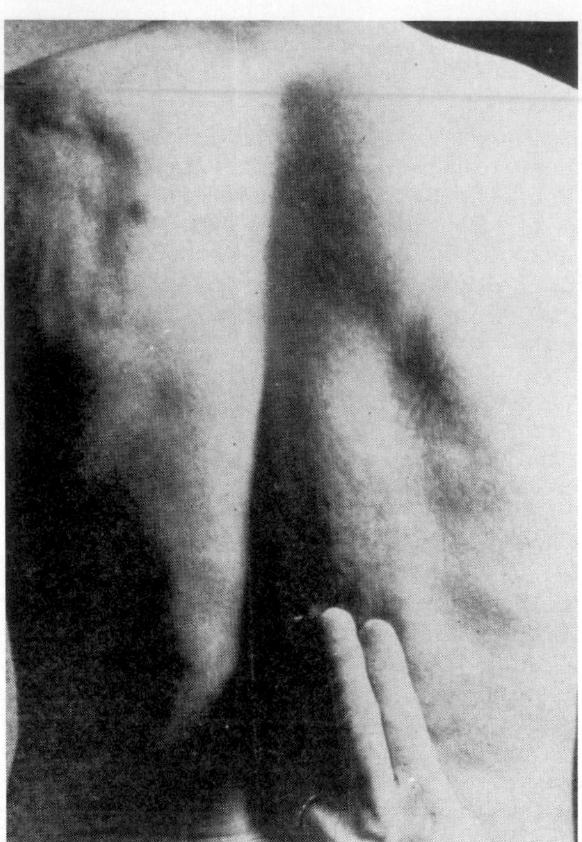

FIGURE 23. Amyloid myopathy, with generalized muscle enlargement. (From Lange, R. K.: *Primary amyloidosis of muscle.* South Med J 63:321, 1974, with permission.)

lymphocytes or plasma cells in the three patients reported by Fitting and associates (1979) and in nine out of the ten patients studied by Trotter and colleagues (1977). In the latter series, seven of eight patients tested had a paraprotein on serum protein electrophoresis: IgG-kappa in five, IgG-lambda in 1, and IgM-lambda in 1. Electrocardiographic abnormalities suggestive of amyloidosis were present in eight of the ten patients.

Pathophysiology. As Trotter and colleagues (1977) have pointed out, there are several resemblances between the polyneuropathy of PGA and the nonamyloid polyneuropathy associated with lytic multiple myeloma. In both conditions, most of the patients are men in middle or late life; sensory disturbance and pain are prominent features; the sensorimotor neuropathy is largely confined to the limbs, with a distal predominance; and the bone marrow shows a proliferation of lymphocytes or plasma cells, which sometimes exhibit immature features. In both conditions axonal degeneration is probably the major pathologic process, though motor nerve conduction velocity is occasionally moderately slow, perhaps as a result of secondary segmental demyelination. The major differences are the predilection for small-diameter sensory and autonomic nerve fibers in amyloidosis, and the more rapid course in myeloma. Because of these similarities, Trotter and colleagues (1977) suggested that both types of neuropathy might be due to toxic effects of immunoglobulins or fragments of immunoglobulins, which are deposited around nerve fibers. Extending that speculation, the tendency to form amyloid and to deposit immunoglobulin material in autonomic nerves may result from overproduction of immunoglobulin components different from those that cause myeloma polyneuropathy. Moreover, there may be subclasses of PGA related to the type of immunoglobulin manufactured, since most patients with primary amyloidosis do not have overt peripheral nerve involvement, and the patients who present with polyneuropathy generally live much longer than other patients with PGA (Trotter et al. 1977; Pruzanski and Katz 1976).

If immunoglobulin overproduction is the basic pathogenic mechanism, it is reasonable to make a vigorous attempt to control this process with cytotoxic chemotherapy. So far, however, there is no report of successful treatment of PGA, with or without neuropathy.

Muscle Enlargement in Amyloidosis

Myopathy is one of the rarest manifestations of primary generalized amyloidosis, and it takes the peculiar form of generalized enlargement and induration of the skeletal muscles (Fig. 23). Muscle weakness and stiffness are accompanied by dysphagia, hoarseness, and enlargement and clumsiness of the tongue. Amyloid is deposited between muscle fibers, without histologic or ultrastructural evidence of damage to muscle or nerve fibers. Serum CPK activity is normal, and EMG shows increased irritability, fibrillations, and myopathic abnormalities (Ringel and Claman 1982; Whitaker et al. 1977).

COLLAGEN-VASCULAR DISEASES

This unsatisfactory designation, used for want of a better term, refers to a group of disorders having several features in common: multisystem involvement, inflammatory pathology, presence of autoantibodies and other immunopathic phenomena, and absence of a specific infectious cause. The disorders that fit these criteria are numerous and have indistinct boundaries, but their neuromuscular complications fall into only a few categories (Table 23).

Polymyositis and Related Disorders

Polymyositis (PM) is a subacute or chronic generalized disorder of skeletal muscle characterized clinically by progressive muscular weakness and pathologically by scattered muscle fiber necrosis and inflammation, without a known infectious cause. In the majority of cases, PM and its close relative dermatomyositis (DM) can be regarded as primary disorders, but in about one fifth of the cases the myopathy is only one of the manifestations of another identifiable collagen-vascular disease. In the UCLA series (Bohan et al. 1977), out of 153 patients with PM there were 12 with scleroderma, 9 with systemic lupus erythematosus, 4 with rheumatoid arthritis, and 3 with Sjögren's syndrome.

PM is an uncommon disease, with an annual incidence between two and eight cases per million population (Medsger et al. 1970; Benbassat et al. 1980). It occurs at all ages, and young women are affected about twice as often as young men. About 40 percent of all patients have cutaneous features of dermatomyositis (Bohan et al. 1977).

CLINICAL FEATURES. The onset is almost always gradual, the muscle weakness increasing over a period of weeks or months before diagnosis. Usually muscle weakness is noticed first in the proximal limb muscles and

TABLE 23. Neuromuscular Manifestations of Collagen-Vascular Diseases

				Nonvasculitic Focal Neuropathy	
Syndrome	Myositis	Mononeuritis Multiplex	Polyneuropathy	Cranial	Spinal
Polymyositis/dermatomyositis	+++	0	±	±	0
Systemic lupus erythematosus	+	±	++	+	±
Mixed connective tissue disease	+++	0	+	++	0
Scleroderma	+	0	+	+	0
Rheumatoid arthritis	+	+	+	0	+
Ankylosing spondylitis	0	0	0	0	+
Hypereosinophilic syndrome and Churg-Strauss syndrome	++	++	+	0	0
Polyarteritis nodosa	0	+++	0	+	0
Wegener's granulomatosis	0	+	+	+	0
Essential cryoglobulinemia	0	+	+	0	0
Giant cell arteritis	0	+	0	+	0

KEY: 0, does not occur; ±, occurs rarely; +, occurs in fewer than 25% of cases; ++, occurs in 25 to 50% of cases; +++, occurs in 50 to 100% of cases.

trunk. Muscle aches or tenderness occur in about half of the patients, though estimates range from 25 percent (Bohan et al. 1977) to 73 percent (DeVere and Bradley 1975). Dysphagia occurs in about 25 percent, Raynaud's phenomenon is present in 10 to 15 percent, and low-grade fever is not uncommon.

In patients with DM, the skin involvement may precede, accompany, or follow the muscle symptoms, but the interval between their appearance is usually not more than a month or two. The most common cutaneous signs are edema of the eyelids; an erythematous or violet discoloration of the eyelids and central face; erythematous, scaly thickening of the skin over the extensor surfaces of the elbows, knees, and knuckles; a ragged, erythematous swelling of the nail beds; and flat, scaly papules on the dorsal surface of the fingers. Less often there is diffuse edema and erythema of the skin. Occasionally muscle involvement remains a minor feature during the entire course of DM.

The pattern of muscle weakness is rather variable. In most patients there is fairly diffuse involvement including the limbs, trunk, neck, and perhaps the swallowing and facial muscles; the limb weakness is greater in the proximal muscles, but distal muscles are not spared. Occasionally there is disproportionate weakness in the neck, the paraspinous muscles, the forearm flexors, or the quadriceps muscles (Bharucha and Morgan-Hughes 1981). In rare cases weakness mainly involves the distal portions of the extremities (Hollinrake 1969; Bates et al. 1973) or mimics the clinical picture of facioscapulohumeral muscular dystrophy (Rothstein et al. 1971).* A few patients have a precipitous course with severe muscle pain and extensive subcutaneous edema (Venables et al. 1982).

Initially the muscles may be slightly swollen, but as the disease progresses, muscular atrophy supervenes and induration becomes more noticeable, reflecting the deposition of fibrous tissue. Musculotendinous contractures are a common complication and may appear within the first 2 or 3 weeks. Muscle stretch reflexes are often depressed in the affected muscles. Pharyngeal weakness produces a nasal voice, nasal regurgitation of liquids, and difficulty swallowing with a tendency to aspirate liquids. Eventually respiratory muscle weakness may be added, and this together with pharyngeal weakness disposes the patient to pulmonary infections, the principal cause of death (except for the complications of treatment).

In patients who do not have an overt collagen-vascular disease, clinical manifestations outside of the skeletal muscles and the skin are uncommon. Actual arthritis has been described (Schumacher et al. 1979) but is probably rare. Diffuse interstitial myocarditis was identified in 30 percent of patients at autopsy (Denbow et al. 1979), and Gottdiener and associates (1978), using a battery of noninvasive diagnostic techniques, were able to detect minor cardiac abnormalities in three fourths of living patients. Congestive heart failure and arrhythmia, however, are rare (Hill and Barrows 1968; Singsen et al. 1976). Interstitial lung disease is present in 5 to 9 percent of patients (Salmeron et al. 1981). Nonproductive cough and dyspnea, which are the leading symptoms of this complication, may precede the onset of PM by as long as 3 years (Schwartz et al. 1976). About 16 cases of ischemic retinopathy with cotton-wool exudates and hemorrhages have been reported in children and adults with DM (Harrison et al. 1973).

*To add to the confusion, patients with genuine facioscapulohumeral muscular dystrophy sometimes have frank inflammatory changes in their muscles, but they do not respond to steroid treatment (Munsat et al. 1972).

Banker and Victor (1966) suggested that childhood DM was an entity distinct from either PM or adult DM, because systemic vasculitis was a major component. However, their findings came from an autopsy series; in clinical series there is little difference in mortality or in the incidence of systemic involvement between childhood and adult cases, except that gastrointestinal ulceration and bleeding are more common in childhood dermatomyositis, occurring in 18 percent of patients (Hill and Wood 1970; Pachman and Cooke 1980).

LABORATORY FINDINGS. Serum CPK activity is almost always increased in untreated patients with clinical weakness and active myositis. Rarely the CPK may be normal in a patient with DM whose skin manifestations precede the muscular symptoms. Bohan and associates (1977) found a normal CPK in 5 percent and DeVere and Bradley (1975) in 36 percent of patients, but the clinical circumstances (such as whether the patients had been treated or not) were not mentioned. EMG shows myopathic motor unit potentials in 90 percent of the cases and fibrillations and irritability in 50 to 75 percent of cases (Devere and Bradley 1975; Bohan et al. 1977). Muscle biopsy shows diffuse or patchy interstitial and perivascular infiltration of lymphocytes, sometimes accompanied by plasma cells, neutrophils, or eosinophils; segmental necrosis of scattered muscle fibers, some of which are undergoing phagocytosis by macrophages; regenerating muscle fibers; and a variable increase of endomysial and perimysial connective tissue (Fig. 24A). True vasculitis is infrequent, though it may be seen in PM, adult DM, and childhood DM, especially the last. There is sometimes selective atrophy of the superficial (perifascicular) muscle fibers, and with oxidative stains a "moth-eaten" appearance of muscle fibers is often noticed. Estimates vary as to how frequent these abnormalities are, but since the diagnosis of PM is based to a considerable degree on the muscle pathology, a "true" incidence cannot be construed. DeVere and Bradley (1975) reported normal findings or nonspecific changes in one third of their cases; the others had either muscle fiber degeneration and regeneration, inflammation, or both. Bohan and associates (1977) found inflammation in 75 percent of muscle biopsies and muscle fiber degeneration in 83 percent; abnormalities were less frequent in patients with DM (in whom the diagnosis could be made by independent criteria).

Other laboratory tests are, for the most part, surprisingly unrevealing. In "pure" PM or DM the erythrocyte sedimentation rate is increased in about half of the cases, the ANA test is rarely positive, and the latex fixation test is abnormal in only 5 percent (Bohan et al. 1977). Minor ECG abnormalities occur in about one fourth of the cases, but arrhythmia, conduction block, and Q waves are uncommon.

CLINICAL VARIANTS. Myositis may present as a localized muscle mass resembling a rhabdomyosarcoma. There are several types of these "pseudotumors" of muscle. *Localized nodular myositis* is an enlarging, usually painful muscle mass that develops over several weeks and resembles a sarcoma at the time of surgery because of its whitish, "fish-flesh" appearance. Histologically it is a focal form of myositis, with muscle fiber degeneration and very active regeneration. In a series of 16 cases there was no recurrence after excision of the mass (Heffner et al. 1977). Cumming and colleagues (1977) reported three patients with focal or multifocal nodular myositis that evolved into generalized polymyositis; they regarded the condition as a variant form of PM. Heffner and Barron (1981) reported six patients with an identical clinical sequence. A somewhat similar clinical picture is presented by *proliferative myositis,* which appears as a single muscle mass that grows rapidly within days or weeks, though it is not usually painful. The mass consists of fibroblasts and basophilic giant cells (thought to be of fibroblastic rather than of myoblastic origin), chiefly involving the perimysium, epimysium and fascia, and separating the muscle bundles, which appear relatively normal (Figs. 24B and C). The growth does not recur after simple excision (Enzinger and Dulcey 1967). A closely related disorder is *pseudomalignant myositis ossificans,* which differs mainly in that the fibroblasts form osteoid, which becomes calcified into bone (Lagier and Cox 1975).

Inclusion-body myositis is a form of PM characterized by painless muscle weakness, often in a distal distribution, which progresses slowly over a period of years and does not respond to steroid therapy. All the patients have been adults of ages 26 to 84 years, and most of them are men. Serum CPK activity may be normal or elevated, and EMG may show a mixture of myopathic and neurogenic abnormalities. A distinctive histologic finding is the presence, within muscle fibers, of small vacuoles containing basophilic granules (Figs. 24D and E); in other respects the light-microscopic picture is similar to that of ordinary PM. Electron microscopy shows whorls of cytomembranes, corresponding to the basophilic granules, within the cytoplasm and in some cases within nuclei (Carpenter et al. 1978). A viral cause has often been postulated, and recently type 2 adenovirus was isolated from the muscle of a patient whose serum contained a high titer of neutralizing antibodies to the virus (Mikol et al. 1982).

The term *granulomatous myositis* has been applied to cases having the histologic features of sarcoid myopathy in the absence of other clinical features of sarcoidosis. Sarcoid myopathy is discussed later in this chapter.

Eosinophilic polymyositis has been reported to occur in some patients with a multisystem disease known as eosinophilic collagen disease or hypereosinophilic syndrome (HES) (Layzer et al. 1977; Stark 1979). The muscle pathology is similar to that of ordinary polymyositis except for the presence of large numbers of eosinophils in the inflammatory infiltrate. Other common manifestations of this syndrome include eosinophilia of the blood (which may reach massive proportions), pancarditis, pulmonary infiltrates, mononeuritis multiplex, and embolic strokes (Chusid et al. 1975). The boundaries of this syndrome are not well defined, and it may merge with true eosinophilic leukemia and with the granulomatous vasculitis of Churg and Strauss. Although HES often takes a fulminating course with a high fatality rate, some patients respond well to corticosteroid therapy, especially those with high serum IgE levels (Bush et al. 1978; Parillo et al. 1978). Patients who do not respond well to corticosteroid therapy can usually be treated effectively with hydroxyurea (Parillo et al. 1978; Fauci 1982).

An eosinophilic form of localized nodular myositis has been reported in a boy with blood eosinophilia and a painless mass within one sternocleidomastoid muscle (Agrawal and Giesen 1981). The authors pointed out that focal eosinophilic myositis is familiar to veterinarians as a disease of domestic animals. No parasitic or other infectious cause has been incriminated in these cases. I have seen a middle-aged woman with a 20-year history of progressive muscular wasting confined to the forearms, without other neuromuscular or systemic symptoms. A muscle biopsy specimen showed typical polymyositis with a predominance of eosinophils in the inflammatory infiltrate.

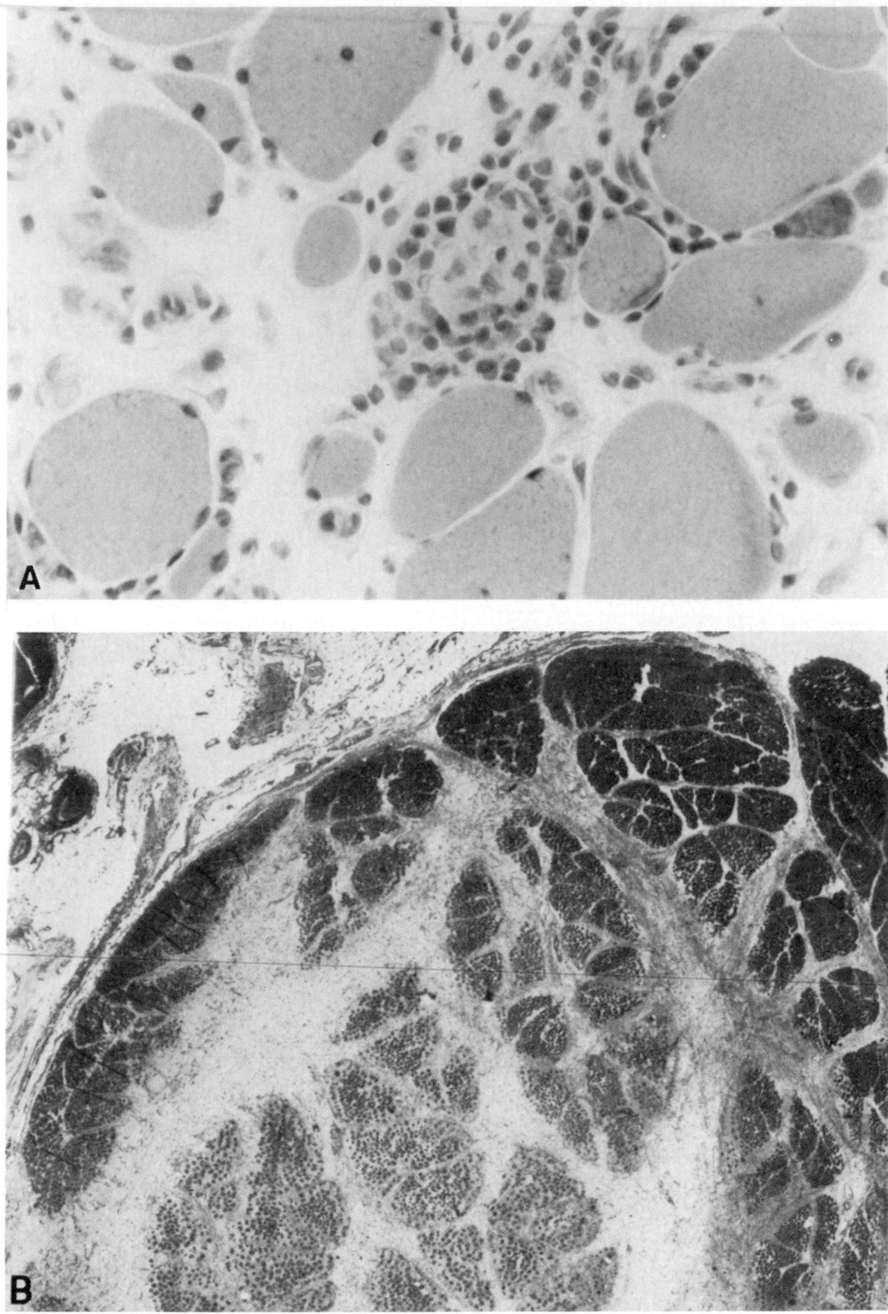

FIGURE 24. Polymyositis and related disorders. (*A*) Polymyositis. In the center, a degenerating muscle fiber, undergoing phagocytosis, is surrounded by an inflammatory infiltrate mainly consisting of small mononuclear cells. Small, rounded muscle fibers and increased endomysial connective tissue are also seen (hematoxylin and eosin). (*B*) In proliferative myositis, the muscle bundles are spread apart by a proliferation of stromal connective tissue.

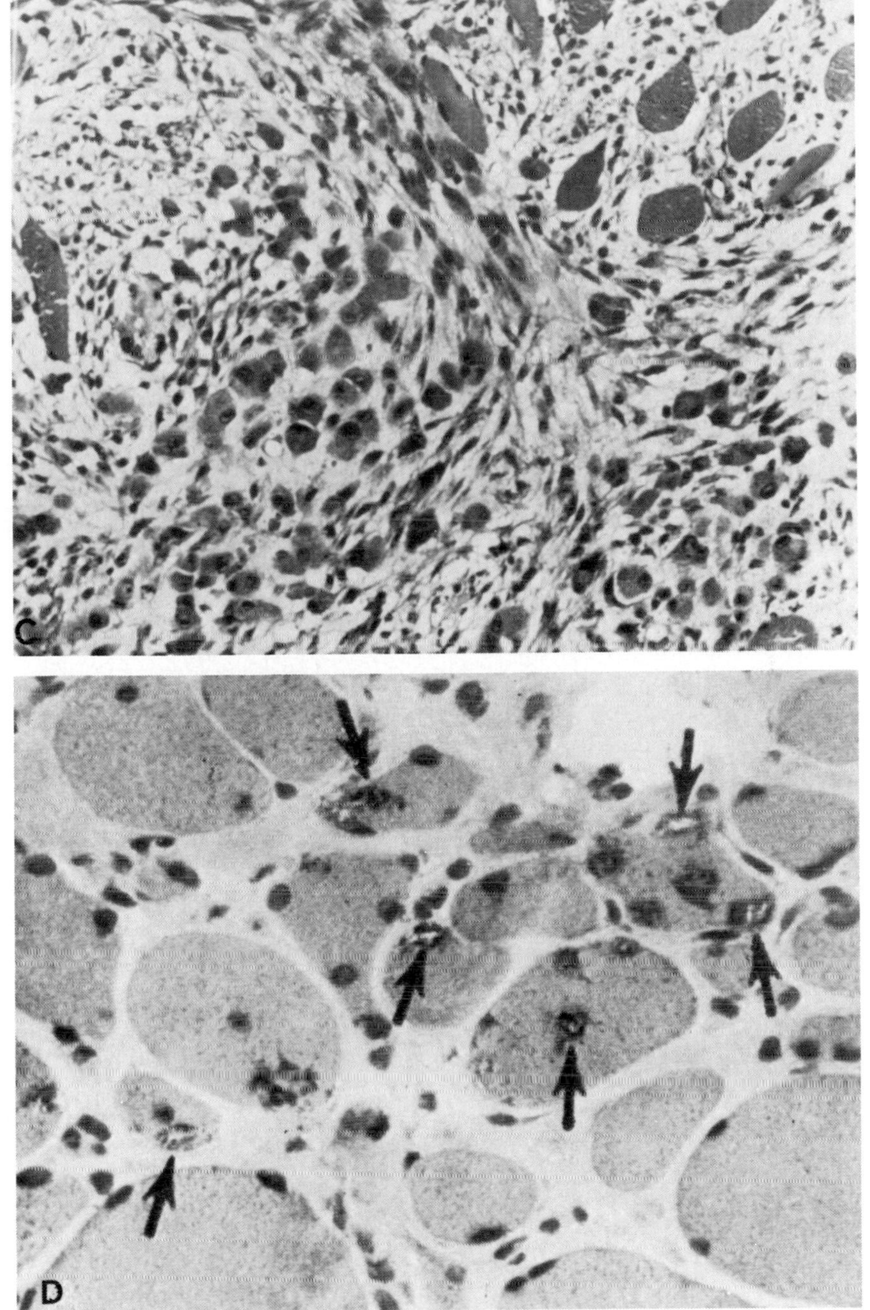

FIGURE 24 *continued.* (*C*) A higher power view of proliferative myositis shows basophilic giant cells closely associated with proliferated fibroblasts (hematoxylin and eosin). (*D*) In inclusion body myositis, single or multiple vacuoles are visible in many muscle fibers (hematoxylin and eosin). (Figure 24 *continues.*)

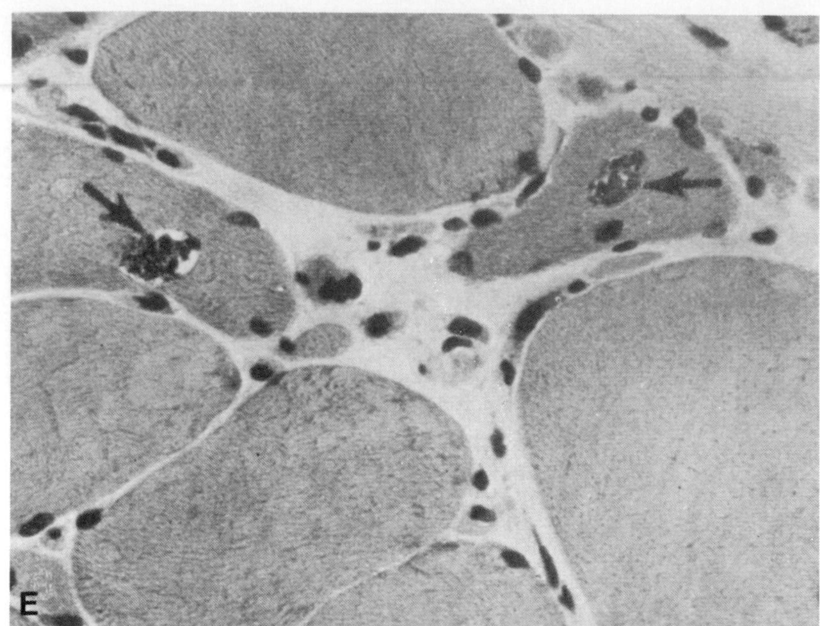

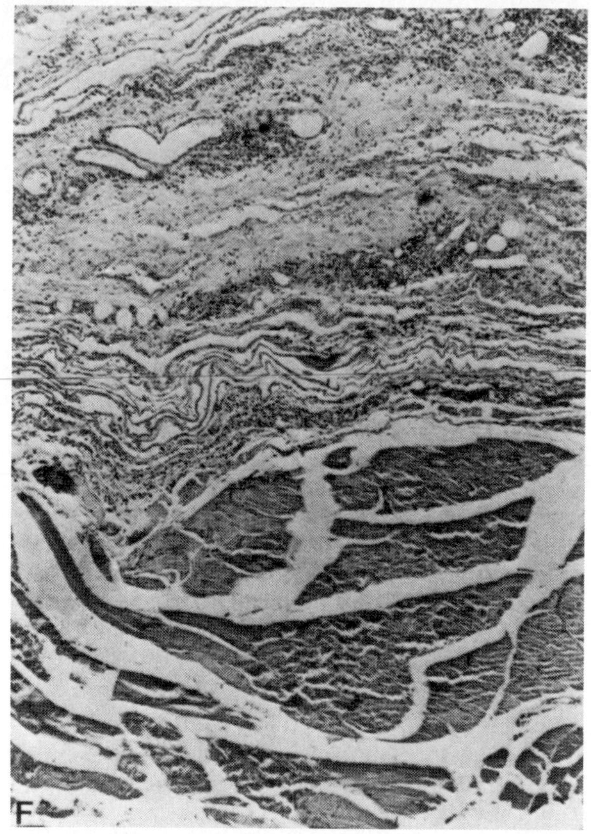

FIGURE 24 *continued.* (*E*) In inclusion body myositis shown under higher power, the vacuoles are seen to be filled with large basophilic granules. Scattered atrophic fibers, nuclear clumps, and increased endomysial connective tissue are also evident (modified trichrome). (*F*) Eosinophilic fasciitis. A portion of an en bloc skin-to-muscle biopsy shows greatly thickened fascia with a large number of mononuclear inflammatory cells (hematoxylin and eosin). (*B* and *C* from Enzinger and Dulcey, 1967, with permission. *D* and *E* from Carpenter et al., 1978, with permission. *F* from Martin, R., et al., J Rheumatol 10:343, 1983, with permission.)

DIFFERENTIAL DIAGNOSIS. *Eosinophilic fasciitis* is a scleroderma-like disorder which should be distinguished from eosinophilic polymyositis and also from dermatomyositis and scleroderma. The syndrome is characterized by swelling and induration of the subcutaneous tissues of the distal extremities, associated with eosinophilia of the blood and hypergammaglobulinemia. The carpal tunnel syndrome is a common complication, but serious systemic complications are rare. The pathologic changes, located primarily in the subcutaneous tissue (panniculus and deep fascia), consist of edema, infiltration with eosinophils and other inflammatory cells, and fibrosis (Fig. 24*F*). Eosinophils are not always found in biopsy specimens, but blood eosinophilia is a constant feature. The inflammation sometimes extends into the perimysium of the underlying skeletal muscle (Barnes et al. 1979; Moutsopoulos et al. 1980; Michet et al. 1981), and numerous mast cells have been seen in the interstitium (Cramer et al. 1982), but clinical and laboratory evidence of myopathy are usually lacking. Recently, however, there have been a few reports of patients with myalgia, mild muscle weakness, and myopathic changes on EMG. The serum enzymes were normal, and muscle fiber changes of atrophy and degeneration were confined to the periphery of fascicles adjacent to the perimysial inflammation—that is, a perimyositis rather than a true myositis (Serratrice et al. 1980; Bjelle et al. 1980; Kaplinsky et al. 1980). Eosinophilic fasciitis may resolve spontaneously, but steroid treatment generally hastens the resolution.

Localized scleroderma (morphea) is a chronic, atrophic process involving skin, subcutaneous tissue, and muscle, which often appears in childhood. The involved area of skin is thin, sunken, and bound down to deeper tissues (Fig. 25), and there may be hyperpigmentation or loss of pigment. The common focal type of morphea often has a linear shape like a saber cut, but the process can be much more extensive, taking the form of facial hemiatrophy (Schwartz et al. 1981), hemiatrophy of the limbs and trunk (Rosenberg and Greenberg 1979; Kesler et al. 1981), or generalized, mutilating morphea (Diaz-Perez et al. 1980). The histologic picture is similar to that of eosinophilic fasciitis except for the absence of eosinophils in the inflammatory infiltrate (Su and Person 1981); there is interstitial myositis with muscle atrophy but little or no muscle fiber necrosis or regeneration. Treatment has been unsatisfactory.

Polymyalgia rheumatica (PMR), one of the clinical forms of giant cell arteritis, is sometimes mistaken for PM, owing to the fact that the painful limitation of movement typical of PMR is easily misinterpreted as muscle weakness. PMR rarely occurs before age 50, with the average age of onset being 65 years. In Göteborg, the incidence is 29 cases per 100,000 in the age group over 50 (Bengtsson and Malmvall 1981). The clinical picture comprises pain and stiffness in the axial and proximal limb muscles, especially the shoulder girdles, causing progressive limitation of activity over a period of weeks or months. The pain occurs with movement but is worsened by inactivity, so that patients find it increasingly difficult to turn over in bed at night or to get out of bed in the morning. The muscles themselves are not tender, and there is no demonstrable muscle weakness when correct technique is used in manual muscle testing. Frank arthritis is infrequent, but the abnormalities demonstrable by pertechnetate joint scintigraphy, roentgenography, and synovial biopsies make it likely that inflammation of the joints is one of the principal causes of pain in PMR (O'Duffy et al. 1980).

Low-grade fever and weight loss occur in the majority of patients. Approximately one fourth of the patients have symptoms of temporal arteritis. The erythrocyte sedimentation rate is almost invariably elevated, usually to a striking degree. The other laboratory findings consist of mild ane-

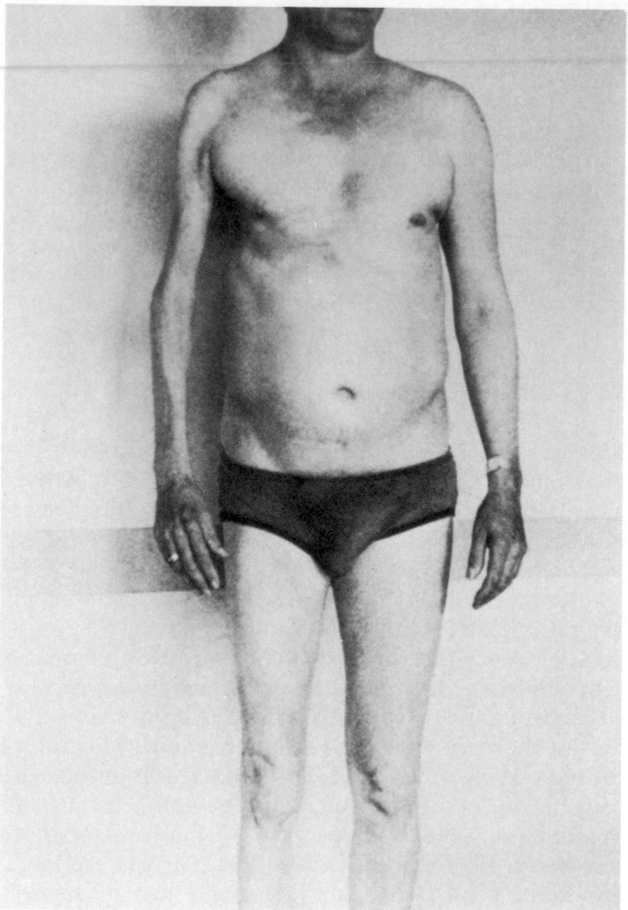

FIGURE 25. Morphea (linear scleroderma). There is hemiatrophy involving the right arm, chest and leg. (From Rosenberg and Greenberg [1979], with permission.)

mia in 15 to 30 percent of patients; elevated serum alkaline phosphatase activity in 12 to 60 percent, with less frequent elevation of other hepatocellular enzyme activities; and increased serum levels of alpha$_2$-globulins and beta-globulins (Goodman 1979). The serum CPK activity is normal, and EMG and muscle biopsy show no diagnostic abnormality. Temporal artery biopsy shows giant cell arteritis in about 30 percent of patients with PMR alone and in 90 percent of PMR patients who have symptoms of temporal arteritis (Bengtsson and Malmvall 1981; Jones and Hazleman 1981).

The rapid clinical response to steroid therapy is so striking that it can serve as a diagnostic test. Most patients obtain considerable relief from pain, stiffness, and constitutional symptoms within 24 to 48 hours, even with only 10 to 15 mg of prednisone daily. When the pain is better, it is easy to demonstrate that the patient has normal strength; the weakness of PM never resolves this rapidly. Unfortunately, low-dose steroid therapy may not prevent the occasional complication of sudden blindness caused by cranial arteritis. A recent study revealed that 42 percent of PMR patients developed temporal arteritis during low-dose steroid therapy, and one fourth of these patients suffered visual or cerebral complications (Jones and Hazleman 1981). However, in several patients the sedimentation rate was not elevated at the time the complication developed, so it is difficult to know whether high-dose steroid therapy would have prevented the complications.

The considerable health risks of high-dose steroid therapy in the elderly suggest that a prudent approach to the management of PMR in patients without cranial symptoms would be to initiate treatment with 10 to 15 mg of prednisone daily. If the sedimentation rate returns to normal within a few weeks, it is probably safe to continue low-dose therapy. Patients with symptoms of temporal arteritis should be started on 40 to 60 mg of prednisone per day, reducing the dose gradually as the symptoms and sedimentation rate are controlled. Most patients require steroid therapy for at least 2 to 3 years (Beevers et al. 1973), and alternate-day therapy is rarely efficacious.

The various *myopathies with high CPK levels* have been confused with polymyositis. The following is a partial list of the causes of this nonspecific syndrome:

Subacute alcoholic myopathy
Chronic potassium deficiency
Drugs: clofibrate, aminocaproic acid
Infection: trichinosis, toxoplasmosis
Myxedema
Genetic diseases: acid maltase deficiency, carnitine deficiency, late-onset phosphorylase or phosphofructokinase deficiency, limb-girdle and Becker muscular dystrophies

The clinical features of most of these disorders are discussed elsewhere in this volume.

Pathophysiology. There is general agreement that immune processes are ultimately responsible for muscle fiber degeneration in the idiopathic inflammatory myopathies, but the nature and origin of the immune disorder are still obscure. One view is that DM in children and young adults is primarily a disease of intramuscular small blood vessels, leading to occlusion and destruction of the vessels and progressive ischemic damage of muscle fibers (Banker and Victor 1966; Banker 1975; Carpenter et al. 1976; Crowe et al. 1982). The proponents of this theory point out that inflammatory infiltration in these cases is primarily located in septa separating muscle fascicles, while in PM and in some adult cases of DM there is interstitial inflammatory infiltration within muscle fascicles, capillary damage is not prominent, and there is scattered necrosis of muscle fibers, perhaps owing to direct inflammatory injury (Carpenter et al. 1976). Not all investigators agree with this analysis, and the clinical differences between the two syndromes are rather vague, especially since skin changes can be slight and fleeting. An increased incidence of HLA-B8 antigen has been reported in both childhood DM and adult PM (Behan et al. 1978).

Nevertheless, it is quite possible that several pathogenic mechanisms are involved in the inflammatory myopathies. Any immune process that is envisaged must account for the localization of the pathology to muscles (or to muscles and skin) in the large majority of cases. Thus, a generalized immune-complex disease like serum sickness, though typically causing vasculitis and endothelial damage, does not fit the requirement for selective tissue involvement. Circulating immune complexes were found in 70 percent of PM patients in one study; the antigens, however, were not identified (Behan et al. 1982). A few patients with adult PM have been reported to have manifestations of immune-complex disease related to hepatitis B antigenemia (Mihas et al. 1978; Damjanov et al. 1980) or to hyperglobulinemic purpura (Ringel et al. 1979), but hepatitis B antigen could not be detected in serum or muscle in 29 patients with DM or PM (Whitaker et al. 1973).

There are several ways that an immune mechanism could affect muscle in a selective fashion. (1) An autoimmune reaction could be directed against a tissue-specific antigen, as in the case of autoimmune thyroiditis or myasthenia gravis. (2)

A chronic, masked infection of muscle could be a repository of antigens provoking immune reactions, as seems to occur in the peripheral nerves of chickens with Marek's disease. (3) Antibody-producing plasma cells in muscle might synthesize immunoglobulins that react with blood-borne antigens, by analogy with rheumatoid arthritis, where autoantibodies against IgG are produced by plasma cells concentrated in synovial tissue.

The first hypothesis, specific autoimmunity to muscle, has received the most attention. An animal model of polymyositis was created by immunizing rats with homogenized muscle mixed with adjuvant (killed tubercle bacilli). An inflammatory, necrotizing myopathy resulted, but interpretaion of the experiments was difficult because adjuvant alone produced similar changes. This difficulty was circumvented by transferring lymphocytes from immunized to unimmunized animals, which then developed myositis (Dawkins 1965; Kakulas 1966). Initial attempts to demonstrate a similar cell-mediated hyperimmunity in patients with inflammatory myopathy appeared to be successful. Lymphocytes from patients with PM and DM had cytotoxic effects on tissue cultures of animal muscle (Dawkins and Mastaglia 1973; Kakulas et al. 1971; Currie et al. 1971) and showed an increased rate of transformation in the presence of a muscle extract (Currie et al. 1971; Esiri et al. 1971). However, these effects were not very specific, and some of them could not be confirmed (Lisak and Zweiman 1975; Iannaccone et al. 1982; DeVere and Bradley 1975; Haas 1980). Meanwhile, attempts to demonstrate autoantibodies against muscle extracts or cellular constituents were mostly unsuccessful (Fessel and Raas 1968; Whitaker and Engel 1972). (A recent case, showing granular deposits of IgA and C3 along the sarcolemma of muscle fibers, was an exception [Alexander et al. 1982]). Because of these developments, the hypothesis of autoimmunity against specific muscle antigens has become less popular.

One finding that emerged from the search for autoantibodies was the presence of deposits of immunoglobulin and complement in the walls of blood vessels of muscles, though not in muscle cells (except for nonspecific adherence). Such deposits were found in most cases of childhood DM and in some adult cases of DM and PM (Whitaker and Engel 1972; Whitaker et al. 1973; Heffner et al. 1979). In a case of myositis associated with hyperglobulinemic purpura, extensive deposits of IgG in the interstitial connective tissue appeared to result from in-situ synthesis of immunoglobulin by large, active plasma cells (Ringel et al. 1979), but this case is exceptional—usually there is no sign of local antibody synthesis. Thus, if the vascular deposits of immunoglobulin and complement are indeed immune complexes, we are still left with the difficult task of explaining why muscle and skin should be selectively involved by an immune-complex vasculitis.

These difficulties are similar to the problem of accounting for chronic synovitis in patients with rheumatoid arthritis. For many years investigators have attempted, without success, to identify a chronic synovial infection in rheumatoid patients; yet infection remains a very attractive hypothesis, especially since in several animal species naturally occurring mycoplasma infections produce a chronic arthritis similar to rheumatoid arthritis. Toxoplasma organisms have been identified in muscle in a few cases of PM and DM, an adenovirus has been isolated from a case of inclusion-body myositis, and virus-like particles are occasionally observed by electron microscopy (see Chapter 4), but aside from these examples there is little direct support for an infectious etiology of the idiopathic inflammatory myopathies. Factors other than infection may be important in children who develop typical DM after immunizations, in older patients who develop DM in association with cancer (see Chapter 6), and in a child who developed PM in a setting of chronic graft versus host disease (Anderson et al. 1982). So far no hypothesis has been able to reconcile the multiplicity of causes that have been incriminated in the clinical syndrome of idiopathic inflammatory myopathy.

TREATMENT. In a retrospective series from the Mayo Clinic, 39 percent of untreated patients with PM or DM recovered without treatment (Winkelman et al. 1968), but 29 percent of the untreated patients died. Although no controlled study of steroid treatment has ever been carried out, there is general agreement that early treatment with high-dose prednisone can achieve full control of the inflammatory process in most patients with PM, DM, or the myositis of collagen-vascular disease. Early treatment is desirable, because muscle fibrosis interferes with the restoration of normal strength, and high-dose treatment is preferred because of the general impression that the damage caused by chronic, "smoldering" inflammation eventually becomes impossible to reverse. The usual approach is to start with prednisone, 1 to 2 mg per kg daily, changing to an alternate-day schedule as the patient's muscle strength improves and the serum CPK activity returns toward normal. Clinical improvement is usually not evident until the patient has been treated for at least 2 to 3 weeks. In one followup study, half of the patients still required therapy after 2½ years (DeVere and Bradley 1975), and few patients can be successfully released from steroid therapy in less than a year.

Unfortunately, a significant minority of patients either do not respond satisfactorily to steroids or encounter serious side effects from the treatment, including steroid myopathy. In many such patients, addition of a cytotoxic drug like azathioprine, intravenous methotrexate, or cyclophosphamide has produced gratifying responses (Metzger et al. 1974; Arnett et al. 1973; Malaviya et al. 1968; Currie and Walton 1971; Benson and Aldo 1973; McFarlin and Griggs 1968; Jacobs 1977). Eventually it was possible to reduce the dose of prednisone considerably or to maintain control with a cytotoxic drug alone. In a few cases plasmapheresis appeared to be beneficial when added to steroid and cytotoxic therapy (Brewer et al. 1980; Dau and Bennington 1981; Anderson and Ziter 1981; Dau 1981), but it is not clear from these reports whether plasmapheresis was effective independent of the potent drug therapy.

In view of the high incidence of steroid side effects and the need for prolonged treatment in many cases, it may be appropriate to initiate treatment with a combination of prednisone and a cytotoxic drug in patients with severe disease or with a high risk of steroid complications, such as diabetics and postmenopausal women. In a prospective study of azathioprine and prednisone therapy, Bunch and associates (1980) found no advantage of combined therapy over prednisone alone after 3 months of treatment, but longer followup (Bunch 1981) revealed far greater improvement and lower requirements for prednisone in the patients receiving both drugs.

Subcutaneous calcification develops in about a third of children who recover from DM and occasionally develops in young persons with PM who do not have a history of skin rash. (Calcinosis of the skin may occur without myositis in patients with SLE or scleroderma.) The calcification often regresses spontaneously after a number of years (Chalmers et al. 1982), but in a few patients it is very extensive, painful, and disabling. Treatment with diphosphonates is only occasionally helpful (Uttley et al. 1975), and no other form of treatment has been of value. One patient developed an osteosarcoma within ossified deposits of intramuscular calcification, 28 years after recovering from DM (Eckhardt et al. 1981).

MYOSITIS IN OTHER COLLAGEN-VASCULAR DISEASES. As shown in Table 23, typical polymyositis occurs with variable frequency in several collagen-vascular diseases. In such cases, the response to steroid treatment is generally similar to that obtained in "pure" PM. However, in most of the collagen-vascular diseases, other causes of muscle weakness are more common than myositis—myopathy from steroid therapy or potassium depletion, for instance, and various types of neuropathy.

One syndrome, *mixed connective tissue disease,* does have a high incidence of myositis, which has been reported to occur in 35 to 72 percent of patients (Sharp et al. 1972; Bennett et al. 1978; Singsen et al. 1977). This syndrome, which is identified by the presence of extremely high serum titers of antibody to ribonucleoprotein, has cutaneous features of both DM and scleroderma and thus may account for some of the cases previously referred to as "sclerodermatomyositis".

In *systemic lupus erythematosus,* overt myositis has been reported to occur in 5 to 12 percent of cases (Estes and Christian 1971; Borenstein et al. 1978; Foote et al. 1982; Tsokos et al. 1981). Many of these patients also have myocarditis and have high titers of antibody to ribonucleoprotein (Borenstein et al. 1978). Grigor and colleagues (1978) found CPK elevations in only 2 of 50 SLE patients who were tested frequently during a period averaging 2½ years. By contrast, about 20 percent of SLE patients complain of myalgia and asthenia at a typical outpatient visit (Fries and Holman 1975). At autopsy the muscles of SLE patients show perivascular inflammation in 24 percent of cases, but severe muscle fiber changes are present in only 2 percent of cases (Ropes 1976).

In *generalized scleroderma* about 12 percent of patients develop typical polymyositis. Most of the remaining patients have mild, nonprogressive muscle weakness, a normal CPK, and histologic changes of interstitial fibrosis in muscle, without muscle fiber degeneration or inflammation. The latter patients do not require, or benefit from, steroid therapy (Clements et al. 1978). As in SLE, there appears to be some association between the occurrence of myocarditis and myositis in generalized scleroderma (West et al. 1981).

Focal inflammatory changes are found in 60 percent of muscle biopsy specimens taken from patients with *rheumatoid arthritis,* yet overt polymyositis appears to be infrequent, and myopathic EMG abnormalities are mainly found in steroid-treated patients (Yates 1963). Only 2.6 percent of patients with PM had rheumatoid arthritis in the series of Bohan and associates (1977), though there are about 1000 patients with rheumatoid arthritis for every patient with PM.

In *Sjögren's syndrome,* myalgia and mild muscle weakness have been reported in 33 percent of patients, but overt myositis appears to be uncommon. Muscle biopsy specimens revealed deposits of immunoglobulin and complement in four Sjögren patients with clinical polymyositis or dermatomyositis, and there was ultrastructural evidence of major microvascular alterations and of tuboreticular inclusions (Ringel et al. 1982). Another patient with Sjögren's syndrome had the clinical and pathologic features of inclusion-body myositis, with tuboreticular inclusions in capillary endothelial cells (Chad et al. 1982a).

Among the diseases primarily characterized by vasculitis, typified by *polyarteritis nodosa,* polymyositis is rarely encountered. Published statements to the contrary are generally explained by failure of the authors to distinguish between true polymyositis and the pathologic findings of vasculitis, perivascular inflammation, and muscle infarction in muscles of patients with neurogenic weakness caused by mononeuritis multiplex.

Mononeuritis Multiplex Caused by Systemic Vasculitis

Vascular lesions are found in all types of collagen-vascular disease, but ischemic neuropathies occur in only a few types. The diameter of the affected blood vessels appears to be one of the determining factors; mononeuritis multiplex occurs when arteritis involves small and medium-sized arteries (periarteritis nodosa, Churg-Strauss syndrome, Wegener's granulomatosis) but is rare in diseases that involve mainly large arteries (temporal arteritis, Takayasu's disease) or arterioles and venules (SLE, dermatomyositis, rheumatoid arthritis, mixed connective tissue disease, and scleroderma) (Fauci et al. 1978; Fan et al. 1980). About 1 percent of patients with rheumatoid arthritis develop systemic necrotizing arteritis after an average of 9 years of joint disease. Most of these patients have subcutaneous nodules and high serum titers of rheumatoid factor. The pathologic and clinical features of this arteritis are much like those of polyarteritis nodosa (Schmid et al. 1961). Patients with SLE may develop similar complications (Johnson and Richardson 1968) but this occurs rarely—no instances of mononeuritis were observed among 75 patients followed closely with regular neurologic examinations in a prospective study that lasted 15 years (Tay and Khoo 1971). During the same period of time, 5 patients (7 percent) developed a distal symmetric polyneuropathy.

Mononeuritis multiplex occurs in about 50 percent of patients with *polyarteritis nodosa* (Conn and Dyck 1975), in 40 to 70 percent of patients with *necrotizing rheumatoid arteritis* (Schmid et al. 1961; Scott et al. 1981), in 70 percent of patients with *allergic granulomatosis* (Churg and Strauss 1951), in 15 percent of patients with *Wegener's granulomatosis* (Drachman 1963; Fauci and Wolff 1973), and in fewer than 8 percent of patients with "essential" mixed *cryoglobulinemia* (Gorevic et al. 1980; Brouet et al. 1974; Konishi et al. 1982). Mononeuritis multiplex is often a presenting feature of these diseases or, in the case of rheumatoid arthritis, the first indication that a relatively benign disorder has entered a more malignant phase.

In a detailed postmortem study of a patient with necrotizing rheumatoid arteritis, Dyck and coworkers (1972) showed that ischemic nerve lesions were mainly located in the proximal nerve trunks of the upper arms and thighs, though vasculitis of the small arteries and arterioles was distributed throughout the length of the nerves. The authors postulated that the areas of ischemic nerve degeneration were probably watershed zones with poor perfusion, and they suggested that vascular occlusions must be numerous and widespread before nerve function is affected, because of the extensive collateral circulation of peripheral nerves (Conn and Dyck 1975).

The clinical picture is distinctive and easily recognized. It consists of a series of acute neuropathies of major peripheral nerves, manifest as sudden weakness or complete paralysis of a group of muscles supplied by a major nerve, deep aching or shooting pain in the limb, and numbness or painful dysesthesia in the cutaneous territory of the nerve. Occasionally the onset of the neuropathy seems to be gradual, reaching a maximum in a few hours or days, but generally the deficit is maximal at onset and remains the same unless another lesion of the same nerve suddenly increases the deficit. Cranial nerves may be affected but spinal nerve roots are rarely, if ever, involved. Wasting and fasciculation of the paralyzed muscles develop in time as a result of Wallerian degeneration of the infarcted nerve fibers. For the same reason, recovery of function is often delayed and protracted, although nerves that are only mildly ischemic can recover within a few weeks. Neuralgic pain can persist for weeks or months.

The CSF protein remains normal in most cases, since the nerve lesions are extraspinal. EMG eventually shows denervation in the paralyzed muscles; nerve stimulation may reveal slowed conduction or conduction block across the sites of ischemic lesions, but the most consistent finding, which can be detected after 2 weeks, is a reduced amplitude of the muscle response to motor nerve stimulation, with little change in conduction velocity. Unaffected nerves show no abnormality, since this is not a diffuse polyneuropathy. Sural nerve biopsy specimens may show vasculitis, but the yield is small (Parry et al. 1981) since the patchy vascular pathology cannot be predicted by clinical examination or electrodiagnostic testing, despite claims to the contrary (Wees et al. 1981). Random muscle biopsy probably has a better chance of showing vasculitis; it is positive in about 45 percent of patients with polyarteritis nodosa (Frohnert and Sheps 1967). EMG sampling has been recommended as a guide to choosing the site for muscle biopsy, but this makes no sense: the EMG would only detect clinically obvious neurogenic paralysis, which has no direct relation to the arterial lesions in the muscle. In practice it is convenient to biopsy both sural nerve and muscle through a single incision in the lower calf.

Aside from the other injurious effects of systemic vasculitis, which may be life-threatening, mononeuritis multiplex itself should be regarded as a neurologic emergency. Vascular injury to major nerve trunks can result in flaccid quadriplegia, a prolonged and painful convalescence, and permanent disablement. It is necessary to act quickly in order to prevent the appearance of new nerve lesions. Often the pace of the disease is leisurely at first and then accelerates rapidly; ideally treatment should be initiated before the accelerated phase begins. In a patient with rheumatoid arthritis who has rheumatoid nodules and a high titer of serum rheumatoid factor, the onset of mononeuritis multiplex is virtually diagnostic of necrotizing arteritis; necrotic skin lesions and digital ischemia may provide additional clues but are not required for diagnosis. In other diseases diagnosis may be unclear at first and it may be necessary to perform laboratory tests, muscle and nerve biopsies, or angiography of the visceral arteries; even so, it is important to pay close attention to the pace of the neuropathy, retaining the option of starting treatment immediately if the patient's course is unfavorable.

Moore and Fauci (1981) have reported that cyclophosphamide, in a dose of 2 mg per kg daily, gives excellent results in the treatment of systemic necrotizing vasculitis. Cyclophosphamide was also effective in five patients with severe rheumatoid vasculitis, and remission of symptoms correlated with a fall of serum levels of rheumatoid factor and immune complexes (Abel et al. 1980). A combination of cyclophosphamide and prednisone appears to be the treatment of choice in Wegener's granulomatosis complicated by mononeuritis multiplex (Fauci et al. 1978). In all these disorders remission has been maintained with low doses of cyclophosphamide alone. In mixed cryoglobulinemia the response to treatment with steroids and cytotoxic drugs has been poor, but there has not been sufficient evaluation of the use of aggressive cytotoxic therapy and plasmapheresis (Geltner et al. 1981).* In fact, it is reasonable to initiate plasmapheresis therapy in any vasculitis syndrome in which circulating immune complexes are present, since the response would probably be faster than with chemotherapy alone; in this category are polyarteritis nodosa and its variants (Bletry et al. 1982), necrotizing rheumatoid arteritis (Brubaker and Winkelstein 1981), and cryoglobulinemia.

Subacute and Chronic Polyneuropathy

The polyneuropathies associated with systemic lupus erythematosus and other collagen-vascular diseases have not been studied as carefully as have

*In judging the response to therapy, success should be defined as the prevention of new nerve lesions, since previously damaged nerves cannot be expected to recover quickly.

the idiopathic inflammatory polyneuropathies discussed earlier. Clinical descriptions are often sparse, electrophysiologic data are almost entirely lacking, and CSF immunoglobulins have not been analyzed. Nevertheless, it appears that there are probably two or three distinct varieties of polyneuropathy in SLE, the disease about which the most information is available.

In three prospective series of cases, the incidence of polyneuropathy in SLE has been found to be 5 to 7 percent (Tay and Khoo 1971; Estes and Christian 1971; Grigor et al. 1978), mostly in the form of a distal sensory polyneuropathy. The incidence of sensory polyneuropathy in mixed connective disease is about 10 percent (Bennett et al. 1978). In rheumatoid arthritis the incidence of polyneuropathy is difficult to deduce because most articles do not distinguish between polyneuropathy, compression neuropathies, and arteritic neuropathies; polyneuropathy does not appear to be a rare complication, however. The most common type is a distal sensory polyneuropathy predominantly affecting the lower limbs, which was found in 19 (63 percent) of 30 rheumatoid patients with neuropathy (Pallis and Scott 1965). Gordon and Silverstein (1970) found only one case of diffuse sensorimotor polyneuropathy among 130 patients with scleroderma, and Tuffanelli and Winkelmann (1961) did not find any examples of polyneuropathy in 727 cases of scleroderma. Polyneuropathy has occurred in the hypereosinophilic syndrome (Chusid et al. 1975; Layzer et al. 1977) but is rarely encountered in polymyositis or dermatomyositis.

Polyneuropathy has also been reported in various forms of vasculitis, but most of the articles do not provide enough details to distinguish between a true polyneuropathy and a mononeuritis multiplex. It is easy for an unsophisticated examiner to mistake a widespread mononeuropathy multiplex for a diffuse polyneuropathy. Thus, "polyneuritis" was present in 8 percent of the published cases of Wegener's granulomatosis reviewed by Drachman (1963), but close examination of the case reports cited does not support that diagnosis. A gradually progressive, sensorimotor polyneuropathy was reported in 10 percent of 86 patients with cryoglobulinemia (Brouet et al. 1974), but the survey included cases of monoclonal gammopathy, lymphoproliferative disorders, and collagen-vascular diseases, all of which may cause polyneuropathy without the presence of cryoglobulinemia. Most of the case histories of polyneuropathy in essential cryoglobulinemia appear to be examples of widespread mononeuropathy multiplex (Cream et al. 1974; Logothetis et al. 1968), though genuine symmetric polyneuropathy has been documented (Chad et al. 1982b).

The distal sensory polyneuropathy of SLE and rheumatoid arthritis may evolve subacutely or may pursue an insidious, progressive course, starting in the lower extremities and spreading to the distal upper extremities. Numbness on the tip of the tongue and inside the mouth is a frequent complaint. Touch, vibration, and position sense are most prominently affected, and the distal limb reflexes are depressed (Pallis and Scott 1965). The CSF protein is moderately increased. Postmortem pathologic examination in two patients with this disorder showed an inflammatory sensory ganglionitis with destruction of the sensory neurons and secondary degeneration of the posterior columns of the spinal cord and of the peripheral sensory nerve fibers (Bailey et al. 1956). Thus, this syndrome has much in common with the syndrome of primary sensory neuronitis associated with carcinoma of the lung (Horwich et al. 1977). Recently, IgG antibodies reacting with cultured human neuroblastoma cells have been demonstrated in the CSF of some patients with neurologic manifestations of SLE, including cranial neuropathies. The antibodies were present in much higher titers than were found in lupus patients without neurologic manifestations or in patients with CNS diseases other than lupus (Bluestein et al. 1981). Similar immunologic studies have not been reported in patients with sensory polyneuropathy.

A rarer but more disabling syndrome is a subacute or chronic relapsing polyneuropathy closely resembling idiopathic polyneuritis (Gargour et al. 1964; Scheinberg 1956; Goldberg and Chitanondh 1959). In this syndrome there is severe, diffuse weakness of the limbs, usually sparing respiratory, trunk, and cranial muscles. In several cases there was little or no sensory impairment initially, but the muscle stretch reflexes were all absent. The CSF protein is moderately or markedly increased (up to 1,000 mg per dl), with little or no increase in the number of white blood cells. Muscle weakness waxes and wanes for months or years, with no consistent response to steroid therapy. Motor nerve conduction velocity has been reported in only two cases; in one, a velocity of 30 m per second was recorded from one ulnar nerve (Goldberg and Chitanondh 1959), and in the other there was little or no slowing in several nerves except for a velocity of 29 m per second in one radial nerve (Bloch et al. 1979). No teased nerve fiber studies or other pathologic examinations have been performed. Several patients developed increased intracranial pressure with papilledema, a complication that also occurs in cases of acute and chronic idiopathic polyneuritis and paraproteinemic polyneuropathy. The mechanism of this pseudotumor syndrome has been debated, but it is probably not a straightforward result of increased CSF protein (Fishman 1980). One possibility is that immune complexes present in the CSF are deposited in the arachnoid villi, interfering with CSF absorption in the sagittal sinus.

Finally, some patients have a sensorimotor polyneuropathy that appears to be a mixture of the two preceding syndromes (Lewis 1965) and tends to run a waxing and waning course. The CSF protein is usually moderately increased. Although motor nerve conduction velocities have not been reported, pathologic studies suggest that axonal degeneration is a prominent feature, but whether there is a demyelinative component has not been determined.

The results of treatment have not been very satisfactory, regardless of the clinical features. Most of the reported patients have been treated only with corticosteroids, and the results are difficult to evaluate. In some cases there was no apparent response, while other patients improved slowly but later deteriorated during continued steroid therapy. There is no information about the response of lupus neuropathy to more vigorous treatment with cytotoxic drugs or plasmapheresis.

Miscellaneous Focal Neuropathies

Aside from vasculitic neuropathies, several varieties of focal neuropathy occur in the collagen-vascular diseases. Among these are entrapment neuropathies, neuropathies related to focal granulomatous inflammation, and focal neuropathies of obscure etiology.

Entrapment Neuropathies

Patients with rheumatoid arthritis are particularly vulnerable to the development of focal neuropathies adjacent to inflamed joints and tendons (Nakano 1975; Mäkelä et al. 1979). Compression of the *median nerve* at the wrist (carpal tunnel syndrome) is caused by tenosynovitis of the adjacent flexor tendons in the carpal tunnel. In two series of patients with carpal tunnel syndrome, the incidence of rheumatoid arthritis was 10 to 12 percent

(Czeuz et al. 1966; Frymoyer and Bland 1973). Carpal tunnel syndrome is also an early feature of eosinophilic fasciitis, in two recent series occurring in 11 of 35 patients (Barnes et al. 1979; Michet et al. 1981), and it has also been associated with polymyalgia rheumatica (Ahmed and Braun 1978).

"Tardy" *ulnar nerve* paralysis results from compression of the nerve by elbow-joint synovitis or olecranon bursitis. Less often the ulnar nerve can be compressed by tenosynovitis in the canal of Guyon at the wrist.

The *posterior interosseous nerve,* which is the deep motor branch of the radial nerve, can be compressed by an elbow joint effusion adjacent to the head of the radius. The resulting extensor weakness of the wrist, fingers, and thumb (without sensory deficit) can be distinguished from ruptured extensor tendons of the fingers by demonstrating passive extension of the digits during manual flexion of the wrist (if joint motion permits).

Peroneal nerve paralysis may be related to arthritis of the knee joint or may be due to external pressure in a bedfast patient. Occasionally a Baker's cyst of the popliteal area causes a compression neuropathy of the *peroneal* or *posterior tibial nerve.*

In the foot, entrapment of the *posterior tibial nerve* or its branches produces neuralgic pain, altered sensation of the sole, and weakness of the plantar muscles. The posterior tibial nerve is vulnerable in the tarsal tunnel behind the medial malleolus, while the *medial and lateral plantar nerves* are affected more distally, on the sole of the foot.

In evaluating mononeuropathies, the mode of onset of the paralysis must be established by careful questioning, because the etiologic diagnosis may depend on this information. Chronic entrapment syndromes produce a gradually progressive neuropathy, while in vasculitic neuropathy the paralysis begins abruptly and usually remains stationary afterwards. However, direct compression may also cause an acute neuropathy; this is frequently the case in peroneal palsies, which often result from direct compression, such as when sleeping with the affected leg undermost. Thus, when a patient presents with peroneal palsy of sudden onset, it is often difficult to decide whether the neuropathy is due to trauma or vasculitis, and electrophysiologic tests may not help to distinguish the two causes.

Cauda Equina Syndrome in Ankylosing Spondylitis

During the active stage of ankylosing spondylitis, many patients experience pain in the hips, thighs, and shoulders, and eventually muscle wasting may develop in the shoulder and pelvic girdles. The muscle wasting may be a result of the restricted motion of the joints, but muscle pathology and electrophysiology have not been systematically examined, and it is interesting that during active spondylitis the CSF protein is mildly or moderately increased in 30 to 40 percent of patients (Whitfield 1979). Slight increases of serum CPK activity were reported in one series (Calin 1975), but this finding is of doubtful significance.

A more serious complication is the cauda equina syndrome, of which more than 25 cases have been reported (Whitfield 1979; Milde et al. 1977). Many years after the spondylitis has become inactive, some patients begin to experience slowly progressive loss of bladder and bowel control with a lax anal sphincter, saddle anesthesia, asymmetric weakness and wasting of the muscles supplied by L-5 through S-2 nerve roots, and loss of the ankle reflexes. Neuralgic pain in a dermatomal distribution is present in a few cases, but usually the disorder is painless and the onset insidious and difficult to date. EMG shows denervation in the affected muscles. The CSF is entirely normal, and myelography shows no abnormality except for the presence, in most cases, of a large lumbar sac with multiple posterior diverticula, best demonstrated in the supine position.

The pathogenesis of this syndrome is poorly understood. The findings at operation or at autopsy have varied from a dense, fibrotic arachnoiditis investing the cauda equina and roots, to a large, multicystic arachnoidal sac with atrophy of the overlying dura—the nerve roots either adhering to the arachnoid or lying free. In either case the nerve roots and arachnoid membranes do not show any active inflammation. These findings suggest that the diverticula probably result from atrophy of the dura, permitting a pulsatile expansion of the arachnoidal sac, especially in the region of the nerve root canals; it is unlikely, however, that the diverticula are responsible for the neuropathy.

The most plausible hypothesis is that a radiculomeningitis occurs during the active phase of ankylosing spondylitis, without producing obvious neurologic deficits, and that many years later, when the inflammatory process has subsided, progressive fibrosis slowly damages the nerves and the pachymeninges, presumably by obliterating the microvasculature in those tissues. The main difficulty with this explanation is that the hypothetical radiculomeningitis has not been documented in early spondylitis, except for the frequent finding of an elevated CSF protein. However, rheumatoid arthritis can produce a florid radiculomeningitis, as described below.

Rheumatoid Lumbosacral Radiculomeningitis

Pachymeningitis is a rare complication of rheumatoid arthritis. In a recent case report (Markenson et al. 1979) the inflammatory process was located in the cauda equina and lumbosacral meninges, including the leptomeninges and dura, producing marked deformation of the lumbar sac at myelography. Although CSF block was not complete, the cisternal CSF was normal while the lumbar CSF protein was 421 to 990 mg per dl, the glucose was 5 mg per dl, and the white count ranged up to 470 cells per mm^3, of which 87 percent were neutrophils. The spinal fluid contained IgM and IgG rheumatoid factors, low molecular weight IgM, and immune complexes, and a comparison with serum immunoglobulin concentrations suggested that immunoglobulins were being synthesized intrathecally. Biopsy of the dura revealed necrotic debris with chronic inflammation and multinucleated giant cells, resembling a rheumatoid nodule. The clinical deficits (a typical cauda equina syndrome) and the CSF abnormalities both resolved on high-dose prednisone therapy.

A similar picture has been described in a patient with mixed connective tissue disease, but in that case only the dura was involved, and the CSF was normal (Kappes and Bennett 1982).

Cranial Neuropathies

Polyarteritis nodosa and related disorders sometimes produce cranial neuropathies as part of a vascular mononeuritis multiplex. Paralysis of the extraocular muscles, sparing the pupillary reactions, is sometimes observed in giant cell (temporal) arteritis. In the only case that has been examined postmortem, there were extensive ischemic lesions of the ocular muscles without any apparent damage to the ocular nerves (Barricks et al. 1977). This finding confounds earlier assumptions that the ocular palsies of temporal arteritis are of neurogenic origin. In SLE, paralysis of the ocular and other cranial nerves is usually caused by small brainstem infarcts rather than by peripheral nerve lesions (Johnson and Richardson 1968).

A painless, slowly progressive, often bilateral trigeminal sensory neuropathy occurs in patients with scleroderma, SLE, mixed connective tissue disease, rheumatoid arthritis, and Sjögren's syndrome (Teasdale et al. 1980; Ashworth and Tait 1971; Lundberg and Werner 1972; Bennett et al. 1978; Searles et al. 1978; Farrell and Medsger 1982). The motor functions of the trigeminal nerve, however, are almost always spared. Facial weakness occurs occasionally in patients with scleroderma, either in a slowly progressive fashion or as a sudden, unilateral paralysis (Teasdale et al. 1980); the pathogenesis is unknown, but the insidious type could be similar to trigeminal sensory neuropathy, which appears to derive from a low-grade inflammatory process involving the trigeminal ganglion and its roots.

In Wegener's granulomatosis, an extradural granuloma may involve the region of the jugular foramen, causing unilateral paralysis of the ninth, tenth, and eleventh cranial nerves, and a leptomeningeal granuloma may cause unilateral involvement of cranial nerves 7 through 12 (Drachman 1963).*

Orbital and retro-orbital inflammatory lesions (which were discussed in Chapter 3) have an important relation to the collagen-vascular diseases. *Orbital pseudotumor* is sometimes associated with polyarteritis nodosa or Wegener's granulomatosis (Jellinek 1969; Cassan et al. 1970). In a series of 140 cases of orbital pseudotumor, Blodi and Gass (1968) encountered 6 cases of Wegener's granulomatosis, and Jellinek (1969) listed 1 case of polyarteritis and 1 of Wegener's granulomatosis in 16 cases of orbital pseudotumor. Looked at the other way, among 29 cases of Wegener's granulomatosis there were ocular manifestations in 14 patients, including 7 with orbital pseudotumor—an incidence of 24 percent (Haynes et al. 1977). Although the pathology of retro-orbital granulomas is less well documented, it is likely that some cases of "painful ophthalmoplegia" also are related to systemic vasculitis. In that syndrome, a granulomatous lesion in the superior orbital fissure or the cavernous sinus surrounds the ophthalmic division of the trigeminal nerve (causing pain in the eye and forehead); the third, fourth, and sixth cranial nerves (causing ptosis and ophthalmoplegia); and the ocular sympathetic nerves. In contrast to orbital pseudotumor, there is little or no proptosis. Mathew and Chandy (1970) found LE cells in five out of eight cases, but antinuclear antibodies were not present and there were no other features of SLE. In most cases there is no evidence of a collagen-vascular disease (Aron-Rosa et al. 1979); however, a case of painful ophthalmoplegia has been reported in a patient with SLE (Evans and Lexow 1978). Treatment with corticosteroids was effective in that case and in other patients with idiopathic painful ophthalmoplegia (Mathew and Chandy 1970). Haynes and associates (1977) used both steroids and cytotoxic drugs in patients with orbital pseudotumor caused by Wegener's granulomatosis.

MISCELLANEOUS CHRONIC INFLAMMATORY DISEASES OF UNKNOWN CAUSE

Sarcoidosis

The neuromuscular manifestations of sarcoidosis include multiple cranial nerve palsies, various forms of peripheral neuropathy, and focal and gen-

*Cranial and spinal radiculoneuropathies are frequent in the syndrome of lymphomatoid granulomatosis, which resembles both Wegener's granulomatosis and malignant lymphoma (see Chapter 6).

eralized myopathies. All of these are associated with direct granulomatous involvement of the affected tissues. A neuromuscular syndrome may be the presenting feature of sarcoidosis, at a time when there is little or no clinical evidence of sarcoidosis elsewhere in the body. This subject was elegantly reviewed by Matthews (1979).

Myopathy

Asymptomatic granulomas are detectable in about 55 percent of random samples of muscle taken from patients with generalized sarcoidosis (Wallace et al. 1958). The ease with which these lesions can be found implies that the majority of patients have extensive involvement of skeletal muscle, so it is difficult to explain why *symptomatic* sarcoid myopathy is so rare. In two large series of patients with sarcoidosis, progressive muscle weakness owing to a generalized myopathy occurred in only 0.3 to 0.4 percent of patients (Silverstein and Siltzbach 1969; Douglas et al. 1973).

CLINICAL FEATURES. Occasionally the presentation is subacute, with myalgia, muscle swelling, tenderness, and weakness that may be generalized or restricted in distribution. The calf muscles are especially likely to show focal induration and tenderness (Fig. 26) (Cameron 1981). The serum

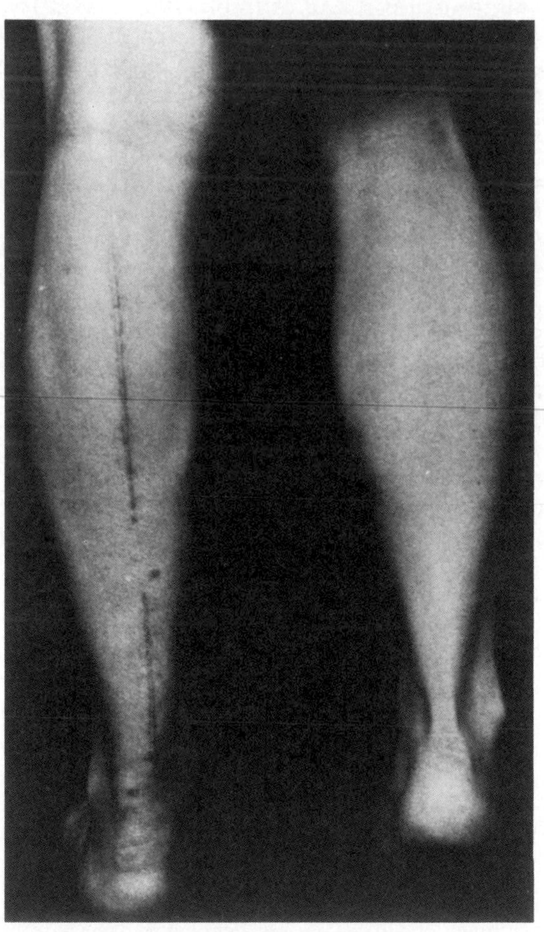

FIGURE 26. Sarcoidosis causing focal enlargement of the right medial gastrocnemius muscle. (From Cameron, 1981, with permission.)

CPK activity may be normal or increased, and EMG may show typical myopathic changes that usually are not accompanied by fibrillations. This picture is more frequent in young patients. Older patients generally manifest a slowly progressive myopathy characterized by widespread, painless muscular weakness and atrophy, sometimes accompanied by muscle induration and contractures. The muscle stretch reflexes are often absent. The CPK is usually normal, but EMG shows myopathic abnormalities. Patients with this clinical picture are often postmenopausal women. The least common muscle syndrome is the appearance of painless masses in the muscles caused by localized sarcoid granulomas. Any form of sarcoid myopathy may be accompanied by peripheral neuropathy, so that it may not be possible to determine how much of the muscle weakness is caused by myopathy and how much by neuropathy.

PATHOLOGY. In asymptomatic patients, muscle specimens may show typical sarcoid granulomas adjacent to atrophic muscle fibers that are otherwise unaffected. In myopathic patients there are in addition scattered muscle fibers undergoing degeneration and atrophy, sometimes accompanied by interstitial lymphocytic infiltration. Muscle fiber necrosis, phagocytosis, and regeneration are usually inconspicuous or absent. In chronic cases there may be extensive fibrosis. The same pathologic features have been described in patients said to have "granulomatous polymyositis," a designation chosen because there was no other evidence of sarcoidosis. In several such cases, however, systemic involvement by sarcoid was eventually demonstrated, either at medical followup or at autopsy.*

TREATMENT. Patients with a subacute myopathy may improve spontaneously, and they tend to respond well to moderate doses of corticosteroids. The insidious, slowly progressive, atrophic form may be totally unresponsive to steroids or cytotoxic drugs. A trial of steroids is warranted but if there is no response in a month or two treatment should not be continued, especially in older women who are at great risk of developing osteoporotic fractures. If patients respond to steroid therapy it is sometimes possible to discontinue treatment without a relapse of symptoms, but some patients may require maintenance therapy for many years.

Neuropathy

In most large surveys of patients with sarcoidosis, nervous system involvement was present in fewer than 5 percent of patients, though a recent series revealed an incidence of 9 percent (Delaney 1977). The majority of these cases consist of cranial and spinal neuropathies. The nerve lesions either are radicular, in which case there is leptomeningeal involvement, or they are located peripheral to the leptomeninges. Leptomeningeal involvement is a prominent feature of CNS sarcoidosis; the granulomatous lesions have a predilection for the basal cisterns and the region of the optic chiasm, but they may be scattered through the spinal and cranial leptomeninges, involving cranial and spinal nerve roots and in places extending into the substance of the brain or spinal cord. The nature of the peripheral nerve lesions has not been established, though granulomas have been seen in sural nerve biopsy specimens.

*Giant cell myositis associated with thymoma has also been loosely termed "granulomatous" (see Chapter 6).

CLINICAL FEATURES. Among the cranial neuropathies, the seventh nerve is involved most frequently (Wiederholt and Siekert 1965). Facial weakness is sometimes bilateral, but the two sides of the face are not usually affected simultaneously. The onset may be as rapid as it is in Bell's palsy, or it may be gradual, the weakness fluctuating in severity for several months. Often there are different degrees of paralysis in separate branches of the facial nerve. Taste sensation may be impaired, pointing to intracranial involvement of the facial nerve in some cases. Deafness and bulbar palsy caused by lower cranial nerve involvement may accompany the facial weakness, producing the picture of cranial polyneuropathy; the nerves controlling ocular movements, however, are rarely affected. Spinal and peripheral nerve involvement may take the form of a generalized mononeuropathy multiplex or a diffuse radiculoneuropathy (Matthews 1979), but usually there are features of both processes. The evolution of these nerve symptoms may be rapid or slow, but the progressive and often fluctuating course distinguishes this disorder from the mononeuropathy multiplex of systemic vasculitis. Distal branches of sensory or motor nerves may be involved—another finding which is uncommon in necrotizing vasculitis. Some patients have pain and cutaneous sensory loss over large areas of the trunk (Matthews 1979), similar to patients with diabetic thoracoabdominal neuropathy.

LABORATORY FINDINGS. Inflammatory changes in the CSF are frequent but are not always present, even in patients with cranial neuropathies. This may be because the granulomatous meningitis is restricted in location, or it may mean that the nerves are involved peripheral to the leptomeninges. When CSF abnormalities are present, the protein level is usually less than 200 mg per dl, and the spinal fluid usually contains between 10 and 100 mononuclear cells per mm^3. The CSF glucose concentration is low—in the range of 30 to 40 mg per dl—in about one fifth of the cases (Fishman 1980). Motor nerve conduction velocity may be reduced or normal, presumably reflecting the multifocal character of the nerve pathology; normal conduction would be expected in cases with purely radiculomeningeal disease or in the unaffected nerves of patients with peripheral mononeuropathy multiplex.

DIAGNOSIS. Among 23 cases of neurosarcoidosis analyzed by Delaney (1977), neurologic dysfunction was the presenting feature in 15 cases and was the sole clinical manifestation in 7 cases. Cranial and peripheral neuropathies in particular tend to appear early in the course of the disease. In such cases the differential diagnosis will focus on other diseases that cause cranial and peripheral neuropathies accompanied by a sterile meningitis: Wegener's granulomatosis, Lyme disease, Behçet's syndrome, and infiltration of the leptomeninges by lymphoma or carcinoma. Unfortunately there are no reliable, specific laboratory tests for sarcoidosis. In patients with active systemic sarcoidosis, biopsy of muscle, lymph nodes, or liver is frequently positive, gallium scans show disseminated lesions, and serum levels of angiotensin-converting enzyme are elevated; whether this is true of patients with neurosarcoidosis is not known. Careful ocular examination for evidence of uveitis, lacrimal gland enlargement, or conjunctival infiltration may provide early diagnostic clues.

TREATMENT. The cranial and peripheral neuropathies may resolve spontaneously; isolated facial paralysis is especially likely to recover. Steroid treatment is often dramatically effective, but the response may be transient, and some patients deteriorate relentlessly despite steroid therapy. Since no alternative treatment is available, however, a trial of steroid therapy is indicated if the symptoms warrant it.

Behçet's Syndrome

This multisystem disease is defined by the triad of oral ulcers, genital ulcers, and uveitis and occurs in a chronic, relapsing, and remitting fashion, with clinical and pathologic evidence of vasculitis involving veins, venules, and capillaries (Alema 1978). There is growing evidence that circulating immune complexes are involved in the pathogenesis (Gamble et al. 1978). CNS symptoms occur in perhaps 10 percent of patients, usually in the form of meningoencephalitis and ischemic lesions of the brain or spinal cord; these are accompanied by CSF abnormalities consisting of elevated protein, lymphocytic pleocytosis, and increased gamma globulin (Schotland et al. 1963).

Peripheral neuropathy has rarely been reported. O'Duffy and associates (1971) reported a patient with bilateral facial weakness and distal sensory neuropathy in the legs. Lobo-Antunes (1972) described a patient with unilateral facial numbness and distal sensory loss in the limbs; the CSF was normal, EMG suggested chronic partial denervation of the muscles, and motor nerve conduction velocities were normal except for distal slowing. In a patient reported by Arkin and coworkers (1980) the lower extremity nerves were inexcitable, motor conduction velocity was moderately slow in the median and ulnar nerves, and sensory nerves were inexcitable; this patient was said to have normal strength, however, and the reflexes and sensation were not described. A few other patients may have had a motor polyneuropathy or a mononeuropathy multiplex, but the clinical information was inadequate (Afifi et al. 1980; Alema 1978). Isolated cranial nerve palsies have been mentioned (Arkin et al. 1980), but these were usually associated with signs of an ischemic brainstem lesion (Schotland et al. 1963).

Overt myopathy has not been reported. One patient (Arkin et al. 1980) had a marked increase of serum CPK activity, but a random muscle biopsy was normal. At autopsy a sample of muscle (from an arm swollen by thrombophlebitis) showed muscle necrosis with acute and chronic inflammation; the authors interpreted this as "myositis," but the published photomicrograph looks more like infarction. Afifi and colleagues (1980) performed random muscle biopsies in seven patients with clinical or CPK evidence of myopathy; light- and electron-microscopy revealed only minor, nonspecific abnormalities.

Lyme Disease

This newly recognized tick-borne disease causes a distinctive skin lesion, recurrent oligoarthritis, and striking neurologic disturbances. In the United States the disorder is concentrated in small geographic areas of New England inhabited by the tick vector; a few cases have also appeared in California. A tick-borne meningopolyneuritis, with the same type of skin lesion but without arthritis, has been recognized in Europe for several decades (Reik et al. 1979). Recently a treponema-like spirochete has been incriminated as the postulated infectious agent (Burgdorfer et al. 1982).

CLINICAL FEATURES. The illness usually begins between May and November (Reik et al. 1979). At the site of a tick bite (not always remembered) a red macule or papule appears on the skin and gradually widens to form a large, annular area of erythema with partial central clearing, referred to as *erythema chronicum migrans.* There may be several skin lesions of this type. Neurologic symptoms appear as the rash is fading or soon after it disappears in 11 percent of patients. The symptoms include fever, headache, backache, myalgia, meningitis, encephalitis, multiple cranial neuritis (especially facial paralysis), multiple neuritis of one limb, mononeuropathy multiplex, and radiculoneuritis. These complications tend to occur in successive episodes, and if no treatment is given the symptoms may wax and wane for a number of months. Most of the neurologic deficits resolve spontaneously, but the neuropathies may proceed to the stage of axonal degeneration, with the consequence of delayed and incomplete recovery. Brief, recurrent attacks of oligoarthritis develop in many patients at various intervals after the skin lesion appears, sometimes many months afterwards.

LABORATORY FINDINGS. The CSF shows increased protein, a predominantly mononuclear pleocytosis, normal or borderline glucose, and a raised concentration of IgG. The only other noteworthy abnormality is the presence of cryoglobulins in the serum early in the course of the neurologic symptoms in 83 percent of patients; circulating immune complexes have also been demonstrated. Reik and colleagues (1979) suggested that many of the neurologic symptoms could be due to an immune-complex disease resembling serum sickness, but features such as meningoencephalitis are unusual in classic serum sickness, and another possible explanation is a persistent infection of the CNS, with secondary hyperimmune reactions.

TREATMENT. The meningeal symptoms usually respond rapidly to steroid therapy. The cranial and other neuropathies respond incompletely, perhaps reflecting varying degrees of reversibility at the time treatment was begun; if this is the correct explanation, treatment should be begun early in order to avoid residual damage or protracted convalescence. Steroid treatment can usually be tapered and discontinued within a few months.

REFERENCES

ABEL, T, ANDREWS, BS, CUNNINGHAM, PH, ET AL: *Rheumatoid vasculitis: Effect of cyclophosphamide on the clinical course and levels of circulating immune complexes.* Ann Intern Med 93:407–413, 1980.

ADAROS, HL AND HELD, JR: *Guillain-Barré syndrome associated with immunization against rabies: Epidemiological aspects.* Proc Assoc Res Nerv Ment Dis 49:178–185, 1971.

ADOUR, KK, BELL, DN AND HILSINGER, RF, JR: *Herpes simplex virus in idiopathic facial paralysis (Bell palsy).* JAMA 233:527–530, 1975.

ADOUR, KK, BYL, FM, HILSINGER, RL, JR, ET AL: *The true nature of Bell's palsy: Analysis of 1,000 consecutive patients.* Laryngoscope 88:787–801, 1978.

ADOUR, KK AND DOTY, HE: *Electronystagmographic comparison of acute idiopathic and herpes zoster facial paralysis.* Laryngoscope 83:2029–2034, 1973.

AFIFI, AK, FRAYHA, RA, BAHUTH, NB, ET AL: *The myopathology of Behçet's disease. A histochemical, light-, and electronmicroscopic study.* J Neurol Sci 48:333–342, 1980.

AGRAWAL, BL AND GIESEN, PC: *Eosinophilic myositis. An unusual cause of pseudotumor and eosinophilia.* JAMA 246:70–71, 1981.

AHMED, T AND BRAUN, AI: *Carpal tunnel syndrome in polymyalgia rheumatica.* Arthritis Rheum 21:221–223, 1978.

ALEKSIC, SN, LIEBERMAN, A AND GEORGE, AE: *Idiopathic diaphragmatic paralysis and neuralgic amyotrophy.* Europ Neurol 10:243–249, 1973.

ALEMA, G: *Behçet's disease.* In VINKEN, PJ AND BRUYN, GW (EDS): *Handbook of Clinical Neurology, vol. 34.* North-Holland Publishing, Amsterdam, 1978, pp 485–512.

Alexander, CB, Croker, BP and Bossen, EH: *Dermatomyositis associated with IgA deposition.* Arch Pathol Lab Med 106:449–451, 1982.

Aminoff, MJ: *Bell's palsy and its treatment.* Postgrad Med J 49:46–51, 1973.

Anderson, BA, Young, PV, Kean, WF, et al: *Polymyositis in chronic graft vs host disease. A case report.* Arch Neurol 39:188–190, 1982.

Anderson, L and Ziter, FA: *Plasmapheresis via central catheter in dermatomyositis: A new method for selected pediatric patients.* J Pediatr 98:240–241, 1981.

Andersson, T and Sidén, A: *A clinical study of the Guillain-Barré syndrome.* Acta Neurol Scand 66:316–327, 1982.

Arkin, CR, Rothschild, BM, Florendo, NT, et al: *Behçet syndrome with myositis. A case report with pathologic findings.* Arthritis Rheum 23:600–604, 1980.

Arnason, BGW: *Neuropathy of serum sickness.* In Dyck, PJ, Thomas, PK and Lambert, EH (eds): *Peripheral Neuropathy.* WB Saunders, Philadelphia, 1975a, pp 1104–1109.

Arnason, BGW: *Inflammatory polyradiculoneuropathies.* In Dyck, PJ, Thomas, PK and Lambert, EH (eds): *Peripheral Neuropathy.* WB Saunders, Philadelphia, 1975b, pp 1104–1109.

Arnett, FC, Whelton, JC, Zizie, TM, et al: *Methotrexate therapy in polymyositis.* Ann Rheum Dis 32:536–546, 1973.

Aron-Rosa, D, Dayan, D, Salamon, G, et al: *Tolosa-Hunt syndrome.* Ann Ophthalmol 10:1161–1168, 1979.

Asbury, AK, Arnason, BG and Adams, RD: *The inflammatory lesion in idiopathic polyneuritis. Its role in pathogenesis.* Medicine 48:173–215, 1969.

Ashworth, B and Tait, GBW: *Trigeminal neuropathy in connective tissue disease.* Neurology 21:609–614, 1971.

Åström, KE and Waksman, BH: *The passive transfer of experimental allergic encephalomyelitis and neuritis with living lymphoid cells.* Pathol Bacteriol 83:89–106, 1962.

Bailey, AA, Sayre, GP and Clark, EC: *Neuritis associated with systemic lupus erythematosus. A report of five cases with necropsy in two.* Arch Neurol Psychiatry 75:251–259, 1956.

Banker, BQ: *Dermatomyositis of childhood: Ultrastructural alterations of muscle and intramuscular blood vessels.* J Neuropathol Exp Neurol 34:46–75, 1975.

Banker, BQ and Victor, M: *Dermatomyositis (systemic angiopathy) of childhood.* Medicine 45:261–289, 1966.

Bardos, V and Somodska, V: *Epidemiologic study of a brachial plexus neuritis outbreak in Northeast Czechoslovakia.* World Neurol 2:973–977, 1961.

Bardwick, PA, Zvaifler, NJ, Gill, GN, et al: *Plasma cell dyscrasia with polyneuropathy, organomegaly, endocrinopathy, M protein, and skin changes: The POEMS syndrome. Report on two cases and a review of the literature.* Medicine 59:311–322, 1980.

Barnes, L, Rodman, GP, Medsger, TA, Jr, et al: *Eosinophilic fasciitis. A pathologic study of twenty cases.* Am J Pathol 96:493–518, 1979.

Barricks, ME, Trairesa, DB and Glaser, JS: *Ophthalmoplegia in cranial arteritis.* Brain 100:209–221, 1977.

Bates, D, Stevens, JC and Hudgson, P: *"Polymyositis" with involvement of facial and distal musculature. One form of the facioscapulohumeral syndrome?* J Neurol Sci 19:105–108, 1973.

Bayer, AS, Galpin, JE, Theofilopoulos, AN, et al: *Neurologic disease associated with* Mycoplasma pneumoniae *pneumonitis. Demonstration of viable* Mycoplasma pneumoniae *in cerebrospinal fluid and blood by radioisotopic and immunofluorescent tissue culture techniques.* Ann Intern Med 94:15–20, 1981.

Becker, WJ, Watters, GV and Humphreys, P: *Fisher syndrome in childhood.* Neurology 31:555–560, 1981.

Beevers, DG, Harpur, JE and Turk, KAD: *Giant cell arteritis—the need for prolonged treatment.* J Chron Dis 26:571–584, 1973.

Behan, WMH, Barkas, MH and Behan, PO: *Detection of immune complexes in polymyositis.* Acta Neurol Scand 65:320–334, 1982.

Behan, WMH, Behan, P and Dick, HA: *HLA-B8 in polymyositis.* N Engl J Med 298:1260–1261, 1978.

Benbassat, J, Geffel, D and Zlotnick, A: *Epidemiology of polymyositis-dermatomyositis in Israel, 1960–76.* Isr J Med Sci 16:197–200, 1980.

Bengtsson, B-A, and Malmvall, B-E: *The epidemiology of giant cell arteritis including temporal arteritis and polymyalgia rheumatica.* Arthritis Rheum 24:899–904, 1981.

BENNETT, RM, BONG, DM AND SPARGO, BH: *Neuropsychiatric problems in mixed connective tissue disease.* Am J Med 65:955–962, 1978.

BENSON, MD AND ALDO, MA: *Azathioprine therapy in polymyositis.* Arch Intern Med 132:547–551, 1973.

BENSON, MD, BRANDT, KD, COHEN, AS, ET AL: *Neuropathy, M components, and amyloid.* Lancet i:10–12, 1975.

BERGER, JR, AYYAR, R AND SHEREMATA, WA: *Guillain-Barré syndrome complicating acute hepatitis B. A case with detailed electrophysiological and immunological studies.* Arch Neurol 38:366–368, 1981.

BERRY, H AND BLAIR, RL: *Isolated vagus nerve palsy and vagal mononeuritis.* Arch Otolaryngol 106:333–338, 1980.

BESINGER, UA, TOYKA, KV, ANZIL, AP, ET AL: *Myeloma neuropathy: Passive transfer from man to mouse.* Science 213:1027–1030, 1981.

BHARUCHA, NE AND MORGAN-HUGHES, JA: *Chronic focal polymyositis in the adult.* J Neurol Neurosurg Psychiatry 44:419–425, 1981.

BJELLE, A, HENRIKSSON, K-G AND HOFER, P-A: *Polymyositis in eosinophilic fasciitis. Review and case report.* Eur Neurol 19:128–137, 1980.

BLAU, JN AND KAPADIA, R: *Idiopathic palsy of the recurrent laryngeal nerve: A transient cranial mononeuropathy.* Br Med J 4:259–261, 1972.

BLETRY, O, BUSSEL, A, BADELON, I, ET AL: *Intérêt des échanges plasmatiques au cours des angéites nécrosantes.* Nouv Presse Méd 11:2827–2831, 1982.

BLOCH, SL, JARRETT, MP, SEDLOW, M, ET AL: *Brachial plexus neuropathy as the initial manifestation of systemic lupus erythematosus.* Neurology 29:1633–1634, 1979.

BLODI, FC AND GASS, JDM: *Inflammatory pseudotumor of the orbit.* Br J Ophthalmol 52:79–93, 1968.

BLONQUIST, HK AND BJORKSTEN, B: *Poliomyelitis-like illness associated with asthma.* Arch Dis Child 55:61–74, 1980.

BLUESTEIN, HG, WILLIAMS, GW AND STEINBERG, AD: *Cerebrospinal fluid antibodies to neuronal cells: Association with neuropsychiatric manifestations of systemic lupus erythematosus.* Am J Med 70:240–246, 1981.

BOHAN, A, PETER, JB, BOWMAN, RL, ET AL: *A computer-assisted analysis of 153 patients with polymyositis and dermatomyositis.* Medicine 56:255–286, 1977.

BOONGIRD, P AND VEJJAJIVA, A: *Electrophysiologic findings and prognosis in Bell's palsy.* Muscle Nerve 1:461–466, 1978.

BORENSTEIN, DG, FYE, WB, ARNETT, FC, ET AL: *The myocarditis of systemic lupus erythematosus. Association with myositis.* Ann Intern Med 89:619–624, 1978.

BOSCH, EP, ANSBACHER, LE, GOEKEN, JA, ET AL: Peripheral neuropathy associated with monoclonal gammopathy. Studies of intraneural injections of monoclonal immunoglobulin sera. J Neuropathol Exp Neurol 41:446–459, 1982.

BRETTLE, RP, GROSS, M, LEGG, NJ, ET AL: *Treatment of acute polyneuropathy by plasma exchange.* Lancet ii:1100, 1978.

BREWER, EJ, GIANNINI, EH, ROSSEN, RD, ET AL: *Plasma exchange therapy of a childhood onset dermatomyositis patient.* Arthritis Rheum 23:509–513, 1980.

BROSTOFF, S, BURNETT, P, LAMPERT, P, ET AL: *Isolation and characterization of a protein from sciatic nerve myelin responsible for experimental allergic neuritis.* Nature (New Biology) 235:210–212, 1972.

BROUET, J-C, CLAUVEL, J-P, DANON, F, ET AL: *Biologic and clinical significance of cryoglobulins. A report of 86 cases.* Am J Med 57:775–788, 1974.

BRUBAKER, DB AND WINKELSTEIN, A: *Plasma exchange in rheumatoid vasculitis.* Vox Sang 41:295–301, 1981.

BRUNET, P, BINET, JL, DE SAXCE, H, ET AL: *Neuropathies au cours de la lymphadenopathie angio-immunoblastique.* Rev Neurol 137:503–515, 1981.

BUNCH, TW: *Prednisone and azathioprine for polymyositis. Long-term followup.* Arthritis Rheum 24:45–48, 1981.

BUNCH, TW, WORTHINGTON, JW, COMBS, JJ, ET AL: *Azathioprine with prednisone for polymyositis. A controlled, clinical trial.* Ann Intern Med 92:365–369, 1980.

BURGDORFER, W, BARBOUR, AG, HAYES, SF, ET AL: *Lyme disease—a tick-borne spirochetosis?* Science 216:1317–1319, 1982.

BUSH, RK, GELLER, M, BUSSE, WW, ET AL: *Response to corticosteroids in the hypereosinophilic syndrome. Association with increased serum IgE levels.* Arch Intern Med 138:1244–1246, 1978.

CALIN, A: *Raised serum creatine phosphokinase activity in ankylosing spondylitis.* Ann Rheum Dis 34:244–248, 1975.

CAMERON, HU: *Symmetrical muscle contractures in tumorous sarcoidosis: Report of a case.* Clin Orthop 155:108–110, 1981.

CARPENTER, S, KARPATI, G, HELLER, I, ET AL: *Inclusion body myositis: A distinct variety of idiopathic inflammatory myopathy.* Neurology 28:8–17, 1978.

CARPENTER, S, KARPATI, G, ROTHMAN, S, ET AL: *The childhood type of dermatomyositis.* Neurology 26:952–962, 1976.

CASSAN, SM, DIVERTIE, MB, HOLLENHORST, RW, ET AL: *Pseudotumor of the orbit and limited Wegener's granulomatosis.* Ann Intern Med 72:687–693, 1970.

CHAD, D, GOOD, P, ADELMAN, L, ET AL: *Inclusion body myositis associated with Sjögren's syndrome.* Arch Neurol 39:186–188, 1982a.

CHAD, D, PARISER, K, BRADLEY, WG, ET AL: *The pathogenesis of cryoglobulinemic neuropathy.* Neurology 32:725–729, 1982b.

CHALMERS, A, SAYSON, R AND WALTERS, K: *Juvenile dermatomyositis: Medical, social and economic status in adulthood.* Can Med Assoc J 126:31–33, 1982.

CHAZOT, G, BERGER, B, CARRIER, H, ET AL: *Manifestations neurologiques des gammapathies monoclonales.* Rev Neurol 132:195–212, 1976.

CHURG, J AND STRAUSS, L: *Allergic granulomatosis, allergic angiitis and periarteritis nodosa.* Am J Pathol 27:277–301, 1951.

CHUSID, MJ, DALE, DC, WEST, BC, ET AL: *The hypereosinophilic syndrome: Analysis of fourteen cases with review of the literature.* Medicine 54:1–27, 1975.

CLEMENTS, PJ, FURST, DE, CAMPION, DS, ET AL: *Muscle disease in progressive systemic sclerosis. Diagnostic and therapeutic considerations.* Arthritis Rheum 21:62–71, 1978.

CLERF, LH: *Unilateral vocal cord paralysis.* JAMA 151:900–903, 1953.

COHEN, AS AND BENSON, MD: *Amyloid neuropathy.* In DYCK, PJ, THOMAS, PK AND LAMBERT, EH (EDS): *Peripheral Neuropathy.* WB Saunders, Philadelphia, 1975, pp 1067–1091.

COMROE, JH, WOOD, FC, KAY, CF, ET AL: *Motor neuritis after tetanus antitoxin with involvement of the muscles of respiration.* Am J Med 10:786–789, 1951.

CONN, DL AND DYCK, PJ: *Angiopathic neuropathy in connective tissue diseases.* In DYCK, PJ, THOMAS, PK, AND LAMBERT, EH (EDS): *Peripheral Neuropathy.* WB Saunders, Philadelphia, 1975, pp 1149–1165.

CONTAMIN, F, SINGER, B, MIGNOT, B, ET AL: *Polyneuropathie à rechutes, évoluant depuis 19 ans, associée à une gammapathie monoclonale IgG bénigne. Effet favorable de la corticothérapie.* Rev Neurol 132:741–762, 1976.

COOK, JD, TINDALL, RAS, WALKER, J, ET AL: *Plasma exchange as a treatment of acute and chronic idiopathic autoimmune polyneuropathy: Limited success.* Neurology 30:361–362, 1980.

COOK, SD AND DOWLING, PC: *The role of autoantibody and immune complexes in the pathogenesis of Guillain-Barre syndrome.* Ann Neurol 9 (suppl):70–79, 1981.

COTTERILL, JA AND SHAPIRO, H: *Dermatomyositis after immunization.* Lancet ii:1158–1159, 1978.

CRAMER, SF, KENT, L, ABRAMOWSKY, C, ET AL: *Eosinophilic fasciitis. Immunopathology, ultrastructure, literature review, and consideration of its pathogenesis and relation to scleroderma.* Arch Pathol Lab Med 106:85–91, 1982.

CREAM, JJ, HERN, JEC, HUGHES, RAF, ET AL: *Mixed or immune complex cryoglobulinemia and neuropathy.* J Neurol Neurosurg Psychiatry 37:82–87, 1974.

CROWE, WE, BOVE, KE, LEVINSON, JE, ET AL: *Clinical and pathogenetic implications of histopathology in childhood polydermatomyositis.* Arthritis Rheum 25:126–139, 1982.

CUMMING, WJK, WEISER, R, TEOH, R, ET AL: *Localised nodular myositis: A clinical and pathological variant of polymyositis.* Q J Med 46:531–546, 1977.

CURRIE, S, SAUNDERS, M, KNOWLES, M, ET AL: *Immunological aspects of polymyositis. The in vitro activity of lymphocytes on incubation with muscle antigen and with muscle cultures.* Q J Med 40:63–84, 1971.

CURRIE, S AND WALTON, JN: *Immunosuppressive therapy in polymyositis.* J Neurol Neurosurg Psychiatry 34:447–452, 1971.

CZEUZ, KA, THOMAS, JE, LAMBERT, EH, ET AL: *Long-term results of operation for carpal tunnel syndrome.* Mayo Clin Proc 41:232–241, 1966.

DALAKAS, MC AND ENGEL, WK: *Immunoglobulin and complement deposits in nerves of patients with chronic relapsing polyneuropathy.* Arch Neurol 37:637–640, 1980.

DALAKAS, MC AND ENGEL, WK: *Chronic relapsing (dysimmune) polyneuropathy: Pathogenesis and treatment.* Ann Neurol 9(suppl):134–145, 1981a.

DALAKAS, MC AND ENGEL, WK: *Polyneuropathy with monoclonal gammopathy: Studies of 11 patients.* Ann Neurol 10:45–52, 1981b.

DALAKAS, MC, HOUFF, SA, ENGEL, WK, ET AL: *CSF "monoclonal" bands in chronic relapsing polyneuropathy.* Neurology 30:864–867, 1980.

DAMJANOV, ID, MOSER, RL, KATZ, SM, ET AL: *Immune complex myositis associated with viral hepatitis.* Hum Pathol 11:478–481, 1980.

DANTA, G: *Electrophysiological study of amyotrophy associated with acute asthma (asthmatic amyotrophy).* J Neurol Neurosurg Psychiatry 38:1016–1021, 1975.

DAU, PC: *Plasmapheresis in idiopathic inflammatory myopathy. Experience with 35 patients.* Arch Neurol 38:544–552, 1981.

DAU, PC AND BENNINGTON, JL: *Plasmapheresis in childhood dermatomyositis.* J Pediatr 98:237–240, 1981.

DAVIS, JK, CASSELL, GH, MINION, FC, ET AL: *Mycoplasma host-cell interactions resulting in chronic inflammation: Acquisition of host antigens and other mechanisms.* Isr J Med Sci 17:633–636, 1981.

DAWKINS, RL: *Experimental myositis associated with hypersensitivity to muscle.* J Pathol Bacteriol 90:619–625, 1965.

DAWKINS, RL AND MASTAGLIA, FL: *Cell-mediated cytotoxicity to muscle in polymyositis. Effect of immunosuppression.* N Engl J Med 288:434–438, 1973.

DELANEY, P: *Neurologic manifestations in sarcoidosis. Review of the literature with a report of 23 cases.* Ann Intern Med 87:336–345, 1977.

DELAUCHE, MC, CLAUVEL, JP AND SELIGMANN, M: *Peripheral neuropathy and plasma cell neoplasias: A report of 10 cases.* Br J Hematol 48:383–392, 1981.

DENBOW, CE, LIE, JT, TANCREDI, RG, ET AL: *Cardiac involvement in polymyositis. A clinicopathologic study of 20 autopsied patients.* Arthritis Rheum 22:1088–1092, 1979.

DEVATHASAN G AND TONG, HI: *Neuralgic amyotrophy: Criteria for diagnosis and a clinical with electromyographic study of 21 cases.* Aust NZ J Med 10:188–191, 1980.

DEVERE, R AND BRADLEY, WG: *Polymyositis: Its presentation, morbidity and mortality.* Brain 98:637–666, 1975.

DIAZ-PEREZ, JL, CONNOLLY, SM, AND WINKELMANN, RK: *Disabling pansclerotic morphea of children.* Arch Dermatol 116:169–173, 1980.

DJUPESLAND, G, BERDAL, P, JOHANNESSEN, A, ET AL: *Viral infection as a cause of acute peripheral facial palsy.* Arch Otolaryngol 102:403–406, 1976.

DJUPESLAND, G, DEGRE, M, STIEN, R, ET AL: *Acute peripheral facial palsy. Part of a cranial polyneuropathy?* Arch Otolaryngol 103:641–644, 1977.

DOUGLAS, AC, MCLEOD, JG AND MATTHEWS, JC: *Symptomatic sarcoidosis of muscle.* J Neurol Neurosurg Psychiatry 36:1034–1040, 1973.

DOWLING, PC AND COOK, SD: *Role of infection in Guillain-Barré syndrome: Laboratory confirmation of herpes viruses in 41 cases.* Ann Neurol 9(suppl):44–55, 1981.

DOWLING, P, MENONNA, J AND COOK, S: *Cytomegalovirus complement fixation in Guillain-Barré syndrome.* Neurology 27:1153–1156, 1977.

DOYLE, JB: *Neurologic complications of serum sickness.* Am J Med Sci 185:484–492, 1933.

DRACHMAN, DA: *Neurological complications of Wegener's granulomatosis.* Arch Neurol 8:145–155, 1963.

DRACHMAN, DA, PATERSON, PY, BERLIN, BS, ET AL: *Immunosuppression and the Guillain-Barré syndrome.* Arch Neurol 23:385–393, 1970.

DRIEDGER, H AND PRUZANSKI, W: *Plasma cell neoplasia with peripheral neuropathy. A study of five cases and a review of the literature.* Medicine 59:301–310, 1980.

DUCHOWNEY, M, CAPLAN, L AND SIBER, G: *Cytomegalovirus infection of the adult nervous system.* Ann Neurol 5:458–461, 1979.

DYCK, PJ, CONN, DL AND OKAZAKI, H: *Necrotizing angiopathic neuropathy. Three-dimensional morphology of fiber degeneration related to sites of occluded vessels.* Mayo Clin Proc 47:461–475, 1972.

DYCK, PJ, LAIS, AC, OHTA, M, ET AL: *Chronic inflammatory polyradiculoneuropathy.* Mayo Clin Proc 50:621–637, 1975.

ECKHARDT, JJ, IVINS, JC, PERRY, HO, ET AL: *Osteosarcoma arising in heterotopic ossification of dermatomyositis: Case report and review of the literature.* Cancer 48:1256–1261, 1981.

EHRENGUT, W: *Dermatomyositis and vaccination.* Lancet i:1040–1041, 1978.

EISEN, A AND HUMPHREYS, P: *The Guillain-Barré syndrome. A clinical and electrodiagnostic study of 25 cases.* Arch Neurol 30:438–443, 1974.

ELIZAN, TS, SPIRE, JP, ANDIMAN, RM, ET AL: *Syndrome of acute idiopathic ophthalmoplegia with ataxia and areflexia.* Neurology 21:281–292, 1972.

ENZINGER, FM AND DULCEY, F: *Proliferative myositis. Report of thirty-three cases.* Cancer 20:2213–2223, 1967.

ESIRI, MM, MACLENNON, KM AND HAZLEMAN, BL: *Lymphocyte sensitivity to skeletal muscle in patients with polymyositis and other disorders.* Clin Exp Immunol 14:25–35, 1971.

ESTES, D AND CHRISTIAN, CL: *The natural history of systemic lupus erythematosus by prospective analysis.* Medicine 50:85–95, 1971.

EVANS, OB AND LEXOW, SS: *Painful ophthalmoplegia in systemic lupus erythematosus.* Ann Neurol 4:584–585, 1978.

FAN, PT, DAVIS, JA, SOMER, T, ET AL: *A clinical approach to systemic vasculitis.* Semin Arthritis Rheum 9:248–304, 1980.

FARRELL, DA AND MEDSGER, TA, JR: *Trigeminal neuropathy in progressive systemic sclerosis.* Am J Med 73:57–62, 1982.

FAUCI, AS (Moderator): *The idiopathic hypereosinophilic syndrome: Clinical, pathophysiologic, and therapeutic considerations.* Ann Intern Med 97:78–92, 1982.

FAUCI, AS, HAYNES, BG AND KATZ, P: *The spectrum of vasculitis. Clinical, pathologic, immunologic, and therapeutic considerations.* Ann Intern Med 89 (Part 1):660–676, 1978.

FAUCI, AS AND WOLFF, JM: *Wegener's granulomatosis: Studies in eighteen patients and a review of the literature.* Medicine 52:535–561, 1973.

FEASBY, TE, HAHN, AF AND GILBERT, JJ: *Passive transfer studies in Guillain-Barré polyneuropathy.* Neurology 32:1159–1167, 1982.

FESSEL, WJ AND RAAS, MC: *Autoimmunity in the pathogenesis of muscle disease.* Neurology 18:1137–1139, 1968.

FISHER, CM: *An unusual variant of acute idiopathic polyneuritis (syndrome of ophthalmoplegia, ataxia, and areflexia).* N Engl J Med 255:57–65, 1956.

FISHMAN, RA: *Cerebrospinal Fluid in Diseases of the Nervous System.* WB Saunders, Philadelphia, 1980.

FITTING, JW, BISCHOFF, A, REGLI, F, ET AL: *Neuropathy, amyloidosis, and monoclonal gammopathy.* J Neurol Neurosurg Psychiatry 42:193–202, 1979.

FOOTE, RA, KIMBROUGH, SM AND STEVENS, JC: *Lupus myositis.* Muscle Nerve 5:65–68, 1982.

FRIES, JF AND HOLMAN, HR: *Systemic Lupus Erythematosus: A Clinical Analysis.* WB Saunders, Philadelphia, 1975.

FROHNERT, PP AND SHEPS, SG: *Long-term follow-up study of periarteritis nodosa.* Am J Med 43:8–14, 1967.

FRYMOYER, JW AND BLAND, J: *Carpal-tunnel syndrome in patients with myxedematous arthropathy.* J Bone Joint Surg 55A:78–82, 1973.

GAMBLE, CN, WIESNER, KB, SHAPIRO, RF, ET AL: *The immune complex pathogenesis of glomerulonephritis and pulmonary vasculitis in Behçet's disease.* Am J Med 66:1031–1039, 1978.

GARGOUR, G, MACGAFFREY, K, LOCKE, S, ET AL: *Anterior radiculopathy and lupus erythematosus cells: Report of a case.* Br Med J 2:799–801, 1964.

GELTNER, D, KOHN, RW, GOREVIC, P, ET AL: *The effect of combination therapy (steroids, immunosuppressives, and plasmapheresis) on 5 mixed cryoglobulinemia patients with renal, neurologic, and vascular involvement.* Arthritis Rheum 24:1121–1127, 1981.

GOLDBERG, M AND CHITANONDH, H: *Polyneuritis with albuminocytologic dissociation in the spinal fluid in systemic lupus erythematosus. Report of a case with review of pertinent literature.* Am J Med 27:342–350, 1959.

GOLDSCHMIDT, B, MENONNA, J, FORTUNATO, J, ET AL: *Mycoplasma antibody in Guillain-Barré syndrome and other neurological disorders.* Ann Neurol 7:108–112, 1980.

GOODALL, JAD, KOSMIDIS, JC AND GEDDES, AM: *Effect of corticosteroids on course of Guillain-Barré syndrome.* Lancet i:524–526, 1974.

GOODMAN, BW: *Temporal arteritis.* Am J Med 67:839–852, 1979.

GORDON, RM AND SILVERSTEIN, A: *Neurologic manifestations in progressive systemic sclerosis.* Arch Neurol 22:126–134, 1970.

GOREVIC, PD, KASSAB, HJ, LEVO, Y, ET AL: *Mixed cryoglobulinemia: Clinical aspects and long-term follow-up of 40 patients.* Am J Med 69:287–308, 1980.

GOTTDIENER, JS, SHERBER, HS, HAWLEY, RJ, ET AL: *Cardiac manifestations in polymyositis.* Am J Cardiol 41:1141–1149, 1978.

GRIGOR, R, EDMONDS, J, LEWKONIA, R, ET AL: *Systemic lupus erythematosus. A prospective analysis.* Ann Rheum Dis 37:121–128, 1978.

GROSS, MLP AND THOMAS, PK: *The treatment of chronic relapsing and chronic progressive idiopathic inflammatory polyneuropathy by plasma exchange.* J Neurol Sci 52:69–78, 1981.

HAAS, DC: *Absence of cell-mediated cytotoxicity to muscle cultures in polymyositis.* J Rheumatol 7:671–676, 1980.

HARRISON, SM, FRENKEL, M, GROSSMAN, BJ, ET AL: *Retinopathy in childhood dermatomyositis.* Am J Ophthalmol 76:786–790, 1973.

HAUSMANOWA-PETRUSEWICZ, I, EMERYK, B, ROWINSKA-MARCINSKA, K, ET AL: *Nerve conduction in the Guillain-Barré-Strohl syndrome.* J Neurol 220:169–184, 1979.

HAYNES, BF, FISHMAN, ML, FAUCI, AS, ET AL: *The ocular manifestations of Wegener's granulomatosis. Fifteen years experience and review of the literature.* Am J Med 63:131–141, 1977.

HEFFNER, RR, JR, ARMBRUSTMACHER, VW AND EARLE, KM: *Focal myositis.* Cancer 40:301–306, 1977.

HEFFNER, RR, JR AND BARRON, SA: *Polymyositis beginning as a focal process.* Arch Neurol 38:439–442, 1981.

HEFFNER, RR, BARRON, SA, JENIS, EH, ET AL: *Skeletal muscle in polymyositis. Immunohistochemical study.* Pathol Lab Med 103:310–313, 1979.

HESSELVIK, M: *Neuropathological studies on myelomatosis.* Acta Neurol Scand 45:95–108, 1969.

HILL, DL AND BARROWS, HS: *Identical skeletal and cardiac muscle involvement in a case of fatal polymyositis.* Arch Neurol 19:545–551, 1968.

HILL, RH AND WOOD, WS: *Juvenile dermatomyositis.* Can Med Assoc J 21:1152–1156, 1970.

HOKKANEN, E, HALTIA, T AND MYLLYLÄ, VV: *Recurrent multiple cranial neuropathies.* Eur Neurol 17:32–37, 1978.

HOLLINRAKE, K: *Polymyositis presenting as distal muscle weakness. A case report.* J Neurol Sci 8:479–484, 1969.

HOPKINS, IJ: *A new syndrome: Poliomyelitis-like illness associated with acute asthma in childhood.* Aust Paediatr J 10:273–276, 1974.

HORWICH, MS, CHO, L, PORRO, RS, ET AL: *Subacute sensory neuropathy: A remote effect of carcinoma.* Ann Neurol 2:7–19, 1977.

HUGHES, RAC, NEWSOM-DAVIS, JM, PERKIN, GD, ET AL: *Controlled trial of prednisolone in acute polyneuropathy.* Lancet ii:750–753, 1978.

IANNACCONE, ST, BOWEN, DE AND SAMAHA, FJ: *Cell-mediated cytotoxicity and childhood dermatomyositis.* Arch Neurol 39:400–402, 1982.

ILETT, SJ, PUGH, RJ AND SMITHELLS, RW: *Poliomyelitis-like illness after acute asthma.* Arch Dis Child 52:738–740, 1977.

IQBAL, A, OGER, JJF AND ARNASON, BGW: *Cell-mediated immunity in idiopathic polyneuritis.* Ann Neurol 9(suppl):65–69, 1981a.

IQBAL, A, OGER, JJF AND ARNASON, BGW, ET AL: *Absence of antibodies to P_2 protein in idiopathic polyneuritis.* Neurology 31(2):156, 1981b.

IWASHITA, H, OHUISHI, A, ASADA, M, ET AL: *Polyneuropathy, skin hyperpigmentation, edema, and hypertrichosis in localized osteosclerotic myeloma.* Neurology 27:675–681, 1977.

JACOBS, JC: *Methotrexate and azathioprine treatment of childhood dermatomyositis.* Pediatrics 59:212–218, 1977.

JELLINEK, EH: *The orbital pseudotumour syndrome and its differentiation from endocrine exophthalmos.* Brain 92:35–58, 1969.

JOHNSON, RT AND RICHARDSON, EP: *The neurological manifestation of systemic lupus erythematosus. A clinical-pathological study of 24 cases and review of the literature.* Medicine 47:337–369, 1968.

JONES, JG AND HAZLEMAN, BL: *Prognosis and management of polymyalgia rheumatica.* Ann Rheum Dis 40:1–5, 1981.

KAHN, SN, RICHES, PG AND KOHN, J: *Paraproteinemia in neurological disease: Incidence, associations, and classification of monoclonal immunoglobulins.* J Clin Pathol 33:617–621, 1980.

KAKULAS, BA: *Destruction of differentiated muscle cultures by sensitised lymphoid cells.* J Pathol Bacteriol 91:495–503, 1966.

KAKULAS, BA, SHUTE, GH AND LECLERE, ALF: *In vitro destruction of human fetal muscle cultures by peripheral blood lymphocytes from patients with polymyositis and lupus erythematosus.* Proc Aust Assoc Neurol 8:85–92, 1971.

KAPLINSKY, N, REVACH, M AND KATZ, WA: *Eosinophilic fasciitis: Report of a case with features of connective tissue disease.* J Rheumatol 7:536–540, 1980.

KAPPES, J AND BENNETT, RM: *Cauda equina syndrome in a patient with high titer anti-RNP antibodies.* Arthritis Rheum 25:349–352, 1982.

Karnes, WE: *Diseases of the seventh cranial nerve.* In Dyck, PJ, Thomas, PK and Lambert, EH, (eds): *Peripheral Neuropathy.* WB Saunders, Philadelphia, 1975, pp 570–603.

Kåss, E, Straume, S and Munthe, E: *Dermatomyositis after BCG vaccination.* Lancet i:772, 1978.

Kearsley, JH: *Vocal cord paralysis (VCP)—an aetiological review of 100 cases over 20 years.* Aust NZ J Med 11:663–666, 1981.

Kelly, JJ, Jr, Kyle, RA, Miles, JM, et al: *The spectrum of peripheral neuropathy in myeloma.* Neurology 31:24–31, 1981a.

Kelly, JJ, Kyle, RA, O'Brien, PC, et al: *Prevalence of monoclonal protein in peripheral neuropathy.* Neurology 31:1480–1483, 1981b.

Kennedy, RH, Danielson, MA, Mulder, DW, et al: *Guillain-Barré syndrome. A 42 year epidemiologic and clinical study.* Mayo Clin Proc 53:93–99, 1978.

Kesler, RW, McDonald, TD, Balasubramanian, M, et al: *Linear scleroderma in children.* Am J Dis Child 135:738–740, 1981.

Kimura, J: *Proximal versus distal slowing of motor nerve conduction velocity in the Guillain-Barré syndrome.* Ann Neurol 3:344–350, 1978.

Knox, DL, Clark, DB and Schuster, FF: *Benign VI nerve palsies in children.* Pediatrics 40:560–564, 1967.

Kohn, J: *Benign paraproteinemias.* J Clin Pathol 28(suppl 6):77–82, 1974.

Konishi, T, Saida, K, Ohnishi, A, et al: *Perineuritis in mononeuritis multiplex with cryoglobulinemia.* Muscle Nerve 5:173–177, 1982.

Kreitzer, SM, Feldman, NT, Saunders, NA, et al: *Bilateral diaphragmatic paralysis with hypercapneic respiratory failure. A physiologic assessment.* Am J Med 65:89–95, 1978.

Lagier, R and Cox, JN: *Pseudomalignant myositis ossificans.* Human Pathol 6:653–665, 1975.

Latov, N, Sherman, WH, Gross, R, et al: *Monoclonal antibodies to peripheral nerve in patients with polyneuritis and plasma cell dyscrasia.* Neurology 31(2):155, 1981.

Latov, N, Sherman, WH, Nemni, R, et al: *Plasma-cell dyscrasia and peripheral neuropathy with a monoclonal antibody to peripheral-nerve myelin.* N Engl J Med 303:618–621, 1980.

Layzer, RB, Shearn, MA and Satya-Murti, S: *Eosinophilic polymyositis.* Ann Neurol 1:65–71, 1977.

Levy, RL, Newkirk, R and Ochoa, J: *Treatment of chronic relapsing Guillain-Barré syndrome by plasma exchange.* Lancet ii:741, 1979.

Lewis, DC: *Systemic lupus and polyneuropathy.* Arch Intern Med 116:518–522, 1965.

Lewis, RA, Sumner, AJ, Brown, MJ, et al: *Multifocal demyelinating neuropathy with persistent conduction block.* Neurology 32:958–964, 1982.

Liebeschuetz, HJ: *Poliomyelitis-type illness associated with severe asthma in a child.* J R Soc Med 74:71–72, 1981.

Link, H: *Immunoglobulin abnormalities in Guillain-Barre syndrome.* J Neurol Sci 18:11–23, 1973.

Lisak, RP and Zweiman, B: *Mitogen and muscle extract induced in vitro proliferative responses in myasthenia gravis, dermatomyositis and polymyositis.* J Neurol Neurosurg Psychiatry 38:521–524, 1975.

Lobo-Antunes, J: *Behçet's disease.* Ann Intern Med 76:332–333, 1972.

Löffel, NB, Rossi, LN, Mumenthaler, M, et al: *The Landry-Guillain-Barré syndrome. Complications, prognosis and natural history in 23 cases.* J Neurol Sci 33:71–79, 1977.

Logothetis, J, Kennedy, WR, Ellington, A, et al: *Cryoglobulinemic neuropathy. Incidence and clinical characteristics.* Arch Neurol 19:389–397, 1968.

Low, PA, Schmelzer, JD and Dyck, PJ: *Results of endoneurial injection of Guillain-Barré serum in Lewis rats.* Mayo Clin Proc 57:360–364, 1982.

Lubetzki Korn, I and Abramsky, O: *Myasthenia gravis following viral infection.* Eur Neurol 20:435–439, 1981.

Luijten, JAFM and Baart de la Faille-Kuyper, EH: *The occurrence of IgM and complement factors along the myelin sheaths of peripheral nerves: An immunochemical study of the Guillain-Barré syndrome.* J Neurol Sci 15:219–224, 1972.

Lundberg, PO and Werner, I: *Trigeminal sensory neuropathy in SLE.* Acta Neurol Scand 48:330–340, 1972.

Mäkelä, A-L, Lang, H and Sillanpää, M: *Neurological manifestations of rheumatoid arthritis.* In Vinken, PJ and Bruyn, GW (eds): *Handbook of Clinical Neurology, vol. 38.* North-Holland Publishing, Amsterdam, 1979, pp 479–503.

Malaviya, AN, Many, A and Schwartz, RS: *Treatment of dermatomyositis with methotrexate.* Lancet ii:485–488, 1968.

Mamoli, B, Neumann, H and Ehrmann, L: *Recurrent Bell's palsy. Etiology, frequency, prognosis.* J Neurol 216:119–125, 1977.

Manson, JI and Thong, YH: *Immunological abnormalities in the syndrome of poliomyelitis-like illness associated with acute bronchial asthma (Hopkins' syndrome).* Arch Dis Child 55:26–32, 1980.

Mark, B, Hurwitz, BJ, Olanow, CW, et al: *Plasmapheresis in idiopathic inflammatory polyradiculoneuropathy.* Neurology 30:361, 1980.

Markenson, JA, McDougal, JS, Tsairis, P, et al: *Rheumatoid meningitis: A localized immune process.* Ann Intern Med 90:786–789, 1979.

Marks, JS and Halpin, TJ: *Guillain-Barré syndrome in recipients of A/New Jersey influenza vaccine.* JAMA 243:2490–2494, 1980.

Martin, WA and Kraft, GH: *Shoulder girdle neuritis: A clinical and electrophysiological evaluation.* Military Med 139:21–25, 1974.

Mathew, NT and Chandy, J: *Painful ophthalmoplegia.* J Neurol Sci 11:243–256, 1970.

Matthews, WB: *Neurosarcoidosis.* In Vinken, PJ and Bruyn, GW (eds): *Handbook of Clinical Neurology, vol. 38.* North-Holland Publishing, Amsterdam, 1979, pp 521–542.

McFarlin, DE and Griggs, RC: *Treatment of inflammatory myopathies with azathioprine.* Trans Am Neurol Assoc 93:244–246, 1968.

McLeod, JG: *Electrophysiological studies in the Guillain-Barré syndrome.* Ann Neurol 9(suppl):20–27, 1981.

McLeod, JG and Walsh, JC: *Neuropathies associated with paraproteinemias and dysproteinemias.* In Dyck, PJ, Thomas, PK and Lambert, EH (eds): *Peripheral Neuropathy.* WB Saunders, Philadelphia, 1975, pp 1012–1029.

McLeod, JG, Walsh, JC, Prineas, JW, et al: *Acute idiopathic polyneuritis. A clinical and electrophysiologic follow-up study.* J Neurol Sci 22:145–162, 1976.

McQuillen, MP: *Idiopathic polyneuritis—Serial studies of nerve and immune functions.* J Neurol Neurosurg Psychiatry 34:607–615, 1971.

Medsger, TA, Dawson, WN, Jr and Masi, AT: *The epidemiology of polymyositis.* Am J Med 48:715–723, 1970.

Metzger, AL, Bohan, A, Goldberg, LS, et al: *Polymyositis and dermatomyositis: Combined methotrexate and corticosteroid therapy.* Ann Intern Med 81:182–189, 1974.

Michet, CJ, Doyle, JA and Ginsburg, WW: *Eosinophilic fasciitis. Report of 15 cases.* Mayo Clin Proc 56:27–34, 1981.

Mihas, AA, Kirby, JD and Kent, SP: *Hepatitis B antigen and polymyositis.* JAMA 239:221–222, 1978.

Mikol, J, Felton-Papaiconomou, A, Ferchal, F, et al: *Inclusion-body myositis: Clinicopathological studies and isolation of an adenovirus type 2 from muscle biopsy specimen.* Ann Neurol 11:576–581, 1982.

Milde, E-J, Aarli, J and Larsen, JC: *Cauda equina lesions in ankylosing spondylitis.* Scand J Rheumatol 6:118–122, 1977.

Miyoshi, T and Oh, SJ: *Proximal slowing of nerve conduction in the Guillain-Barré syndrome.* Electromyogr Clin Neurophysiol 17:287–296, 1977.

Moore, PM and Fauci, AS: *Neurologic manifestations of systemic vasculitis. A retrospective and prospective study of the clinicopathologic features and response to therapy in 25 patients.* Am J Med 71:517–524, 1981.

Morgan, DJR and Gawler, J: *Severe peripheral neuropathy complicating legionnaire's disease.* Br Med J 283:1577–1578, 1981.

Moutsopoulos, HM, Webber, BL, Pavlidis, NA, et al: *Diffuse fasciitis with eosinophilia. A clinicopathologic study.* Am J Med 68:701–709, 1980.

Munsat, TL, Piper, D, Cancilla, P, et al: *Inflammatory myopathy with facioscapulohumeral distribution.* Neurology 22:335–347, 1972.

Nakano, KK: *The entrapment neuropathies of rheumatoid arthritis.* Orthop Clin North Am 6:837–860, 1975.

Nemni, R, Galassi, G, Latov, N, et al: *Peripheral neuropathy and plasma-cell dyscrasia: The range of pathological findings in peripheral nerve.* Neurology 31(2):155, 1981.

Newsom-Davis, J: *Diaphragm function and alveolar hypoventilation.* Q J Med 45:87–100, 1976.

Nyland, H and Aarli, JA: *Guillain-Barré syndrome: Demonstration of antibodies to peripheral nerve tissue.* Acta Neurol Scand 58:35–43, 1978.

Nyland, H, Matre, R and Mørk, S: *Immunological characterization of sural nerve biopsies from patients with Guillain-Barré syndrome.* Ann Neurol 9(suppl): 80–86, 1981.

O'DUFFY, JD, CARVEY, JA AND DEODHAR, S: *Behçet's disease. Report of 20 cases, 3 with new manifestations.* Ann Intern Med 75:561–570, 1971.

O'DUFFY, JD, HUNDER, GG AND WAHNER, HW: *A follow-up study of polymyalgia rheumatica: Evidence of chronic axial synovitis.* J Rheumatol 7:685–693, 1980.

O'DUFFY, JD, WAHNER, HW AND HUNDER, GG: *Joint imaging in polymyalgia rheumatica.* Mayo Clin Proc 51:519–524, 1976.

OH, SJ: *Subacute demyelinating polyneuropathy responding to corticosteroid treatment.* Arch Neurol 35:509–516, 1978.

PACHMAN, LM AND COOKE, N: *Juvenile dermatomyositis: A clinical and immunologic study.* J Pediatr 96:226–234, 1980.

PALLIS, CA AND SCOTT, JT: *Peripheral neuropathy in rheumatoid arthritis.* Br Med J 1:1141–1147, 1965.

PARILLO, JE, FAUCI, AS AND WOLFF, SM: *Therapy of the hypereosinophilic syndrome.* Ann Intern Med 89:167–172, 1978.

PARRY, GJ, BROWN, MJ AND ASBURY, AK: *Diagnostic value of nerve biopsy in mononeuritis multiplex.* Neurology 31(2):129–130, 1981.

PARSONAGE, MJ AND TURNER, JWA: *Neuralgic amyotrophy: The shoulder-girdle syndrome.* Lancet i:973–978, 1948.

PATTON, WF AND LYNCH, JP: *Lymphomatoid granulomatosis. Clinicopathologic study of four cases and literature review.* Medicine 61:1–12, 1982.

PENNER, E, MAIDA, E, MAMOLI, B, ET AL: *Serum and cerebrospinal fluid immune complexes containing hepatitis B surface antigen in Guillain-Barré syndrome.* Gastroenterology 82:576–580, 1982.

PEPOSE, JS: *A theory of virus-induced demyelination in the Landry-Guillain-Barré syndrome.* J Neurol 227:93–97, 1982.

PHILIPSZOON, AJ: *Nystagmus and Bell's palsy.* Pract Otorhinolaryngol (Basel) 24:233, 1962.

PHILLIPS, TM, QUENN, W, BALLANTI, J, ET AL: *Cross-reactive antibodies to influenza vaccine and peripheral nerve in Guillain-Barré syndrome (GBS).* Neurology 31(2):154, 1981.

PRINEAS, JW: *Polyneuropathies of undetermined cause.* Acta Neurol Scand (Suppl 44) 46:1–72, 1970.

PRINEAS, JW: *Pathology of the Guillain-Barré syndrome.* Ann Neurol 9(Suppl):6–19, 1981.

PRINEAS, JW AND MCLEOD, JG: *Chronic relapsing polyneuritis.* J Neurol Sci 27:427–458, 1976.

PROCTOR, B, CORGILL, DA AND PROUD, G: *The pathology of Bell's palsy.* Trans Am Acad Ophthalmol Otolaryngol 82:ORL-70–ORL-80, 1976.

PRUZANSKI, W AND KATZ, A: *Clinical and laboratory findings in primary generalized and multiple-myeloma-related amyloidosis.* Can Med Assoc J 114:906–909, 1976.

QUAST, U, HENNESSEN, W AND WIDMARK, RM: *Mono- and polyneuritis after tetanus vaccination (1970–1977).* Dev Biol Stand 43:25–32, 1979.

READ, DJ, VANHEGAN, RI AND MATTHEWS, WB: *Peripheral neuropathy and benign IgG paraproteinemia.* J Neurol Neurosurg Psychiatry 41:215–219, 1978.

READ, D AND WARLOW, C: *Peripheral neuropathy and solitary plasmacytoma.* J Neurol Neurosurg Psychiatry 41:177–184, 1978.

REIK, L, STURE, AC, BARTENHAGEN, NH, ET AL: *Neurologic abnormalities of Lyme disease.* Medicine 58:281–294, 1979.

RINGEL, SP AND CLAMAN, HN: *Amyloid-associated muscle pseudohypertrophy.* Arch Neurol 39:413–417, 1982.

RINGEL, SP, FORSTOT, JZ, TAN, EM, ET AL: *Sjögren's syndrome and polymyositis or dermatomyositis.* Arch Neurol 39:157–163, 1982.

RINGEL, SP, THORNE, EG, PHANUPHAK, P, ET AL: *Immune complex vasculitis,polymyositis, and hyperglobulinemic purpura.* Neurology 29:682–689, 1979.

ROPES, MW: *Systemic Lupus Erythematosus.* Harvard University Press, Cambridge, MA, 1976.

ROPPER, AH, SHAHANI, B AND HUGGINS, CE: *Improvement in 4 patients with acute Guillain-Barré syndrome after plasma exchange.* Neurology 30:361, 1980.

ROSENBERG, R AND GREENBERG, J: *Linear scleroderma as a cause for hemiatrophy.* Ann Neurol 5:307, 1979.

ROTHSTEIN, TL, CARLSON, CB AND SUMI, SM: *Polymyositis with facioscapulohumeral distribution.* Arch Neurol 25:313–319, 1971.

ROWLAND, LP, DEFENDINI, R, SHERMAN, W, ET AL: *Macroglobulinemia with peripheral neuropathy simulating motor neuron disease.* Ann Neurol 11:532–536, 1982.

RUMPL, E, MAYR, U, GERSTENBRAND, F, ET AL: *Treatment of Guillain-Barré syndrome by plasma exchange.* J Neurol 225:207–217, 1981.

SAFMAN, BL: *Bilateral pathology in Bell's palsy.* Arch Otolaryngol 93:55–57, 1971.

SAIDA, T, SAIDA, K, LISAK, RP, ET AL: In vivo *demyelinating activity of sera from patients with Guillain-Barré syndrome.* Ann Neurol 11:69–75, 1982.

SALMERON, G, GREENBERG, D AND LIDSKY, MD: *Polymyositis and diffuse interstitial lung disease. A review of the pulmonary histopathologic findings.* Arch Intern Med 141:1005–1010, 1981.

SANDER, JE AND SHARP, FR: *Lumbosacral plexus neuritis.* Neurology 31:470–473, 1981.

SCHEINBERG, L: *Polyneuritis in systemic lupus erythematosus. Revew of the literature and report of a case.* N Engl J Med 255:416–421, 1956.

SCHMID, FR, COOPER, NS, ZIFF, M, ET AL: *Arteritis in rheumatoid arthritis.* Am J Med 30:56–83, 1961.

SCHMITZ, H AND ENDERS, G: *Cytomegalovirus as a frequent cause of Guillain-Barré syndrome.* J Med Virol 1:21–27, 1977.

SCHOENBERGER, LB, HURWITZ, ES, KATONA, P, ET AL: *Guillain-Barré syndrome: Its epidemiology and associations with influenza vaccination.* Ann Neurol 9(Suppl):31–38, 1981.

SCHOTLAND, DL, WOLF, SM, WHITE, HH, ET AL: *Neurologic aspects of Behçet's disease. Case report and review of the literature.* Am J Med 34:544–553, 1963.

SCHUMACHER, HR, SCHIMMER, B, GORDON, GV, ET AL: *Articular manifestations of polymyositis and dermatomyositis.* Am J Med 67:287–292, 1979.

SCHWARTZ, MI, MATTHAY, RA, SAHN, SA, ET AL: *Interstitial lung disease in polymyositis and dermatomyositis: Analysis of six cases and review of the literature.* Medicine 55:89–104, 1976.

SCHWARTZ, RA, TEDESCO, AS, STERN, LZ, ET AL: *Myopathy associated with sclerodermal facial hemiatrophy.* Arch Neurol 38:592–594, 1981.

SCOTT, DGI, BACON, PA AND TRIBE, CR: *Systemic rheumatoid vasculitis: A clinical and laboratory study of 50 cases.* Medicine 60:288–297, 1981.

SEARLES, RP, MLADINICH, EK AND MESSNER, RP: *Isolated trigeminal sensory neuropathy: Early manifestation of mixed connective tissue disease.* Neurology 28:1286–1289, 1978.

SERRATRICE, G, PELLISIER, J-F, CROS, D, ET AL: *Relapsing eosinophilic perimyositis.* J Rheumatol 7:199–205, 1980.

SERVER, AC, LEFKOWITZ, J, BRAINE, H, ET AL: *Treatment of chronic relapsing inflammatory polyradiculoneuropathy by plasma exchange.* Ann Neurol 6:258–261, 1979.

SEWELL, HF, MATTHEWS, JB, GOOCH, E, ET AL: *Autoantibody to nerve tissue in a patient with a peripheral neuropathy and an IgG paraprotein.* J Clin Pathol 34:1163–1166, 1981.

SHAPIRO, GG, CHAPMAN, JT, PIERSON, WE, ET AL: *Poliomyelitis-like illness after acute asthma.* J Pediatr 94:767–768, 1979.

SHARP, GC, IRVIN, WS, TAN, EM, ET AL: *Mixed connective tissue disease—an apparently distinct rheumatic disease syndrome associated with a specific antibody to an extractable nuclear antigen (ENA).* Am J Med 52:148–159, 1972.

SHERMAN, WH, LATOV, N, HAYS, AP, ET AL: *Monoclonal IgM_k antibody precipitating with chondroitin sulfate C from patients with axonal polyneuropathy and epidermolysis.* Neurology 33:192–201, 1983.

SHERMAN, WH, OSSERMAN, EF, LATOV, N, ET AL: *Peripheral neuropathy, plasma cell dyscrasia, and hot blood.* Ann Neurol 12:3, 1982.

SILVERSTEIN, A AND SILTZBACH, LE: *Muscle involvement in sarcoidosis. Asymptomatic, myositis and myopathy.* Arch Neurol 21:235–241, 1969.

SINGSEN, BH, BERNSTEIN, HB, KORNREICH, HK, ET AL: *Mixed connective tissue disease in childhood. A clinical and serologic survey.* J Pediatr 90:893–900, 1977.

SINGSEN, B, GOLDREYER, B, STANTON, R, ET AL: *Childhood polymyositis with cardiac conduction defects.* Am J Dis Child 130:72–74, 1976.

SPECTOR, RH AND SCHWARTZMAN, RJ: *Benign trigeminal and facial neuropathy.* Arch Intern Med 135:992–993, 1975.

SPILLANE, JO AND WELLS, CEC: *The neurology of Jennerian vaccination.* Brain 87:1–44, 1964.

STARK, RJ: *Eosinophilic polymyositis.* Arch Neurol 36:721–722, 1979.

STECK, AJ, MURRAY, N, MEIER, C, ET AL: *Demyelinating neuropathy and monoclonal IgM antibody to myelin-associated glycoprotein.* Neurology 33:19–23, 1983.

STEELE, JC AND VASUVAT, A: *Recurrent multiple cranial nerve palsies: A distinctive syndrome of cranial polyneuropathy.* J Neurol Neurosurg Psychiatry 33:828–832, 1970.

STEVENS, JG, PEPOSE, JS AND COOK, ML: *Marek's disease: A natural model for the Landry-Guillain-Barré syndrome.* Ann Neurol 9(Suppl):102–106, 1981.

STEWART, GJ, POLLARD, JD, MCLEOD, JG, ET AL: *HLA antigens in the Landry-Guillain-Barré syndrome and chronic relapsing polyneuritis.* Ann Neurol 4:285–298, 1978.

SU, WP AND PERSON, JR: *Morphea profunda. A new concept and a histopathologic study of 23 cases.* Am J Dermatopath 3:251–260, 1981.

SUMNER, A, SAID, G, IDY, I, ET AL: *Syndrome de Guillain-Barré. Effets électrophysiologiques et morphologiques du sérum humain introduit dans l'espace endoneural du nerf sciatique du rat. Résultats préliminaire.* Rev Neurol 138:17–24, 1982.

SWIFT, TR, LESHNER, RT AND GROSS, JA: *Arm-diaphragm synkinesis: Electrodiagnostic studies of aberrant regeneration of phrenic motor neurons.* Neurology 30:339–344, 1980.

TAVERNER, D, COHEN, SB AND HUTCHINSON, BC: *Comparison of corticotrophin and prednisone in treatment of idiopathic facial paralysis (Bell's palsy).* Br Med J 4:20–22, 1971.

TAVERNER, D, KEMBLE, F AND COHEN, SB: *Prognosis and treatment of idiopathic facial (Bell's) palsy.* Br Med J 4:581–583, 1967.

TAY, CH AND KHOO, OT: *Neurological involvement in systemic lupus erythematosus.* Singapore Med J 12:18–23, 1971.

TAY, CH, TAN, YT, CHEAH, JS, ET AL: *Ocular palsies of obscure origin in South East Asia.* J Neurol Neurosurg Psychiatry 37:739–744, 1974.

TAYLOR, RA: *Heredofamilial mononeuritis multiplex with brachial predilection.* Brain 83:113–137, 1960.

TEASDALE, RD, FRAYHA, RA AND SHULMAN, LE: *Cranial nerve involvement in systemic sclerosis (scleroderma): A report of 10 cases.* Medicine 59:149–159, 1980.

TOVI, F, SIDI, J, HAIKIN, H, ET AL: *Viral infection and acute peripheral facial palsy. A study with herpes simplex and varicella zoster viruses.* Isr J Med Sci 16:576–580, 1980.

TROTTER, JL, ENGEL, WK AND IGNACZAK, TF: *Amyloidosis with plasma cell dyscrasia. An overlooked cause of adult onset sensorimotor neuropathy.* Arch Neurol 34:209–214, 1977.

TSAIRIS, P, DYCK, PJ AND MULDER, DW: *Natural history of brachial plexus neuropathy. Report on 99 patients.* Arch Neurol 27:109–117, 1972.

TSOKOS, GC, MOUTSOPOULOS, HM AND STEINBERG, AO: *Muscle involvement in systemic lupus erythematosus.* JAMA 246:766–768, 1981.

TUFFANELLI, DL AND WINKELMANN, RK: *Systemic scleroderma. A clinical study of 727 cases.* Arch Derm 84:359–371, 1961.

UTTLEY, WS, BELTON, NR, SYME, J, ET AL: *Calcium balance in children treated with diphosphonates.* Arch Dis Child 50:187–190, 1975.

VALENSTEIN, E, WATSON, RT AND PARKER, JL: *Myokymia, muscle hypertrophy and percussion "myotonia" in chronic recurrent polyneuropathy.* Neurology 28:1130–1134, 1978.

VENABLES, GS, BATES, D, CARTLIDGE, NEF, ET AL: *Acute polymyositis with subcutaneous edema.* J Neurol Sci 55:161–164, 1982.

WAKSMAN, BH AND ADAMS, RD: *Allergic neuritis: Experimental disease of rabbits induced by the injection of peripheral nervous tissue and adjuvants.* J Exp Med 102:213–235, 1955.

WALLACE, SL, LATTES, R, MALIA, JP, ET AL: *Muscle involvement in Boeck's sarcoid.* Ann Intern Med 48:497–511, 1958.

WALSH, JC: *The neuropathy of multiple myeloma. An electrophysiological and histological study.* Arch Neurol 25:404–414, 1971.

WEES, SJ, SUNWOO, IN AND OH, SJ: *Sural nerve biopsy in systemic necrotizing vasculitis.* Am J Med 71:525–532, 1981.

WEST, SG, KILLIAN, PJ AND LAWLESS, OJ: *Association of myositis and myocarditis in progressive systemic sclerosis.* Arthritis Rheum 24:662–667, 1981.

WEXLER, I: *Serial sensory and motor conduction measurement in Guillain-Barré syndrome.* Electromyogr Clin Neurophysiol 20:87–103, 1980.

WHEELER, SD AND OCHOA, J: *Poliomyelitis-like syndrome associated with asthma. A case report and review of the literature.* Arch Neurol 37:52–53, 1980.

WHITAKER, JN AND ENGEL, WK: *Vascular deposits of immunoglobulin and complement in idiopathic inflammatory myopathy.* N Engl J Med 286:333–338, 1972.

WHITAKER, JN, HASHIMOTO, K AND QUINONES, M: *Skeletal muscle pseudohypertrophy in primary amyloidosis.* Neurology 27:47–54, 1977.

WHITAKER, JN, HOLLAND, PV, ALTER, HJ, ET AL: *Idiopathic inflammatory myopathy. Failure to detect hepatitis B antigen in serum and muscle.* Arch Neurol 28:410–411, 1973.

WHITFIELD, AGW: *Neurological complications of ankylosing spondylitis.* In VINKEN, PJ AND BRUYN, GW (EDS): *Handbook of Clinical Neurology, vol. 38.* North-Holland Publishing, Amsterdam, 1979, pp 505–520.

Wiederholt, WC and Siekert, RC: *Neurological manifestations of sarcoidosis.* Neurology 15:1147–1154, 1965.

Williams, RG: *Idiopathic recurrent laryngeal nerve paralysis.* J Laryngol 73:161–166, 1959.

Wilson, G and Hadden, SB: *Neuritis and multiple neuritis following serum therapy.* JAMA 98:123–125, 1932.

Winkelmann, RK, Mulder, DW, Lambert, EH, et al: *Dermatomyositis-polymyositis: Comparison of untreated and cortisone-treated patients.* Mayo Clin Proc 43:545–556, 1968.

Wolf, SM, Wagner, JH, Jr, Davison, S, et al: *Treatment of Bell palsy with prednisone: A prospective, randomized study.* Neurology 28:158–161, 1978.

Yates, DAH: *Muscular changes in rheumatoid arthritis.* Ann Rheum Dis 22:342–347, 1963.

Chapter 6

NEOPLASTIC DISEASES

DIRECT INVOLVEMENT OF NERVES AND MUSCLE BY CANCER

Metastasis to Muscle

Considering the abundant blood supply of skeletal muscle, and the fact that it constitutes approximately 40 percent of the body's weight, it is surprising that metastasis of cancer to muscle is seen so rarely in clinical practice. Pearson (1959), in a thorough search at autopsy, found muscle metastases in 6 of 38 patients (16 percent), though 3 of the patients had lymphosarcoma or leukemia, tumors that are especially likely to be widely disseminated. From that study it appears that tumors metastasize to skeletal muscle more frequently than clinical experience would suggest, but that subsequent growth of the tumor is discouraged. We do not know why the muscle environment is so inhospitable to metastatic cancer.

A few cases of symptomatic metastasis to muscle have been reported (Adams 1975), and a recent patient presented with masses of lymphomatoid granulomatosis in several different muscles (Schmalzl et al. 1982). Two patients with a subacute generalized myopathy were found to have diffuse infiltration of the muscles by metastatic carcinoma (Doshi and Fowler 1983). The muscles were not swollen; in fact, one patient actually had wasted muscles. The CPK was normal, and EMG showed myopathic abnormalities without irritable features. One of the patients, who had breast cancer, regained muscle strength following treatment with tamoxifen.

Compression and Invasion of Nerves

In order to focus treatment on the correct anatomic site, it is important to determine whether nerves are involved within the leptomeningeal space, at a dural or extradural location (within the skull or spine), or in the periphery. In each of these locations, the neurologic symptoms grow steadily and inexorably worse unless the tumor is successfully treated.

Leptomeningeal Metastasis

Diffuse infiltration of the leptomeninges by cancer produces a characteristic syndrome of headache, altered mentation, signs of meningeal irritation, and multiple deficits of the cranial and spinal nerves. The spinal nerve symptoms consist of radicular pain, focal muscle weakness and atrophy, fasciculation, sensory loss in a dermatomal distribution, and depressed reflexes. When the lumbosacral nerve roots are affected the signs are usually bilateral, asymmetric, and patchy; the muscle weakness has a radicular distribution, and straight leg-raising usually evokes radicular pain. Eventually control of the bladder and rectal sphincters is lost. Examination of the CSF usually reveals abnormalities such as raised pressure, an increased concentration of protein, a low concentration of glucose, or a lymphocytic pleocytosis, and in the majority of cases malignant cells can be identified in the CSF by cytologic examination, especially if several lumbar punctures are done (Olson et al. 1974). CSF levels of β-glucuronidase are often increased in patients with leptomeningeal carcinoma but not in those with meningeal lymphoma (Schold et al. 1980). Computed tomography may show obliteration of the basal cisterns and increased enhancement by contrast material of the leptomeninges and ventricular lining; in a recent series about half of 50 proven cases were positive by this technique (Ascherl et al. 1981).

The early stages of leptomeningeal metastasis may be much more difficult to verify. Focal deposits of tumor may involve a cranial or a spinal nerve root and the adjacent leptomeninges without producing any abnormality in the routine CSF analysis, though cytologic examinations have not been reported in this situation. After some time has elapsed, leptomeningeal metastases will usually spread to the cranial or spinal nerves, and the diagnosis will then be apparent. If the nerve signs remain localized in one region, a dural or a more peripheral metastasis should be suspected. In the series reported by Posner and his colleages (Olson et al. 1974), which did not include patients with leukemia or primary intracranial tumor, 90 percent of the cases of leptomeningeal cancer were caused by four tumors: breast carcinoma (36 percent), lymphoma (28 percent), lung carcinoma (16 percent), and melanoma (10 percent). There is no clinical difference in the neurologic manifestations produced by different tumors, except that lymphoma has a tendency to invade peripheral nerves as well as the meninges and nerve roots. Leptomeningeal spread occurs in only 2 percent of patients with Hodgkin's disease but occurs in more than 25 percent of patients with malignant lymphomas (diffuse histiocytic and undifferentiated types), probably spreading to the meninges from the bone marrow in most cases (Bunn 1976; Cairncross and Posner 1980). Meningeal lymphomatosis occasionally presents with a progressive or fluctuating cranial polyneuropathy, with little or no evidence of lymphoma elsewhere in the body. The CSF protein is elevated, but the cell count may be normal initially; such cases may be mistakenly diagnosed as idiopathic polyneuritis (Teoh et al. 1980).

Lymphomatoid granulomatosis is a disseminated granulomatosis in which necrotizing angiitis is combined with pathologic features of a lymphoreticular malignancy. The syndrome resembles Wegener's granulomatosis but shows a greater predilection for involvement of the lungs, skin, and nervous system (Israel et al. 1977; Patton and Lynch 1982). The brain, leptomeninges, cranial nerves, and peripheral nerves may be directly invaded by the lymphoreticular tissue, and ischemic strokes occur as a result of the necrotizing angiopathy (Calatayud et al. 1980). A distinctive feature of lymphomatoid granulomatosis is a peculiar leprosy-like picture, with scattered patches of numbness where the skin is infiltrated by the tumor (Garcia et al. 1978; Hogan et al. 1981). The disorder carries a high mortality rate and is particularly resistant to therapy (Patton and Lynch 1982).

At present the incidence of leptomeningeal involvement in patients with acute leukemia approximates 50 percent. This high incidence is a direct consequence of the success of modern chemotherapy, which prolongs survival but has only limited access to the CNS and meninges. In lymphoblastic leukemia, this complication occurs in 2 to 4 percent of patients per month; the incidence is lower in patients with myeloblastic leukemia. Both leukemic and lymphomatous leptomeningitis are apt to be associated with diffuse invasion of the peripheral nerves.

Radiation of the neuraxis, and intrathecal chemotherapy with methotrexate, frequently lead to gratifying remissions in patients with leukemia, less often in patients with lymphoma, and rarely in patients with other types of cancer. Apparent cure has been reported in rare instances (Olson et al. 1974; Cairncross and Posner 1980; Yuill 1980).

Dural and Extradural Involvement by Tumor

Distant metastasis to the dura is uncommon, occurring mainly with lymphoma and with carcinoma of the breast or prostate. The tumor may spread subdurally and infiltrate one or several adjacent nerve roots, but the clinical signs remain relatively focal and the CSF is usually normal. More often the tumor spreads to the dura from adjacent bone, compressing and infiltrating nerves of the extradural space, or enters the spine by spreading along nerve sheaths from a paravertebral focus.

SPINAL NERVE ROOTS. Compression of a spinal nerve root as a result of vertebral metastasis produces pain, weakness, atrophy, and sensory loss. There may be pain in the spine, local bone tenderness, and paraspinous muscle spasm, and motion of the spine may aggravate the local and radicular pains. The tumor may spread epidurally to adjacent nerve roots, or it may compress the spinal cord. Plain x-rays or tomography of the spine will usually disclose the bony metastasis; if these are negative, myelography may reveal an extradural mass.

CRANIAL NERVES. Greenberg and colleagues (1981) have recently outlined five anatomic syndromes related to metastatic involvement of cranial nerves at the base of the skull (Fig. 27). Breast carcinoma accounted for 40 percent of the cases, the remainder being due to carcinoma of the lung and prostate, head and neck tumors, lymphoma, and other malignancies. Metastasis to the *occipital condyle* causes a severe, constant headache in the occipital or temporal region, with weakness, atrophy, and fasciculation of one half of the tongue. Skull metastases near the *jugular foramen* cause headache behind the ear, hoarseness, dysphagia, and sometimes eleventh or twelfth cranial nerve symptoms. In the *middle fossa,* compression of the trigeminal ganglion causes numbness of the middle and lower face; facial pain is sometimes present, but the masticatory muscles are usually spared. The sixth, fourth, and third cranial nerves may also be involved. Metastasis to the *cavernous sinus* causes unrelenting pain and sensory loss in the eye and fore-

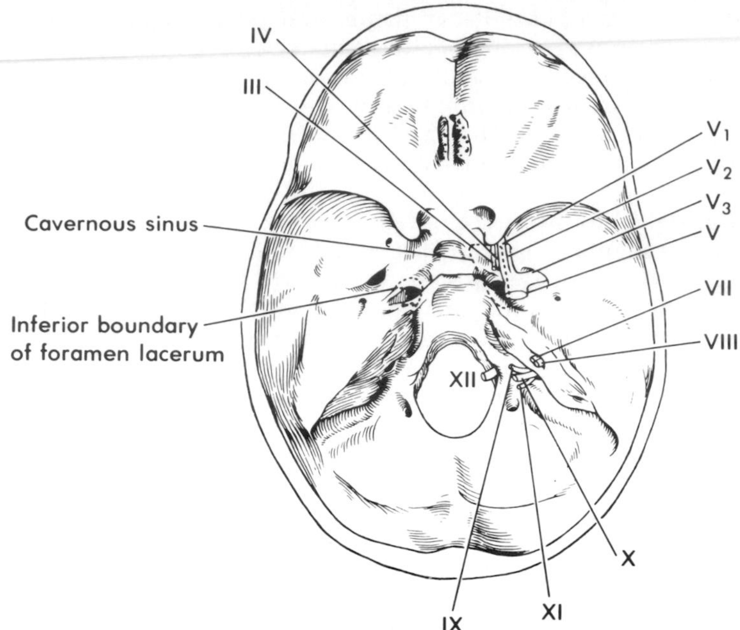

FIGURE 27. The floor of the cranial cavity, showing relation of cranial nerves to dura mater. Focal deposits of cancer in dura or bone may compress adjacent cranial nerves. The most common sites are the occipital condyle (twelfth nerve); the jugular foramen (ninth, tenth, and eleventh nerves); the middle fossa (second and third divisions of the fifth nerve); the cavernous sinus (third, fourth, and sixth nerves and first division of fifth nerve); and the orbit (third, fourth, and sixth nerves, first division of fifth nerve, and optic nerve).

head with progressive paralysis of the three ocular cranial nerves. *Orbital* metastasis produces proptosis and variable paralysis of the orbital muscles and nerves, depending on where the tumor is located, but the optic nerve is usually spared. Plain x-rays of the base of the skull are positive in 28 percent of these cases; computed tomography with bone windows is positive in 53 percent; and hypocycloidal tomography is positive in 74 percent (Greenberg et al. 1981). High-resolution computed tomography may now be the procedure of choice, however. If radiography is negative the CSF should be examined for evidence of leptomeningeal involvement; in the cavernous sinus syndrome carotid angiography and orbital phlebography may be revealing (Unsold et al. 1980). In patients with known cancer, radiation therapy can be given on the basis of the clinical diagnosis alone.

Tumors of the head and neck involve the cranial nerves by direct extension or by lymphatic spread. Carcinomas of the paranasal sinuses and plasmacytomas arising from the region of the sella turcica or the clivus extend upward into the extradural space to compress and invade various cranial nerves, especially those that traverse the cavernous sinus (Spaar 1980; Weisberger and Dedo 1977). The cranial nerve signs are usually unilateral. In this location the most frequent tumor is nasopharyngeal carcinoma, which involves cranial nerves in about half of the cases (Turgman et al. 1978). About 16 percent of patients with nasopharyngeal carcinoma present with neurologic symptoms; the diagnosis is often difficult to establish because there are no signs of nasopharyngeal tumor or cervical adenopathy. The reason is that carcinoma arising in the lateral nasopharyngeal wall (the fossa of Rosenmüller) tends to extend upward to the base of the skull, where it can pass directly through the foramen lacerum into the middle cranial fossa and cavernous sinus (Fig. 28). Here the fifth and sixth cranial nerves are likely to be involved, with pain and numbness of the face and diplopia; the third and fourth cranial nerves are also accessible. The lower cranial nerves are more likely to be involved extracranially, either by direct extension of the tumor or by metastasis to regional lymph nodes; cranial nerves 9 through 12 are usually compressed by nodes in the retroparotidean space, and the seventh nerve may be involved in the neck outside the stylomastoid foramen (Thomas and Waltz 1965). In the large majority of cases, the multiple cranial nerve signs are unilateral.

For the diagnosis of nasopharyngeal carcinoma, computed tomography efficiently demonstrates both the soft-tissue tumor mass and the bony destruction at the base of the skull (Carter 1980). However, at an early stage some tumors still escape detection, and blind biopsy of the retropharyngeal tissue has a low yield. Thus, it is sometimes necessary to wait and repeat the x-rays periodically. The CSF is normal except in rare instances when the tumor crosses the dura and invades the leptomeninges.

Invasion or Compression of Peripheral Nerves

The peripheral nerves can be compressed or infiltrated by cancer in several ways: (1) by direct extension of a primary tumor; (2) via lymph node metastasis of a carcinoma or sarcoma, or a lymph node focus of lymphoma; (3) within bony canals or foramina, from bone metastases or infiltrated bone marrow; and (4) rarely, by diffuse infiltration, in patients with lymphoma, leukemia, and myeloma.

CRANIAL NERVES. Lymph node metastases of nasopharyngeal carcinoma can compress cranial nerves 9 through 12 in the region of the carotid sheath

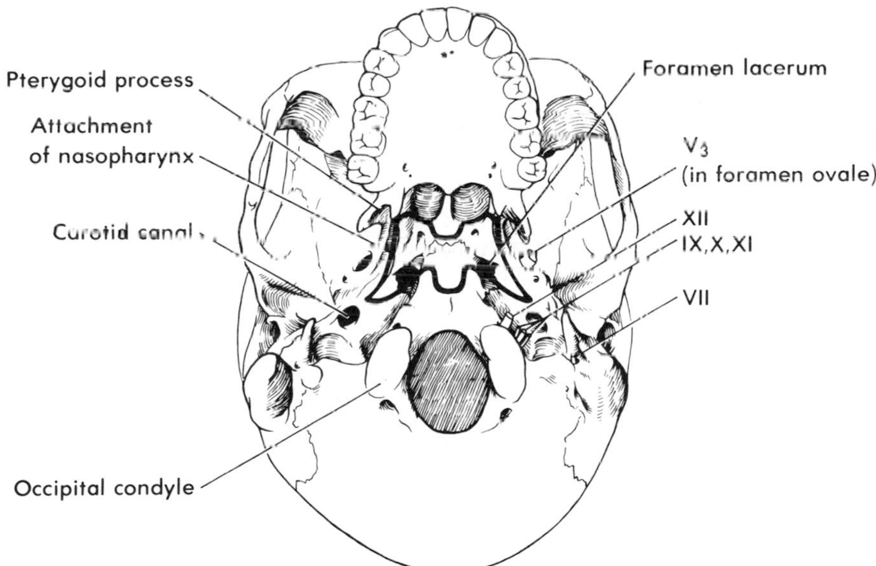

FIGURE 28. The base of the skull from below, showing the attachment of the nasopharynx (heavy solid line). At the apex of the fossa of Rosenmüller, or lateral pharyngeal recess, lies the foramen lacerum, which is covered by a fibrocartilaginous membrane. Nasopharyngeal carcinoma can penetrate this membrane to enter the cavernous sinus or middle fossa, compressing the third, fourth, fifth, and sixth cranial nerves. (See also Figure 27.)

underneath the parotid gland, and involve the seventh nerve near the stylomastoid foramen. Carcinoma of the paranasal sinuses is prone to involve supraorbital or infraorbital sensory branches of the trigeminal nerve. Squamous or basal cell carcinomas of the face or oral mucosa have a tendency to invade branches of the trigeminal and facial nerves, and to spread within nerve sheaths to distant sites, even to the brain (Dodd et al. 1970). Parotid gland tumors may present with facial weakness, and submandibular and sublingual salivary gland tumors may invade the lingual branch of the trigeminal nerve and the hypoglossal nerve. Rhabdomyosarcoma of the tongue may present with unilateral or bilateral paralysis and atrophy of the tongue. The initial manifestation of aggressive thyroid cancer may be hoarseness caused by invasion of the nearby recurrent laryngeal nerve. More often this nerve is compressed by tumor-filled lymph nodes in the mediastinum, where the phrenic nerve is also vulnerable. These two nerves, as well as the spinal accessory nerve, can also be compressed by lymph nodes in the neck. Patients with bone marrow involvement by histiocytic or undifferentiated lymphoma may present with facial numbness or weakness caused by involvement of cranial nerves within bony canals or foramina of the face (Cairncross and Posner 1980; Nobler 1969).

SPINAL NERVES. In certain locations, tumor masses can produce a distinctive anatomic syndrome by involving a group of adjacent peripheral nerves. The most important locations are the paravertebral gutter, the brachial plexus, and the lumbosacral plexus. Because the tumor is often difficult to demonstrate in these locations, diagnosis and treatment are frequently delayed for a long time while the patient suffers increasing and unremitting pain.

Paravertebral Tumor. This usually arises from lymph nodes involved by lymphoma or by lymphatic spread of cancer of the lung, digestive tract, or pelvic organs. The tumor then spreads longitudinally in the "gutter," invading the intercostal and sympathetic nerves and giving rise to segmental, unilateral pain and numbness, excessive or deficient sweating, and increased redness and warmth of the skin. At the lower thoracic levels one sees abdominal muscle weakness and loss of the abdominal reflexes, while at the lumbar level leg weakness occurs.

When cancer arises near the pleural surface at the apex of the lung, it may grow outward and posteriorly into the paravertebral space and posterior chest wall. The resulting symptoms are referred to as the *Pancoast syndrome* (Pancoast 1932; Hepper et al. 1966; Paulson 1975 and 1979).*

It is important to recognize this syndrome, because early treatment gives a much higher rate of cure than is possible in other types of lung cancer. The neurologic symptoms result from direct invasion of the extraspinal nerve roots, from C-8 to T-3, and of the sympathetic chain and stellate ganglion that overlie the costovertebral joints (Fig. 29). The tumor also invades the necks of the first three ribs and the transverse processes and bodies of C-7 through T-3 vertebrae; eventually it may even invade the spinal canal, compressing the spinal cord. However, the tumor is often a

---

*It is a common misconception that this syndrome refers to involvement of the brachial plexus in the supraclavicular space by upward extension of carcinoma of the lung apex. Actually, the Pancoast or superior sulcus tumor involves the extraspinal nerve roots in the paravertebral gutter, proximal to the brachial plexus.

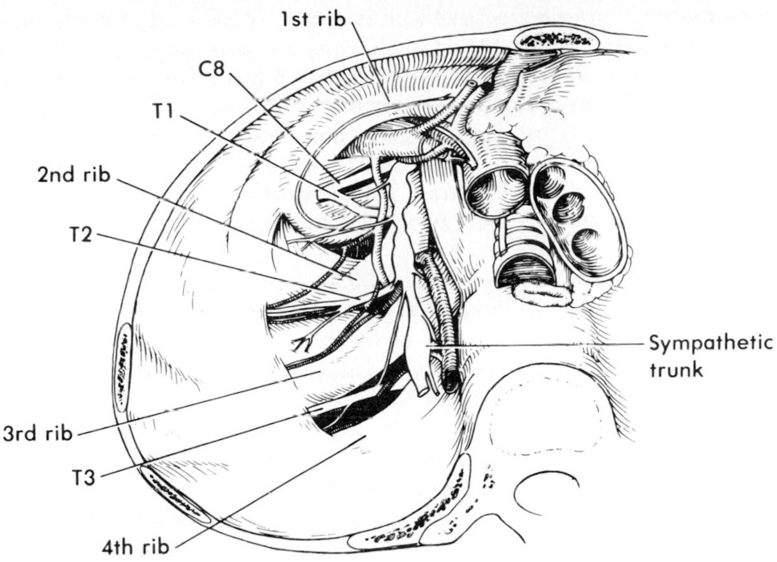

FIGURE 29. Apex of the right thoracic cavity, seen from below. The Pancoast tumor, arising in the apex of the lung near the pleural surface, extends posteriorly toward the costovertebral joints, invading the sympathetic chain and the paravertebral nerves from C-8 to T-3.

low-grade epidermoid carcinoma that grows slowly and metastasizes late, so that cure is possible even after the chest wall and spine have been invaded.

The sterotyped clinical picture begins with aching pain in the shoulder, followed by pain in the upper anterior chest and medial scapular border. Over a period of weeks or months, localizing neurologic symptoms appear: (1) pain and numbness down the inner aspect of the arm, forearm, and hand, owing to involvement of the sensory portions of T-1 and C-8 extraspinal nerve roots; (2) weakness and wasting of the intrinsic hand muscles (motor portions of C-8 and T-1); and (3) sympathetic hypoactivity (warm, dry arm and Horner's syndrome), caused by involvement of the sympathetic chain derived from the T-1 and T-2 nerve roots. There may be spasm of the upper paravertebral and suprascapular muscles, and abduction of the arm is likely to elicit radiating pain and paresthesias in a C-8, T-1 distribution. Most patients do not have pulmonary symptoms, venous distension, paralysis of the phrenic or recurrent laryngeal nerves, or involvement of the scalene nodes.

Once the physician has grasped the anatomic significance of the signs and symptoms, diagnostic studies should be pursued doggedly. Plain chest x-rays may show an obvious apical tumor, but in up to 40 percent of cases x-rays show only apical pleural thickening, which may even be present on old radiographs; the tumor tends to be plaque-like and is thought to arise in areas of old subpleural scarring. Computed tomography and radionuclide bone scan will demonstrate the tumor in almost every case if the radiologist directs his attention to the correct anatomic area. A soft-tissue mass between the lung and the bony structures is especially well seen by computed tomography. Bronchoscopy and sputum cytology are not usually helpful.

Paulson (1975, 1979) has obtained good results with a radical surgical approach to treatment. Mediastinoscopy is performed to detect mediastinal lymph node metastases, and palpable scalene nodes are biopsied. About two thirds of patients are free of overt metastasis; these patients are offered a two-stage approach to curative treatment, consisting of preoperative radiation (3000 rads over 12 days), followed in 3 to 4 weeks by en block resection of the posterior chest wall and superior lobe of the lung. The 5-year survival rate is over 40 percent, and most of the survivors are cured. When complete resection is not possible, palliative radiation (Attar et al. 1979) and neurosurgical procedures (Batzdorf and Brechner 1979) have been used, but unfortunately the pain is often very hard to control.

Tumor in the Brachial Plexus. The brachial plexus becomes involved by cancer when metastases to the axillary or cervical lymph nodes compress or infiltrate nerves in the neck, axilla, or upper arm. The pattern of neurologic signs and symptoms depends on the location of the involved nodes. For patients with carcinoma of the breast, the most frequent avenue into the plexus is via the axillary nodes, which lie adjacent to the axillary vein along the anteromedial aspect of the brachial plexus, at the level of the medial cord and the medial cutaneous nerves of the arm and forearm (Fig. 30). Pain, dysesthesia, and sensory loss thus tend to be located initially along the medial aspect of the arm, forearm, or hand, and weakness affects the intrinsic hand muscles first, as in the Pancoast syndrome. The ocular sympathetic nerves are not involved, however, and pain does not radiate into the paravertebral and suprascapular areas. The median and ulnar nerves can also be involved directly in the distal plexus, but the musculocutaneous and radial nerves are usually spared. Metastatic cancer in the deep cervical nodes at the root of the neck involves the upper brachial plexus at the level of the nerve trunks or roots, and in this location the cervical sympathetic chain may be involved. Primary or metastatic cancer in the apex of the lung can spread to either the axillary or the deep cervical lymph nodes.

Once tumor invades the plexus it can spread proximally along the nerves, through the neural foramina, and into the spinal canal, where it can extend longitudinally to involve other nerve roots in the epidural space. These vagaries can foil attempts at precise localization, even when undertaken by experienced examiners.

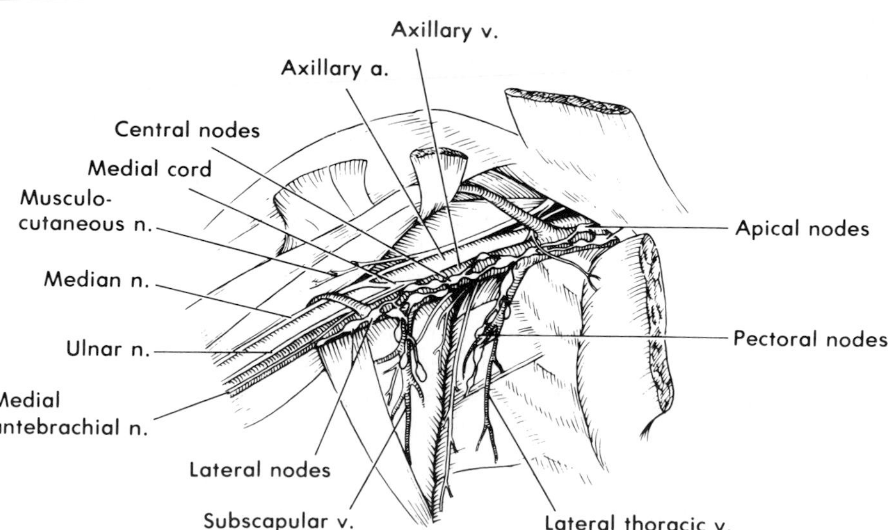

FIGURE 30. Relation of axillary lymph nodes to the brachial plexus. Lymphatic spread of breast carcinoma tends to involve the medial cord of the plexus and the proximal portions of the ulnar and median nerves.

Recently Kori and colleagues (1981) reviewed their experience with 78 cases of cancer in the brachial plexus: 70 percent of the cases were due to carcinoma of the lung or breast, in about equal proportion; 8 percent were caused by lymphoma; and the remaining cases were contributed by eight other forms of cancer, the majority of which had metastasized to the upper lobe of the lung before spreading to the plexus. They found that 80 percent of the patients presented with pain in the shoulder and arm, 54 percent had a Horner's syndrome, and 75 percent had neurologic signs of a lesion of the lower trunk or of the C-8 and T-1 nerve roots. (It is not clear whether patients with the Pancoast syndrome were included in the series; myelography showed epidural spread of tumor in 25 patients, 19 of whom had lung cancer, and in these cases the tumor may have extended directly from the lung to the paravertebral area.)

Brachial plexus metastases can turn up many years after treatment of the original cancer; this is especially true of breast cancer, in which the latent period can be as long as 16 years (Thomas and Colby 1972). For patients who received radiation treatment in the supraclavicular area, the principal diagnostic problem is to distinguish metastatic involvement from radiation-induced neuropathy. This topic is discussed fully in Chapter 10, but it should be mentioned here that Kori and colleagues (1981) found only two instances of radiation neuropathy in a consecutive series of 45 cancer patients with brachial plexus neuropathy, although nearly half of the patients had received radiotherapy. Thus, the great majority of cancer patients who develop progressive brachial plexus neuropathy will be found to have metastatic disease. Surgical exploration and biopsy is the accepted method of confirming the diagnosis, but confirmation is not required unless the diagnosis is in doubt. Moreover, surgical exploration is negative in about one fifth of the cases (Kori et al. 1981). If the clinical diagnosis is secure, palliative radiation therapy may be given without pathologic confirmation. This treatment provides at least temporary relief of pain in most patients with breast cancer (Nisce and Chu 1968) but is less effective in other types of cancer.

Tumor in the Lumbosacral Plexus. Tumors of the pelvic organs spread by direct extension or via lymph channels to involve the pelvic and lower abdominal nerves. Carcinomas of the cervix, prostate, bladder, and rectum spread to the internal and external iliac lymph node chains. In the former location, tumor may invade the sacral plexus, including the nerves to the gluteal muscles, the sciatic nerve, and the posterior cutaneous nerve of the thigh; in the latter situation the tumor is more anteriorly placed on the lateral wall and brim of the pelvis, where it can involve the obturator nerve, the psoas muscle, and the adjacent femoral and genitofemoral nerves (Fig. 31). Tumors of the testis and ovary follow lymph channels to the lower aortic lymph nodes, where they may contact the lower lumbar nerve roots. Ovarian carcinoma may also extend directly into the subjacent obturator nerve or may seed the peritoneal cavity to involve nerves in the iliac fossa. Sometimes the picture of retroperitoneal fibrosis is produced by infiltrating carcinomas and lymphomas. Surgical biopsies may initially be negative for tumor, an ambiguous finding since idiopathic retroperitoneal fibrosis can also cause plexopathy (Thomas and Chisholm 1973; McKinney 1973).

Late recurrences of carcinoma of the rectum (especially squamous cell carcinoma) may present with unilateral invasion of the sacral plexus and the obturator nerve, offering a diagnostic problem similar to that of late recurrence of breast carcinoma in the brachial plexus. Many years after an abdominal-perineal resection, the patient experiences a constant, deep pain

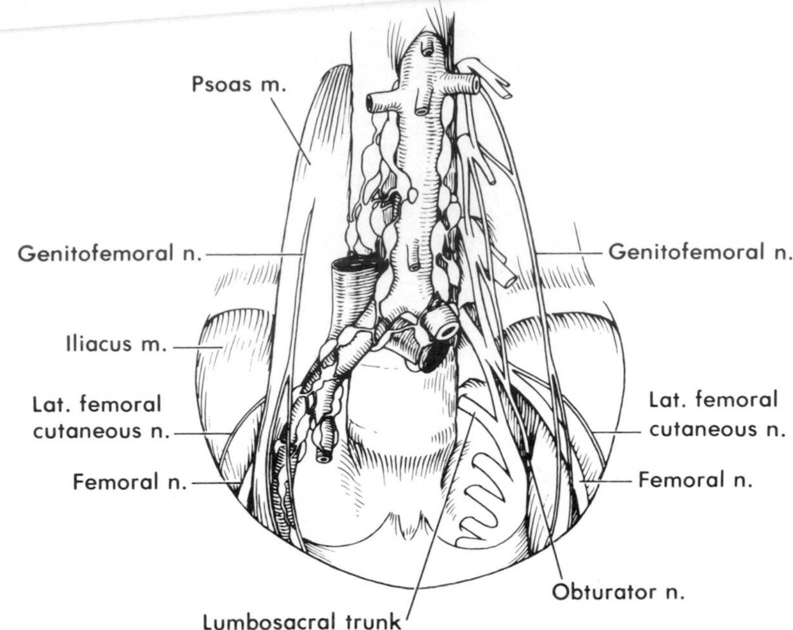

FIGURE 31. Relation of abdominal and pelvic lymph nodes to the lumbar and sacral nerve plexuses.

in the hip and posterolateral thigh, increasing instability of the hip, and wasting of the gluteal muscles. Surgical exploration may be negative or may show only retroperitoneal fibrosis. Radiography and bone scan eventually reveal destruction of bone in the lateral or posterior wall of the pelvis. In such cases it is reasonable to give radiation treatment before reaching a definitive diagnosis, in the hope of controlling the relentless pain and progressive paralysis.

Lymphoma arising in the lower aortic nodes may compress or infiltrate the lower lumbar nerve roots; in the iliac nodes along the pelvic brim, lymphoma may invade the femoral or obturator nerves. Retroperitoneal sarcoma is also likely to compress or invade portions of the lumbar and sacral plexuses.

Tumor in the Mediastinum and Root of the Neck. In these locations the recurrent laryngeal nerves and phrenic nerves are subject to encroachment by a primary tumor or by lymph nodes enlarged by cancer. The right recurrent laryngeal nerve, which loops around the subclavian artery at the apex of the lung, is less vulnerable within the mediastinum than the left, which loops around the arch of the aorta adjacent to the carinal lymph nodes (Fig. 32). The left recurrent laryngeal nerve is paralyzed twice as often as the right, usually by bronchial carcinoma of the left lung metastatic to the carinal nodes (Ballenger 1977). The right recurrent laryngeal nerve is sometimes involved by spread of a Pancoast tumor into the apex of the superior sulcus, and either nerve can be compressed by lymph node masses at the root of the neck. The left phrenic, vagus, and recurrent laryngeal nerves pass close to each other on the anterior aspect of the aortic arch, while the right phrenic nerve lies about 1 cm away from the recurrent laryngeal nerve adjacent to the subclavian artery. Consequently, combined paralysis of the left phrenic and recurrent laryngeal nerves probably indicates a

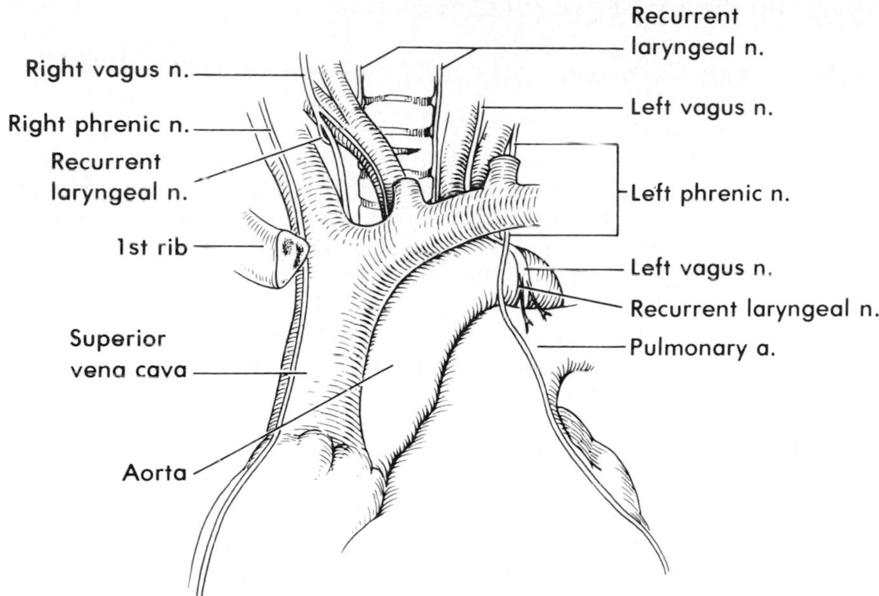

FIGURE 32. Root of the neck and superior mediastinum. On the left side, the recurrent laryngeal nerve is frequently involved by metastases in the carinal lymph nodes. The left phrenic nerve may also be involved as it crosses the aorta near the vagus and recurrent laryngeal nerves. On the right side, the phrenic, vagus, and recurrent laryngeal nerves are near each other in the root of the neck.

lesion in the mediastinum, while on the right side this combination suggests a lesion at the root of the neck.

Diffuse Invasion of the Peripheral Nerves

Direct infiltration of the peripheral nerves has been recorded in cases of multiple myeloma, leukemia, myeloid metaplasia, and lymphoma (Barron et al. 1960; Spaar 1980; Cairncross and Posner 1980; Yuill 1980). In some cases the path of entry is probably the vasa nervorum, since the nerves show multiple foci of perivascular infiltration. In other cases the tumor may have seeded the leptomeninges and spread centrifugally or may have invaded the nerves from adjacent sites of bony or soft tissue infiltration. Within the nerves the tumor spreads longitudinally in the perinourium and interfascicular connective tissue, producing focal degeneration of myelin and axons.

While these pathologic features are well established, their clinical counterpart has received little mention. Barron and associates (1960) claimed that some patients presented with a picture of symmetric polyneuropathy, but in their report the neurologic findings were poorly documented, so it is possible that these were multiple neuropathies that resembled polyneuropathies in the advanced stage of disease. If the nerve infiltration is entirely peripheral, the CSF would be normal and nerve conduction tests might show slowed conduction velocities compatible with the myelin degeneration observed pathologically, but this has not been reported. Although thorough microscopic examination of the peripheral nervous system has not often been undertaken in autopsies of patients with reticulosis and polyneuropathy, it appears that direct infiltration of nerves is a rare cause of this syndrome compared with the paraneoplastic mechanisms described below.

REMOTE EFFECTS OF CANCER

Asthenia and Cachexia

Asthenia is one of the major symptoms of cancer. Present in nearly all patients with advanced malignancy, it is an early complaint in patients with certain types of cancer, especially carcinomas of lung and gastrointestinal tract. Easy fatigue and a disinclination for both mental and physical effort are the main attributes of this poorly understood disorder. Muscle strength, as tested clinically, remains normal, and there is no direct evidence that a biochemical disorder of muscle energy metabolism is responsible for this type of fatigue (Theologides 1982). Generalized weight loss with prominent muscle wasting (cachexia), another poorly understood remote effect of cancer, is discussed in Chapter 9.

Carcinomatous Neuromyopathy

An association between dermatomyositis and cancer was commented on by many authors in the early years of this century, but delineation of the other paraneoplastic syndromes began after 1950, when English neurologists described various neurologic disorders that Brain and Henson (1958) termed collectively "carcinomatous neuromyopathy." The central nervous system disorders resembled neuronal "system degenerations," while the motor unit disorders consisted of polyneuropathies and of cases of proximal weakness having features of both motor neuron degeneration and myopathy (Henson et al. 1954; Brain and Henson 1958). In the ensuing years, the application of modern diagnostic procedures helped to delineate a number of distinct neuromuscular disorders in patients with cancer, but some patients with proximal weakness show mixed features of both neurogenic and myopathic pathogenesis.

Croft and Wilkinson (1965) examined 1476 untreated patients with various types of carcinoma. Of these patients 103 (7 percent) had neurologic abnormalities that did not appear to be of metastatic origin, and of these 90 percent were disorders of the motor unit. The incidence of motor unit disorders was highest (14 percent) in patients with lung or ovarian carcinoma. The commonest abnormality, present in 72 patients, was proximal weakness and muscle wasting, with preservation of distal strength and depressed knee or ankle jerks. EMG, serum enzymes, and muscle biopsy findings were not reported.

There have been several subsequent surveys of the neuromuscular findings in patients with cancer, but the results have been contradictory, and none of the studies attempted to correlate electrophysiologic abnormalities with serum enzyme measurements, muscle histochemistry, or pathologic examination of nerves and spinal cord. Consequently, the nature of the neuromuscular disorder originally described by Brain and Henson remains uncertain. Trojaborg (1969) examined 55 consecutive patients with early lung carcinoma; three patients had clinical and electrophysiologic evidence of a sensorimotor polyneuropathy, and one patient had proximal weakness and atrophy, myopathic EMG abnormalities, and mild interstitial myositis on biopsy. Seventeen patients (31 percent) had asymptomatic EMG abnormalities consisting mainly of fibrillations in *distal* muscles. In contrast, Campbell and Paty (1974) found *proximal* weakness in 53 percent of 30 unselected patients with lung carcinoma; EMG showed myopathic abnormalities in proximal muscles often accompanied by fibrillations and fasciculations.

Nerve conduction was normal, but one patient had the Lambert-Eaton syndrome. These authors considered the "neuromyopathy" to be an expression of lower motor neuron disease.

Paul and colleagues (1978) surveyed 195 Indian patients with untreated cancer of many types, all of whom underwent neurologic examination and detailed electrophysiologic testing. Muscle weakness was a prominent symptom in only seven patients (3.6 percent), but on examination muscle weakness and wasting of nonmetastatic origin were judged to be present in 42 patients (22 percent). The muscle weakness, which was severe in 10 patients, was diffusely distributed in two thirds of the patients, while one third of the patients had mainly proximal weakness. Electrophysiologic testing revealed that the generalized muscle weakness and wasting was nearly always neurogenic in character; EMG showed denervation in 75 percent of those patients and myopathic abnormalities in only 3.6 percent, while nerve conduction abnormalities were present in 39 percent, suggesting that peripheral neuropathy was a significant cause. Among the patients with proximal weakness and wasting, myopathic EMG abnormalities (with or without fibrillations) were found in 72 percent, while the remainder had a neurogenic EMG. Among clinically normal patients, only 1.3 percent had myopathic EMG changes, but 17 percent had neurogenic EMG changes. There were no abnormalities of neuromuscular transmission in the entire group of patients. Of the 25 patients with lung cancer, 12 percent had proximal weakness and wasting and 27 percent had generalized weakness and wasting; 12 percent had a myopathic EMG, 14 percent had a neurogenic EMG, and 64 percent had nerve conduction abnormalities.

Finally, Lenman and colleagues (1981) compared 50 unselected patients with lung cancer with 50 unselected controls. On clinical examination there were no definite cases of nonmetastatic neuromuscular disease; EMG showed myopathic abnormalities in two patients (with fibrillations in one), and fibrillations or fasciculations were present in 13 patients. Serum CPK was slightly elevated in only 5 patients and motor and sensory nerve conduction tests showed mild abnormalities in only a few patients.

Thus, despite discrepancies, there does seem to be a distinct syndrome consisting of proximal muscle weakness and wasting, depressed reflexes, myopathic EMG abnormalities with frequent fibrillation and fasciculation, and normal or mildly elevated CPK levels, without a definite abnormality of motor nerve conduction or neuromuscular transmission. It is convenient to refer to this syndrome as "carcinomatous neuromyopathy" (Campbell and Paty 1974), altering the original, more general usage of the term (Brain and Henson 1958). The nature of this proximal muscular disorder remains uncertain, since pathologic data are lacking, but it seems to be more frequent than any of the better-characterized syndromes described below. It is probably not a myopathy, but it could be an unusual variety of motor neuronopathy in which loss of function in nerve terminals produces the EMG picture of "depleted" motor units, namely, the "myopathic" EMG. Morphologic abnormalities of the intramuscular motor nerves have been observed by electron microscopy (Barron and Heffner 1978).

Disorders of Muscle

Dermatomyositis

Several retrospective studies since 1916 have disclosed a high incidence of cancer in older patients with dermatomyositis (Rowland and Schotland

1965). In one study, more than half of dermatomyositis patients over the age of 40 had known or occult cancer (Arundell et al. 1960). Nevertheless, some authors have recently argued that the relation between cancer and dermatomyositis has been greatly exaggerated, if it exists at all (Bohan et al. 1977). Furthermore, the specific association of cancer with dermatomyositis (rather than polymyositis) has been questioned, perhaps because polymyositis has been confused with the poorly understood "neuromyopathy" syndrome discussed above.

There are no prospective data on the incidence of cancer in myositis, but recent retrospective data confirm the early claims that about half of dermatomyositis patients over the age of 40 have cancer, and that the incidence of cancer is much lower in older patients with polymyositis. There is no association with cancer in childhood dermatomyositis. The genuine association of adult dermatomyositis with cancer has been blurred in several previous studies by failure to exclude younger patients with dermatomyositis, patients without a skin rash, and patients with collagen-vascular diseases.

De Vere and Bradley (1975), reviewing the cases of polymyositis seen at Newcastle over a period of 20 years, recorded 21 cases of dermatomyositis and 97 cases of polymyositis. Of the 15 patients with dermatomyositis who were older than 39, 6 patients (40 percent) had cancer, while only 3.4 percent of the older patients with polymyositis had cancer. Callen and coworkers (1980) carried out a followup study of patients with dermatomyositis and polymyositis seen between 1956 and 1975. Their ages ranged from 22 to 80, and patients with other collagen-vascular diseases were excluded. Cancer was associated in 7 (26 percent) of the 27 patients with dermatomyositis but in only 1 (3.2 percent) of the 31 patients with polymyositis. Of the 8 patients with cancer, 6 were women, and the tumors found were adenocarcinoma of the colon (2), adenocarcinoma of the breast (2), Hodgkin's disease (1), and metastatic malignancy of unknown origin (3).

I have reviewed the inpatient records of 20 patients over the age of 40 with well-documented dermatomyositis who were admitted to the University of California Medical Center, San Francisco, during the period 1970 to 1978. Of these patients, 11 (9 of whom were women) proved to have cancer, an incidence of 55 percent. The tumors were carcinomas of the lung (4), endometrium (2), ovary (3), colon (1), and breast (1). The symptoms of dermatomyositis preceded the diagnosis of cancer in 8 patients by intervals of 2 to 36 months; in 4 of these cases the initial cancer workup was negative 4 to 5 months after the onset of dermatomyositis, and the diagnosis of cancer was made 4 to 42 months later. Interestingly, there were atypical diagnostic features in 4 of the 9 patients without cancer. One patient had minimal skin findings; another's rash was more suggestive of systemic lupus erythematosus than of dermatomyositis; a third had the sicca (Sjögren's) syndrome with a high titer of rheumatoid factor; and a fourth developed polyarthritis, pulmonary fibrosis, digital vasculitis, and a cerebral infarction.

In a recent review, Barnes (1976) found that women represented 63 percent of the published cases of combined cancer and dermatomyositis; 77 percent of the patients were over 45, and 97 percent were over 30 years of age. Cancer of the stomach and ovary were more frequent than in the general population. In 60 percent of the cases muscle symptoms preceded the diagnosis of cancer, usually by less than 1 year (mean interval 11 months); in 10 percent of the cases the two conditions appeared simultaneously; and in 30 percent the diagnosis of cancer preceded the onset of dermatomyositis by a mean interval of 16 months.

Moss and Hanelin (1977) argued that radiologic screening for occult malignancy was of no value, even in older patients with dermatomyositis. They found only 2 cases of cancer in 28 patients with dermatomyositis, 18 of whom were over 40 years of age. Since their report came from my own institution and covered approximately the same period of time that I reviewed, I doubt the validity of their data, which differ markedly from my own. It is true that in many cases the occult cancer was discovered by routine screening tests or by investigation of suspicious bodily symptoms. It is also true that, even when cancer was discovered soon after the onset of dermatomyositis, it was usually not curable. Nevertheless, given a 50 percent incidence of cancer in older patients with dermatomyositis, it would be callous not to make a vigorous search for cancer, in the hope of curing a few of them. If no cancer is found, one should maintain close surveillance of the patients for at least 2 years. The number of patients in question is too small for clinicians to quibble over the "cost-benefit ratio" of a thorough cancer workup.

Many articles report improvement of dermatomyositis after treatment of the cancer, but a recent report described three patients who developed dermatomyositis, with a fatal outcome in two cases, during tamoxifen treatment for breast cancer. The myopathy appeared as the tumor was regressing, and the authors suggested that tamoxifen treatment might somehow have provoked the emergence of the inflammatory disorder (Harris et al. 1982). Ninety-one percent of cancer-dermatomyositis patients improve under steroid treatment (Barnes 1976), certainly as good a response as in patients without cancer, though the mortality rate in the former is a good deal higher than in the latter.

Other Myopathies

Barbara Smith (1969) drew attention to a *noninflammatory, necrotizing myopathy* in two patients with carcinoma, and subsequently two similar cases have been reported (Urich and Wilkinson 1970; Swash 1974). The distinctive pathology consisted of extensive muscle fiber necrosis, which often involved entire fascicles; degeneration of the internal contents of myofibers with preservation of the sarcolemma and a thin rim of cytoplasm; regeneration within the empty sarcolemmal tubes; the presence of endomysial edema; and infrequent phagocytosis.

One of the patients also had an acute polyneuropathy characterized by Wallerian degeneration, and another patient had cutaneous signs of a small-vessel vasculopathy, but none had typical dermatomyositis. The clinical picture consisted of subacute or fulminating muscle weakness and pain with a moderate increase of serum enzyme levels. There was no response to steroid therapy, and two patients died as a result of severe weakness, although another patient recovered after excision of a breast cancer. Smith (1969) pointed out that necrosis of muscle fibers from within, as seen in these cases, implies a different pathogenesis from that in polymyositis, where the interstitial inflammatory process appears to attack the myocytes from the outside. Swash (1974) did not detect any immunoglobulin deposits in muscle sections, and the pathogenesis of this unusual muscle lesion remains unknown. It is also unclear how rare this type of necrosis is. Muscle necrosis with little or no inflammation was mentioned in many older reports of polymyositis and dermatomyositis associated with cancer, and it occurs in dermatomyositis without cancer. Further pathologic studies are needed to clarify these questions.

Heffner (1971) reported three patients with a unique syndrome of *migratory embolic muscle infarction* caused by nonbacterial thrombotic endocarditis. All three patients had a mucinous adenocarcinoma of the colon or pancreas. The clinical picture consisted of sudden focal muscle pain, swelling, tenderness, and weakness that appeared in scattered muscles, one after the other. The discomfort and swelling subsided in a few days but the weakness took longer to resolve. Heffner characterized the picture as a "migrating monomyositis multiplex" by analogy with mononeuritis multiplex. Embolic strokes, a much more common manifestation of marantic endocarditis (Rosen and Armstrong 1973), also occurred in two of the three cases.

Disorders of Neuromuscular Transmission

The Lambert-Eaton Syndrome

The Lambert-Eaton syndrome (LES)* is associated with cancer in about 70 percent of cases. The neoplasm is almost invariably a bronchogenic carcinoma, usually of the oat-cell type. It is perhaps the most widely known of the paraneoplastic neuromuscular disorders, yet in overt form it is quite rare; there were no examples of LES among 450 unselected lung cancer patients in the four series cited previously (Croft and Wilkinson 1963; Trojaborg et al. 1969; Campbell and Paty 1974; Lenman et al. 1981). There has been little comment on the clinical background of the patients who did not have cancer, but a few have had autoimmune diseases such as Sjögren's syndrome, hypothyroidism, pernicious anemia, vitiligo, and celiac disease (Gutmann et al. 1972; Lang et al. 1981).

CLINICAL FEATURES. (Elmqvist and Lambert 1968; Lambert and Rooke 1965). Most of the patients are men, including those without lung cancer. The chief complaint is weakness and easy fatigability of the legs, causing difficulty in walking, rising from a chair, and climbing stairs. Some patients complain of aching muscles. Cranial muscle symptoms are rarely prominent, but some patients report mild ptosis, blurred vision, mild dysphagia, hoarseness, or dysarthria. Respiratory muscle weakness is rarely a spontaneous complaint, though it occurs after anesthesia. Symptoms of parasympathetic autonomic insufficiency, which are common, include dry mouth, impotence, and inability to focus on near objects. Half of the patients complain of distal paresthesias.

Neurologic examination shows limb muscle weakness with little or no atrophy, concentrated in the pelvic girdle, thighs, neck, and trunk. There are no fasciculations. Muscle strength improves during sustained effort; likewise, the muscle stretch reflexes are initially depressed or absent but can be restored by a few seconds of strong voluntary contraction. The sensory system is usually intact, and there are usually no signs of other nonmetastatic neurologic complications.

*The first article on this subject was by Lambert, Eaton, and Rooke (1956), the second by Eaton and Lambert (1957). I have chosen to preserve the original order of the names, in view of Lambert's primary role in the subsequent elucidation of the disorder, though most authors refer to the Eaton-Lambert syndrome. Neither eponym does justice to the contribution of Rooke. Lambert himself consistently avoids the eponymic designation, referring simply to the "myasthenic syndrome," but this term is excessively ambiguous.

Like patients with myasthenia gravis, patients with LES are extremely susceptible to paralysis by neuromuscular blocking drugs. In the early 1950s, before the disorder was clearly defined, it was recognized that lung cancer patients without overt neuromuscular symptoms sometimes exhibited prolonged postoperative apnea following the administration of long-acting neuromuscular blocking drugs like d-tubocurarine. However, patients with myasthenia gravis are abnormally resistant to the paralyzing action of decamethonium, while LES patients are abnormally sensitive to that agent.

LABORATORY FINDINGS. CSF composition and serum CPK activity are normal, and in most cases muscle biopsy is unrevealing. The important abnormalities are found with electrophysiologic testing (Lambert and Rooke 1965; McQuillen and Johns 1967; Elmqvist and Lambert 1968; Sanders et al. 1980). Needle EMG may show no abnormality or may show excessive variation in the amplitude of individual motor unit potentials, or low-amplitude, short-duration motor unit potentials (myopathic type). There is usually no increase of spontaneous activity at rest. Nerve conduction testing gives normal results except for reduced amplitude of the compound action potential recorded from the muscle surface, averaging one fifth of the normal mean. Repetitive motor nerve stimulation shows a characteristic abnormality: at slow rates of stimulation (3 Hz) there is often a decrement in the already small amplitude of the compound muscle action potential, while at faster rates of stimulation (10 to 50 Hz) there is an incrementing response that may reach 20 times the initial amplitude. This facilitation persists for 15 to 30 seconds after delivery of a train of tetanic stimulation or after a 10-second period of forceful voluntary contraction ("post-activation facilitation"). The muscle tension evoked by motor nerve stimulation parallels the electrical responses, being weak initially and increasing during tetanic stimulation. However, even muscles that appear clinically normal usually show the electrophysiologic defects.

Pathophysiology. Studies with intracellular microelectrodes reveal a defect in the release of acetylcholine from nerve terminals, rather similar to that produced by high magnesium concentration (Elmqvist and Lambert 1968; Sanders et al. 1980). The amplitude and frequency of spontaneous miniature end-plate potentials (mepps) are normal, indicating that the postsynaptic response to a single packet of acetylcholine is normal, and that the packets have a normal content of acetylcholine. In contrast, the end-plate potentials (epps) produced by motor nerve stimulation have a very low amplitude, and the epp amplitude varies widely, so that some nerve impulses produce no epp at all. Analysis of the epps shows that they are produced by only 3 to 10 packets of acetylcholine, the normal number being about 50. The size of the epps is increased by rapid, tetanic nerve stimulation and also by an increased extracellular concentration of calcium ions at the nerve terminals.

These findings suggest that the defect in LES, like that in botulism, may involve the calcium-mediated release of acetylcholine in the nerve terminals. Normally, when an action potential invades a nerve terminal the depolarization produces an influx of calcium ions, and the raised internal concentration of ionic calcium somehow triggers the release of acetylcholine from synaptic vesicles close to the surface membrane. Repetitive nerve stimulation at a high frequency produces a relatively long-lasting increase in internal calcium concentration, and this fact probably explains the phenomenon of postactivation facilitation. 4-Aminopyridine improves neuromuscular transmission in both botulism and LES (Sanders et al. 1980; Lundh et al. 1977); by prolonging the negative after-potential in the nerve terminals, the drug increases the influx of calcium ions. Botulism and LES are not identical, however. In botulism there is a marked reduction in the spontaneous release of acetylcholine quanta (mepps), and facilitation by repetitive stimulation is much less striking than in LES, but it lasts much longer—several minutes as opposed to 15 to 30 seconds.

Oat-cell carcinomas are especially apt to cause paraneoplastic syndromes by secreting peptide hormones such as ACTH, ADH, and MSH. It is tempting, therefore, to speculate that a peptide substance resembling botulinum toxin may be responsible for LES. Ishikawa and colleagues (1977) reported that an extract of a lung tumor from a patient with LES had in-vitro effects on neuromuscular transmission, but the resemblance of those effects to the defect in LES was not convincing. Newsom-Davis and colleagues (1982) found a presynaptic defect of neuromuscular transmission in mice given repeated injections of immunoglobulins obtained from seven patients with LES, five of whom had no underlying cancer. These findings, as well as apparent responses to immunosuppressive and plasma-exchange therapy, led the authors to postulate an autoimmune etiology for both neoplastic and non-neoplastic LES.

TREATMENT. Anticholinesterase drugs produce at best modest improvement of strength. Guanidine hydrochloride has been moderately effective in many patients; the action of the drug is not entirely understood, but it facilitates the calcium-mediated release of acetylcholine from nerve terminals (McQuillen and Johns 1967; Elmqvist and Lambert 1968). The effective dosage of guanidine is 15 to 35 mg per kg per day in divided doses; unfortunately, this often causes side-effects such as gastrointestinal irritation, paresthesias, perioral numbness, tremors, and muscle twitching. In addition, there are occasional instances of serious toxic reactions, including kidney damage and bone-marrow suppression (Norris et al. 1974). A combination of pyridostigmine and guanidine seems to be more effective in some patients and may permit a lower dose of guanidine to be used. 4-Aminopyridine, a much more effective agent, is too toxic to be useful (Lundh et al. 1977), but 3,4-diaminopyridine appears to be both safe and effective (Lundh et al. 1983).

Surgical removal or irradiation of a lung tumor has sometimes resulted in dramatic improvement of the neuromuscular disorder, and recurrence of the tumor may revive the neuromuscular symptoms (Lambert and Rooke 1965; Norris et al. 1965). Plasma exchange and treatment with prednisolone and azathioprine have been reported to be helpful in some non-neoplastic cases (Newsom-Davis et al. 1982; Dau and Denys 1982), but many patients are not sufficiently disabled to warrant such powerful immunosuppressive measures.

Thymoma, Myasthenia Gravis, and Polymyositis

About one third of patients with thymoma have myasthenia gravis, while 10 to 15 percent of patients with myasthenia gravis have a thymoma (Namba et al. 1978). Almost all of the patients with this combination are between 20 and 70 years of age; patients under the age of 20 compose only 1.7 percent of the cases (Slater et al. 1978). Men and women are represented about equally. Most of the tumors are composed of lymphoid or epithelial elements or a mixture of both; about two thirds of the tumors are encapsulated and one third are invasive (Wilkins et al. 1966; Slater et al. 1978; Namba et al. 1978). Invasive thymomas may extend into the mediastinal fat or may invade adjacent structures such as pleura, pericardium, lung, diaphragm, phrenic nerve, innominate vein, or superior vena cava. The tumor may also seed within the thoracic cavity (Bergh et al. 1978). Lymph node metastasis occurs in 3 percent of cases and distant metastasis in only 1 percent (Namba et al. 1978); in the few reported cases, distant metastases were found in lungs, liver, bones, leptomeninges, spleen, and kidneys (Guillan et al. 1971; Butterworth et al. 1973). The histology of the tumor does not seem to have any bearing on its invasive or metastatic propensities; the diagnosis of "malignancy" is based on the gross findings at operation.

PROGNOSIS. Myasthenic patients with thymoma have a worse prognosis following thymectomy than those without thymoma (Bernatz et al. 1973; Wilkins et al. 1966), but it is unclear whether this applies to all thymomas or only to invasive tumors. At the Mt. Sinai Hospital in New York, the 5-year survival was about 50 percent for myasthenic patients with invasive tumors and 70 percent for those with noninvasive tumors (Slater et al. 1978); at the same institution, the 5-year survival was 86 percent in nonthymomatous myasthenia (Papatestas et al. 1971). The rate of remission of myasthenia following thymectomy was very low in the thymoma patients, regardless of tumor invasiveness. However, in a much smaller sample Emeryk and Strugalska (1976) observed remission or marked improvement after thymectomy in 9 of 12 cases of benign thymoma, the same proportion as in nonthymoma patients, while none of the 8 patients with invasive thymoma improved, and 4 of them died. My own experience suggests that the prognosis after total thymectomy for patients with benign thymoma and for patients without thymoma is similar.

ONSET OF MYASTHENIA GRAVIS AFTER REMOVAL OF A THYMOMA. Myasthenia sometimes begins *after* total removal of a thymoma and of all adjacent thymic tissue. This subject was recently reviewed by Namba and associates (1978), who found 7 instances among 28 of their own patients, and 42 cases in the literature. These cases represent about 10 percent of all reported myasthenic patients with thymoma. The interval between the operation and the onset of myasthenic symptoms can be weeks, months, or years. Nine such patients subsequently had a thorough examination of the mediastinum at autopsy, and 1 had a repeat thoracotomy; in 2 of the 10 cases microscopic thymic tissue was found, and a third patient had a visible thymic remnant. Namba and associates were impressed by the 7 patients who did not appear to have residual thymic tissue and concluded that the thymus gland itself was not responsible for the delayed myasthenia. It is remarkable, however, that residual thymic tissue was discovered in 30 percent of the patients who were supposed to have undergone *total* removal of all thymic tissue; it is quite possible that residual thymic tissue went undetected in the remaining 70 percent. The boundaries of the thymus gland are peculiarly indeterminate; about 20 percent of normal persons are said to have atopic cervical thymic tissue (Papatestas et al. 1975), and mediastinal adipose tissue adjacent to the thymus gland, not routinely removed by some surgeons, contains thymic tissue in 72 percent of myasthenic patients (Masaoka et al. 1975).

DIAGNOSIS OF THYMOMA. There is general agreement that thymomas should be removed because even encapsulated tumors may eventually become invasive. The growth of these tumors is usually slow, so that a tumor may be present for several years before the onset of myasthenic symptoms; symptoms attributable to the tumor itself are present in only 10 percent of patients (Namba et al. 1978). Routine anteroposterior and lateral chest radiograms prior to thymectomy will detect about 70 percent of thymomas in myasthenic patients, and if thymectomy is going to be done anyway there is no need to search for a small thymoma, especially if the transsternal approach is used. The question of detecting a small thymoma arises when early thymectomy is not part of the therapeutic plan—for instance, with patients over the age of 60, or those who decline the operation. In such patients, detection of a thymoma may change the therapeutic plan or may influence the patient to accept thymectomy. Computed tomography of the chest detects almost all thymomas, but unfortunately cannot distinguish between normal or hyperplastic thymic tissue and tumor in many cases (Fon et al. 1982; Moore et al. 1982). Radionuclide selenium scans do not distinguish between thymic hyperplasia and tumor (Testa and Angelini 1979), and radionuclide gallium scans are negative in about one fourth of thymomas, though they are not likely to give a false positive result (Swick et al. 1976). A useful ancillary test is measurement of the serum titer of antibodies to striated muscle. The titer is increased in nearly all myasthenic patients with thymoma but in only 11 percent of myasthenic patients without thymoma (Oosterhuis et al. 1976). A negative result therefore provides strong evidence against the presence of a thymoma (Keesey et al. 1980).

Paraneoplastic syndromes are remarkably frequent in patients with thymoma. At the Mayo Clinic, 74 percent of 146 cases of thymoma were associated with one or more of the following disorders (Souadjian et al. 1974):

Myasthenia gravis
Nonthymic cancer
Aplastic anemia, leukopenia, and thrombocytopenia
Hypogammaglobulinemia
Polymyositis and dermatomyositis
Giant cell polymyositis
Chronic mucocutaneous candidiasis
Pemphigus
Autoimmune thyroid disease
Systemic lupus erythematosus, scleroderma, rheumatoid arthritis, Sjögren's syndrome
Pernicious anemia, Addison's disease
Regional ileitis, ulcerative colitis
Vitiligo, alopecia
Severe infections
Cushing's syndrome

By far the largest group of disorders are those regarded as having an autoimmune pathogenesis. Antinuclear antibody has been found in about 50 percent of thymoma patients with or without myasthenia gravis, in 18 percent of myasthenic patients without thymoma, and in 4 percent of matched controls (Oosterhuis et al. 1976). Almost all the disorders listed above have been associated with myasthenia gravis in a few cases, but some syndromes are particularly linked with myasthenia. Five of eight reported cases of thymoma with *pemphigus* were associated with myasthenia gravis (Krain 1974). *Chronic mucocutaneous candidiasis* starting after the third decade, a syndrome in which thymoma is regularly found, has been associated with myasthenia gravis in 10 of 28 cases (Kirkpatrick and Windhorst 1979). *Idiopathic giant cell polymyositis* is a distinctive disorder regularly linked to thymoma; 7 of the 13 reported cases have also been associated with myasthenia gravis, and almost all were associated with myocarditis, which may be the presenting feature. The polymyositis is pathologically similar to ordinary lymphocytic polymyositis (which also occurs with thymoma), except for the presence of multinucleated giant cells of myogenous type; granulomas of sarcoid type are not seen. These cases respond poorly to steroid and immunosuppressive therapy, and all the patients have died within 4 years after the onset of skeletal muscle or cardiac symptoms, the median survival being only 9 months (Namba et al. 1974).

PATHOPHYSIOLOGY. There is reason to suspect that most of the disorders associated with thymoma are related to defects of lymphocyte function (one exception is Cushing's syndrome, which is due to secretion of ACTH or a similar peptide). Three fourths of the patients with chronic candidiasis have some impairment of cell-mediated immunity, and 35 percent evince cellular anergy to multiple antigens (Kirkpatrick and Windhorst 1979). In some patients with thymoma, thymus-derived lymphocytes appear to suppress the maturation of immunoglobulin-producing B-cells and of erythroid precursors (Litwin and Zanjani 1977). The high incidence of autoimmune and neoplastic disorders could result from failure to suppress antibody production, from abnormal susceptibility to chronic infections, or from failure to eliminate harmful lymphocyte clones (Souadjian et al. 1974).

It is interesting that young female patients with myasthenia and thymic hyperplasia have a high incidence of the HLA-B8 phenotype, while thymoma, male sex, and older age at onset are associated with a normal or low frequency of HLA-B8 (Fritze et al. 1976; Oosterhuis et al. 1976). The HLA-B8 phenotype is strongly associated with Graves' disease and other autoimmune disorders, and some of the same diseases are associated with thymoma, so that different genetic factors seem to lead to the same autoimmune tendency. The relation between neoplasia of the thymus and autoimmunity is completely unknown; it is possible that both the thymoma and the diseases associated with it are a result of some underlying disorder of lymphocyte function.

Peripheral Neuropathies

The polyneuropathies associated with carcinoma, lymphoma, and leukemia fall into several categories (Table 24) that are sufficiently different in their clinical and pathologic features to suggest that their pathogeneses may also differ (McLeod 1975; McLeod and Walsh 1975). In clinical practice, however, it is not always easy to differentiate these syndromes from each other. The polyneuropathies associated with multiple myeloma and other B-cell dyscrasias are described in Chapter 5.

Incidence

Prineas (1970) found that an occult malignancy eventually came to light in 9 percent of 91 consecutive patients referred for inpatient workup of a polyneuropathy of undetermined cause. Excluded from this study were patients in whom the cause of the neuropathy was easily ascertained by the primary physicians. The underlying cancer was discovered within 2 years in all cases.

TABLE 24. Peripheral Neuropathies Indirectly Associated with Cancer

Syndrome	Type of Cancer
Subacute sensory neuropathy	Lung (oat-cell); rarely, Hodgkin's disease
Guillain-Barré syndrome	Hodgkin's disease, angioimmunoblastic lymphadenopathy; rarely, carcinomas
Subacute or chronic sensorimotor polyneuropathy	Carcinoma (many types), lymphoma, B-cell malignancy
Amyloid neuropathy	B-cell malignancy

In contrast, overt polyneuropathy is uncommon in patients with carcinoma. Croft and Wilkinson (1963) found polyneuropathy in 1.6 percent of patients with carcinoma of the lung and in 1.0 percent of patients with all types of carcinoma. In other surveys of lung cancer the incidence of overt neuropathy ranged from 0 to 5 percent (Trojaborg et al. 1969; Campbell and Paty 1974; Lenman et al. 1981). Surprisingly, in unselected patients with lymphoma Walsh (1971) found an 8 percent incidence of clinically evident neuropathy and a 35 percent incidence of nerve conduction abnormalities.

Subacute Sensory Neuropathy (Ganglioradiculitis)

This rare but distinctive disorder was originally described by Denny-Brown (1948). According to Horwich and colleagues (1977), the most important clinical and pathologic alterations involve the sensory system, but mild muscle weakness occurs in about half of the patients. In three fourths of the patients the onset of sensory symptoms precedes the discovery of cancer by up to 46 months. The initial symptoms are pain, paresthesia, dysesthesia, and numbness of the extremities, usually in a distal distribution but not always symmetric. The trunk and face are occasionally affected. The sensory symptoms spread proximally over the course of several weeks, producing a sensory ataxia of gait and incoordination of the limbs. The muscle stretch reflexes become unobtainable, and all modalities of sensation become severely depressed, especially vibration and position sense. Occasionally there are also signs and symptoms attributable to a diffuse polioencephalomyelopathy (carcinomatous encephalomyelitis), such as dementia, nystagmus, ocular palsy, pupillary paralysis, and other cranial nerve disturbances. Mild, distal muscle weakness and atrophy may supervene in the later stages. There are usually no autonomic symptoms other than bladder dysfunction. The course of the neuropathy is usually not affected by treatment of the tumor, and the symptoms grow progressively worse for several months before becoming static. Death occurs at an average of 14 months after onset of the sensory symptoms.

The CSF protein is elevated to the range of 100 to 200 mg per dl in two thirds of the cases, and the immunoglobulin concentration may be increased (Croft et al. 1965). The CSF cell count is usually normal, but a mild lymphocytic pleocytosis is sometimes found. Motor nerve conduction velocities are normal or slightly reduced, while sensory nerve responses are reduced or unobtainable.

At autopsy, the principal finding is a severe degeneration of sensory neurons in the dorsal root ganglia, which are infiltrated by lymphocytes, plasma cells, and macrophages. The inflammatory process is remarkably restricted, showing little extension into the nerve roots, and older, "burnt out" cases show fibrosis with little or no active inflammation. In cases with CNS involvement there are scattered foci of neuronal degeneration and lymphocytic infiltration of the brain, spinal cord, and meninges.

The striking and selective inflammatory pathology suggests one of two possible mechanisms: an autoimmune process with organ-specific antibodies to sensory ganglion cells, or infection by an organism having a predilection for those neurons. The latter mechanism is perhaps more consistent with the fact that in many cases the disease process comes to a halt after a few months. It is also pertinent that a disorder with similar clinical and pathologic features has been described in patients with systemic lupus erythematosus (Chapter 5), and one of the patients with subacute sensory neuropathy described by Horwich and colleagues (1977) had Sjögren's syndrome without a known malignancy. At any rate, attempts to demonstrate either an autoimmune or an infectious etiology have been no more successful than in the other paraneoplastic syndromes collectively termed carcinomatous polioencephalomyelitis. Croft and coworkers (1965) found antibrain antibodies in four cases, but Horwich and colleagues (1977) could not confirm this in two other cases.

Guillain-Barré Syndrome

Although rare instances of typical Guillain-Barré syndrome (GBS) have been recorded in patients with carcinoma (McLeod 1975), this association may be coincidental. Thus, one patient with lung carcinoma developed GBS in a setting of penicillin allergy (Croft et al. 1967, case 11). However, patients with Hodgkin's disease or angioimmunoblastic lymphadenopathy do seem to have an increased incidence of GBS (Cameron et al. 1958; Klington 1965; Lisak et al. 1977; Brunet et al. 1981), although only one case of GBS was detected in a retrospective survey of 210 cases of Hodgkin's disease (Currie et al. 1970). Most of the patients make a good recovery, but some die in the acute phase of the paralysis.

PATHOPHYSIOLOGY. Patients with Hodgkin's disease often have deficiencies of cell-mediated immunity at various times during the course of their disease. Lisak and associates (1977) speculated that an immune deficiency may predispose to the occurrence of GBS, pointing out that temporary depression of immune function is also a feature of pregnancy, the postoperative state, viral infections, and organ transplantation—conditions that have been linked to the occurrence of GBS. Patients with partial immune deficiencies have a propensity to develop autoimmune diseases and cancer, especially lymphoproliferative disorders, and this susceptibility could be the reason for the association of GBS and Hodgkin's disease in some patients. A persistent viral infection has been postulated in both disorders but remains entirely hypothetical.

Subacute, Chronic, and Relapsing Polyneuropathies

These cases constitute the largest category of the paraneoplastic polyneuropathies. The onset of neuropathy precedes the diagnosis of cancer about half of the time, usually by a few months but occasionally by one or several years. Among the 22 cases analyzed by Croft and coworkers (1967), half were related to carcinoma of the lung (especially the oat-cell type), the others to lymphoma and carcinoma of the breast, colon, stomach, pancreas, endometrium, and cervix. Other authors have reported this type of neuropathy in association with carcinoma of the kidney, thyroid, prostate, and testis (McLeod 1975), and with angioimmunoblastic lymphadenopathy (Brunet et al. 1981). A few cases of angiofollicular lymph node hyperplasia have been complicated by polyneuropathy; one such patient had a monoclonal gammopathy, suggesting a link with the paraproteinemic neuropathies (Hineman et al. 1982). (Conspicuously absent from this list is carcinoma of the ovary, which is strongly associated with dermatomyositis and with subacute cerebellar degeneration.)

The clinical picture is far from uniform, and there may well be more than one pathogenesis in this syndrome. The course is rapid (weeks) or slow (months), with diffuse sensory and motor deficits in the extremities, not always symmetric or strictly distal in distribution, and sometimes affecting the arms more than the legs. Pain may be a prominent feature or may be completely absent. Some patients improve spontaneously, and some of these later relapse. Symptoms of an associated polioencephalomyelitis may also be present.

The CSF cell count is normal; the protein is elevated in two thirds of the cases, up to 800 mg per dl, and the globulin content is elevated in about one third of cases. Oligoclonal bands of IgG have not been looked for. Nerve conduction velocity may be mildly, moderately, or markedly slow. At autopsy the nerves show demyelination, axonal degeneration, proliferation of Schwann cells, and endoneurial fibrosis. The demyelination appears to be a primary process and is usually more extensive than the axonal degeneration. Sparse endoneurial and perineurial lymphocytic infiltration is seen in fewer than one third of the cases.

The resemblance of many of these cases to subacute and chronic idiopathic polyneuritis is readily apparent. There is some indication that the carcinomatous cases, like the idiopathic ones, may respond to steroid therapy (Croft et al. 1967). These similarities emphasize the fact that the diagnosis of chronic idiopathic polyneuritis must be made by exclusion in older patients, and neither a fluctuating course nor a favorable response to steroids excludes an underlying malignancy. The pathogenesis of the carcinomatous cases, as of the idiopathic disorder, remains unknown.

Motor Neuron Disease

In their early papers on the nonmetastatic neurologic disorders associated with carcinoma, Henson and colleagues (1954) and Brain and Henson (1958) mentioned that autopsies of patients with cerebral signs and symptoms often showed patchy degeneration of the motor neurons in the ventral horns of the spinal cord. Subsequent reports of patients with subacute carcinomatous cerebellar degeneration or encephalomyelitis likewise made note of pathologic and clinical involvement of the upper and lower motor neurons (Henson et al. 1965; Brain and Wilkinson 1965). Brain suggested the term "diffuse polioencephalopathy" to emphasize the patchy and variable involvement of many neuronal structures throughout the CNS, but a more accurate term would be polioencephalomyelitis, since there is often an inflammatory component, and the spinal gray matter and dorsal root ganglia are often involved. There is a spectrum of clinical syndromes, the details of which depend on the severity of the neuronal disease in different portions of the neuraxis. The most common manifestations are a pancerebellar syndrome, dementia, sensory neuropathy, patchy upper and lower motor neuron signs, and brainstem disturbances such as ocular palsy, nystagmus, and bulbar palsy. The progressive course of these disorders over a period of weeks or months sometimes becomes arrested, but substantial improvement is unusual. The CSF may be normal, but in some cases there is a slight excess of lymphocytes and the protein and IgG levels are mildly elevated. Cases of this kind are mainly associated with carcinoma of the lung, ovary, or breast, but other neoplasms have been found, including lymphoma.

In a few reported cases, lower motor neuron degeneration has dominated the clinical picture, though there were signs of a more widespread neuronal disorder (Case Records of the Massachusetts General Hospital 1970). When typical amyotrophic lateral sclerosis occurs in a patient with cancer, however, the possibility of a coincidental association must be considered. Norris and Engel (1965) found 13 patients with a major cancer in 130 consecutive cases of clinically diagnosed amyotrophic lateral sclerosis;

one was later shown to have polymyositis, but even without this case the association was greater than in the matched controls with stroke, 1 percent of whom had cancer.

Brain and Wilkinson (1965) described 11 patients with upper and lower motor neuron signs associated with cancer. The clinical picture was indistinguishable from that of ordinary amyotrophic lateral sclerosis, but at autopsy degenerative changes were present in the dorsal root ganglia and posterior columns to a greater extent than is usual in idiopathic amyotrophic lateral sclerosis. Nevertheless, many would continue to regard an association between clinically typical amyotrophic lateral sclerosis and cancer as fortuitous unless there is autopsy evidence of pathologic changes different from those of the classical disease. Recently, however, Mitchell and Olczak (1979) reported on a 54-year-old man who developed patchy, moderately severe upper and lower motor neuron signs together with pulmonary osteoarthropathy and gynecomastia. A large-cell carcinoma of the lung was discovered, and following pneumonectomy there was nearly complete remission of the neurologic signs and symptoms during 6 months of observation. This case lends plausibility to the contention that cancer may cause a small proportion of cases of amyotrophic lateral sclerosis.

A third type of lower motor neuron disorder, *subacute motor neuronopathy*, has been described in patients with lymphoma, especially Hodgkin's disease (Schold et al. 1979). The patients manifest patchy muscle weakness, atrophy, and fasciculations, primarily affecting the lower extremities. There are no upper motor neuron signs, but minor sensory symptoms and signs may be present. The neuromuscular symptoms progress for several months but tend to improve spontaneously and may resolve completely 1 to 3 years after the onset, without any relation to treatment of the tumor. Radiation therapy is not the sole cause, since some of the patients did not receive radiation. The CSF is usually normal except for a mild increase in protein concentration, and motor nerve conduction velocities are normal or slightly reduced. The findings at autopsy consist of noninflammatory degeneration of the anterior horn neurons, patchy demyelination and gliosis of the white matter tracts of the cord, patchy segmental demyelination of the spinal roots and of the brachial and lumbar plexuses, and proliferation of bizarrely formed Schwann cells.

A similar lower motor neuron syndrome in a patient with Waldenstrom's macroglobulinemia remitted after treatment with chlorambucil, although the neurologic disorder had already been present for 5 years (Peters and Clatanoff 1968). The patient succumbed to the neoplasm 4 years later without recurrence of the weakness, suggesting that the motor neuron disease had "burnt out" and was not dependent on the bulk of the malignant cells. As Schold and colleagues (1979) speculated, an infectious cause would most easily account for all these clinical observations, but no direct evidence for an infectious agent has been discovered by electron microscopy or viral culture.

REFERENCES

ADAMS, RD: *Diseases of Muscle. A Study in Pathology*, ed 3. Harper & Row, New York, 1975.

ARUNDELL, FD, WILKINSON, RD AND HASERICK, JR: *Dermatomyositis and malignant neoplasms in adults.* Arch Dermatol 82:772–775, 1960.

ASCHERL, GF, JR, HILAL, SK AND BRISMAN R: *Computed tomography of disseminated meningeal and ependymal malignant neoplasms.* Neurology 31:567–574, 1981.

Attar, S, Miller, JE, Satterfield, J, et al: *Pancoast's tumor: Irradiation or surgery?* Ann Thorac Surg 28:578–586, 1979.

Ballenger, JJ: *Diseases of the Nose, Throat and Ear*, ed. 12. Lea & Febiger, Philadelphia, 1977, pp 444–477.

Barnes, BE: *Dermatomyositis and malignancy. A review of the literature.* Ann Intern Med 84:68–76, 1976.

Barron, KD, Rowland, LP and Zimmerman, HM: *Neuropathy with malignant tumor metastases.* J Nerv Ment Dis 131:10–31, 1960.

Barron, SA and Heffner, RR: *Weakness in malignancy: Evidence for a remote effect of tumor on distal axons.* Ann Neurol 4:268–274, 1978.

Batzdorf, U and Brechner, VL: *Management of pain associated with the Pancoast syndrome.* Am J Surg 137:638–646, 1979.

Bergh, NP, Gatzinsky, P, Larsson, S, et al: *Tumors of the thymus and thymic region: I. Clinicopathological studies on thymomas.* Ann Thorac Surg 25:91–98, 1978.

Bernatz, PE, Khonsari, S, Harrison, EG, jr, et al: *Thymoma: Factors influencing prognosis.* Surg Clin North Am 53:885–892, 1973.

Bohan, A, Peter, JB, Bowman, RL, et al: *A computer-assisted analysis of 153 patients with polymyositis and dermatomyositis.* Medicine 56:255–286, 1977.

Brain, WR and Henson, RA: *Neurological syndromes associated with carcinoma.* Lancet 2:971–975, 1958.

Brain, WR and Wilkinson, M: *Subacute cerebellar degeneration associated with neoplasms.* Brain 88:465–478, 1965.

Brain, WR, Croft, PB and Wilkinson, M: *Motor neuron disease as a manifestation of neoplasm.* Brain 88:479–500, 1965.

Brunet, P, Binet, JL, de Saxce H, et al: *Neuropathies au cours de la lymphadenopathie angioimmunoblastique.* Rev Neurol 137:503–515, 1981.

Bunn, PA, jr, Schein, PS, Banks, PM, et al: *Central nervous system complications in patients with diffuse histiocytic and undifferentiated lymphoma: Leukemia revisited.* Blood 47:3–10, 1976.

Butterworth, STG, Newell, JE and Stack, HRB: *Malignant thymoma with central nervous system metastases.*Br J Dis Chest 67:141–145, 1973.

Cairncross, JG and Posner, JB: *Neurological complications of malignant lymphoma.* In Vinken, PJ and Bruyn, GW (eds): *Handbook of Clinical Neurology*, Vol. 39. North-Holland Publishing, Amsterdam, 1980, pp 27–62.

Calatayud, T, Vallejo, AR, Dominguez, L, et al: *Lymphomatoid granulomatosis manifesting as a subacute polyradiculoneuropathy. A case report and review of the neurological manifestations.* Eur Neurol 19:213–223, 1980.

Callen, JP, Hyla, JF, Bole, GG, jr, et al: *The relationship of dermatomyositis and polymyositis to internal malignancy.* Arch Dermatol 116:295–298, 1980.

Cameron, DG, Howell, DA and Hutchinson, JL: *Acute peripheral neuropathy in Hodgkin's disease.* Neurology 8:575–577, 1958.

Campbell, MJ and Paty, DW: *Carcinomatous neuromyopathy.* J Neurol Neurosurg Psychiatry 37:131–141, 1974.

Carter, BL: *Computed tomographic scanning in head and neck tumors.* Otolaryngol Clin North Am 13:449–457, 1980.

Case Records of the Massachusetts General Hospital (Case 42-1970). N Engl J Med 283:806–814, 1970.

Croft, PB and Wilkinson, M: *Carcinomatous neuromyopathy. Its incidence in patients with carcinoma of the lung and carcinoma of the breast.* Lancet i:184–188, 1963.

Croft, PB, and Wilkinson, M: *The incidence of carcinomatous neuromyopathy with special reference to carcinoma of the lung and the breast.* In Brain, WR and Norris, FH, jr (eds): *The Remote Effects of Cancer on the Nervous System.* Grune & Stratton, New York, 1965, pp 44–54.

Croft, PB, Henson, RA, Urich, H et al: *Sensory neuropathy with bronchogenic carcinoma: A study of four cases showing serological abnormalities.* Brain 88:501–514, 1965.

Croft, PB, Urich, H and Wilkinson, M: *Peripheral neuropathy of sensorimotor type associated with malignant disease.* Brain 90:31–66, 1967.

Currie, S, Henson, RA, Morgan, HG et al: *The incidence of the nonmetastatic neurological syndromes of obscure origin in the reticuloses.* Brain 93:629–640, 1970.

Dau, PC and Denys, EH: *Plasmapheresis and immunosuppressive drug therapy in the Eaton-Lambert syndrome.* Ann Neurol 11:570–575, 1982.

De Vere, R and Bradley, WG: *Polymyositis: Its presentation, morbidity and mortality.* Brain 98:637–666, 1975.

Dodd, GD, Dolan, PA, Ballantyne, AJ, et al: *The dissemination of tumors of the head and neck via the cranial nerves.* Radiol Clin North Am 8:445–461, 1970.

Doshi, R and Fowler, T: *Proximal myopathy due to discrete carcinomatous metastases to muscle.* J Neurol Neurosurg Psychiatry 46:358–360, 1983.

Eaton, LM and Lambert, EH: *Electromyography and electric stimulation of nerves in diseases of the motor units.* JAMA 163:1117–1124, 1957.

Elmqvist, D and Lambert, EH: *Detailed analysis of neuromuscular transmission in a patient with the myasthenic syndrome sometimes associated with bronchogenic carcinoma.* Mayo Clin Proc 43:689–713, 1968.

Emeryk, B and Strugalska, MH: *Evaluation of results of thymectomy in myasthenia gravis.* J Neurol 211:155–168, 1976.

Fon, GT, Bein, ME, Mancuso, AA, et al: *Computed tomography of the anterior mediastinum in myasthenia gravis. A radiologic-pathologic correlative study.* Radiology 142:135–141, 1982.

Fritze, D, Herrmann, C, jr, Naeim, F, et al: *The biologic significance of HL-A antigen markers in myasthenia gravis.* Ann NY Acad Sci 274:440–450, 1976.

Garcia, CA, Hackett, ER and Kirkpatrick, LL: *Multiple mononeuropathy in lymphomatoid granulomatosis: Similarity to leprosy.* Neurology 28:731–733, 1978.

Greenberg, HS, Deck, MDF, Vikram, B, et al: *Metastasis to the base of the skull: Clinical findings in 43 patients.* Neurology 31:530–537, 1981.

Guillan, RA, Zelman, S, Smalley, RL, et al: *Malignant thymoma associated with myasthenia gravis, and evidence of extrathoracic metastases. An analysis of published cases and report of a case.* Cancer 27:827–830, 1971.

Gutmann, L, Crosby, TW, Takamori, M, et al: *The Eaton-Lambert syndrome and autoimmune disorders.* Am J Med 53:354–356, 1972.

Harris, AL, Smith, IE and Snaith, M: *Tamoxifen-induced tumour regression associated with dermatomyositis.* Br J Med 284:1674–1675, 1982.

Heffner, RR, jr: *Myopathy of embolic origin in patients with carcinoma.* Neurology 21:840–846, 1971.

Henson, RA, Russell, DS and Wilkinson, M: *Carcinomatous neuropathy and myopathy.* Brain 77:82–121, 1954.

Henson, RA, Hoffman, HL and Urich, H: *Encephalomyelitis with carcinoma.* Brain 88:449–464, 1965.

Hepper, NGG, Herskovic, T, Witten, DM, et al: *Thoracic inlet tumors.* Ann Intern Med 64:979–989, 1966.

Hineman, VL, Phyliky, RL and Banks, PM: *Angiofollicular lymph node hyperplasia and peripheral neuropathy. Association with monoclonal gammopathy.* Mayo Clin Proc 57:379–382, 1982.

Hogan, PJ, Greenberg, MK and McCarty, GE: *Neurologic complications of lymphomatoid granulomatosis.* Neurology 31:619–620, 1981.

Horwich, MS, Cho, L, Porro, RS, et al: *Subacute sensory neuropathy: A remote effect of carcinoma.* Ann Neurol 2:7–19, 1977.

Ishikawa, I, Engelhardt, JK, Fujisawa, T, et al: *A neuromuscular transmission block produced by a cancer tissue extract derived from a patient with the myasthenic syndrome.* Neurology 27:140–143, 1977.

Israel, HL, Patchefsky, AS and Saldana, MJ: *Wegener's granulomatosis, lymphomatoid granulomatosis and benign lymphocytic angiitis and granulomatosis of lung.* Ann Intern Med 87:691–699, 1977.

Keesey, J, Bein, M, Mink, J, et al: *Detection of thymoma in myasthenia gravis.* Neurology 30:233–239, 1980.

Kirkpatrick, CH and Windhorst, DB: *Neurocutaneous candidiasis and thymoma.* Am J Med 66:939–945, 1979.

Klington, GH: *The Guillain-Barre syndrome associated with cancer.* Cancer 18:157–163, 1965.

Kori, SH, Foley, KM and Posner, JB: *Brachial plexus lesions in patients with cancer: 100 cases.* Neurology 31:45–50, 1981.

Krain, LS: *The association of pemphigus with thymoma or malignancy: A critical review.* Br J Derm 90:397–405, 1974.

Lambert, EH and Rooke, ED: *Myasthenic state and lung cancer.* In Brain, WR and Norris, FH, jr

(EDS): *The Remote Effects of Cancer on the Nervous System.* Grune & Stratton, New York, 1965, pp 67–80.

LAMBERT, EH, EATON, LM AND ROOKE, ED: *Defect of neuromuscular transmission associated with malignant neoplasms.* Am J Physiol 187:612–613, 1956.

LANG, B, WRAY, D, NEWSOM-DAVIS, J, ET AL: *Autoimmune aetiology for myasthenic (Eaton-Lambert) syndrome.* Lancet ii:224–226, 1981.

LENMAN, JAR, FLEMING, AM, ROBERTSON, MAH, ET AL: *Peripheral nerve function in patients with bronchial carcinoma. Comparison with matched controls and effects of treatment.* J Neurol Neurosurg Psychiatry 44:54–61, 1981.

LISAK, RP, MITCHELL, M, ZWEIMAN, B, ET AL: *Guillain-Barre syndrome and Hodgkin's disease: Three cases with immunological studies.* Ann Neurol 1:72–78, 1977.

LITWIN, SD AND ZANJANI, ED: *Lymphocytes suppressing both immunoglobulin production and erythroid differentiation in hypogammaglobulinemia.* Nature 266:57–58, 1977.

LUNDH, H, NILSSON, O AND ROSEN, I: *4-Aminopyridine—A new drug tested in the treatment of Eaton-Lambert syndrome.* J Neurol Neurosurg Psychiatry 40:1109–1112, 1977.

LUNDH, H, NILSSON, O AND ROSEN, I: *Novel drug of choice in Eaton-Lambert syndrome.* J Neurol Neurosurg Psychiatry 46:684–685, 1983.

MASAOKA, A, NAGAOKA, Y AND KOTAKE Y: *Distribution of thymic tissue at the anterior mediastinum. Current procedures in thymectomy.* J Thorac Cardiovasc Surg 70:747–754, 1975.

MCKINNEY, AS: *Neurologic findings in retroperitoneal mass lesions.* South Med J 66:862–864, 1973.

MCLEOD, JG: *Carcinomatous neuropathy.* In DYCK, PJ, THOMAS, PK, LAMBERT, EH (EDS): *Peripheral Neuropathy.* WB Saunders, Philadelphia, 1975, pp 1301–1313.

MCLEOD, JG AND WALSH, JC: *Peripheral neuropathy associated with lymphomas and other reticuloses.* In DYCK, PJ, THOMAS, PK AND LAMBERT, EH (EDS): *Peripheral Neuropathy.* WB Saunders, Philadelphia, 1975, pp 1314–1325.

MCQUILLEN, MP AND JOHNS, RJ: *The nature of the defect in the Eaton-Lambert syndrome.* Neurology 17:527–536, 1967.

MITCHELL, DM AND OLCZAK, SA: *Remission of a syndrome indistinguishable from motor neurone disease after resection of bronchial carcinoma.* Br Med J 2:176–177, 1979.

MOORE, AV, KOROBKIN, M, POWERS, B ET AL: *Thymoma detection by mediastinal CT: Patients with myasthenia gravis.* AJR 138:217–222, 1982.

MOSS, AA AND HANELIN, LG: *Occult malignant tumors in dermatologic disease. The futility of radiological search.* Radiology 123:69–71, 1977.

NAMBA, T, BRUNNER, NG AND GROB D: *Idiopathic giant cell polymyositis. Report of a case and review of the syndrome.* Arch Neurol 31:27–30, 1974.

NAMBA, T, BRUNNER, NG AND GROB, D: *Myasthenia gravis in patients with thymoma, with particular reference to onset after thymectomy.* Medicine 57:411–433, 1978.

NEWSOM-DAVIS, J, MURRAY, N, WRAY, D, ET AL: *Lambert-Eaton myasthenic syndrome: Electrophysiological evidence for a humoral factor.* Muscle Nerve 5:S17–S20, 1982.

NISCE, LZ AND CHU, FC: *Radiation therapy of brachial plexus syndrome from breast cancer.* Radiology 91:1022–1025, 1968.

NOBLER, MP: *Mental nerve palsy in malignant lymphoma.* Cancer 24:122-127, 1969.

NORRIS, FH, JR AND ENGEL, WK: *Carcinomatous amyotrophic lateral sclerosis.* In BRAIN, WR AND NORRIS, FH, JR (EDS): *The Remote Effects of Cancer on the Nervous System.* Grune & Stratton, New York, 1965, pp 24–34.

NORRIS, FH, JR, IZZO, AJ AND GARVEY, PH: *Brief report: Tumor size and Lambert-Eaton syndrome.* In BRAIN, WR AND NORRIS, FH, JR (EDS): *The Remote Effects of Cancer on the Nervous System.* Grune & Stratton, New York, 1965, pp 81–82.

NORRIS, FH, JR, EATON, JM AND MIELKE, CH: *Depression of bone marrow by guanidine.* Arch Neurol 30:184–185, 1974.

OLSON, ME, CHERNIK, NL AND POSNER, JB: *Infiltration of the leptomeninges by systemic cancer. A clinical and pathologic study.* Arch Neurol 30:122–137, 1974.

OOSTERHUIS, HJGH, FELTKAMP, TEW, VAN ROSSUM, AL, ET AL: *HL-A antigens, autoantibody production, and associated diseases in thymoma patients, with and without myasthenia gravis.* Ann NY Acad Sci 274:468–474, 1976.

PANCOAST, HK: *Superior pulmonary sulcus tumor. Tumor characterized by pain, Horner's syndrome, destruction of bone and atrophy of hand muscles.* JAMA 99:1391–1396, 1932.

PAPATESTAS, AE, ALPERT, LI, OSSERMAN KE, ET AL: *Studies in myasthenia gravis: Effects of thymectomy. Results on 185 patients with nonthymomatous and thymomatous myasthenia gravis, 1941–1969.* Am J Med 50:465–474, 1971.

PAPATESTAS, AE, GENKINS, G, KORNFELD, P, ET AL: *Transcervical thymectomy in myasthenia gravis.* Surg Gynecol Obst 140:535–540, 1975.

PATTON, WF, AND LYNCH, JP, III: *Lymphomatoid granulomatosis. Clinicopathologic study of four cases and literature review.* Medicine 61:1–12, 1982.

PAUL, T, KATIYAR, BC, MISRA, S, ET AL: *Carcinomatous neuromuscular syndromes. A clinical and quantitative electrophysiological study.* Brain 101:53–63, 1978.

PAULSON, DL: *Carcinomas in the superior pulmonary sulcus.* J Thorac Cardiovasc Surg 70:1095–1103, 1975.

PAULSON, DL: *Carcinomas in the superior pulmonary sulcus.* Ann Thorac Surg 28:3–4, 1979.

PEARSON, CM: *The incidence and type of pathologic alterations observed in muscles in a routine autopsy survey.* Neurology 9:757–766, 1959.

PETERS, HA AND CLATANOFF, DV: *Spinal muscular atrophy secondary to macroglobulinemia. Reversal of symptoms with chlorambucil therapy.* Neurology 18:101–108, 1968.

PRINEAS, J: *Polyneuropathies of undetermined cause.* Acta Neurol Scand (Suppl 44) 46:1–72, 1970.

ROSEN, P AND ARMSTRONG, D: *Nonbacterial thrombotic endocarditis in patients with malignant neoplastic diseases.* Am J Med 54:23–29, 1973.

ROWLAND, LP AND SCHOTLAND, DL: *Neoplasms and muscle disease.* In BRAIN, WR AND NORRIS, FH, JR (EDS): *The Remote Effects of Cancer on the Nervous System.* Grune & Stratton, New York, 1965, pp 83–97.

SANDERS, DB, KIM, YI, HOWARD, JF JR, ET AL: *Eaton-Lambert syndrome: A clinical and electrophysiological study of a patient treated with 4-aminopyridine.* J Neurol Neurosurg Psychiatry 43:978–985, 1980.

SCHMALZL, F, GASSER, RW, WEISER, G, ET AL: *Lymphomatoid granulomatosis with primary manifestation in the skeletal muscular system.* Klin Wochenschr 60:311–316, 1982.

SCHOLD, SC, CHO, ES, SOMASUNDARAM, M, ET AL: *Subacute motor neuronopathy: A remote effect of lymphoma.* Ann Neurol 5:271–287, 1979.

SCHOLD, SC, WASSERSTROM, WR, FLEISHER, M, ET AL: *Cerebrospinal fluid biochemical markers of central nervous system metastases.* Ann Neurol 8:597–604, 1980.

SLATER, G, PAPATESTAS, AE, GENKINS, G, ET AL: *Thymomas in patients with myasthenia gravis.* Ann Surg 188:171–174, 1978.

SMITH, B: *Skeletal muscle necrosis associated with carcinoma.* J Pathol 97:207–210, 1969.

SOUADJIAN, JV, ENRIQUEZ, P, SILVERSTEIN, MN, ET AL: *The spectrum of diseases associated with thymoma.* Arch Intern Med 134:374–379, 1974.

SPAAR, FW: *Paraproteinemias and multiple myeloma.* In VINKEN, PJ AND BRUYN, GW (EDS): *Handbook of Clinical Neurology,* Vol 39. North-Holland Publishing, Amsterdam, 1980, pp 131–179.

SWASH, M: *Acute fatal carcinomatous neuromyopathy.* Arch Neurol 30:324–326, 1974.

SWICK, HM, PRESTON, DF AND MCQUILLEN, MP: *Gallium scans in myasthenia gravis.* Ann NY Acad Sci 274:536–554, 1976.

TEOH, R, BARNARD, RO AND GAUTIER-SMITH, PC: *Polyneuritis cranialis as a presentation of malignant lymphoma.* J Neurol Sci 48:399–412, 1980.

TESTA, GF AND ANGELINI, C: *Assessment of the value of thymic scan in myasthenia gravis.* J Neurol 220:21–29, 1979.

THEOLOGIDES, A: *Asthenia in cancer.* Am J Med 73:1–3, 1982.

THOMAS, JE AND WALTZ AG: *Neurological manifestations of nasopharyngeal malignant tumors.* JAMA 192:103–106, 1965.

THOMAS, JE AND COLBY, MY, JR: *Radiation-induced or metastatic brachial plexopathy? A diagnostic dilemma.* JAMA 222:1392–1395, 1972.

THOMAS, MH AND CHISHOLM, GD: *Retroperitoneal fibrosis associated with malignant disease.* Br J Cancer 28:453–458, 1973.

TROJABORG, W, FRANTZEN, E AND ANDERSEN, J: *Peripheral neuropathy and myopathy associated with carcinoma of the lung.* Brain 92:71–82, 1969.

TURGMAN, J, BRAHAM, J, MODAN, B, ET AL: *Neurological complications in patients with malignant tumors of the nasopharynx.* Eur Neurol 17:149–154, 1978.

UNSOLD, R, SAFRAN, AB, SAFRAN, E, ET AL: *Metastatic infiltration of nerves in the cavernous sinus.* Arch Neurol 37:59–61, 1980.

URICH, H AND WILKINSON, M: *Necrosis of muscle with carcinoma: Myositis or myopathy?* J Neurol Neurosurg Psychiatry 33:398–407, 1970.

WALSH, JC: *Neuropathy associated with lymphoma.* J Neurol Neurosurg Psychiatry 34:42–50, 1971.

Wilkins, EW, Edmunds, H, jr and Castleman, B: *Cases of thymoma at the Massachusetts General Hospital.* J Thorac Cardiovasc Surg 52:322–328, 1966.

Weisberger, EC and Dedo, H: *Cranial neuropathies in sinus disease.* Laryngoscope 87:357–363, 1977.

Yuill, GM: *Leukaemia: Neurological involvement.* In Vinken, PJ and Bruyn, GW (eds): *Handbook of Clinical Neurology,* Vol 39. North-Holland Publishing, Amsterdam, 1980, pp 1–26.

Chapter 7

RENAL DISORDERS

DISORDERS OF MUSCLE

Although myopathic muscle weakness is not common in patients with renal disease, several different causes have been identified (Table 25). All but two of these are discussed in Chapters 2 and 3.

Iron Overload and Hemodialysis Patients

Recently Bregman and colleagues (1980) described 10 patients who developed proximal muscle weakness while on maintenance hemodialysis and were found to have iron overload without hemochromatosis. They had been given the usual oral iron supplements during hemodialysis, which had been in effect for periods of 1 to 8 years. Serum ferritin levels were elevated, and bone marrow iron stores were excessive. All 10 patients were said to have chronic proximal muscle weakness, the clinical features of which were not described. EMG and CPK were normal, but motor nerve conduction velocity was moderately reduced in most of the patients. Type 2 atrophy was seen in four out of seven muscle biopsy specimens, with a mild degree of muscle fiber necrosis in two cases and mild denervation changes in two cases. All of the biopsies showed iron deposition in macrophages or in muscle fibers.

The authors attributed the muscle weakness to a myopathy caused by iron deposition, but the data presented do not really demonstrate that the weakness was due to a myopathy, much less one caused by iron toxicity. As the authors themselves pointed out, iron deposition in muscle, without weakness, is a frequent finding in hemosiderosis and hemochromatosis. It is possible that these patients had other causes of muscle weakness, and that the iron deposition was unrelated or was a consequence rather than a cause of muscle injury, although two of the patients improved after iron supplements were withdrawn. Clearly, more clinical and laboratory information is needed before accepting the concept of "iron-overload myopathy."

TABLE 25. Causes of Myopathy in Chronic Renal Failure

Type	Cause
Chronic myopathy with normal serum enzymes	Uremic (osteomalacia) myopathy Aluminum intoxication Chronic phosphorus depletion Iron overload (?)
Subacute myopathy with high serum enzymes or myoglobinuria	Chronic potassium deficiency Azotemic vasculopathy
Acute, reversible paralysis	Chronic potassium deficiency with acute hypokalemia

Ischemic Myopathy in Azotemic Hyperparathyroidism

Patients with chronic renal failure and secondary hyperparathyroidism have a tendency to develop arterial calcification and ischemic gangrene of the digits. Occasionally, the occlusive arterial changes lead to the appearance of large patches of ischemic skin necrosis in the lower extremities (Anderson et al. 1968; Mallick and Berlyne 1968). In 1969, Richardson and coworkers (1969) drew attention to a syndrome of subacute necrotizing myopathy, myoglobinuria, and ischemic ulceration of skin in patients with azotemic hyperparathyroidism. The small arteries of the subcutaneous tissues and muscles were severely narrowed by calcification and fibrous intimal hyperplasia, while arteries in other organs were largely unaffected.

Several similar cases have been reported since then (Chazan et al. 1970; Goodhue et al. 1972). Peterson (1978) found radiologic evidence of extensive arterial calcification in 12 (9 percent) of 131 patients who had functioning kidney grafts; 5 of these patients had muscle symptoms, associated in 3 cases with extensive cutaneous gangrene.

The myopathy develops subacutely with proximal muscle pain and weakness, at first occurring mainly during exercise (as might be expected from the ischemic cause) but soon progressing to muscle pain at rest, with incapacitating muscle weakness and tenderness, greater in the proximal limbs and trunk. Serum enzymes are moderately or markedly increased, EMG shows myopathic abnormalities, and myoglobinuria may occur. Extensive necrosis of the skin and subcutaneous tissues usually develops around the same time; the skin lesions are located primarily on the buttocks and thighs and sometimes appear on the trunk (Fig. 33). The onset of skin necrosis may be heralded by livedo reticularis, which develops into large, dark-red, tender patches that soon become gangrenous ulcers covered by black eschars. At this stage the disorder is likely to be fatal. Other patients present with peripheral vascular ischemic symptoms: gangrene of the toes or fingers, or even of the whole limb, sometimes necessitating amputation (Conn et al. 1973). For some reason patients with distal ischemic symptoms do not usually have proximal muscle and skin necrosis.

The vascular calcifications may be apparent on soft-tissue x-rays (Fig. 34), but they are seen to best advantage by means of magnified fine-grain radiography, by which bone changes can be simultaneously evaluated. With this technique, Meema and associates (1976) observed calcifications of distal limb arteries in 30 to 50 percent of patients with severe chronic renal disease; the incidence increased with age. Serial studies demonstrated a progressive increase of calcification in 36 percent of nondialyzed patients, in 13 percent of post-transplantation patients, and in 8 percent of hemodi-

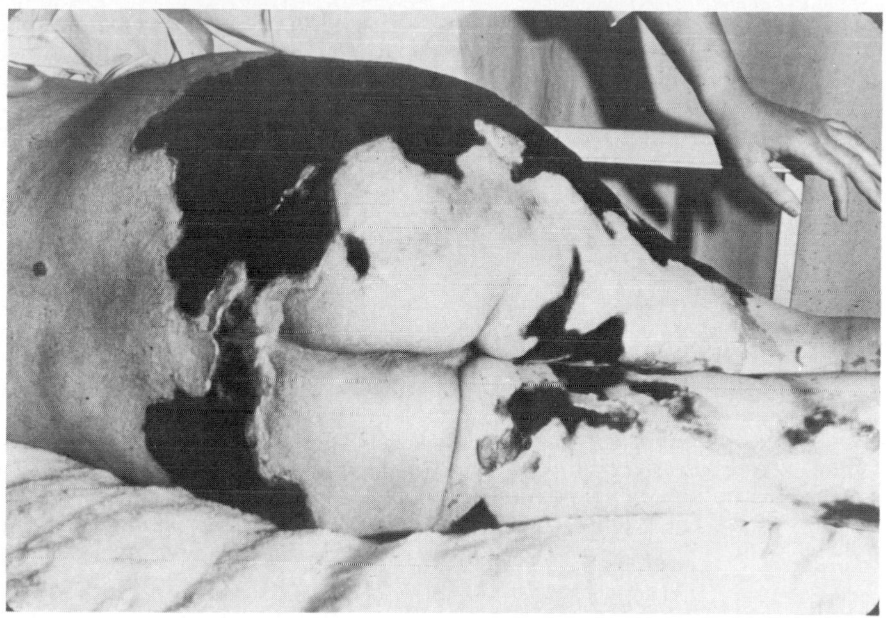

FIGURE 33. A patient with ischemic necrosis of skin and muscle owing to azotemic hyperparathyroidism. (From Richardson et al., 1969, with permission.)

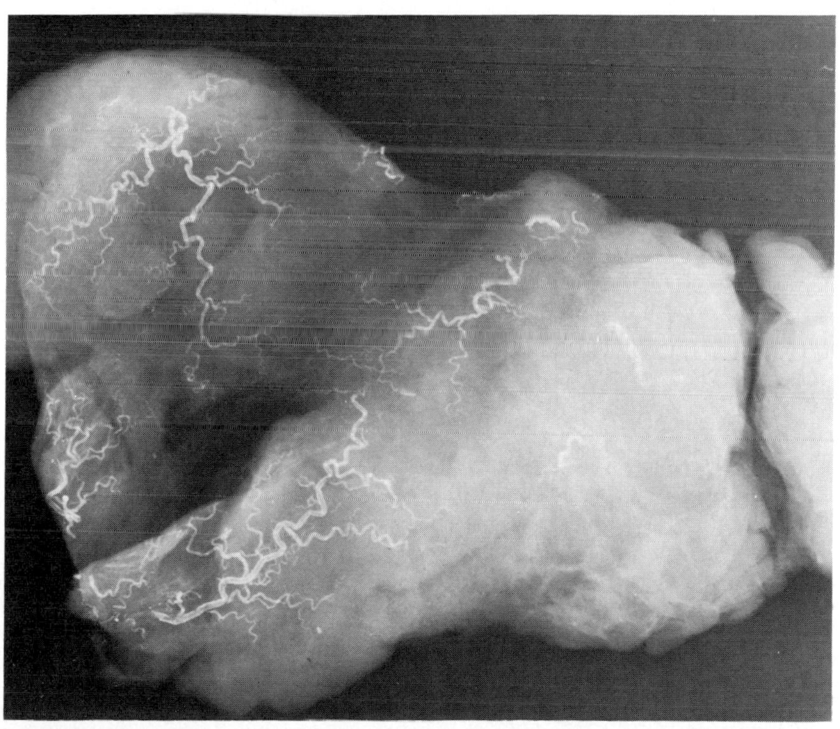

FIGURE 34. Calcification of muscular arteries in azotemic hyperparathyroidism. Postmortem radiograph of pectoral muscle. (From Richardson et al., 1969, with permission.)

alyzed patients. When arterial calcification is observed in the proximal limb muscles, the likelihood of ischemic myopathy developing is probably much greater than when only distal arterial calcification is present.

Microscopic examination of skin and muscle shows striking changes in arterioles and small arteries, consisting of medial calcification and occlusive fibrous intimal proliferation (Fig. 35). The affected muscle shows the typical changes of ischemia and infarction. The viscera usually show little or no vascular or ischemic changes.

Pathophysiology. There is convincing evidence that secondary hyperparathyroidism is responsible for the metastatic calcification that occurs in some persons with chronic renal failure. A high serum calcium-phosphorus product increases the risk that calcium phosphate will be deposited in soft tissues, and treatment with vitamin D must therefore be monitored carefully to keep the calcium-phosphorus product below 75 (Mallick and Berlyne 1968). However, arterial calcification can occur in patients whose serum calcium and calcium-phosphorus product are normal; therefore, simple precipitation of calcium phosphate probably does not account for the vascular lesions. The vascular changes have been likened to the experimental syndrome of "calciphylaxis" described by Selye (1962), but the precise mechanism

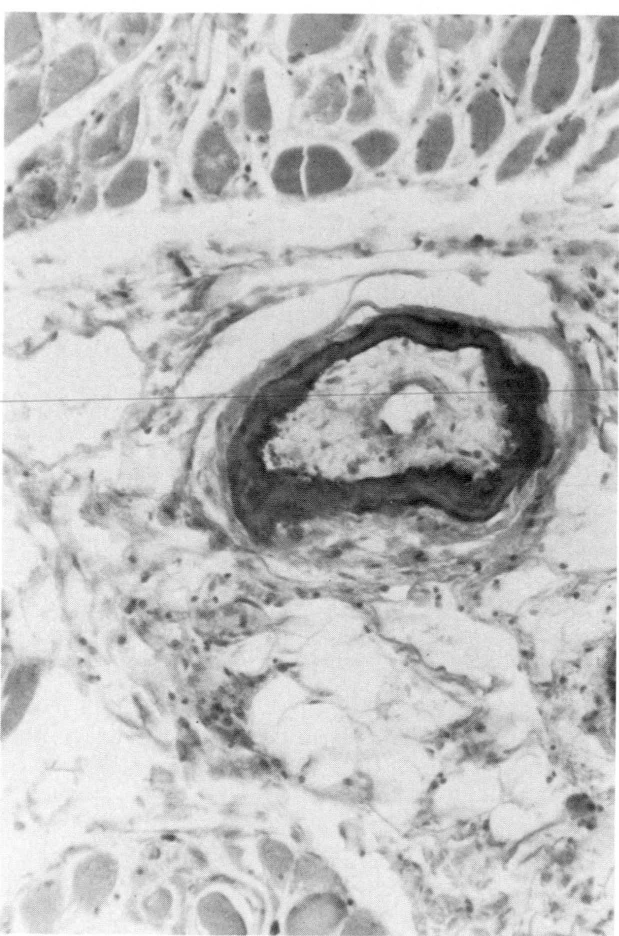

FIGURE 35. A muscular artery from a patient with azotemic hyperparathyroidism, showing fibrous intimal proliferation and medial calcification.

remains unclear. Similar arterial lesions in uremic rats (Ejerblad et al. 1979) appeared to begin with necrosis of smooth muscle cells in the media of large arteries; this was followed by calcification of the middle zone of the media. In smaller arteries, degeneration of the internal elastic lamina appeared to precede calcium deposition in the inner zone of the media and was often accompanied by fibrous intimal proliferation. Parathyroidectomy reduced the severity of these changes but did not prevent them entirely. From these experiments it appears that biochemical changes in the arterial media may precede overt calcification; the nature of this biochemical abnormality and its relation to hyperparathyroidism remain to be elucidated.

The recorded experience with several fatal cases suggests that aggressive measures should be undertaken to control hyperparathyroidism in patients with progressive vascular calcification, preferably before overt signs of ischemia appear. (Another reason for concern is that hyperparathyroidism causes deterioration of renal function in transplant patients.) Patients on hemodialysis should be considered for renal transplantation, while post-transplantation patients may require subtotal parathyroidectomy.

DISORDERS OF NEUROMUSCULAR TRANSMISSION

Spontaneous myasthenic weakness has not been reported as a direct consequence of uremia, but drugs with weak neuromuscular blocking activity may induce overt myasthenia-like weakness in patients with renal insufficiency. The principal examples are the aminoglycoside antibiotics (see Chapter 10), but recently D,L-carnitine was found to cause bulbar and limb weakness in 4 of 20 patients on maintenance hemodialysis. This effect appeared to be due to the D isomer, since L-carnitine was subsequently administered without ill effects. (L-carnitine, the natural isomer, is depleted by chronic hemodialysis; the resulting impairment of long-chain fatty acid metabolism causes hypertriglyceridemia, which is reversed by treatment with L-carnitine.) Electrophysiologic studies demonstrated a defect of neuromuscular transmission resembling the presynaptic block caused by hemicholinium, a substance that depletes cholinergic nerve terminals of acetylcholine, by inhibiting the uptake of choline (De Grandis et al. 1980; Bazzato et al. 1981).

High blood levels of D-carnitine or the aminoglycoside antibiotics partly account for their toxicity in uremic patients. A low serum calcium concentration may also contribute, by reducing the amount of acetylcholine released by nerve impulses. It is also possible that uremia alters the function of peripheral nerve terminals and renders them especially sensitive to drugs that act on the presynaptic side of the neuromuscular junction. For the same reasons, magnesium salts should be administered very cautiously to azotemic patients.

PERIPHERAL NERVE DISORDERS

Uremic Polyneuropathy

In 1963, Asbury and associates (1963) drew attention to a distal, symmetric, sensorimotor polyneuropathy in several patients with advanced chronic renal disease. Hitherto unrecognized, uremic polyneuropathy is now known to be an important cause of disability in patients maintained on hemodialysis, and the development of neuropathy has become one of the principal criteria for recommending renal transplantation.

Clinical Features

The clinical picture is fairly uniform (Thomas et al. 1971; Nielsen 1971a, 1971b; Asbury 1975). Sensory and motor symptoms begin in the distal lower extremities and ascend as the neuropathy worsens, always remaining more severe in the legs than in the arms. Sensory symptoms generally outweigh motor symptoms. Paresthesia (tingling or pins and needles) and dysesthesia begin in the toes and feet and are soon symmetrically distributed, slowly creeping up the legs over the course of months or years. Burning feet and other spontaneous pains occur in fewer than one fourth of patients. Muscle weakness, rarely appearing before the sensory complaints, likewise starts in the toes and ankles and ascends gradually. The neuropathy is mild or moderately severe in most patients, but a few patients develop severe, generalized weakness and wasting, with a distal predominance, and become bedridden. Although the course is usually gradual, rapid worsening sometimes occurs; this may be largely motor in character, and it has been suggested that such cases may result from a coincidental attack of acute idiopathic polyneuritis (Bolton 1980; Dyck et al. 1979).

The signs of neuropathy are more prevalent than the symptoms, if muscle cramps and restless legs are excluded from consideration. Depression of ankle jerks and impairment of vibration sense in the toes and feet are the earliest signs. Sensory loss is distal and symmetric and mainly involves the large nerve fiber functions of vibration sense, position sense, and touch. Distal weakness and atrophy are less common and initially are confined to toe and ankle movements. Signs of autonomic nerve involvement are rarely seen.

Incidence

In one series of undialyzed patients (Nielsen 1971a; 1971b), 40 percent of the patients had sensory complaints and 51 percent had signs of neuropathy. These patients had been azotemic for 29 to 42 months at the time of examination. In a more recent series of patients referred for hemodialysis, Thomas (1978) found sensory symptoms in only 8 percent, reduced ankle jerks in 14 percent, diminished vibration sense in 9 percent, and weakness in 3 percent; overall, about 25 percent of the patients had some signs of neuropathy. The low incidence of clinical abnormalities in this series probably reflects a practice of earlier referral of patients for hemodialysis. Males were affected more often than females in the early reports, but in Nielsen's series (1971a) this was not the case.

In general, neuropathy does not appear until the glomerular filtration rate has fallen below 20 ml per minute and the plasma creatinine level has risen above 6 mg per dl (Savazzi et al. 1980). In a prospective study of 14 uremic patients whose mean serum creatinine level was 6.4 mg per dl initially and who were followed without dialysis therapy for an average of 13 months, only the 2 patients with the highest final serum creatinine levels (13.5 mg per dl and 18 mg per dl) developed polyneuropathy (Jebsen et al. 1967). Likewise, Nielsen (1974a) observed a reduction of vibration perception (assessed by a quantitative technique) in 8 of 13 patients with severe uremia who were followed for a mean of 5 months before dialysis, by which time the creatinine clearance was 1.0 to 4.2 ml per minute. The vibration threshold tended to remain stable for several months and then to rise abruptly over the course of a few weeks, and other signs of neuropathy soon followed.

Laboratory Findings

The spinal fluid protein is increased in 50 to 60 percent of uremic patients, usually to less than 100 mg per dl (Fishman 1980), but there is no indication that this occurs more frequently in patients with neuropathy. Motor nerve conduction velocities and distal motor latencies are reduced to a mild or moderate degree in patients with clinical neuropathy. Nerve conduction slowing generally precedes the onset of clinical symptoms or signs, a finding that points to a "preclinical" stage of neuropathy. In one study, 22 (73 percent) of 30 uremic patients had reduced motor nerve conduction velocities in the peroneal nerves, though neuropathy was detected clinically in only 4 patients (Hansen and Ballantyne 1978). The earliest changes are likely to be detected in the distal lower extremity nerves, which are the longest in the body. As in other axonal polyneuropathies, there is only a rough, inverse correlation between conduction velocity and clinical severity (Thomas et al. 1971; Nielsen 1974a). Sensory nerve responses are often small or unobtainable, and sensory latencies are prolonged, even in the upper limbs. EMG shows changes of chronic denervation in distal muscles, mainly in patients with clinical weakness.

Using a computer-assisted method for estimating the total of motor units (i.e., axons) in the motor nerves, Hansen and Ballantyne (1978) found a reduced number of motor units in the extensor digitorum brevis muscle (peroneal nerve) in 40 percent of uremic patients, the majority of whom did not have clinical weakness. Thus, loss of functioning motor axons appears to precede the appearance of clinically detectable weakness. Hansen and Ballantyne (1978) also found indications that collateral sprouting from surviving axons was impaired compared with that of patients with diabetic neuropathy.

Pathology

The major finding is a distal degeneration of axons, with secondary degeneration of myelin sheaths, the longest nerves being most severely affected (Asbury 1975). This is the picture of a "dying-back" axonal neuropathy. The large-diameter nerves appear to be most severely affected. Secondary paranodal demyelination also occurs, as in other axonal neuropathies. The slowing of motor nerve conduction velocity is partly due to the predominant affection of large-diameter nerves, which have the fastest conduction velocities; secondary demyelination is probably another factor. The preferential impairment of large-fiber sensory functions (especially vibration sense) can also be understood on this basis. The ultrastructural abnormalities are similar to those found in other axonal neuropathies and do not offer obvious clues to the pathogenesis.

Effects of Hemodialysis and Renal Transplantation

Successful renal transplantation has a striking beneficial effect on uremic neuropathy. Patients with mild neuropathy recover completely, and patients with moderate or severe neuropathy show substantial improvement. In Nielsen's prospective study (1974b), eight of ten patients with moderate or severe clinical neuropathy recovered completely within 1 year of successful transplantation, and the other two patients were much improved; seven patients with mild neuropathy recovered completely within 3 months. The course of recovery was biphasic, with rapid improvement in the first few months followed by slow improvement during the ensuing 1 to 2 years. Motor and sensory nerve conduction abnormalities also improved in a biphasic fashion, but the electrical abnormalities persisted longer than the clinical signs (Nielsen 1974c).

The response to hemodialysis has been more variable. In most patients sensory symptoms (paresthesia and pain) improve quickly during the first several weeks, and vibration perception improves for several months, but other clinical signs of neuropathy tend to persist or to improve very slowly, and nerve conduction velocities generally show little improvement (Nielsen 1974a; Bolton 1980). A few patients deteriorate; switching to a more efficient dialyzer or increasing the frequency or duration of dialysis may reverse or stabilize the neuropathy, but these measures are not consistently successful (Bolton 1980). Thus, renal transplantation is still the most effective treatment for moderate or severe uremic neuropathy. If effective dialysis is begun early enough, disabling neuropathy can usually be prevented (Thomas 1978; Chan and Eng 1979). Peritoneal dialysis was initially thought to be more effective than hemodialysis in preventing the development of neuropathy, but recent experience suggests that neuropathy worsens slowly during chronic peritoneal dialysis (Bolton 1980).

The rapid, early improvement of sensory complaints and vibration-sense threshold following institution of regular hemodialysis implies a very labile disturbance of nerve metabolism. Indeed, electrophysiologic improvement has been demonstrated on the day after dialysis (Lang and Forsstrom 1977) and even within an hour of completing dialysis (Stanley et al. 1977). The improvement was mainly evident in the amplitude of responses, not in the conduction velocities. It is possible that the factors responsible for these labile fluctuations of nerve function are not the same as those responsible for lasting nerve damage in uremia.

Electrophysiologic Measurements as a Guide to Therapy

In the early years of hemodialysis there was much enthusiasm for using motor nerve conduction tests to gauge the adequacy of a dialysis regimen. However, there is only a rough correlation between the clinical severity of the neuropathy and the degree of slowing of nerve conductions, and there is a temporal dissociation between electrophysiologic and clinical improvement or worsening (Nielsen 1974a). Dyck and colleagues (1979) were unable to distinguish a clearly inadequate short-dialysis program from an adequate long-dialysis program by changes in motor or sensory nerve conduction, comparing either conduction velocity or amplitude of responses; five of nine patients on the short program developed non-neurologic uremic complications, while the thirteen patients on the long program remained asymptomatic. Even predialysis levels of urea and creatinine were not reliable indications of the need for dialysis. Attempts have been made to improve the prognostic value of electrophysiologic testing by combining several parameters (Savazzi et al. 1980) or by using research techniques (Hansen and Ballantyne 1978), but these are unlikely to be widely applicable. It seems, therefore, that the adequacy of a dialysis regimen must continue to be judged by clinical status and standard blood chemistries rather than by nerve conduction tests.

Pathophysiology. It is hard to escape the presumption that uremic polyneuropathy is caused by the accumulation of some unidentified toxins that are less effectively removed by hemodialysis than by the normal kidney. Scribner and colleagues suggested that, since small molecules like urea and creatinine pass dialysis membranes easily, the putative toxins are in the "middle molecule" range of 500 to 2000 daltons (Milutinovic et al. 1978). The toxic mechanism might be an indirect one, such as failure to absorb an essential nutrient, or might involve a more direct interference with neuronal function. So far no specific substance has been convincingly identified as toxic to peripheral nerves.

Instead of looking for the "middle molecule," it might be more fruitful to elucidate the pathophysiology of the dying-back phenomenon in uremic neuropathy. The fact that the longest axons are affected at their most distal extremities strongly suggests a deficiency of one or more essential metabolites that are manufactured in the nerve cell body and are transported down the axon to the nerve terminals. A preliminary study of axonal transport in nerve biopsy samples from 4 uremic patients suggested that an abnormality might be present (Brimijoin and Dyck 1979), but more information is needed before any conclusions are drawn. The effect of uremia on the various components of axoplasmic transport has not yet been examined in experimental animals.

Focal Neuropathies

Compression Neuropathies

Clinical experience suggests that uremic patients may be more than normally susceptible to nerve compression palsies. Ulnar nerve compression at the elbow, peroneal nerve compression at the head of the fibula, and carpal tunnel syndrome are the most frequently encountered focal neuropathies, as they are in nonuremic patients (Thomas 1978; Nielsen 1971a). The carpal tunnel syndrome is especially liable to occur in a limb with a Cimino-Brescia fistula of the forearm. Warren and Otieno (1975) elicited carpal tunnel symptoms on the side of a forearm shunt in 23 out of 36 dialysis patients, 4 of whom went on to carpal tunnel surgery. In addition to the usual nocturnal exacerbation of pain and paresthesias, these patients commonly experience increased symptoms during hemodialysis, and occlusion of the radial artery below the fistula may lesson the symptoms, suggesting that ischemia owing to vascular steal by the shunt may be a factor (Harding and Le Fanu 1977). There is also evidence that increased venous pressure and edema of the wrist and hand play a role; the hand volume is greater on the affected side and it increases during dialysis (Warren and Otieno 1975). Soft-tissue edema and ischemia are known to be important causative factors in the ordinary carpal tunnel syndrome.

The shunt itself can cause a compression neuropathy; this may be the explanation of an anterior interosseous nerve paralysis reported after placement of a forearm shunt (Adams 1981).

Ischemic Neuropathies

A vascular steal mechanism appears to be the major factor responsible for the occurrence of painful neuropathies distal to an upper-arm shunt between the brachial artery and the cephalic vein (Bolton et al. 1979). The median, ulnar, and radial nerves all tend to be involved, each to a different degree; painful dysesthesia, numbness, and weakness are greater in the distal portion of the limb, as would be expected from an ischemic mechanism. The sensory and motor symptoms may appear immediately upon placement of the shunt or may begin later, worsening transiently with each dialysis. Ischemic skin changes may be associated. Sudden worsening may occur spontaneously and may not resolve when the shunt is closed, suggesting that the nerve has undergone ischemic degeneration. Bolton and colleagues (1979) speculated that nerve injury may be more frequent with upper arm shunts because of the relatively precarious blood supply of nerves at that level. However, they also demonstrated that upper arm shunts cause more severe vascular steal phenomena in the hand than are usual in forearm shunts, so the degree of distal ischemia may simply be more severe in upper arm shunts. Some authors have attributed these neuropathies to entrapment, perhaps related to increased venous pressure and engorgement of the tissues surrounding the nerves (Delmez et al. 1982).

Mononeuritis Multiplex Following Rapid Ultrafiltration Dialysis

Meyrier and coworkers (1972) reported three patients who developed acute, asymmetric neuropathies in several limbs a few weeks after ultrafiltration was added to their hemodialysis regimen for the purpose of reducing edema. It appeared that a marked reduction of blood volume, resulting from the rapid fluid removal, may have caused ischemic damage to nerves already sensitized by uremia. None of the patients had diabetes mellitus, but all three had severe hypertension and manifested fluctuating hypotension during ultrafiltration dialysis.

Retroperitoneal Hemorrhage

In a recent survey, Milutinovich and colleagues (1977a) found that 3 percent of patients on chronic hemodialysis had suffered a spontaneous retroperitoneal hemorrhage. Both the bleeding diathesis of uremia and the use of heparin and other anticoagulants during hemodialysis probably contribute to the high incidence of the complication. When retroperitoneal hemorrhage involves the psoas or iliac muscle, it often presents with an acute femoral neuropathy (Vanichayakornkul et al. 1974). Compression neuropathies caused by intramuscular hematomas are discussed in Chapter 8.

SYMPTOMS OF UNCERTAIN PATHOGENESIS

Acute Hyperkalemic Paralysis

Patients with persistent hyperkalemia caused by chronic renal failure sometimes develop acute, generalized weakness resembling an acute polyneuropathy. The serum potassium level rises during the paralytic episode, and treatment that lowers the potassium level helps to reverse the paralysis. This syndrome is discussed in Chapter 2.

Restless Legs Syndrome

This curious syndrome, which is described in Chapter 1, occurs in 17 to 50 percent of patients with advanced renal failure (Nielson 1971a; Thomas 1978; Bolton 1980). It tends to appear at a late stage of uremia, but it is unclear whether it is related to uremic neuropathy. Nielsen (1971a) found that the complaint was just as frequent in patients without neuropathy as in those with neuropathy, while Thomas (1978) elicited a history of restless legs syndrome in 20 percent of patients with clinical or subclinical neuropathy, compared with only 5 percent of patients without neuropathy.

The relation of restless legs syndrome to uremic neuropathy is at most an indirect one and is not influenced by the severity of the neuropathy.

Thomas (1978) found no change in the incidence of restless legs syndrome before and after a long period on maintenance hemodialysis, although the incidence of distal lower extremity paresthesia fell from 7 percent to 0. Restless legs syndrome occurs in other types of polyneuropathy, especially diabetic neuropathy, but the great majority of patients with restless legs syndrome do not have neuropathy or any other predisposing illness. Although the symptom is often mentioned together with cramps, there appears to be no particular association between these symptoms (Nielsen 1971a).

There was no treatment for restless legs syndrome until Matthews (1979) found that clonazepam was highly effective in the idiopathic disorder. Read and associates (1981) confirmed the efficacy of clonazepam in 14 out of 15 uremic patients, most of whom had failed to respond to diazepam and other medications. The dosage of clonazepam was 0.5 mg twice a day; in patients with mainly nocturnal symptoms, the first dose was given at 6 PM and the second dose a half hour before retiring.

Muscle Cramps

Painful nocturnal leg cramps, which may appear well before any clinical evidence of neuropathy, are frequent complaints in uremic patients. In Nielsen's (1971a, 1971b) series, they were present in 50 percent of the patients and were not significantly associated with the presence or absence of neuropathy. Many patients also experience flexion cramps in the hands. Vigorous diuretic treatment is sometimes a precipitating factor.

Muscle cramps are an especially troublesome problem during hemodialysis treatments. In a prospective study (Neal et al. 1981), over a period of 6 weeks fully one third of 36 patients experienced muscle cramps during dialysis; 4 patients had one episode of cramping, 4 patients had two episodes, and 4 patients had three or more episodes. The cramps tend to appear toward the end of the dialysis session and they correlate with higher ultrafiltration rates and greater loss of weight. Surface EMG monitoring has shown that dialysis cramps, like ordinary cramps, are accompanied by high-voltage EMG activity. After 1 or 2 hours of dialysis there is a gradual increase of "tonic" EMG activity, culminating in outright cramps after about 4 hours of dialysis (Howe et al. 1978).

The standard dialysis fluid is slightly hypotonic, with a sodium concentration around 130 mEq per liter. This suggests that either plasma volume contraction or hyponatremia could be responsible for dialysis cramps. Stewart and colleagues (1972) attempted to prevent cramps by increasing the dialysate sodium concentration to 145 mEq per liter. The frequency of cramps was reduced from 49 to 23 percent of dialysis episodes, but the patients complained of thirst and gained weight between dialyses. Catto and coworkers (1973) gave patients 140 mEq of oral slow-release sodium before and during each dialysis, reducing the frequency of cramps from 55 to 41 percent. Other nephrologists chose to treat the cramps as they occurred, by intravenous injection of some type of hypertonic solution. Gotloib and Servadio (1972) and Jenkins and Dreher (1975) reported that rapid injection of hypertonic sodium chloride (35 to 105 mEq of sodium) relieved cramps within 2 to 3 minutes. Acchiardo and associates (1975), in a double-blind trial, injected 20 ml of various solutions as an intravenous bolus; 23.5-percent sodium chloride (70 mEq of sodium) was effective in 83 percent of cramp episodes, compared with 13 percent relief of cramps from a 5-percent glucose placebo, while 0.9-percent sodium chloride, 20-percent glucose, and mannitol were effective in 40 to 50 percent of episodes. Milutinovich and colleagues (1977b) and Neal and coworkers (1981) found that 50-percent glucose was effective in 65 to 89 percent of episodes, in a dose of 50 ml or 1 ml per kg.

These observations suggest that hyponatremia is not the cause of dialysis cramps, and that either extracellular volume contraction or hypo-osmolarity is responsible. Dialysis cramps thus seem comparable to the cramps precipitated by vigorous diuretic therapy, profuse perspiration, diarrhea, or vomiting in nonuremic persons.

PATHOPHYSIOLOGY. As discussed in Chapter 1, the pathophysiology of muscle cramps is poorly understood, but EMG data indicate that they involve high-frequency discharges of motor nerves, a fact ignored by authors who speculate about the relation of muscle metabolism to dialysis cramps (Jenkins and Dreher 1975; Chillar and Desforges 1972). The site of origin of this spontaneous neural activity is still unknown, and the relation between extracellular volume contraction or hypo-osmolarity and peripheral nerve hyperactivity is equally obscure. Dialysis patients may, in fact, provide an excellent opportunity to learn more about the mechanism of muscle cramps; such studies would benefit not only uremic patients but the large number of healthy persons who suffer frequent and distressing leg cramps.

REFERENCES

ACCHIARDO, SR, SKOUTAKIS, VA AND HATCH, FE: *Management of muscle cramps in hemodialysis patients. Controlled prospective study.* Proc Dial Trans Forum 5:6–8, 1975.

ADAMS, JP: *Arteriovenous shunts and nerve damage.* Lancet i:211, 1981.

ANDERSON, DC, STEWART, WK AND PIERCY, DM: *Calcifying panniculitis with fat and skin necrosis in a case of uraemia with autonomous hyperparathyroidism.* Lancet ii:323–325, 1968.

ASBURY, AK: *Uremic neuropathy.* In DYCK, PJ, THOMAS, PK AND LAMBERT, EH (EDS): *Peripheral Neuropathy.* WB Saunders, Philadelphia, 1975, pp 982–992.

ASBURY, AK, VICTOR, M AND ADAMS, RD: *Uremic polyneuropathy.* Arch Neurol 8:413–428, 1963.

BAZZATO, G, COLI, U, LANDINI, S, ET AL: *Myasthenia-like syndrome after D,L- but not L-carnitine.* Lancet i:1209, 1981.

BOLTON, CF: *Peripheral neuropathies associated with chronic renal failure.* Can J Neurol Sci. 7:89–96, 1980.

BOLTON, CF, DRIEDGER, AA AND LINDSAY, RM: *Ischaemic neuropathy in uraemic patients caused by bovine arteriovenous shunt.* J Neurol Neurosurg Psychiatry 42:810–814, 1979.

BREGMAN, H, WINCHESTER, JF, KNEPSHIELD, JH, ET AL: *Iron-overload-associated myopathy in patients on maintenance haemodialysis: A histocompatibility-linked disorder.* Lancet ii:882–885, 1980.

BRIMIJOIN, S AND DYCK, PJ: *Axonal transport of dopamine-β-hydroxylase and acetylcholinesterase in human peripheral neuropathy.* Exp Neurol 66:467–478, 1979.

CATTO, GRD, SMITH, FW AND MACLEOD, M: *Treatment of muscle cramps during maintenance haemodialysis.* Br Med J 3:389–390, 1973.

CHAN, JC AND ENG G: *Long-term hemodialysis and nerve conduction in children.* Pediat Res 13:591–593, 1979.

CHAZAN, JA, AMBLER, M, KALDERON, A, ET AL: *Vascular deposits causing ischemic myopathy in uremia. Two brothers with hereditary nephritis.* Ann Intern Med 73:73–79, 1970.

CHILLAR, RK AND DESFORGES, JF: *Muscular cramps during maintenance haemodialysis.* Lancet ii:285, 1972.

CONN, J, JR, KRUMLOVSKY, FA, DEL GRECO, F, ET AL: *Calciphylaxis: Etiology of progressive vascular calcification and gangrene?* Ann Surg 177:206–210, 1973.

DE GRANDIS, D, MEZZINA, C, FIASCHI, A, ET AL: *Myasthenia due to carnitine treatment.* J Neurol Sci 46:365–371, 1980.

DELMEZ, JA, HOLTMANN, B, SICARD, GA, ET AL: *Peripheral nerve entrapment syndromes in chronic hemodialysis patients.* Nephron 30:118–123, 1982.

DYCK, PJ, JOHNSON, WJ, LAMBERT, EH, ET AL: *Comparison of symptoms, chemistry, and nerve function to assess adequacy of hemodialysis.* Neurology 29:1361–1368, 1979.

Ejerblad, S, Eriksson, I and Johansson, H: *Uraemic arterial disease. An experimental study with special reference to the effect of parathyroidectomy.* Scand J Urol Nephrol 13:161–169, 1979.

Fishman, RA: *Cerebrospinal Fluid in Diseases of the Nervous System.* WB Saunders, Philadelphia, 1980, pp 303–304.

Goodhue, WW, Davis, JN and Porro, RS: *Ischemic myopathy in uremic hyperparathyroidism.* JAMA 221:911–912, 1972.

Gotloib, L and Servadio, C: *Muscle cramps during maintenance haemodialysis.* Lancet ii:877, 1972.

Hansen, S and Ballantyne, JP: *A quantitative electrophysiological study of uraemic neuropathy. Diabetic and renal neuropathies compared.* J Neurol Neurosurg Psychiatry 41:128–134, 1978.

Harding, AE and Le Fanu, J: *Carpal tunnel syndrome related to antebrachial Cimino-Brescia fistula.* J Neurol Neurosurg Psychiatry 40:511–513, 1977.

Howe, RC, Wombolt, DG and Michil, DD: *Analysis of tonic muscle activity and muscle cramps during hemodialysis.* J Dialysis 2:85–99, 1978.

Jebsen, RH, Tenckhoff, H and Honet, JC: *Natural history of uremic polyneuropathy and effects of dialysis.* N Engl J Med 277:327–332, 1967.

Jenkins, PG and Dreher, WH: *Dialysis-induced muscle cramps: Treatment with hypertonic saline and theory as to etiology.* Trans Am Soc Artif Intern Organs 21:479–481, 1975.

Lang, AH and Forsstrom, J: *Transient changes of sensory nerve functions in uraemia.* Acta Med Scand 202:495–500, 1977.

Mallick, NP and Berlyne, GM: *Arterial calcification after vitamin-D therapy in hyperphosphataemic renal failure.* Lancet ii:1316–1319, 1968.

Matthews, WB: *Treatment of the restless legs syndrome with clonazepam.* Br Med J 1:751, 1979.

Meema, HE, Oreopoulos, DG and de Veber, GA: *Arterial calcification in severe chronic renal disease and their relationship to dialysis treatment, renal transplantation and parathyroidectomy.* Radiology 121:315–321, 1976.

Meyrier, A, Fardeau, M and Richet, G: *Acute asymmetrical neuritis associated with rapid ultrafiltration dialysis.* Br Med J 2:252–254, 1972.

Milutinovic, J, Babb, AL, Eschback, JW, et al: *Uremic neuropathy: Evidence of middle molecule toxicity.* Artif Organs 2:45–51, 1978.

Milutinovich, J, Follette, WC and Scribner, BH: *Spontaneous retroperitoneal bleeding in patients on chronic hemodialysis.* Ann Intern Med 86:189–192, 1977a.

Milutinovich, J, Graefe, U, Follette, WC, et al: *Effect of hypertonic glucose on the muscular cramps of hemodialysis.* Ann Intern Med 90:926–928, 1977b.

Neal, CR, Resnikoff, E and Unger, AM: *Treatment of dialysis-related muscle cramps with hypertonic dextrose.* Arch Intern Med 141:171–173, 1981.

Nielsen, VK: *The peripheral nerve function in chronic renal failure. I. Clinical symptoms and signs.* Acta Med Scand 190:105–111, 1971a.

Nielsen, VK: *The peripheral nerve function in chronic renal failure. II. Intercorrelation of clinical symptoms and signs and clinical grading of neuropathy.* Acta Med Scand 190:113–117, 1971b.

Nielsen, VK: *The peripheral nerve function in chronic renal failure. VII. Longitudinal course during terminal renal failure and regular hemodialysis.* Acta Med Scand 195:155–162, 1974a.

Nielsen, VK: *The peripheral nerve function in chronic renal failure. VIII. Recovery after renal transplantation. Clinical aspects.* Acta Med Scand 195:163–170, 1974b.

Nielsen, VK: *The peripheral nerve function in chronic renal failure. IX. Recovery after renal transplantation. Electrophysiological aspects (sensory and motor nerve conductions).* Acta Med Scand 195:171–180, 1974c.

Peterson, R: *Small vessel calcification and its relationship to secondary hyperparathyroidism in the renal homotransplant patient.* Radiology 126:627–633, 1978.

Read, DJ, Feest, TG and Nassim, MA: *Clonazepam: Effective treatment for restless legs syndrome in uremia.* Br Med J 283:885–886, 1981.

Richardson, JA, Herron, G, Reitz, R, et al: *Ischemic ulcerations of skin and necrosis of muscle in azotemic hyperparathyroidism.* Ann Intern Med 71:129–138, 1969.

Savazzi, GM, Migone, L and Cambi, V: *The influence of glomerular filtration rate on uremic polyneuropathy.* Clin Nephrol 13:64–72, 1980.

Selye, H: *Calciphylaxis.* University of Chicago Press, Chicago, 1962.

Stanley, E, Brown, JC and Pryor, JS: *Altered peripheral nerve function resulting from haemodialysis.* J Neurol Neurosurg Psychiatry 40:39–43, 1977.

STEWART, WK, FLEMING, LW AND MANUEL, MA: *Muscle cramps during maintenance haemodialysis.* Lancet i:1049–1051, 1972.

THOMAS, PK: *Screening for peripheral neuropathy in patients treated by chronic hemodialysis.* Muscle Nerve 1:396–399, 1978.

THOMAS, PK, HOLLINRAKE, K, LASCELLES, RG, ET AL: *The polyneuropathy of chronic renal failure.* Brain 94:761–780, 1971.

VANICHAYAKORNKUL, S, CIOFFI, RF, HARPER, E, ET AL: *Spontaneous retroperitroneal hematoma. A complication of hemodialysis.* JAMA 230:1164–1165, 1974.

WARREN, DJ AND OTIENO, LS: *Carpal tunnel syndrome in patients on intermittent haemodialysis.* Postgrad Med J 51:450–452, 1975.

Chapter 8

CIRCULATORY DISORDERS

SUDDEN OCCLUSION OF A MAJOR LIMB ARTERY

Tourniquet Ischemia

Since the pioneering experiments of Sir Thomas Lewis in the 1930s there has been continuing interest in the effects of tourniquet ischemia on nerve and muscle function. Tourniquet experiments serve as a model for the study of circulatory arrest produced by embolism and thrombosis, but they have a practical application as well, for they furnish precise information about the length of time that a tourniquet can be safely applied during limb surgery.

As a model of disease, the tourniquet has certain drawbacks. It produces total circulatory arrest in the limb, whereas in spontaneous arterial occlusion ischemia is usually incomplete and venous return is not prevented. Furthermore, the pressure from a pneumatic cuff, though far less injurious than the outmoded ligature, directly compresses the underlying nerves, especially at the edges of the cuff, and the resulting mechanical deformation causes local nerve injury that may persist long after the rapidly reversible effects of simple ischemia (Ochoa et al. 1972). Cuff pressures of 500 to 1000 torr are generally required to produce this injury in primate experiments (Fowler et al. 1972). To minimize such injury during limb surgery, the width of the cuff should exceed the diameter of the limb by 20 percent, and the pneumatic pressure should be set 50 to 75 torr above systolic blood pressure, using a reliable pressure gauge (Klenerman 1980).

Nerve Conduction

When the tourniquet is inflated above systolic pressure, a well-defined sequence of physiologic changes occurs in the nerves distal to the tourniquet. The earliest change is a decline in electrical threshold (a rise in excitability) of the peripheral nerves that begins a few seconds after the onset of ischemia, reaches a nadir at about 3 minutes, and returns to normal after 10 to 12 minutes of ischemia. The subject experiences tingling in the distal digits as a result of spontaneous discharge of large-diameter sensory nerve fibers (Kugelberg 1946). After about 15 minutes of ischemia, conduction begins to fail in the large-diameter, longest sensory nerves, causing numbness in the tips of the fingers or toes. Anesthesia spreads proximally at a rate of 3 to 4 cm per minute, and there is dysesthesia of the hypesthetic skin because the function of small-diameter pain nerves is preserved. Conduction of pain and temperature impulses is abolished somewhat later.

Loss of motor function likewise spreads centripetally from the most distal portions of the limb. Both failure of neuromuscular transmission and blockade of motor nerve conduction contribute to the paralysis, but neuromuscular transmission usually fails in 5 to 20 minutes, at a time when nerve conduction is retained and the muscle still responds to direct stimulation. The duration of ischemia required to abolish neuromuscular transmission depends on the motor nerve activity: the greater the activity, the sooner transmission will fail, about 3500 to 7000 impulses being transmissible before total neuromuscular block occurs. This suggests that synaptic block occurs because the stores of acetylcholine in the nerve terminals are exhausted, with resynthesis having been prevented by the ischemia (Dahlbäck et al. 1970).

When the tourniquet is released after ½ hour of ischemia, nerve function returns in 30 to 60 seconds; after 2 hours of ischemia it returns in a few minutes. As sensation returns there is unpleasant tingling and dysesthesia of the skin, probably caused both by spontaneous discharges of sensory nerves and by an earlier return of function in pain nerves than in large-diameter sensory nerves. As the period of ischemia is increased to 4 and 6 hours, recovery after release of the tourniquet is more delayed, and some nerve fibers are irreversibly damaged, eventually undergoing Wallerian degeneration. After 8 hours of ischemia all of the nerves are irreversibly damaged. However, the nerves beneath the cuff suffer earlier and more severe damage because of the combined effects of compression and ischemia (Lundborg 1970). Thus, from the standpoint of nerve damage, the safe period for tourniquet compression is about 2 hours, but with respect to ischemia alone the safe period is 4 to 6 hours.

Although nerves are irreversibly damaged by ischemia lasting 8 hours or longer, release of the tourniquet restores good blood flow in the microcirculation of nerves even after 10 to 16 hours of ischemia. After 6 to 8 hours of ischemia, however, the nerve capillaries become increasingly leaky to albumin and other large molecules, and there is extravasation of fluid resulting in endoneurial edema, which Lundborg (1980) considered to be mainly responsible for the irreversibility of ischemic nerve damage. These changes are more severe and appear earlier directly under the pneumatic tourniquet.

Muscle Function

During ischemia, muscle excitability persists until well after nerve conduction ceases. If the muscle remains inactive, little or no pain will be felt in the limb, because analgesia occurs within 30 minutes, before muscle pain begins. However, if the muscle is exercised before the onset of ischemic paralysis, a deep, continuous, aching pain develops within a few minutes and persists until the circulation is restored or until the pain nerves cease to function. This phenomenon, like ischemic myocardial pain and the pain of intermittent claudication, is presumably caused by metabolites produced by working muscle. Lewis (1946) observed that when a cuff is inflated around the upper arm, pain develops in the forearm flexor muscles and hand after the fist is strongly clenched 30 to 40 times, and after 60 to 90 contractions the pain is so intense that it is impossible to continue voluntary muscle work.

The substances responsible for this pain have never been identified. Rodbard (1975) postulated that they are large molecules because they are somewhat slow to diffuse away when circulation is restored; although the pain subsides in a few seconds, pain returns quickly if exercise is resumed within 5 to 10 minutes after release of the cuff. It has been suggested that lactic acid is not responsible because patients with muscle phosphorylase also experience severe pain during ischemic exercise even though no lactic acid is produced; however, in these patients the pain could be attributable to muscle contracture, while in normal subjects the painful muscle remains relaxed.

Paradoxically, although muscle function persists longer than nerve function during ischemia, muscle damage occurs earlier. Although no histologic signs of muscle fiber damage were observed in human hand muscles sampled immediately after 2 hours of tourniquet ischemia (Józsa et al. 1980), animal experiments have shown that signs of muscle damage appear several hours after the circulation is restored. In the rabbit hind limb, even 2 hours of ischemia is followed by a delayed rise of serum CPK activity, which begins 4 to 8 hours after circulation is restored and reaches a peak in 24 to 48 hours. Much larger, but still delayed CPK elevations followed tourniquet applications lasting 4 to 6 hours. Cooling the limb during the ischemia prevents the CPK elevation almost completely (Presta and Ragnotti 1981). Tourniquet ischemia of 30 minutes causes necrosis of a few scattered muscle fibers, while 2 hours of ischemia leads to moderately extensive degeneration of muscle fibers, the majority of which are type 1, the type of muscle fibers that depend heavily on oxidative metabolism as a source of energy (Dahlbäck 1970). If ischemia is maintained for 6 to 8 hours without artificial cooling, complete muscle necrosis will usually result.

In practice, 1 hour of tourniquet ischemia is probably safe for both muscle and nerve, and longer periods of tourniquet ischemia can probably be employed if the tourniquet is released periodically. Dog experiments have shown that the rise of CPK activity in the venous effluent of muscle after 3 hours of tourniquet ischemia can be prevented by releasing the tourniquet for 15 minutes after each hour (Chiu et al. 1976).

Pathophysiology of Muscle Damage. The remarkably delayed rise of serum CPK activity suggests that most of the muscle damage occurs during reperfusion and is more closely related to the events that follow the restoration of circulation than to the metabolic changes present during ischemia. In various mammals, ischemia lasting up to 3 hours produces a steady decline in the muscle membrane potential, a marked increase in muscle lactate content, a 50-percent drop in creatine phosphate levels, but little or no reduction in ATP concentration (Enger et al. 1978; Jennische et al. 1979; Miller et al. 1979). Similar changes have been observed in the lower limbs of children (Haljamäe and Enger 1975) and of adults (Larsson and Hultman 1979). Considering that the energy charge hardly changes during or after ischemia, that the creatine phosphate levels are restored within 5 minutes after release of the tourniquet, and that the lactate levels and membrane potential return to normal within an hour (Enger et al. 1978), one would expect the effects of 2 to 3 hours of ischemia to be quite inocuous. However, the time course of metabolic changes observed in dog muscle (Enger et al. 1978) suggests that the heterogeneous metabolic properties of muscle fibers must be taken into account. Creatine phosphate and ATP levels decline maximally in the first hour and then remain stable during 2 more hours of ischemia, while lactate content rises at a steady rate. This may mean that low-glycolytic type 1 muscle fibers are metabolically exhausted during the first hour of ischemia, while high-glycolytic type 2 fibers maintain their high energy phosphate levels and continue to produce lactate until their glycogen stores are exhausted, in about 2 hours (Stock et al. 1971). Thus, Jennische and colleagues (1979) showed that the decline of high energy phosphates during ischemia is much greater in cat soleus muscle (mostly type 1) than in muscles with predominantly type 2 fibers. These differences may explain why type 1 fibers are much more readily damaged by ischemia and why hypothermia prevents this, by reducing the rate of ATP utilization.

Assuming that a serious depletion of cellular high energy phosphate content during ischemia is a necessary preliminary to cell damage, what is the difference between reversible and irreversible ischemic injury, and why does most of the cell necrosis occur after reperfusion of the tissue? There is now considerable evidence that raised intracellular calcium-ion levels are primarily responsible for both phenomena (Farber et al. 1981). The evidence comes from recent experimental studies of anoxic-ischemic cell injury in liver and heart. These tissues are much more dependent on aerobic metabolism than either red or white skeletal muscle. During the first 15 minutes of ischemia creatine phosphate stores are rapidly exhausted, and the ATP content falls steadily thereafter; after 60 minutes of ischemia, when glycolysis comes to a halt, the ATP content has fallen to less than 10 percent of normal, and mitochondrial function is markedly impaired (Jennings and Reimer 1981). Yet these changes are completely reversed by aerobic reperfusion, and there is no increase in cellular or mitochondrial calcium levels. After longer periods of ischemia, however, aerobic reperfusion is followed by a threefold to fourfold increase in tissue and mitochondrial calcium levels. The mitochondria, damaged by a high calcium content, are unable to regenerate ATP, and cell necrosis follows (Farber et al. 1981).

The key role of calcium in this sequence was shown in several ways. Lowering the calcium content of the perfusate during the first 5 minutes of reperfusion prevented the influx of calcium; mitochondrial calcium levels and ATP generation remained normal, and necrosis did not occur (Shine 1981; Nayler 1981). Pretreatment with chlorpromazine also prevented calcium influx, mitochondrial overload with calcium, and cell necrosis (Farber et al. 1981). Treatment with verapamil, in contrast, did not prevent excessive calcium influx during reperfusion but did prevent both mitochondrial overload with calcium and cell necrosis (Nayler 1981). Thus, the critical biochemical alteration during reperfusion appears to be irreversible mitochondrial damage by calcium overload (Fig. 36). If the tissue is permitted to resume aerobic metabolism while protected for only a few minutes from calcium overload, it will recover sufficiently to be immune to re-exposure to calcium.

What is the reason for the marked influx of calcium during reperfusion? Experimental data suggest that it results from a progressive loss of phospholipids from the plasma membrane during ischemia, a loss that can be prevented by chlorpromazine (Farber et al. 1981). A "detergent" action of long-chain lipid esters (which accumulate because anaerobiosis blocks their oxidation) and activation of endogenous phospholipases by calcium have been suggested as agents that possibly cause loss of phospholipids from mitochondrial and plasma membranes (Neely and Fenvray 1981; Farber et al. 1981).

Although these biochemical mechanisms have not been examined in the same detail in skeletal muscle, it is very likely that they apply, because they account for the delayed onset of muscle necrosis during reperfusion and the patchy necrosis of type 1 muscle fibers following ischemia of intermediate duration. Some authors have suggested that postischemic failure of oxidative metabolism may be caused by impaired microcirculation owing to capillary injury or to edema and raised tissue pressure (Enger et al. 1978; Miller et al. 1979), but these factors probably play only a minor part except in muscles situated in a closed fascial compartment. The fact that muscle lactate levels fall very slowly during aerobic reperfusion after several hours of ischemia is probably due not to inadequate microcirculation but to mitochondrial malfunction.

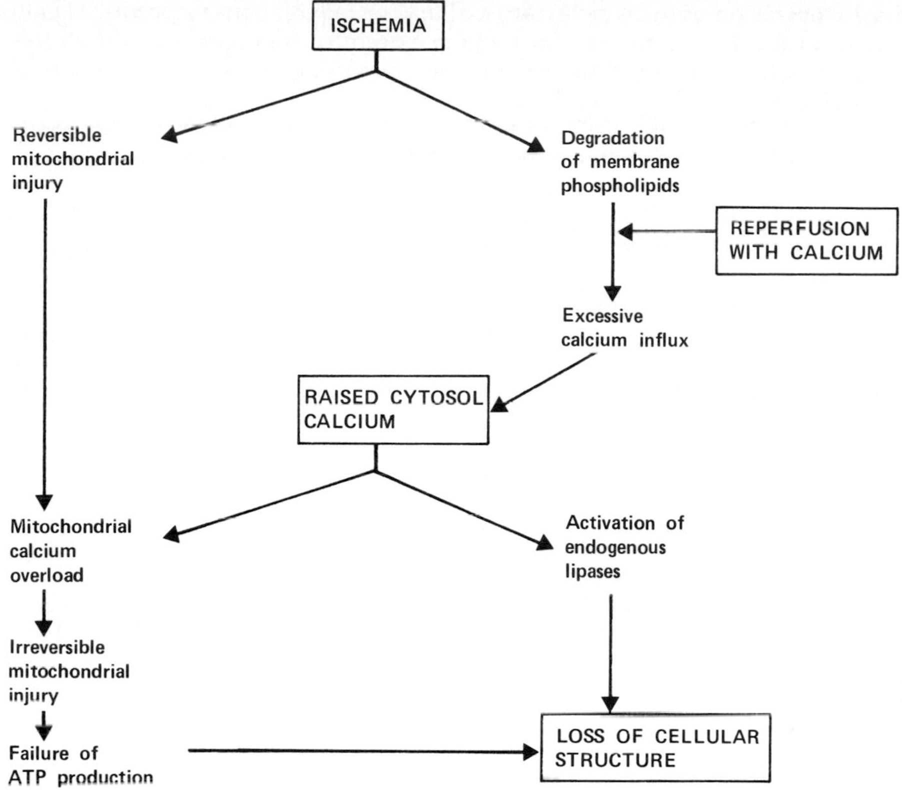

FIGURE 36. Hypothetical pathophysiology of ischemic muscle necrosis. (Adapted from Nayler, 1981, and Farber et al., 1981).

Embolism and Thrombosis of Major Limb Arteries

Clinical Features

The signs and symptoms of sudden occlusion of a major limb artery are well known (Lewis 1946; Slaney and Hamer 1973). Pallor and coolness of the skin gradually spread from the digits up the limb, and the distal pulses are lost. Numbness (with loss of touch sensation before pain sensation) and muscle weakness likewise spread in a centripetal direction toward the point of occlusion. Pins and needles paresthesias are more commonly experienced than in the circumstance of complete circulatory arrest produced by a tourniquet. Muscle pain occurs if the muscles are actively used before pain sensation is lost; as was mentioned previously, this pain continues either until circulation is restored or until analgesia supervenes during continuing ischemia. If the muscles remain inactive during the entire period of ischemia, however, pain may be minor or absent. The location of the arterial occlusion can be roughly correlated with the location of pain and the upper level of sensory loss. With obstruction of the aortic bifurcation pain may be present in any muscles of the legs, thighs, or hips, and the sensory and motor disturbances can rise to the mid-thighs or hips; one leg is often more affected than the other. Occlusion of the common femoral bifurcation, the commonest location, causes pain in the muscles below the knee, with numbness and weakness ascending to the knee. Occlusion of the popliteal artery causes pain, numbness, and weakness in the foot and lower leg. Similarly, occlusion of the subclavian, axillary, or brachial artery produces pain in any of the distal muscles of the upper extremity, together with numbness and weakness starting in the fingers and spreading proximally to the level of occlusion (Savelyev et al. 1977).

Occlusion of the distal aorta sometimes causes sudden, flaccid weakness of the lower extremities in a patchy, asymmetric distribution. Although motor findings may predominate, bladder and bowel function may be impaired and there may be patchy sensory loss in the legs without a sensory level on the trunk. The clinical signs of arterial insufficiency may be subtle and easily overlooked in patients with chronic atherosclerosis who have extensive collateral circulation to the lower extremities. The mechanism of the paralysis is uncertain, though the abrupt onset suggests a spinal cord location, and ischemia of the lumbosacral cord can lead to selective degeneration of the ventral gray matter containing the motor neurons (Herrick and Mills 1971).

Postischemic Muscle Swelling and Necrosis

Upon relief of prolonged occlusion of a major limb artery, marked hyperemia develops owing to the peripheral vasodilation produced by metabolic products escaping from the muscle. Some degree of muscle swelling is usual, reflecting interstitial edema caused both by increased filtration pressure at the arterial end of the capillaries and by anoxic injury to the capillaries, which become more permeable to colloids (Holden 1979). The edema usually clears uneventfully over the next 24 hours or so. Occasionally, however, after circulation has been occluded for several hours, postischemic swelling assumes a malignant form. This much-feared complication, which begins several hours after circulation is restored, is characterized by severe pain, rigidity, and swelling of the muscles, followed by hyperkalemia, hypocalcemia, myoglobinuria, and oliguria (Haimovicci 1979). The complication carries a high mortality rate, and amputation of the limb is necessary in many of the patients who survive. This sequence of events probably represents a calcium-dependent reperfusion syndrome. Presumably there is a large influx of calcium into muscle cells, leading to muscle contracture, which causes intense pain and rigidity of the limb, exhausts the remaining cellular stores, and initiates muscle necrosis. The resulting swelling further compromises capillary circulation, especially in the fascial compartments of the distal limb. Massive muscle necrosis leads to an outpouring of potassium and myoglobin, and myoglobinuria causes oliguria or anuria. As in other forms of rhabdomyolysis, hypocalcemia and hyperkalemia tend to occur, and ventricular fibrillation may result. Serum CPK activity is extremely high, as it is in other types of myoglobinuria.

This syndrome has occurred after embolectomy, thromboendarterectomy, or arterial bypass surgery performed on the aorta, the iliac artery, and the femoral artery. It is more likely to occur in a limb that has been ischemic for 8 hours or more, especially if it is already painful and rigid before surgery. In one series, 10 cases were encountered in 200 patients operated on for acute arterial occlusions (an incidence of 5 percent), and 75 percent of the postoperative deaths from this type of surgery are attributed to this cause (Haimovicci 1979).

Lesser degrees of postoperative muscle swelling, pain, and tenderness are more common, have a favorable outcome, and probably represent less extensive cellular injury or necrosis. Following temporary femoral artery occlusion during cardiopulmonary bypass surgery, massive edema requiring fasciotomies of the leg compartments occurred in 12 (10 percent) of 120 patients, and 24 other patients developed less serious leg swelling. The complication began 8 to 24 hours after bypass procedures lasting 2½ to 4 hours (Fisher et al. 1970).

Repair of Ischemic Muscle Necrosis

Skeletal muscle has the ability to regenerate rapidly and effectively after ischemic necrosis, provided that the microcirculation and venous channels are not thrombosed, so that effective circulation can be restored. In rat experiments, complete necrosis of the devascularized soleus muscle, left in situ, was followed by muscle regeneration beginning in a few days and proceeding to restoration of normal mechanical and histochemical properties within 30 days (Hanzlikova and Gutmann 1979). The more usual result of arterial occlusion, either in animal experiments in which the aorta is ligated (Karpati et al. 1974) or in human patients with temporary arrest of arterial circulation to a limb, is a patchy necrosis of small groups of muscle fibers, which are quickly replaced by regenerating muscle fibers. The major obstacle to successful repair of ischemic muscle necrosis is the perpetuation of ischemia by swelling within a tight fascial compartment. This problem is discussed next.

Compartment Syndromes

In certain portions of a limb, postischemic muscle swelling is restricted by osteofascial septa, which divide the limb into relatively rigid compartments. As a result of these restrictions, an elevated interstitial pressure may impede capillary circulation within the muscle, producing further ischemic swelling of the muscle—a vicious circle eventually causing ischemic muscle necrosis. Major nerve trunks running through the compartment also suffer compression and circulatory embarrassment. In contrast, distal arterial pulses are usually preserved, and clinical signs of ischemia are not observed in the digits, so that the damage taking place within the compartment is often unsuspected until it is irreversible. The end result is Volkmann's contracture: fibrotic shortening of the muscle, accompanied by sensorimotor paralysis distal to the compartment.

Compartment syndromes classically affect the forearm and foreleg; complete fascial confinement of muscles and nerves is not an anatomic feature of the thigh or upper arm. Experimental injection of saline within muscles produces a steep rise of interstitial pressure in the distal limbs but only a modest rise of pressure in the thigh or upper arm (Holden 1979). The muscle compartments of the leg and forearm are illustrated in Figure 37. In the leg there are four compartments: the *anterior tibial,* containing the deep peroneal nerve; the *peroneal,* containing the superficial peroneal nerve; the *deep posterior,* containing the posterior tibial nerve; and the *superficial posterior,* containing the sural nerve. In the forearm the *volar* compartment contains the anterior interosseous, median, and ulnar nerves, and the *dorsal* compartment contains the posterior interosseous and radial nerves. The deep posterior compartment of the leg and the volar compartment of the forearm are the ones most associated with ischemic muscle and nerve damage.

The clinical features of the compartment syndrome are increasing muscle pain aggravated by stretching, tense swelling of the muscles, and numbness and paralysis of the hand or foot in the distribution of the com-

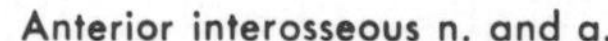

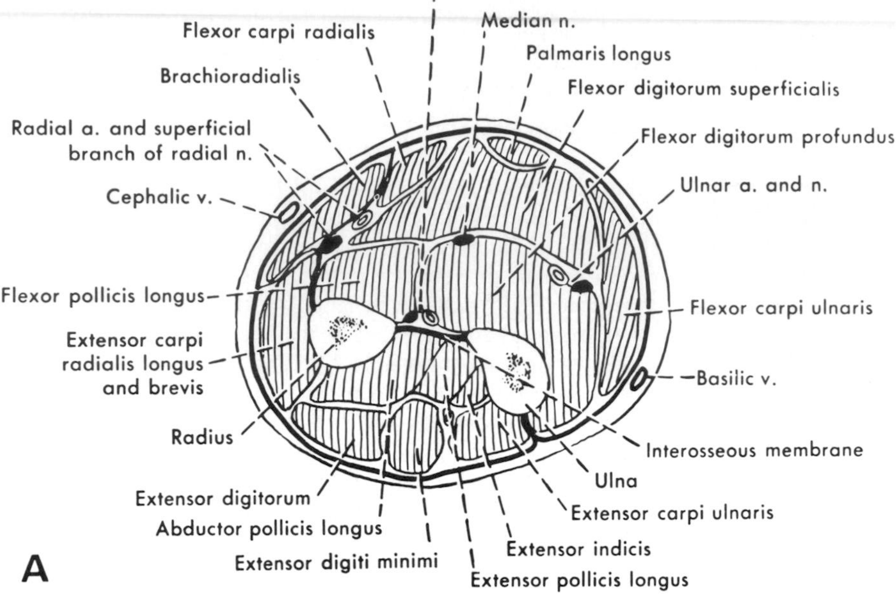

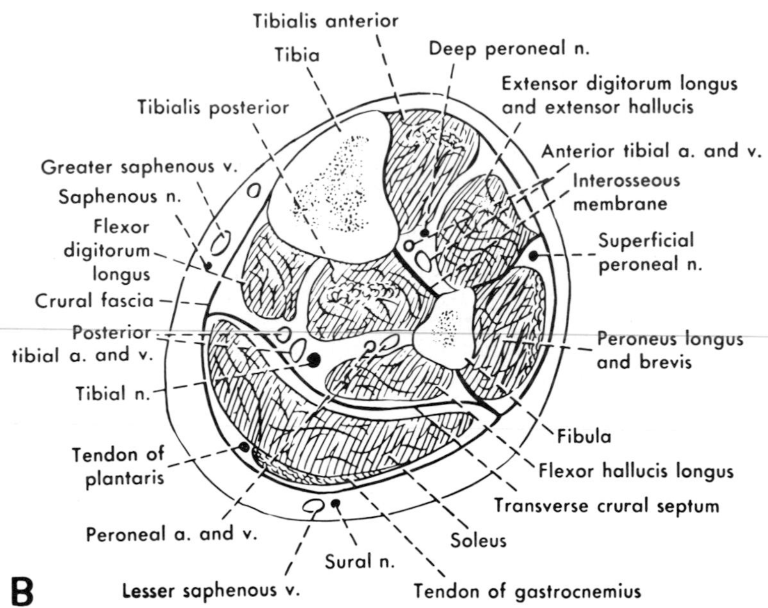

FIGURE 37. Cross sections through (*A*) the upper third of the forearm and (*B*) the lower part of the leg. The major fascial compartments are enclosed by heavy lines. (From Hollinshead, W.H.: *Anatomy for Surgeons*, ed. 3. Harper & Row, New York, 1982, with permission.)

promised nerves. The distal pulse is rarely absent, and the color and temperature of the hand or foot are usually unaffected. Early diagnosis can be obtained by inserting a wick catheter through a needle cannula to measure intracompartmental pressures; the catheter can be left in place to provide a series of pressure measurements during the critical period of observation. A pressure greater than 8 torr is considered to be elevated, and 30 torr is likely to impede capillary circulation (Mubarak et al. 1978). In animal experiments, muscle damage results from pressures of 34 torr maintained for 8 hours (Hargens et al. 1981).

When there is clinical evidence of muscle or nerve ischemia in a tight compartment, thorough decompression should be carried out by performing subcutaneous fasciotomies. In some cases skin closure can be achieved without undue rise in compartment pressure, while in others closure must be delayed until the muscle edema subsides (Mubarak et al. 1978). Mubarak and his colleagues recommend prophylactic fasciotomy, before clinical signs appear, if the compartment pressure is 30 torr or greater, but other authorities set a higher limit, up to 50 to 70 torr (Mubarak and Hargens 1981). The higher the pressure, presumably, the sooner muscle infarction can be expected to occur. Systemic hypotension appears to reduce the safe compartment pressure still further (Zweifach et al. 1980).

Compartment syndromes occur in several different clinical settings. Closed arterial injury caused by fractured bones or penetrating trauma are the classical precipitating factors, but tourniquet ischemia, arterial clamping during surgery, cardiac bypass operations, intramuscular hematomas, and crush injuries of the soft tissues have also been incriminated. Excessive leg exercise may precipitate an anterior tibial compartment syndrome (Mubarak and Hargens 1981).

Owen and associates (1979) postulate that the occurrence of myoglobinuria in patients rendered comatose by drug overdose or carbon monoxide poisoning results from high compartment pressures in limbs compressed by the weight of the patient's body. They showed that in normal subjects lying on a hard surface, mean interstitial pressures up to 100 torr will register in the forearm and up to 142 torr in the anterior tibial compartment, when the tissues are directly compressed by the head or torso. This explanation is probably an oversimplification of a complicated problem. There is little doubt that direct compression of muscles, arteries, and nerves causes muscle ischemia and nerve injury in a setting of hypotension, anoxia, and metabolic derangement, as pointed out by Penn and coworkers (1972) (Fig. 38). However, the thigh and gluteal muscles are predominantly affected, rather than the foreleg and forearm muscles, and usually the sciatic nerves are injured in the gluteal region, not below the knee. While soft-tissue pressure may have been quite high during the period of limb compression, there is little evidence that the vicious circle of a true compartment syndrome occurs in the thighs and buttocks, despite a description of a "gluteal compartment syndrome" (Owen et al. 1978). Mubarak and his colleagues (Mubarak et al. 1978; Owen et al. 1978) report good results from fasciotomy and epimysiotomy of deltoid, biceps, gluteal, and thigh muscles in such cases, but the intramuscular pressures in many of their patients were only moderately elevated, and they do not report the results of conservative treatment. Because of these uncertainties, there is still disagreement as to whether fasciotomy of the proximal limb muscles should be performed routinely in cases of this sort.

Neuropathy Caused by Acute Arterial Occlusion

Sunderland (1945) was the first to point out that the lateral popliteal (peroneal) nerve is especially vulnerable to ischemic damage by compression. In the popliteal region, where its superficial location exposes it to direct trauma, the nerve receives only a single nutrient artery. In contrast, the medial popliteal nerve has a rich anastomotic circulation derived from multiple arterial branches of the gluteal and femoral arteries.

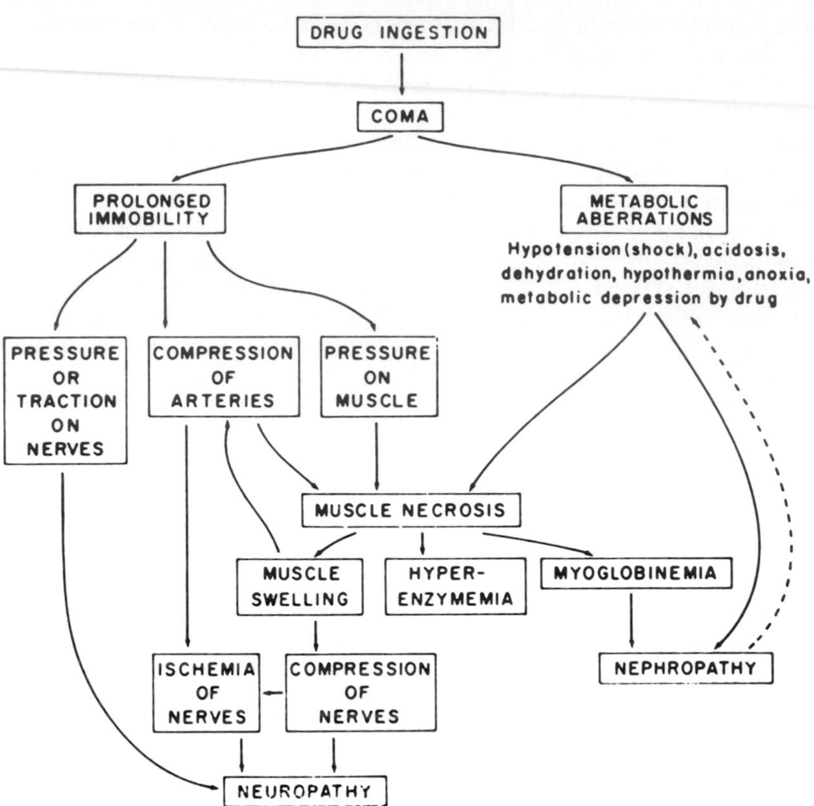

FIGURE 38. Pathophysiology of muscle necrosis and nerve trunk injuries in coma caused by drug overdose. (From Penn et al., 1972, with permission.)

For the same reason, paralysis of the lateral popliteal nerve may develop acutely following embolism or thrombosis of the femoral or popliteal artery (Ferguson and Liversedge 1954; Welti et al. 1961; Eames and Lange 1967). The usual clinical picture consists of a sudden pain in the calf or foot, coolness of the foot, foot drop, and loss of the pedal pulses. Superficial numbness may be present but is generally minor and confined to distal portions of the peroneal dermatome. In some cases there is also mild flexor weakness of the ankle and toes, and the ankle jerk is lost, indicating that the medial popliteal nerve is not entirely spared. Improvement can be expected over the next several months, and fairly good recovery of function is the rule.

Welti and associates (1961) reported the occurrence of an acute femoral neuropathy following embolic occlusion of the aortic bifurcation. In another case, embolism of the brachial artery caused paralysis of the radial nerve and of the thenar branch of the median nerve.

Temporary Aortic Occlusion During Surgery

When the infrarenal aorta is crossed-clamped during reconstructive surgery, the blood flow to the lower extremities is reduced by 50 to 65 percent (Eklöf et al. 1981a; Sjöström et al. 1982). The collateral arterial pathways that provide this surprisingly good circulation are better developed in older patients with atherosclerosis and intermittent claudication than in normal persons. After 1 to 2 hours of clamping, muscle lactate is markedly elevated, but ATP levels are unchanged, phosphocreatine levels have declined by only 30 percent, and the energy charge remains constant (Andersson et al. 1979). Following release of the aortic clamp, however, there is a paradoxical deterioration of muscle energy metabolism. There is an immediate, large increase of muscle blood flow, sometimes causing dangerous systemic hypotension; these hemodynamic changes result from vasodilation in the leg muscles and can be prevented by administration of alpha-adrenergic and $beta_1$-adrenergic blocking agents during surgery (Eklöf et al. 1981a). At the same time, muscle levels of ATP fall slightly, and the creatine and adenylate pools decline substantially, suggesting that these important metabolites are escaping from damaged muscle cells. Moreover, the muscle lactate level is still markedly elevated 20 minutes after declamping, indicating that oxidative function is significantly impaired (Eklöf et al. 1981b; Sjöström et al. 1982). This finding is especially remarkable when compared with the prompt restoration of normal metabolite levels after total tourniquet ischemia of similar duration.

The clinical significance of these changes is uncertain, since most patients are able to walk a day or two after surgery (Andersson et al. 1979). Even so, the potential for delayed muscle necrosis exists, especially after longer periods of aortic clamping. Eklöf and colleagues (1981b) were able to prevent these metabolic abnormalities in patients undergoing reconstructive arterial surgery by infusing low-molecular-weight dextran intravenously before and during the operation. They postulated that the beneficial effect of dextran resulted from improved microcirculation in the muscles; dextran has also been shown to improve capillary reperfusion after shock. If this explanation is correct, it implies that the primary cause of postischemic metabolic derangements in muscle is impairment of the microcirculation. Why this impairment should be greater after partial ischemia than after tourniquet ischemia is puzzling. It would be interesting to know whether infusion of low-molecular-weight dextran would improve the results of emergency embolectomy or thromboendarterectomy in major limb arteries.

Major Venous Occlusion

Sudden occlusion of the major venous drainage of a limb leads to massive swelling, induration, pain, and cyanosis—a condition known as *phlegmasia cerulea dolens.* It appears that elevated venous pressure and interstitial edema, combined with systemic hypovolemia, impede arterial flow and capillary perfusion in the muscle, leading to a type of compartment syndrome that may result in ischemic muscle necrosis. Fasciotomy has been advocated in the management of this rare disorder; it has been shown to be effective in animal experiments (Mubarak and Hargens 1981), but human experience is limited.

In a recently reported case, ligation of the inferior vena cava produced rhabdomyolysis and myoglobinuric renal failure, ending fatally (Olivero and Ayus 1978). The clinical picture closely resembled bilateral phlegmasia cerulea dolens, and aortography showed a sharp diminution of blood flow below the mid-thighs, the level to which swelling had ascended. Oliguria occurs in about a third of patients 24 hours after ligation of the inferior vena cava; this has been attributed to hypovolemia and renal hypoperfusion, but evidence of muscle necrosis and myoglobinuria may not have been looked for.

CHRONIC ARTERIAL INSUFFICIENCY OF THE LOWER EXTREMITIES

In contrast to the dramatic effects of acute occlusion of a major limb artery, chronic atherosclerotic occlusion of the arteries of the lower extremities is a slowly progressive, multifocal process in which there is time for a collateral circulation to develop to its maximal extent. Symptoms of vascular insufficiency may occur episodically as new occlusions develop and lead to new patterns of collateral circulation. Prominent among these symptoms are two neuromuscular syndromes: intermittent claudication and ischemic neuropathy.

Intermittent Claudication

Exercise of skeletal muscle becomes painful if the contractions are repeated for a long period of time. Pain appears sooner if the work load is increased or if contraction is sustained instead of intermittent. Pain is induced still more quickly if exercise is carried out while the arterial circulation is occluded. These commonplace facts account for the clinical syndrome of intermittent claudication, in which exercise of the leg muscles leads to muscle pain that increases rapidly and forces the patient to rest for a few minutes to allow the pain to subside. The pain is generally felt as a dull, aching tightness deep in the muscle, but it may be described as boring, stabbing, squeezing, pulling, or even burning. Although the pain is sometimes referred to as a cramp, there is no actual spasm in the painful muscles. The location of the pain is determined by the site of the major arterial occlusion (Taylor 1973). The most frequent lesion, present in about two thirds of patients, is occlusion of the superficial femoral artery between the groin and the knee, producing calf pain that sometimes radiates to the popliteal region and lower thigh. Aortoiliac occlusive disease induces pain in the gluteal and quadriceps muscles, while occlusion of the popliteal or more distal arteries causes pain in the foot.

In the typical case of superficial femoral artery occlusion, there is a good femoral pulse at the groin, but arterial pulses are absent at the knee and foot, though resting circulation appears to be good in the foot. Following exercise, the patient may complain of numbness of the foot as well as of pain in the calf, and the foot may be cold and pale, an indication that the circulation has been diverted to the arteriolar bed of the leg muscles.

Pathophysiology. The mechanism of the muscle pain generated during ischemic exercise is not fully understood. As was discussed earlier, the clinical experiments carried out by Lewis (1943) and subsequently extended by Rodbard (1975) suggested that an unidentified metabolite, elaborated by working muscle, diffuses into the extracellular space, where it excites the pain-nerve endings. The pain subsides rapidly when the muscle is allowed to rest and the circulation is restored, as if the putative metabolite were being washed away by the flow of fresh blood. If work is resumed immediately, however, pain returns much more quickly than before, implying that the metabolite is still present in high concentration in the muscle. Mense and Schmidt (1977) have identified nociceptive nerves in muscle, belonging to group III and IV afferent fibers, which respond to the application of a variety of chemical substances including bradykinin, serotonin, and histamine, as well as to increased concentrations of phosphate, lactate, potassium ions, and hydrogen ions. Whether any of these substances is responsible for ischemic muscle pain remains unknown, but it is tempting to speculate that ischemic pain represents a chemical signal to the central nervous system that the muscle cannot replenish energy stores fast enough to keep up with energy expenditure, and that cellular injury is about to occur. Usually this protective device is highly effective; voluntary activation of muscle is effectively abolished by ischemic pain, and patients with chronic occlusive peripheral vascular disease do not develop exertional myoglobinuria.

Ischemic Neuropathy

Mild neuropathic abnormalities in the legs are present in many patients with peripheral vascular disease, a fact that has received little clinical attention. Hutchinson and Liversedge (1956) detected signs or symptoms of peripheral nerve disease in over half of 90 nondiabetic patients with intermittent claudication, although only one patient had muscle weakness. Eames and Lange (1967), studying patients with more severe claudication, found weakness of one or both legs in 50 percent of the patients, muscle wasting in 31 percent, and sensory abnormalities in 88 percent. In both surveys the neuropathic findings were more severe in the more ischemic leg, and superficial sensory impairment tended to have a patchy, stocking distribution; less often there were localized areas of numbness within the boundaries of cutaneous nerves. Complaints of paresthesia are common, and a few patients complain of severe, stabbing leg pains reminiscent of the lightning pains of tabes dorsalis. Nevertheless, most patients have little or no neurologic disability, the symptoms of intermittent claudication and of digital ischemia being predominant. The few exceptions tend to be patients with an acute arterial occlusion superimposed on a chronic obliterative process, who develop an acute neuropathy of the lateral popliteal nerve (Hutchinson 1970).

Eames and Lange (1967) have suggested that nerve ischemia may be partly responsible for the ominous resting pain that signals the presence of severe ischemia with impending gangrene. This is a constant pain located in the forefoot and toes, sometimes lessened by placing the foot in a dependent position. However, the immediate cessation of rest pain after surgical restoration of effective circulation (Taylor 1973) favors a different explanation, such as the accumulation in ischemic tissues of chemical substances capable of stimulating nociceptive nerve fibers.

Because of the extensive collateral circulation of peripheral nerves, occlusion of a single artery rarely causes permanent nerve damage (Hess et al. 1979). However, in chronic peripheral vascular disease the accumulation of multiple sites of arterial occlusion and stenosis may eventually cause ischemic degeneration of portions of the nerve trunks. This degeneration is typically patchy in distribution, is more extensive in the central portion of a nerve fascicle than in the periphery, and consists of both Wallerian degeneration and paranodal demyelination (Hess et al. 1979). Eames and Lange (1967) made the interesting observation that small endoneurial arteries in specimens of sural nerve taken from patients with peripheral vascular disease show marked occlusive changes, with intimal thickening and medial degeneration and fibrosis. This finding suggests that, even in nondiabetic patients, chronic obliterative peripheral vascular disease is not confined to large and medium-sized arteries but involves the vasa nervorum as well, contributing to the occurrence of ischemic nerve degeneration.

OCCLUSION OF SMALL ARTERIES IN NERVE AND MUSCLE

We have been considering occlusive disorders of the large limb arteries resulting from atherosclerosis and thromboembolic disease. The neuromuscular manifestations of small-artery occlusive disease are somewhat different, and the pathologic basis of these syndromes is less uniform.

Angiopathic Neuropathies

When the nutritive arteries of peripheral nerve trunks are involved by a generalized occlusive disease, the clinical picture that results is the well-known syndrome of *mononeuropathy multiplex.* Large nerve trunks are affected seriatim in a patchy, seemingly random distribution; each neuropathy usually occurs abruptly, causing partial or complete paralysis of a group of muscles, often accompanied by muscle pain and by superficial sensory loss, dysesthesia, and neuralgia. As fresh vascular insults supervene, the clinical signs and symptoms increase in a stepwise fashion until the deficits come to resemble a diffuse polyneuropathy. If the patient is seen for the first time at this advanced stage of the nerve disorder, the true nature of the underlying vasculopathy can be discerned by careful inquiry into the mode of onset and temporal course of the nerve symptoms, and by scrupulous attention to the asymmetric character of the motor and sensory deficits.

The two pathologic processes that have been identified in this syndrome are vasculitis, which is discussed in Chapter 5, and diabetic angiopathy, which is discussed in Chapter 3.* In diabetes, angiopathic neuropathy usually takes the form of a simple mononeuropathy of the oculomotor, abducens, femoral, sciatic, or peroneal nerves. Occasionally multiple nerves are affected simultaneously in one limb. Contrasting with this picture is the ominous, widespread, subacute course of multiple mononeuropathies caused by polyarteritis nodosa and related vasculitides.

In angiopathic polyneuropathy there is usually little or no external indication of limb ischemia; the peripheral pulses are preserved and the skin is not cold or pale. Thus, the only clinical clues pointing to the vascular etiology of these neuropathies are the abrupt onset, the absence of apparent trauma, and clinical or laboratory signs indicating that nerve damage has occurred in a location remote from common sites of pressure or entrapment. Most often the nerve lesions are located in the middle of the upper arm and in the mid-thigh, where the collateral circulation of the vasa nervorum is most precarious (Dyck et al. 1972). The same distribution of nerve damage has been seen in experimental ischemic neuropathies produced in animals by ligation of multiple large arteries (Korthals and Wisniewski 1975) or by injection of arachidonic acid into the femoral artery (Parry and Brown 1981). In human cases, complete necrosis of a nerve segment is not usually found; instead there is patchy degeneration of axons and myelin sheaths, most marked in the center of nerve fascicles, with Wallerian degeneration distal to the primary site of ischemic degeneration. In the animal experiments of Parry and Brown (1981), thrombosis induced by arachidonic acid caused a true nerve infarct with pancellular necrosis, but the border zones showed the same patchy, centrofascicular nerve degeneration seen in human cases. Large myelinated fibers were relatively less involved than small myelinated and unmyelinated fibers (Parry and Brown 1982). Thus, nerve damage in diffuse, small-vessel angiopathies such as polyarteritis

*Angiopathic neuropathies have occurred in patients with bacterial endocarditis (Jones and Siekert 1968); whether they were caused by embolism or by vasculitis is not known.

nodosa and diabetic microangiopathy is the late result of a widespread vascular occlusive process that eventually culminates in patchy degeneration of nerve fibers in the most severely ischemic fascicles.

Nerve conduction tests performed within a few days after an ischemic nerve insult will show the electrophysiologic picture of conduction block, with preservation of nerve function distal to the lesion. A week or two later, when Wallerian degeneration has occurred, a conduction block will no longer be found, but the motor and sensory responses to nerve stimulation will be absent or reduced in amplitude, without a large reduction of conduction velocity. At this time, EMG will reveal the usual signs of acute denervation. Regeneration of nerves from proximal sites of degeneration takes place slowly over the course of many months and may continue for 2 or 3 years. The longest nerves, as might be expected, are the least likely to recover completely, so that distal weakness and sensory loss are the usual late sequelae. Some degree of muscle function can also be restored by collateral sprouting from preserved intramuscular axons.

Angiopathic Myopathy

Histologic examination of muscle sections from patients with polyarteritis nodosa may reveal small areas of ischemic muscle damage, but overt muscle infarction is extremely uncommon. Why this should be so is not at all evident, because infarction of large volumes of muscle does occur in three arterial diseases that have been described in preceding chapters: infarction of thigh muscles in diabetes mellitus (Chapter 3); necrotizing myopathy in azotemic hyperparathyroidism (Chapter 7); and migratory embolic infarction of muscle in marantic endocarditis (Chapter 6). A curious feature of these syndromes is the absence of ischemic neuropathies in the affected limbs. These disorders are presumably caused by occlusion of somewhat larger arteries than those responsible for angiopathic neuropathies; but arteries of this size are regularly involved in polyarteritis, despite the lack of ischemic muscle symptoms. Exertional muscle pain caused by ischemia has also been described in giant-cell arteritis.

NEUROPATHY CAUSED BY AN ARTERIOVENOUS FISTULA

Ischemic neuropathies of the upper limb may develop distal to a surgically placed arteriovenous shunt in patients undergoing chronic hemodialysis (Chapter 7). Ischemic neuropathy has not been observed in persons with congenital vascular malformations of the limbs, though patients with spinal cord angiomas involving the conus medullaris or cauda equina may have vascular steal symptoms in the lower extremities. One patient with a vascular malformation of the upper extremity that extended into the carpal tunnel developed symptoms of median nerve compression. At operation the angioma appeared to be compressing the median nerve, and division of the transverse carpal ligament relieved the symptoms (Chopra et al. 1979). Traumatic arteriovenous fistula of the upper arm or thigh may be associated with peripheral nerve symptoms, which are usually attributable to direct nerve trauma occurring at the time of the original arterial injury; however, a vascular steal mechanism may add to the impairment of nerve function and may interfere with nerve regeneration (Sunderland 1978).

HEMORRHAGIC DISORDERS

Intraspinal Hematoma

Bleeding into the epidural or subdural space of the lumbar spine may compress the cauda equina and produce flaccid weakness of the legs, areflexia, and loss of sphincter control. In its acute form, this event is a neurologic emergency, because permanent paralysis will usually result unless the cauda equina is decompressed within 12 hours. The onset of bleeding is typically marked by severe pain in the lower back, which may radiate into the buttocks, groin, or lower extremities. The subsequent paraplegia usually appears rapidly but occasionally evolves over a span of days or weeks.

Only about 9 cases of spinal epidural hematoma are reported yearly, and subdural hematoma is still more rare; a total of 25 cases have been reported since 1948 (Edelson 1976; Bruyn and Bosma 1976). Almost all the subdural cases were in patients with a hemorrhagic diathesis caused by anticoagulant therapy or thrombocytopenia, and half of the cases followed a lumbar puncture (Edelson 1976). Epidural hemorrhage, in contrast, often occurs spontaneously or after minor trauma: anticoagulation, hemophilia, and other bleeding diatheses are present in fewer than half of the cases (Bruyn and Bosma 1976), and lumbar puncture is rarely responsible (Laglia et al. 1978; Senelick et al. 1976).

The spinal epidural space is richly supplied with large, thin-walled veins that are part of Batson's plexus, while only minute blood vessels are found on the inner surface of the dura mater, and bridging veins such as occur within the cranial cavity are not present (Edelson 1976). These anatomic differences help to explain why spinal epidural hematoma is so much more frequent than subdural hematoma, but not why lumbar puncture is more likely to cause subdural or subarachnoid hemorrhage than epidural hemorrhage. Edelson and associates (1974) suggested that the major radicular vein accompanying the artery of Adamkiewicz, which accompanies the third, fourth, or fifth lumbar nerve root, may be the usual vessel injured by a spinal needle, and that because of the lateral position of this vessel a true midline lumbar puncture should be relatively safe. However, Breuer and colleagues (1982) argued that nerve roots are commonly brushed or even impaled during a lumbar puncture, and they postulated that laceration of the small radicular arteries and veins that cover each nerve root is the principal cause of traumatic subarachnoid and subdural hemorrhage. These nerves cannot be avoided by a midline lumbar puncture.

Since Edelson and associates (1974) alerted neurologic readers to the hazard of subdural and subarachnoid hemorrhage in thrombocytopenic patients, many practitioners have been understandably apprehensive about performing a lumbar puncture in patients with bleeding disorders. However, in some cases analyzing the CSF is more important than the possible complications. In order to minimize the risk, the spinal puncture should be performed by a skilled physician, using a #22 needle and taking special care to stay in the midline and to minimize trauma. The hemostatic defect should be corrected before the puncture, if possible. Signs and symptoms of spinal hematoma should be watched for closely during the next day or two, in the expectation of performing emergency myelography and laminectomy if necessary.

Bleeding into Muscle

Muscle hemorrhage is rare in normal persons, occurring mainly as a result of contusions, tears, or other muscle injuries. In patients with bleeding disorders, however, muscle hematomas can develop spontaneously or following minor trauma or intramuscular injections. Hemophiliac patients suffer intramuscular bleeding about a fifth as often as bleeding into the joints (Duthie et al. 1972). There are many reports of intramuscular bleeding in patients receiving anticoagulant drugs and in patients undergoing chronic hemodialysis (Milutinovich et al. 1977; Nichol et al. 1958); in these circumstances the most common site of bleeding is retroperitoneal, usually involving the psoas or iliac muscles, which are probably injured by stretching during walking or more vigorous activities. Other common sites of muscle hemorrhage are the buttock, calf, thigh, and arm. About half of these bleeding episodes are complicated by a compression neuropathy, as discussed below.

In the absence of severe trauma, muscle bleeding may develop suddenly or over several days. Pain, muscle shortening, and a firm, tender muscle mass are the usual signs, but the mass is often not palpable in cases of retroperitoneal hemotoma. The pain is intensified by attempts to stretch the muscle, and there is usually involuntary shortening of the muscle, producing limitation of passive motion at the affected joint. The bleeding may be extensive enough to lower the hematocrit, especially when it involves the retroperitoneal space. Diagnosis is not difficult except in the occult iliopsoas hematoma, and this is readily demonstrated by sonography or computed tomography.

There is little place for needle aspiration of blood in the treatment of muscle hematoma. Aspiration not only is ineffective but may cause infection. Conservative treatment is advisable in most cases. External pressure is applied to control the bleeding, and the coagulation defect is treated with measures appropriate to the specific cause. After bleeding has ceased, the muscle and joint are immobilized by a splint and the muscle contracture is gradually corrected by a succession of casts or other measures. Results are usually quite good except in the forearm or calf muscles, where fibrotic contractures sometimes cause permanent deformity despite good management (Duthie et al. 1972). Some of these failures may represent Volkmann's ischemic contracture, and it is appropriate to watch carefully for clinical signs of this complication and to perform a fasciotomy if indicated (Madigan et al. 1981).

Compression of Peripheral Nerves by Hematoma

In hemophilia, 75 to 80 percent of the episodes of nerve compression are caused by muscle hematomas (Duthie et al. 1972; Ehrmann et al. 1981). Peripheral nerve lesions occur in about 11 percent of all hemophiliacs and in 18 percent of severe hemophiliacs. About one third of the neuropathies involve the femoral nerve or lumbar plexus, being due to a psoas or iliac hematoma. Other muscular sites are buttock (sciatic nerve), forearm (radial, median, and ulnar nerves), and calf (posterior tibial nerve). Periarticular hematomas located at the elbow or wrist may compress the median or ulnar nerves, and hematomas of the knee may compress the common peroneal nerve. More than two thirds of the bleeding incidents causing neuropathy are in adult hemophiliacs; iliopsoas hematomas, however, are more common from 15 to 20 years of age.

Chronic anticoagulation therapy can also cause femoral neuropathy owing to iliopsoas hemorrhage (Butterfield et al. 1972; Zarranz and Salisachs 1979; Emery and Ochoa 1978), sciatic neuropathy owing to gluteal hemorrhage (Parkes and Kidner 1970), or carpal tunnel syndrome owing to tenosynovial hemorrhage (Hartwell and Kurtay 1966).

The femoral nerve syndromes have received particular attention recently. Emery and Ochoa (1978) suggested that two syndromes can be distinguished. Psoas hemorrhages tend to be large, involving the L2-4 roots and the femoral nerve, which passes through this muscle, and causing paralysis of the hip flexors, hip adductors, and quadriceps muscle. Sensory loss may involve not only the femoral and saphenous nerves (anterior thigh and medial leg) but also the obturator nerve (medial upper thigh) and the lateral femoral cutaneous nerve (anterolateral thigh). Hemorrhage into the iliacus muscle is said to be more common; it is usually smaller, perhaps because of close confinement by the iliac fascia, and a bulge may be felt in the groin or in the iliac fossa. Only the femoral nerve is compressed, but flexion of the hip is somewhat weak owing to compression of motor branches to the iliacus muscle and the direct effect of the muscle hemorrhage.

In both circumstances, deep pain radiates into the loin, back, and groin, and neuralgic pain may be felt in a cutaneous nerve distribution. At first, motor testing is difficult to perform because of pain, guarding, and spasm of hip flexion. The pattern of sensory involvement and the activity of the quadriceps and thigh adduction reflexes are the most reliable indicators of the extent of nerve involvement. (In a pure femoral neuropathy, the knee jerk is abolished while the adductor reflex is preserved.)

Although the clinical features of iliopsoas hemorrhage are quite distinctive, the diagnosis is frequently missed or delayed because of lack of familiarity with this entity. Fever and leukocytosis may occur, causing confusion with appendicitis or other intra-abdominal infections. Diagnostic confusion may also arise in cases of acute femoral or lumbar plexus neuritis, which is frequently painful. In neuritis, however, involuntary hip flexion is not often seen. Psoas irritation by an intra-abdominal infection such as appendicitis produces spasm of hip flexion but is unlikely to cause femoral neuropathy. Any diagnostic uncertainty is resolved by CT radiography, which shows the muscle hematoma in precise anatomic detail (Fig. 39).

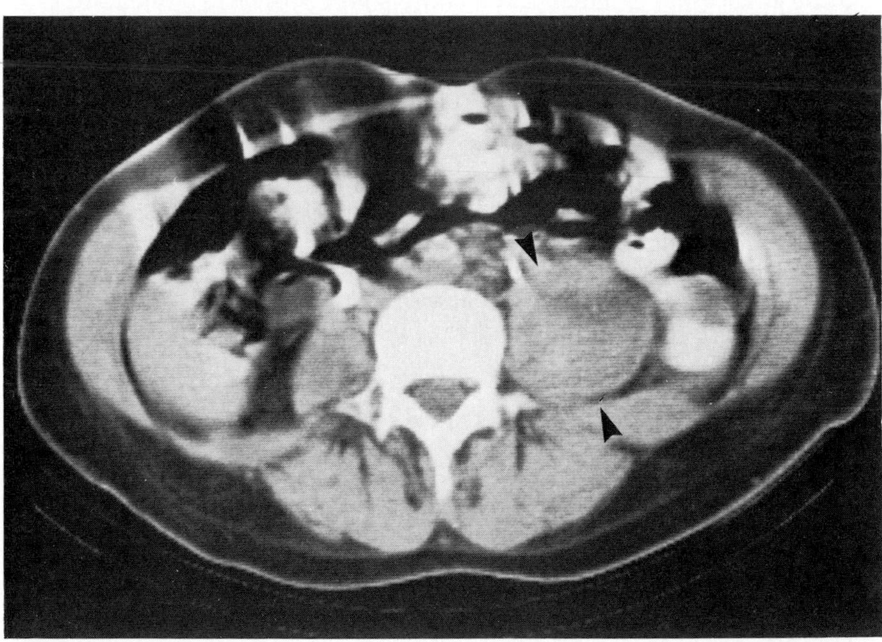

FIGURE 39. CT radiograph of pelvis showing hematoma within psoas muscle *(arrows).*

The treatment of iliopsoas hematoma is controversial. Some authors recommend early surgical exploration, primarily to perform fasciotomy so as to relieve the nerve compression (Young and Norris 1976). However, the natural course of untreated iliopsoas hematomas is not well known. In severe cases, convalescence may be long and painful, with flexion contracture of the hip, weakness of knee extension, and painful dysesthesia of the thigh and leg; yet often a satisfactory recovery occurs eventually. Hemophiliacs usually recover completely from incomplete femoral nerve palsies without surgery (Duthie et al. 1972; Ehrmann et al. 1981). This suggests that surgical treatment, if it is to be performed at all, should be reserved for patients with complete femoral nerve paralysis.

REFERENCES

Andersson, J, Eklöf, B, Neglén, P, et al: *Metabolic changes in blood and skeletal muscle in reconstructive aortic surgery.* Ann Surg 189:283–289, 1979.

Breuer, AC, Tyler, R, Marzewski, DJ, et al: *Radicular vessels are the most probable source of needle-induced blood in lumbar puncture. Significance for the thrombocytopenic cancer patient.* Cancer 49:2168–2172, 1982.

Bruyn, GW and Bosma, NJ: *Spinal extradural haematoma.* In Vinken, PJ and Bruyn, GW (eds): *Handbook of Clinical Neurology, vol 26.* North-Holland Publishing, Amsterdam, 1976, pp 1–30.

Butterfield, WC, Neiraser, RJ and Roberts, MP: *Femoral neuropathy and anticoagulants.* Ann Surg 176:58–61, 1972.

Chiu, D, Wang, HH and Blumenthal, MR: *Creatine phosphokinase release as a measure of tourniquet effect on skeletal muscle.* Arch Surg 111:71–74, 1976.

Chopra, JS, Khanna, SK and Murthy, MK: *Congenital arteriovenous fistula producing carpal tunnel syndrome.* J Neurol Neurosurg Psychiatry 42:815–817, 1979.

Dahlbäck, L-O: *Effects of temporary tourniquet ischemia on striated muscle fibers and motor end-plates. Morphological and histochemical studies in the rabbit and electromyographical studies in man.* Scand J Plast Reconstr Surg Suppl 7, 1970.

Dahlbäck, L-O, Ekstedt, J and Stålberg, E: *Ischemic effects on impulse transmission to muscle fibers in man.* Electroenceph Clin Neurophysiol 29:579–591, 1970.

Duthie, RB, Matthews, JM, Rizza, CR, et al: *The Management of Musculo-skeletal Problems in the Haemophilias.* Blackwell, Oxford, 1972.

Dyck, PJ, Conn, DL and Okazaki, H: *Necrotizing angiopathic neuropathy. Three-dimensional morphology of fiber degeneration related to sites of occluded vessels.* Mayo Clin Proc 47:461–475, 1972.

Eames, RA and Lange, LS: *Clinical and pathological study of ischaemic neuropathy.* J Neurol Neurosurg Psychiatry 30:215–226, 1967.

Edelson, RN: *Spinal subdural hematoma.* In Vinken, PJ and Bruyn, GW (eds): *Handbook of Clinical Neurology, vol 26.* North-Holland Publishing, Amsterdam, 1976, pp 31–38.

Edelson, RN, Chernik, NL and Posner, JB: *Spinal subdural hematomas complicating lumbar puncture.* Arch Neurol 31:134–137, 1974.

Ehrmann, L, Lechner, K, Mamoli, B, et al: *Peripheral nerve lesions in haemophilia.* J Neurol 225:175–182, 1981.

Eklöf, B, Neglén, P and Thomson, D: *Temporary incomplete ischemia of the legs induced by aortic clamping in man. Effects on central hemodynamics and skeletal muscle metabolism by adrenergic block.* Ann Surg 193:89–98, 1981a.

Eklöf, B, Neglén, P and Thomson, D: *Temporary incomplete ischemia of the legs caused by aortic clamping in man. Improvement of skeletal muscle metabolism by low molecular weight dextran.* Ann Surg 193:99–104, 1981b.

Emery, S and Ochoa, J: *Lumbar plexus neuropathy resulting from retroperitoneal hemorrhage.* Muscle Nerve 1:330–334, 1978.

Enger, EA, Jennische, E, Medegård, A, et al: *Cellular restitution after 3 h of complete tourniquet ischemia.* Eur Surg Res 10:230–239, 1978.

Farber, FL, Chien, KR and Mittnacht, S, Jr: *The pathogenesis of irreversible cell injury in ischemia.* Am J Pathol 102:271–281, 1981.

Ferguson, FR and Liversedge, LA: *Ischaemic lateral popliteal nerve palsy.* Br Med J 3:333–335, 1954.

FISHER, RD, FOGARTY, TJ AND MORROW, AG: *Clinical and biochemical observations of transient femoral artery occlusion in man.* Surgery 68:323–328, 1970.

FOWLER, TJ, DANTA, G AND GILLIATT, RW: *Recovery of nerve conduction after a pneumatic tourniquet: Observations on the hind limb of the baboon.* J Neurol Neurosurg Psychiatry 35:638–647, 1972.

HAIMOVICCI, H: *Muscular, renal, and metabolic complications of acute arterial occlusions: Myonephropathic-metabolic syndrome.* Surgery 85:461–468, 1979.

HALJAMÄE, H AND ENGER, E: *Human skeletal muscle energy metabolism during and after complete tourniquet ischemia.* Ann Surg 182:9–14, 1975.

HANZLIKOVA, V AND GUTMANN, E: *Effect of ischemia on contractile and histochemical properties of the rat soleus muscle.* Pflugers Arch 379:209–214, 1979.

HARGENS, AR, SCHMIDT, DA, EVANS, KL, ET AL: *Quantitation of skeletal-muscle necrosis in a model compartment syndrome.* J Bone Jt Surg 63-A:631–636, 1981.

HARTWELL, SW, JR AND KURTAY, M: *Carpal tunnel compression caused by hematoma associated with anti-coagulant therapy.* Cleve Clin Q 33:127–129, 1966.

HERRICK, MK AND MILLS PE, JR: *Infarction of spinal cord. Two cases of selective gray matter involvement secondary to asymptomatic aortic disease.* Arch Neurol 24:228–241, 1971.

HESS, K, EAMES, RA, DARVENIZA, P, ET AL: *Acute ischaemic neuropathy in the rabbit.* J Neurol Sci 44:19–43, 1979.

HOLDEN, CEA: *The pathology and prevention of Volkmann's ischaemic contracture.* J Bone Jt Surg 61B: 296–300, 1979.

HUTCHINSON, EC: *Ischaemic neuropathy and peripheral vascular disease.* In VINKEN, PJ AND BRUYN, GW (EDS): *Handbook of Clinical Neurology, vol 8.* North-Holland Publishing, Amsterdam, 1970, pp 149–153.

HUTCHINSON, EC AND LIVERSEDGE, LA: *Neuropathy in peripheral vascular disease. Its bearing on diabetic neuropathy.* Q J Med 25:267–274, 1956.

JENNINGS, RB AND REIMER, KA: *Lethal myocardial ischemic injury.* Am J Pathol 102:241–255, 1981.

JENNISCHE, E, AMUNDSON, B AND HALJAMÄE, H: *Metabolic responses in feline "red" and "white" skeletal muscle to shock and ischemia.* Acta Physiol Scand 106:39–45, 1979.

JONES, HR, JR AND SIEKERT, RG: *Embolic mononeuropathy and bacterial endocarditis.* Arch Neurol 19:535–537, 1968.

JÓZSA, L, RENNER, A AND SÁNTHA, E: *The effect of tourniquet ischaemia on intact, tenotomized and motor nerve injured human hand muscles.* Hand 12:235–240, 1980.

KARPATI, G, CARPENTER, S, MELMED, C, ET AL: *Experimental ischemic myopathy.* J Neurol Sci 23:129–161, 1974.

KLENERMAN, L: *Tourniquet time—how long?* Hand 12:231–234, 1980.

KORTHALS, JK AND WISNIEWSKI, HM: *Peripheral nerve ischemia, Part I (Experimental model).* J Neurol Sci 24:65–76, 1975.

KUGELBERG, E: *Neurologic mechanism for certain phenomena in tetany.* Arch Neurol Psychiatry 56:507–521, 1946.

LAGLIA, AG, EISENBERG, RL, WEINSTEIN, PR, ET AL: *Spinal epidural hematoma after lumbar puncture in liver disease.* Ann Intern Med 88:515–516, 1978.

LARSSON, J AND HULTMAN, E: *The effect of long-term arterial occlusion on energy metabolism of the human quadriceps muscle.* Scand J Clin Lab Invest 39:257–264, 1979.

LEWIS, T: *Pain.* Macmillan, New York, 1943, pp 96–104.

LEWIS, T: *Vascular Disorders of the Limbs,* ed 2. Macmillan & Co, London, 1946.

LUNDBORG, G: *Ischemic nerve injury. Experimental studies on intraneural microvascular pathophysiology and nerve function in a limb subjected to temporary circulatory arrest.* Scand J Plast Reconstr Surg (Suppl) 6:1–113, 1970.

MADIGAN, RR, HANNA WT AND WALLACE, SL: *Acute compartment syndrome in hemophilia.* J Bone Joint Surg 63A:1327–1329, 1981.

MENSE, S AND SCHMIDT, RF: *Muscle pain: Which receptors are responsible for the transmission of noxious stimuli?* In Rose, FC (ED): *Physiological Aspects of Clinical Neurology.* Blackwell Scientific Publications, Oxford, 1977, pp 265–278.

MILLER, SH, PRICE, G, BUCK, D, ET AL: *Effects of tourniquet ischemia and postischemic edema on muscle metabolism.* J Hand Surg 4:547–555, 1979.

MILUTINOVICH, J, FOLLETTE, WC AND SCRIBNER, BH: *Spontaneous retroperitoneal bleeding in patients on chronic hemodialysis.* Ann Intern Med 86:189–192, 1977.

MUBARAK, SJ AND HARGENS, SR: *Compartment Syndromes and Volkmann's Contracture.* WB Saunders, Philadelphia, 1981.

MUBARAK, SJ, OWEN, CA, HARGENS, AR, ET AL: *Acute compartment syndromes: Diagnosis and treatment with the aid of the wick catheter.* J Bone Joint Surg 60A:1091–1095, 1978.

NAYLER, WG: *The role of calcium in the ischemic myocardium.* Am J Pathol 102:262–270, 1981.

NEELY, JR AND FENVRAY, D: *Metabolic products and myocardial ischemia.* Am J Pathol 102:282–291, 1981.

NICHOL, ES, KEYES, JN, BORG, JF, ET AL: *Long-term anticoagulant therapy in coronary atherosclerosis.* Am Heart J 55:142–152, 1958.

OCHOA, J, FOWLER, TJ AND GILLIATT, RW: *Anatomical changes in peripheral nerves compressed by a pneumatic tourniquet.* J Anat 113:433–455, 1972.

OLIVERO, J AND AYUS, JC: *Rhabdomyolysis and acute myoglobinuric renal failure. Complications of inferior vena cava ligation.* Arch Intern Med 138:1548–1549, 1978.

OWEN, CA, WOODY, PR, MUBARAK, SJ, ET AL: *Gluteal compartment syndromes. A report of three cases and management utilizing the wick catheter.* Clin Orthop 132:57–60, 1978.

OWEN, CA, MUBARAK, SJ, HARGENS AR, ET AL: *Intramuscular pressures with limb compression. Clarification of the pathogenesis of the drug-induced muscle-compression syndrome.* N Engl J Med 300:1169–1172, 1979.

PARKES, JD AND KIDNER, PH: *Peripheral nerve and root lesions developing as a result of hematoma formation during anticoagulation treatment.* Postgrad Med J 46:146–148, 1970.

PARRY, GJ AND BROWN, MJ: *Arachidonate-induced experimental nerve infarction.* J Neurol Sci 50:123–133, 1981.

PARRY, GJ AND BROWN MJ: *Selective fiber vulnerability in acute ischemic neuropathy.* Ann Neurol 11:147–154, 1982.

PENN, AS, ROWLAND, LP AND FRASER, DW: *Drugs, coma, and myoglobinuria.* Arch Neurol 26:336–344, 1972.

PRESTA, M AND RAGNOTTI, G: *Quantification of damage to striated muscle after normothermic or hypothermic ischemia.* Clin Chem 27:297–302, 1981.

RODBARD, S: *Pain in contracting muscle.* In CRUE, BL, JR. (ED): *Pain Research and Treatment.* Academic Press, New York, 1975, pp 183–196.

SAVELYEV, VS, ZATEVAKHIN, II AND STEPANOV, NV: *Artery embolism of the upper limbs.* Surgery 81:367–375, 1977.

SENELICK, RC, NORWOOD, CW AND COHEN, GH: *"Painless" spinal epidural hematoma during anticoagulant therapy.* Neurology 26:213–215, 1976.

SHINE, KI: *Ionic events in ischemia and anoxia.* Am J Pathol 102:256–261, 1981.

SJÖSTRÖM, M, NEGLÉN, P, FRIDÉN, J, ET AL: *Human skeletal muscle metabolism and morphology after temporary incomplete ischemia.* Eur J Clin Invest 12:69–79, 1982.

SLANEY, G AND HAMER, JD: *Arterial embolism.* In BIRNSTINGL, M (ED): *Peripheral Vascular Surgery.* William Heinemann, London, 1973, pp 189–210.

STOCK, W, BOHN HJ AND ISSELHARD, W: *Metabolic changes in rat skeletal muscle after acute arterial occlusion.* Vasc Surg 5:249–255, 1971.

SUNDERLAND, S: *Blood supply of the sciatic nerve and its popliteal divisions in man.* Arch Neurol Psychiatry 54:283–289, 1945.

SUNDERLAND, S: *Nerves and Nerve Injuries,* ed 2. Churchill Livingstone, Edinburgh, 1978, pp 172–173.

TAYLOR, GW: *Chronic arterial occlusion.* In BIRNSTINGL, M. (ED): *Peripheral Vascular Surgery.* William Heinemann, London, 1973, pp 211–234.

WELTI, J-J, MELEKIAN, B AND REVELLAUD, M: *Paralysies périphériques ischémiques (paralysies périphériques provoquées par une embolie artérielle des membres).* Presse Med 69:333–334, 1961.

YOUNG, MR AND NORRIS, JW: *Femoral neuropathy during anticoagulant therapy.* Neurology 26:1173–1175, 1976.

ZARRANZ, JJ AND SALISACHS, P: *Femoral neuropathy due to compression by retroperitoneal haemorrhage. A modern evaluation.* J Neurol Sci 43:479–482, 1979.

ZWEIFACH, SS, HARGENS AR, EVANS, KL, ET AL: *Skeletal muscle necrosis in pressurized compartments associated with hemorrhagic hypotension.* J Trauma 20:941–947, 1980.

Chapter 9

NUTRITIONAL AND GASTROINTESTINAL DISORDERS

STARVATION AND CACHEXIA

The Metabolic Impact of Starvation and Illness on Skeletal Muscle

The initial metabolic response of muscle to starvation is an accelerated degradation of protein; this liberates large amounts of alanine, which is then converted to glucose in the liver. By this means, the brain's appetite for glucose is fueled at the expense of muscle protein. In an average-sized man, muscle protein is consumed at the rate of 60 to 70 g per day, equivalent to a loss of 280 g of whole muscle daily (Brennan 1977). At the same time, muscle sharply reduces its consumption of glucose, and fatty acids are liberated from adipose tissue, elevating plasma levels of free fatty acids and ketone bodies. Within a few days the brain adapts to the use of ketone bodies as an alternate fuel, and the catabolism of protein in muscle and other body tissues is correspondingly reduced. During chronic starvation, therefore, muscle tissue is consumed at a much lower rate (about 20 g of muscle mass per day), and the body's caloric requirements are provided mainly by consumption of stored fat. When fat stores are exhausted, proteolysis again rises sharply, and the individual dies soon afterward of the effects of protein loss from muscle, heart, and other vital organs.

PATHOPHYSIOLOGY. The biochemical mechanisms responsible for a net loss of muscle protein during starvation are only partly understood. There is an increased rate of protein degradation as well as a decreased rate of protein synthesis, the latter being associated with reduced cellular levels of RNA, a lower rate of protein synthesis per unit weight of muscle ribosomes, and low plasma levels of insulin, an anabolic hormone (Li and Goldberg 1976). In rats, the degree of starvation atrophy is greater in white than in red muscle, and in mixed muscles the atrophy is greatest in fast-glycolytic muscle fibers, intermediate in fast-oxidative-glycolytic fibers, and least in slow-oxidative fibers. These changes are consistent with a suppression of glucose utilization in favor of the oxidative catabolism of lipids and ketone bodies. Interestingly, however, the twitch tension and tetanic tension of gastrocnemius muscle do not decline as much as the muscle weight, so that muscle strength does not decline as rapidly as muscle mass (Gardiner et al. 1980).

Major illnesses such as trauma, major surgery, sepsis, or extensive burns impose a catabolic state of even greater magnitude than that caused by acute starvation. Under the influence of raised plasma levels of catabolic hormones such as catecholamines and corticosteroids, skeletal muscle becomes resistant to insulin, protein catabolism and gluconeogenesis increase, and muscle glucose consumption declines despite elevated plasma levels of glucose and insulin (Richards 1980). In this setting, muscle appears to act as a reservoir of fuel (glucose) for other organs of the body, and in extreme instances the loss of muscle mass can amount to 400 to 500 g per day (Brennan 1977). This catabolic state would lead to death by inanition in 2 to 3 weeks if it were not counteracted by vigorous nutritional measures. An important and long-established component of treatment is to reduce sympathoadrenal discharge by means of analgesia, replacement of blood and fluid losses, removal of necrotic tissue, and control of infection. More recently, intravenous hyperalimentation has proved life-saving in patients who are severely malnourished or who are unable to assimilate oral or tube feedings. It has also been suggested that insulin therapy, by overcoming the insulin resistance of muscle, may counteract the hypercatabolism present in such patients (Richards 1980).

Neuromuscular Effects of Starvation and General Debility

The treatment of adult obesity by *total therapeutic starvation* is attended by a number of medical hazards, most importantly the risk of serious cardiac arrhythmia, possibly because of myocardial potassium depletion. Neuromuscular complications have been reported in only three cases, however. One patient (Scobie et al. 1980) lost 48 kg of body weight during a 17-week fast in which potassium and vitamin supplements were given. Nine days after he began to eat again he had several episodes of ventricular arrhythmia, and 6 weeks later he developed proximal muscle weakness with a slight elevation of serum CPK activity; serum potassium and phosphorus values at that time were not mentioned. The weakness resolved in another 7 weeks. Two obese patients who were starved by surgical gastric partitioning developed a severe sensory polyneuropathy of demyelinating type, with extensive accumulation of lipids in neurons and Schwann cells. There was no muscle weakness, although the anterior horn cells were swollen and contained lipid droplets (Feit et al. 1982).

Prolonged *semistarvation* is the most common clinical form of malnutrition. Protein-calorie malnutrition can be the result of food deprivation, as in the victims of famine or in maltreated prisoners; of poor dietary habits as in food faddists and alcoholics; of anorexia owing to a wide variety of illnesses including digestive disorders, advanced congestive heart failure, uremia, tuberculosis, chronic pain, and cancer; of enteric fistula and other major defects of food absorptions; or of deliberate refusal to eat in patients with anorexia nervosa. In adults, the resulting loss of fat and muscle tissue, termed *cachexia*, is often accompanied by apathy, depression, muscle soreness and cramps, and reduced motor activity; muscle weakness is said to be present, sometimes in a proximal distribution (Harriman 1966), but detailed clinical descriptions and electrodiagnostic studies are lacking. My own experience is that most debilitated hospital patients with mild or moderate muscular wasting are not particularly weak as judged by ordinary manual tests of muscle strength. It is well known that patients with anorexia nervosa may be quite active despite an extremely emaciated appearance, and EMG has been reported to be normal in that disorder as well as in patients immobilized in bed for up to 6 months (Buchthal 1970). Likewise, Denny-Brown (1958) remarked, "In severe and prolonged simple starvation . . . [the] muscles may become extraordinarily thin with surprising retention of power of contraction."

While the clinical and electromyographic features of cachectic muscular atrophy have received scant attention, several pathologic studies have been done on patients with such diverse underlying diseases as anorexia nervosa, chronic infection, cancer, Alzheimer's disease, and prolonged immobility owing to coma, arthritis, or other causes. To the naked eye, the muscle has been said to have a brownish tinge, which is not related to the presence of lipofuscin pigment (Harriman 1966). Histologic examination shows atrophic muscle fibers distributed in a scattered fashion; in more severe cases the atrophic fibers may be clustered in small groups, suggesting a possible neurogenic cause (Tomlinson et al. 1969; Lindboe and Torvik 1982; Lindboe et al. 1982). However, motor point biopsies show normal terminal innervation (Harriman 1966), histochemical studies do not show the fiber-type grouping of reinnervation, and the normal EMG findings argue strongly against denervation as the cause of cachectic muscular atrophy.

Many of the patients mentioned above were merely bedridden individuals with no particular systemic disease. In those cases, simple disuse would explain some of the muscle atrophy. *Disuse atrophy* has been extensively studied in experimental models, which were recently reviewed by Mendell (1979). The histologic picture varies with the procedure used to produce immobilization: tenotomy causes selective atrophy of type 1 muscle fibers; cordotomy combined with deafferentation causes type 2 muscle fiber atrophy; and cordotomy alone causes unselective atrophy of all muscle fibers, as does simple joint fixation. The effects of disuse on human muscle likewise vary with the underlying cause. Gluteal muscle from patients with severe degenerative arthritis of the hip showed rather selective type 2 atrophy; leg muscle from patients bedridden by "chronic disease" showed moderate atrophy of type 1 fibers and severe atrophy of type 2 fibers; and leg muscle of paraplegic patients showed equally severe atrophy of both muscle fiber types (Bundscher et al. 1973). Immobilization of the knee joint by a cast for 4 weeks produced selective atrophy of type 1 fibers in the quadriceps muscle (Haggmark and Eriksson 1979), but immobilization for 8 to 30 weeks resulted in similar atrophy of both fiber types (Sargeant et al. 1977). The latter authors observed that the work capacity of the injured leg (measured by one-leg cycling) was reduced by only 15 percent, indicating that, as in starvation atrophy, the degree of functional impairment is much less than the degree of atrophy.

Muscles adjacent to a painful joint undergo so-called *"reflex atrophy,"* which initially progresses even more rapidly than denervation atrophy. In the lower extremity, extensor muscles such as the quadriceps and gastrocnemius-soleus group are predominantly affected. The corresponding muscle stretch reflexes may be transiently reduced or abolished, causing the unwary physician to search for a neurologic cause for the pain.

Pathophysiology. Experimental studies suggest that reflex muscle atrophy is dependent on suprasegmental influences from the central nervous system, since the atrophy is prevented by transection of the spinal cord above the level of the muscle innervation (Hnik et al. 1977). In rat experiments, a painful lesion of the paw produced an equal degree of atrophy of the red soleus and the white plantaris, both muscles being extensors of the ankle (Hnik et al. 1977). The vastus medialis muscle of patients with long-standing unilateral knee joint disease showed predominant atrophy of type 1 muscle fibers in some cases and of type 2 fibers in others, but the average reduction of size was about equal for the two fiber types (Lindboe and Platou 1982).

Neuromuscular Aspects of Malnutrition in Infants and Children

Muscle wasting, hypotonia, weakness, and hyporeflexia are present in a large proportion of children with severe protein-calorie malnutrition (kwashiorkor). The weakness tends to be greater in proximal muscles; some children make use of the Gowers' maneuver to rise from the ground and have a waddling gait, while others are unable to walk (Sachdev et al. 1971). In severe cases there is a 50-percent reduction of motor nerve conduction velocity even when the values are corrected for low skin temperature (Engsner and Woldemariam 1974; Osuntokun 1971). Sensory nerve responses are absent in some cases (Sachdev et al. 1971). EMG shows small motor unit potential amplitudes in proximal muscles and fibrillations in a diffuse distribution, while muscle biopsy shows very small muscle fibers, grouped fiber atrophy, and fragmentation of muscle fibers (Sachdev et al. 1971). The motor nerve conduction velocities return to normal rapidly within 5 weeks during intensive nutritional therapy (Engsner and Woldemariam 1974), indicating that the abnormalities are probably not due to structural nerve damage; in fact, examination of teased nerve fibers from two fatal cases showed no definite abnormality (Osuntokun 1971).

Compared with children with kwashiorkor, infants with marasmus are younger and more severely malnourished, showing severe growth retardation, loss of subcutaneous fat, muscular weakness and wasting, and hypotonia (Singh et al. 1976). However, motor nerve conduction velocities are normal in these cases (Singh et al. 1976; Engsner and Woldemariam 1974), suggesting perhaps that transient biochemical disturbances rather than simple protein-calorie malnutrition are responsible for the nerve conduction abnormalities found in kwashiorkor. Microscopic examination of muscle from infants or children with marasmus or severe kwashiorkor shows uniform atrophy of all muscle fibers, together with a reduction of the total number of muscle fibers (Montgomery 1962; Dastur et al. 1982).

Recently, followup studies have indicated that boys who have suffered from malnutrition in early childhood continue to demonstrate growth retardation, diminished work capacity, and reduced muscle mass in adolescence (Satyanarayana et al. 1979, 1981). However, the adolescent youths in that study still had low body weights, having remained in the same nutritionally poor environment. It is not known whether the neuromuscular defects of malnourished children can be corrected, but experiments in rats have indicated that this can be achieved by a combination of good nutrition and physical exercise (Raju 1977).

Cachexia in Patients with Cancer

The weight loss that is so characteristic of cancer may be due to anorexia, disturbances of digestion and assimilation of food, and energy consumption by the tumor (Costa 1977). However, in some patients weight loss occurs despite normal food intake and at a very early stage of tumor development, when the metabolic demands of the tumor are too small to account for the negative nitrogen balance. Recently, Strain and colleagues (1979) demonstrated striking weight loss in mice with small human hypernephroma grafts, in the absence of a significant reduction of food intake, impairment of food absorption, or increase of the basal metabolic rate. Other implanted human and mouse tumors did not cause weight loss despite much lower food intakes. Thus, as several authors have postulated, it seems likely that some types of cancer secrete humoral substances that cause cachexia in the host by mechanisms that are still unknown.

Some studies have demonstrated an increased basal metabolic rate in cancer patients, but the data are inconclusive (Strain 1979). More consistent evidence points to a state of insulin resistance of skeletal muscle, associated with increased hepatic gluconeogenesis using amino acids derived from muscle protein (Brennan 1977). The rate of protein synthesis was reduced and the activity of lysosomal proteolytic enzymes was increased in muscle biopsy samples from cancer patients (Lundholm et al. 1976). In the same study, the activities of several glycolytic and oxidative enzymes were significantly reduced in muscle tissue, and incorporation of glucose carbon into glycogen, lactate, and carbon dioxide was diminished, suggesting that muscle energy metabolism and anabolic processes were subservient to catabolic processes. In rats with implanted tumors, protein depletion is more extensive in gastrocnemius than in soleus muscle (like the selective atrophy caused by starvation or cortiscosteroid therapy), and there is a striking reduction of protein synthesis by ribosomal preparations obtained from gastrocnemius muscle (Clark and Goodlad 1971; Goodlad and Clark 1972; Clark and Goodlad 1975).

Thus, as Brennan (1977) has pointed out, the metabolism of cancer patients resembles that of patients with burns, trauma, or sepsis. Such patients may require an unusually large caloric intake to reverse their negative nitrogen balance. We still know little of the biochemical mechanisms that cause skeletal muscles to be consumed for the benefit of the diseased parts of the body.

VITAMIN DEFICIENCIES

Thiamine Deficiency

It is accepted that thiamine deficiency causes most cases of Wernicke's encephalopathy and is also capable of causing peripheral neuropathy and high-output cardiomyopathy. There are some puzzling discrepancies, however. Oriental thiamine deficiency (beriberi) was characterized by peripheral neuropathy and congestive cardiomyopathy, but Wernicke's disease was rarely observed in this population. In Western countries, where thiamine deficiency is mainly encountered in alcoholic patients or in patients with protracted vomiting, Wernicke's disease is the usual complication; there are a few cases of congestive cardiomyopathy, but there are no documented examples of thiamine-deficiency neuropathy among nonalcoholic patients. Alcoholic neuropathy has often been attributed to thiamine deficiency (Victor 1975), but this attribution is disputed because in many patients there is no evidence of thiamine deficiency or even of malnutrition.

Also puzzling is the fact that it is difficult to produce thiamine-deficiency neuropathy in mammals, though neuropathy can readily be produced in birds. In a recent study, monkeys with dietary thiamine deficiency developed signs of Wernicke's disease (nystagmus, abducens paralysis, truncal ataxia, and dysmetria), congestive heart failure, and proximal weakness of the lower extremities, but there were no clinical signs of peripheral neuropathy (Mesulam et al. 1979). Thiamine deficiency causes anorexia and weight loss in rats; a minor degree of distal axonal degeneration has been observed in some experiments (Kark 1975; Prineas 1970), but similar changes are found in control animals starved to a comparable degree (Pawlik et al. 1977). Thus, there is no satisfactory experimental model of human thiamine-deficient polyneuropathy.

Polyneuropathy

Beriberi had nearly disappeared from Japan by 1965, but in the early 1970s Japanese physicians began to see young men with polyneuropathy and edema of the face and ankles. Yabuki and associates (1976), reviewing 56 published cases and 24 cases of their own, presented strong evidence that these were examples of thiamine deficiency neuropathy, which had become so rare that the true diagnosis was not suspected. These cases provide the only contemporary record of the clinical and laboratory features of thiamine-deficiency polyneuropathy.

Almost all the patients were teen-age boys and young men; the symptoms came on during the summer, often after a period of strenuous exercise such as a cycling tour or an athletic training program.* Most of the patients had a history of an unbalanced diet deficient in animal protein and fresh vegetables and high in unfortified rice and "instant" foods.

The symptoms came on acutely or subacutely. Most of the patients complained of paresthesia and weakness of the legs while about half of the patients reported stiffness, pain, or cramps in the calf muscles. Edema of the face and ankles was present in 60 percent of the patients, and a few patients experienced exertional dyspnea, palpitation, and fatigue. All showed a stocking-glove disturbance of superficial sensation, consisting of hypesthesia, hypalgesia, and nonpainful dysesthesia, while deep sensation was mildly reduced in only a quarter of the patients. Three fourths of the patients had mild or moderate distal muscular weakness, of which the earliest manifestations were foot drop and weakness of extension of the fingers and wrists. Muscle tenderness or effort spasm was present in 30 percent of the cases. The muscle stretch reflexes were always diminished in the distal lower extremities.

The heart was enlarged in 24 percent and minor ECG abnormalities were present in 36 percent of the patients. Serum CPK activity was increased slightly or moderately in 48 percent. CSF cell counts and protein levels were normal. Motor nerve conduction velocity was slightly reduced in half of the patients, but there were neurogenic abnormalities on EMG in 91 percent. Sural nerve biopsy specimens showed axonal degeneration affecting mainly large, myelinated nerve fibers (Takahashi and Nakamura 1976). Thiamine levels in the blood were undetectable in all cases before treatment, though erythrocyte transketolase activity was not measured.

*Heavy exercise is known to predispose to the development of beriberi. This is because the requirement for thiamine depends on the metabolic rate, the minimum requirement for the vitamin being 0.33 mg per 1000 calories (Hoyumpa 1980).

Following dietary therapy, including administration of multiple vitamins, there was a gradual recovery: the motor disturbances resolved within 6 months and sensory disturbances within 1 year. Edema usually subsided in a few weeks but tended to recur after exercise. The neuropathy often relapsed during the summer in subsequent years.

In summary, the principal features of thiamine-deficiency neuropathy are an acute or subacute course, pain and tenderness in the calf muscles, foot drop and wrist drop, distal loss of superficial sensation without hyperpathia, and peripheral edema. This clinical picture is identical to that described in earlier accounts of beriberi, including the cases that occurred in prisoners of war in Southeast Asia during the Second World War. Denny-Brown (1947, 1958) observed that loss of superficial sensation was much greater than loss of deep sensation and was located in a characteristic distribution over the outer aspects of the legs, on top of the feet, on the thighs, in patches over the abdomen, chest, and forearms, and sometimes on the lips. In severe cases there was hoarseness or aphonia owing to laryngeal nerve paralysis, and deafness developed in rare cases. Thus, thiamine-deficiency neuropathy appears to have features of a multiple mononeuropathy as well as a distal polyneuropathy. According to Platt (1958), weakness may be more severe in one hand when it is used more strenuously than the other hand. The neuropathy is due to axonal degeneration, which explains the slow recovery of motor and sensory function during vitamin therapy.

The so-called dry, atrophic, or chronic form of beriberi consists of a distal sensorimotor polyneuropathy, similar to that described above but unaccompanied by cardiac involvement and often resistant to dietary or vitamin therapy. Not much is known about the origin of this syndrome. It has been attributed to chronic thiamine deficiency or to inadequate treatment of subacute beriberi, but Platt (1958) suggested that in Shanghai, before the Second World War, this form of beriberi was associated with heavy consumption of alcohol and with chronic lead poisoning.

Myopathy

There are some indications that myopathy may also occur in thiamine deficiency. Calf muscle tenderness and elevated serum CPK levels are described in beriberi (Yabuki et al. 1976), although the serum enzyme elevations could be of cardiac origin. Kark (1975) observed mitochondrial abnormalities, lipid accumulation, and a minor degree of muscle fiber degeneration in thiamine-deficient rats, but no myopathic abnormalities were observed in another study (Juntunen et al. 1979). Mesulam and coworkers (1979) observed early and striking proximal lower extremity weakness in thiamine-deficient monkeys, but did not characterize the muscle weakness. These data are incomplete and inconsistent, yet it seems plausible that thiamine deficiency would impair muscle function, since the vitamin is necessary for oxidative metabolism. It is not clear to what extent the high-output state, edema, exertional dyspnea, and tachycardia of beriberi are due to lactic acidosis rather than cardiomyopathy; the same symptoms occur in some patients with mitochondrial myopathies, who generate excessive amounts of lactic acid during exercise.

Causes of Thiamine Deficiency

Aside from dietary lack, the most common causes of thiamine deficiency are alcoholism and malabsorption. In alcoholics, inadequate diet is probably the most important factor, though alcohol and malnutrition also impair the active transport of thiamine across the intestinal mucosa. (Absorption of pharmacologic doses are not impaired, however, since at high luminal concentrations thiamine transport is largely passive and nonsaturable [Hoyumpa 1980].) Severe and protracted vomiting is the only gastrointestinal disorder likely to produce overt neurologic symptoms of thiamine deficiency, and the typical complication is Wernicke's disease, not neuropathy. Some degree of thiamine deficiency is fairly common in various other malabsorption states, but there is little evidence that neurologic complications result (Pallis and Lewis 1974).

Diagnosis of Thiamine Deficiency

Measurement of plasma or serum thiamine levels is technically difficult, and the results do not correlate well with clinical findings. Currently the standard test for thiamine deficiency is to measure erythrocyte transketolase activity, with and without added thiamine pyrophosphate. The degree of enzyme activation by thiamine pyrophosphate is supposed to reflect the degree of deficiency of the coenzyme. The upper limit of normal for the activation ratio (mean value plus two standard deviations) is about 1.20, that is, 20-percent activation by thiamine pyrophosphate (Bayoumi and Rosalki 1976; Langohr et al. 1981). Yet only half of a group of patients with Wernicke's encephalopathy had an elevated activation ratio, compared with 88 percent who had low transketolase activity without added thiamine pyrophosphate (Wood et al. 1977).

Pyridoxine Deficiency

Pyridoxine deficiency causes seizures in infancy, but in adults neurologic symptoms are rarely traceable to lack of pyridoxine, even though there is evidence of pyridoxine deficiency in many patients with cancer (Potera et al. 1977) or celiac disease (Morris et al. 1970), and in uremic patients on maintenance hemodialysis (Teehan 1978). Disorders of pyridoxine metabolism in adults are mainly caused by treatment with isoniazid or other drugs, and peripheral neuropathy is the main complication encountered; seizures, mental disturbance, and optic neuritis occur less frequently.

Isoniazid Neuropathy

Isoniazid inactivates pyridoxal by combining with it to form an isonicotinylhydrazine. Slow inactivators of isoniazid have high plasma concentrations of the drug on standard dosage; without pyridoxine supplementation, 50 percent of such individuals will develop peripheral neuropathy. Hydralazine inactivates pyridoxine by a similar mechanism and is a rare cause of neuropathy, and penicillamine may cause neuropathy by acting as an antimetabolite of pyridoxine. In all of these cases neuropathy can be prevented by concomitant administration of pyridoxine.

The neuropathy begins with numbness and paresthesia in the fingers and toes and progresses slowly over the course of months to produce a stocking-glove pattern of sensory disturbance, distal muscle weakness and wasting, and pain and tenderness in the calves. Fasciculations may be observed. Deep sensation is less impaired than superficial sensation, and spontaneous burning pain is commonly reported. The muscle stretch reflexes are depressed, especially in the distal portions of the extremities.

Motor nerve conduction velocity may be reduced to a slight or moderate extent, mainly in the lower extremities. The pathologic findings consist of Wallerian degeneration of both myelinated and unmyelinated nerves, accompanied by abundant regeneration of nerve fibers. Clinical recovery is very slow and may continue for more than a year, but it is eventually complete except in the most severely affected patients (LeQuesne 1975; Ochoa 1970).

Carpal Tunnel Syndrome

Ellis and colleagues (Ellis et al. 1976, 1977; Folkers et al. 1978) claim to have shown that pyridoxine deficiency is a frequent cause of carpal tunnel syndrome, nocturnal leg cramps, and assorted other symptoms. They reported that patients with these complaints had a low basal activity of erythrocyte glutamicoxaloacetic transaminase with excessive enhancement by pyridoxal phosphate, and that treatment with pyridoxine corrected the biochemical abnormalities and improved the symptoms. These claims cannot be taken very seriously, inasmuch as the diagnosis of carpal tunnel syndrome was not documented by clinical description or electrodiagnostic tests, the biochemical measurements were not performed in a properly controlled fashion, and treatment with pyridoxine was not randomized or controlled in any way.

Vitamin B_{12} Deficiency

Peripheral Neuropathy

The well-known neurologic picture of spinal cord involvement in pernicious anemia includes signs of posterior and lateral column involvement, with sensory ataxia and spasticity in the lower extremities. In recent years, however, a sensorimotor polyneuropathy has come to be recognized as a frequent and early manifestation of vitamin B_{12} deficiency (Pallis and Lewis 1974). The findings consist of impairment of superficial sensation in a stocking-glove distribution, reduction or absence of muscle stretch reflexes, and sometimes distal weakness and wasting of muscles. Vibratory sensation is nearly always reduced, but it is difficult to decide whether this abnormality is due to involvement of the spinal cord, the peripheral nerves, or both. In most cases there is probably simultaneous involvement of the spinal cord and peripheral nerves, so that the term *myeloneuropathy* is an appropriate designation.

Recently, some authors have claimed that clinical signs of neuropathy are encountered more frequently than signs of myelopathy in untreated patients with megaloblastic anemia caused by vitamin B_{12} deficiency (Shorvon et al. 1980; Cox-Klazinga and Endtz 1980). However, the clinical criteria used for diagnosing isolated neuropathy were ambiguous; for example, isolated loss of vibration sense in the legs was said to be evidence for a neuropathy (Shorvon et al. 1980). Even loss of reflexes does not prove that a neuropathy is present, since degeneration of the central limbs of afferent neurons could give the same result (Kosik et al. 1980). Electrophysiologic tests, however, show unequivocal peripheral nerve abnormalities in two thirds of patients with megaloblastic anemia caused by vitamin B_{12} deficiency. The most frequent abnormality is a reduced amplitude of the sensory nerve action potential; less often there is slowing of motor or sensory conduction velocity. All of these findings are more marked in the lower extremities. In patients with neuropathic weakness, electromyographic evidence of denervation is found, and in severe cases the motor nerve trunks may be inexcitable (Kosik et al. 1980).

In a recent study of sural nerve pathology, the main finding was axonal degeneration; there was a small amount of segmental demyelination and nerve fiber regeneration. The predominance of axonal degeneration is compatible with the minor degree of nerve conduction slowing observed electrophysiologically. However, in the spinal cord demyelination of white matter tracts is the primary lesion, both in human cases (Pant et al. 1968) and in monkeys (Agamanolis et al. 1978); axonal degeneration is a late development in severe cases. Torres and colleagues (1971) stated that segmental demyelination was the main peripheral nerve lesion in monkeys with experimental vitamin B_{12} deficiency, although Wallerian degeneration occurred in more severe cases; unfortunately, the authors did not perform electrophysiologic tests, and the study has been criticized because the diets were not precisely defined, so that other vitamin deficiencies could have been present. Agamanolis and associates (1976) did not observe peripheral nerve lesions in their vitamin B_{12}-deficient monkeys; nerve root demyelinative lesions did not extend beyond the leptomeningeal reflection. However, they did not study nerve conduction electrophysiologically and did not use quantitative morphometric techniques in assessing peripheral nerve pathology.

Results of Treatment

Both the peripheral and central nervous system lesions of vitamin B_{12} deficiency are potentially reversible, but following treatment the peripheral nerve lesions generally recover to a greater degree. This is not surprising, since only in the peripheral nervous system can axonal degeneration be repaired by regeneration and terminal sprouting. As a result, the signs of peripheral neuropathy are less apparent in treated cases, and a flaccid paraplegia may be replaced by a spastic paraparesis. Even so, severe neuropathy may leave permanent muscle weakness, muscular atrophy, and sensory loss in the distal lower extremities.

Obstacles to the Diagnosis of Vitamin B_{12} Deficiency

All too often, the diagnosis of vitamin B_{12} deficiency is not made until nervous system damage is far advanced and only partly reversible. The reasons for diagnostic delay are many and various. The onset of neurologic symptoms is usually insidious; vague paresthesias and subjective weakness may be present for months or years before the disease accelerates to produce obvious neurologic abnormalities. In a few patients there may even be a remitting course or a stepwise progression, leading to an erroneous diagnosis of multiple sclerosis. Another misleading feature is the occurrence of Lhermitte's sign in up to 25 percent of cases (Gautier-Smith 1973; Butler et al. 1981); this symptom of posterior column demyelination is sometimes incorrectly assumed to be specific for multiple sclerosis. Loss of erectile potency, upper motor neuron bladder symptoms, and abnormalities of visual, auditory, and somatosensory evoked responses are other consequences of vitamin B_{12} deficiency that are easily misinterpreted as evidence of multiple sclerosis (Krumholz et al. 1981).

Most patients develop a macrocytic, megaloblastic anemia. The erythrocyte mean corpuscular volume (MCV) is often increased for many months before anemia develops. Though accurate MCV results are now provided routinely by automated blood counts, high MCV values often go unnoticed, perhaps because physicians do not scan the red cell indices if anemia is not present, or because other causes of macrocytosis are more common than vitamin B_{12} deficiency (Hall 1981). Furthermore, folic acid therapy can abolish the anemia and the macrocytosis while the neurologic state continues to deteriorate.

Another source of difficulty is a widespread reliance on serum vitamin B_{12} levels for the diagnosis of vitamin B_{12} deficiency. Although inaccuracies of the radioisotopic assays have been publicized recently, the microbiologic assays are just as insensitive, and it has been estimated that 10 to 20 percent of the common vitamin B_{12} deficiency states would not be recognized by either assay (England and Linnell 1980). Most of the cobalamin present in human serum is bound to transcobalamin I and has a half-life of 240 hours; the cobalamin bound to transcobalamin II, which accounts for 10 to 30 percent of the total serum cobalamin assayed by radioisotopic or microbiologic methods, has a half-life of 0.1 hour and is thought to be the metabolically important fraction. Thus, the total serum cobalamin level does not accurately reflect the cobalamin available to the tissues. Furthermore, cobalamins can be inactivated by nitrous oxide, producing myeloneuropathy with normal serum cobalamin levels (Layzer 1978).

England and Linnell (1980) recommend the following approach to the diagnosis of vitamin B_{12} deficiency in a patient with suggestive neurologic symptoms: (1) First take a dietary history. (2) If dietary intake of vitamin B_{12} appears to be inadequate, the patient should be given a therapeutic trial of vitamin B_{12}. (In this context a low serum cobalamin level may be misleading, since the levels are low in 75 percent of vegetarians, most of whom do not have clinical manifestations of vitamin B_{12} deficiency.) (3) If dietary intake is adequate, a Schilling test should be performed. If vitamin B_{12} absorption is defective, a repeat test performed with intrinsic factor will then distinguish addisonian pernicious anemia from other types of malabsorption.

Causes of Vitamin B_{12} Deficiency

According to a recent study, among 50 consecutive patients admitted to a London Hospital with megaloblastic anemia owing to vitamin B_{12} deficiency there were 32 patients with addisonian pernicious anemia, 8 patients with dietary deficiency, and 7 patients with "gastrointestinal disease." The last category was not described further but did not include celiac disease or malabsorption, though these diseases were identified as frequent causes of folate deficiency (Shorvon et al. 1980). The presence of a large Indian vegetarian population in London may explain the high proportion of cases caused by dietary deficiency. Pallis and Lewis (1974) scrutinized 131 published cases of vitamin B_{12} deficiency myelopathy occurring in conditions other than addisonian pernicious anemia. Only 33 cases were accepted as adequately documented. Of these 16 were due to partial gastrectomy and 3 to total gastrectomy; the remaining cases included inadequate diet and various small intestinal disorders such as diverticulosis, fistula, stricture, blind loop, and resection. Gastroenterostomy was a frequently reported cause, but none of the cases were well documented. Neurologic complications are also common in patients with vitamin B_{12} deficiency caused by infestation with the fish tape worm, Diphyllobothrium latum. Thus, the gastrointestinal disorders most often associated with neurologic complications of vitamin B_{12} deficiency are those involving gastric resection and structural alterations of the small intestine. Celiac disease, regional ileitis, and other malabsorption syndromes can interfere with the absorption of vitamin B_{12}, but neurologic complications are unlikely to result (Pallis and Lewis 1974).

Pathophysiology. Only two mammalian enzymes are known to require vitamin B_{12} as a cofactor, but until recently neither enzyme could be clearly implicated in the neurologic disorders associated with vitamin B_{12} deficiency. Current research, however, assigns a central role to the enzyme methionine synthetase, which generates methionine from homocysteine by transferring a methyl group from 5-methyltetrahydrofolate (Fig. 40).

One line of evidence came from an unexpected source. Amess and associates (1978) observed that exposure to nitrous oxide caused megaloblastic bone marrow changes in postoperative patients. Simultaneously, my colleagues and I came upon several cases of peripheral neuropathy and myeloneuropathy in persons heavily exposed to nitrous oxide, either as a "recreational" drug or through contamination of dental operating rooms (Layzer et al. 1978). The peripheral neuropathy could be mild or severe and appeared to involve axonal degeneration, as judged by electrophysiologic testing. The neurologic features of these cases bore a striking resemblance to those of pernicious anemia, though serum vitamin B_{12} levels were normal. Dinn and colleagues (1978, 1980), following up the lead provided by the work of Amess and associates, quickly showed that a myelopathy typical of vitamin B_{12} deficiency could be produced in monkeys by prolonged exposure to nitrous oxide. Meanwhile, several groups of investigators demonstrated that nitrous oxide rapidly and selectively inactivates methionine synthetase, leaving unaffected methylmalonyl-CoA mutase, the other enzyme that requires vitamin B_{12} (Deacon et al. 1978). Nitrous oxide oxidizes the cobalt atom, preventing the formation of methylcobalamin and in the process becoming reduced to nitrogen and oxygen. Thus, the clinical and biochemical effects of nitrous oxide suggested that lack of methionine synthetase activity was responsible for the neurologic complications of vitamin B_{12} deficiency.

Dinn and colleagues (1980) postulated that the neurologic disorder was due to "methyl group deficiency" resulting from deficiency of methionine and its active form, S-adenosyl methionine, a methyl-group donor necessary for a variety of methylation reactions. In support of this hypothesis, they showed that dietary supple-

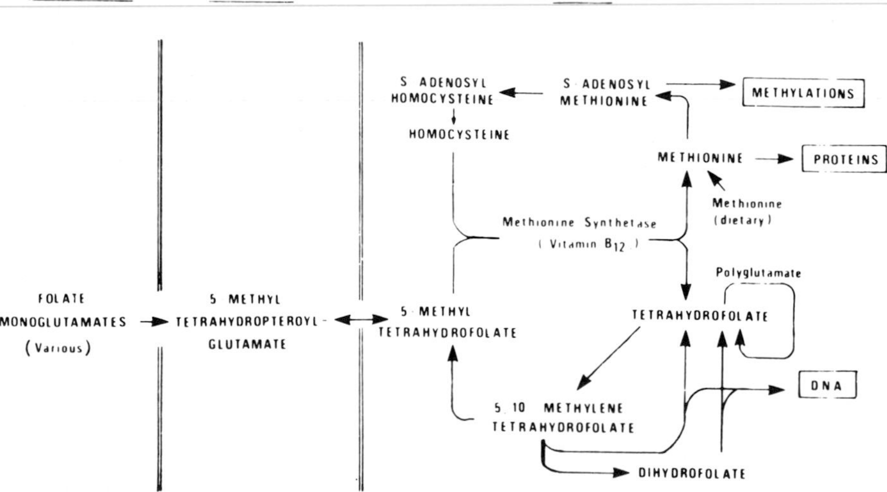

FIGURE 40. The role of B_{12}-dependent methionine synthetase in methylation reactions and DNA synthesis. This key enzyme reaction generates both S-adenosylmethionine, which is thought to be important in nervous system metabolism, and the active forms of folic acid, which are required for hemopoiesis. (From Scott et al., 1981, with permission.)

ments of methionine largely prevented nitrous oxide myeloneuropathy in monkeys (Scott et al. 1981). The fact that methionine deficiency caused by low methionine synthetase activity can be offset by dietary methionine may explain why the severity of neurologic involvement is so variable in patients with pernicious anemia, and why rodents are so resistant to the neurologic complications of vitamin B_{12} deficiency.

Meanwhile, another line of evidence was converging on the same hypothesis. Several years earlier Gandy and coworkers (1973) had induced subacute combined degeneration of the cord in mice by feeding them cycloleucine. This chemical analogue of methionine inhibits the biosynthesis of S-adenosyl methionine, which is not only a methyl donor but is also an essential cofactor for the conversion of homocysteine to methionine by the methionine synthetase reaction. Gandy and coworkers postulated that methylation of myelin constituents might be defective in subacute combined degeneration.

This speculation has been extended by recent evidence showing that cycloleucine inhibits the methylation of myelin basic protein in the spinal cord (Small and Carnegie 1981). However, methylation reactions are numerous and involve phospholipids as well as proteins, so hunting for one crucial methylation reaction may be an overly simple approach. The status of the peripheral nervous system in these speculations remains unclear; peripheral nerve myelin is different from central myelin, and demyelination does not appear to be the dominant abnormality in the peripheral nerve lesions.

Deficiency of Other Water-Soluble Vitamins

After a critical review of the pertinent literature, Pallis and Lewis (1974) concluded that there was no evidence that deficiency of riboflavin, niacin, or pantothenic acid can cause a peripheral neuropathy. Reynolds and coworkers (1973) have frequently suggested that folic acid deficiency causes neurologic symptoms, especially depression and dementia. However, isolated folic acid deficiency is a rare occurrence, because human folate deficiency is almost always due to other diseases such as alcoholism, malabsorption, or nutritional deficiency, which themselves are capable of producing neuropathy (Pallis and Lewis 1974). In a recent investigation of 34 patients with megaloblastic anemia owing to folate deficiency, Reynolds' group reported that peripheral neuropathy was present in 18 percent of the patients (Shorvon et al. 1980), but they did not provide any clinical or electrophysiologic details to substantiate the diagnosis of neuropathy, and they did not mention the age of the patients or their underlying diagnoses. Furthermore, there was no control group of patients with similar underlying diseases but without folate deficiency. In an earlier, better controlled study the incidence of neuropathy in patients with folate deficiency was 58 percent but was not significantly greater than in a control group (Reynolds et al. 1973).

Vitamin E Deficiency

Clinical Features

Although dietary deficiency of vitamin E induces myopathy and other neurologic abnormalities in many animal species, until recently there has been little evidence for the existence of similar disorders in man. Now, however, there are growing indications that prolonged deficiency of vitamin E during childhood and adolescence may be responsible for a distinctive combination of CNS, peripheral nerve, and muscle abnormalities. In most of the reported cases vitamin E deficiency was due to chronic steatorrhea associated with either cholestatic liver disease or cystic fibrosis (Gomez et al. 1972; Tomasi 1979; Rosenblum et al. 1981; Elias et al. 1981; Guggenheim et al. 1982), but in one case there was malabsorption of vitamin E without steatorrhea or any apparent bowel abnormality (Burck et al. 1981). A similar syndrome has been reported, without vitamin E measurements, in a patient with celiac disease (Telerman-Toppet et al. 1969) and in another patient with steatorrhea of undetermined cause (Direkze 1973).

In most of the reported cases, the symptoms developed in childhood or adolescence and progressed slowly for many years. The earliest and most constant findings were loss of reflexes, impaired vibration sense, and sensory ataxia. Position sense was less severely affected, and small diameter nerve fibers conducting pain and temperature sensation were usually spared. Muscle weakness and atrophy developed later and could be diffuse, predominantly distal, or in a myopathic distribution with lordosis, waddling gait, Gowers' sign, and proximal limb weakness. Progressive external ophthalmoplegia was present in about half of the cases, and Babinski's signs were infrequent.

Serum CPK levels were normal or mildly increased. Sensory nerve conduction tests showed reduced or absent responses, while motor nerve conduction was slightly or moderately slow in some patients and normal in others. Examination of the sural nerves by biopsy or autopsy showed a slight reduction of the number of large myelinated fibers. Muscle biopsies showed mainly neurogenic abnormalities, including atrophy of scattered type 1 and type 2 fibers, small-group or large-group fiber atrophy, fiber type grouping, and target fibers. In muscle fibers and Schwann cells there were dense, autofluorescent lipopigment bodies that contained abundant amounts of acid phosphatase and appeared to represent secondary lysosomes. Primary myopathic changes have been negligible or absent. In autopsy cases the primary lesion was a degeneration of large-diameter sensory axons in the posterior columns, sensory roots, and peripheral nerves, with numerous axonal swellings (spheroids) in the gracile and cuneate nuclei, Clarke's column, and posterior columns. Lipopigment was present in neurons of the dorsal root ganglia, anterior horns, and brainstem motor nuclei, and there was mild loss of neurons with reactive astrocytosis in the third and fourth nerve nuclei (Geller et al. 1977; Sung et al. 1980; Rosenblum et al. 1981).

Experimental vitamin E deficiency in rhesus monkeys has recently been reported to cause nearly identical pathologic lesions. It appears that both the spinal cord and peripheral nerve sensory axon degeneration are due to a dying-back axonopathy rather than to degeneration of the dorsal root ganglion cells, which are less severely affected (Nelson et al. 1981). Moreover, these cases bear a striking resemblance to the neurologic picture associated with abetalipoproteinemia (Bassen-Kornzweig disease), a hereditary disease characterized by steatorrhea, malabsorption of fats, and profound vitamin E deficiency (Miller et al. 1980). There are preliminary reports that treatment with vitamin E may improve the neurologic abnormalities in that disease (Herbert et al. 1978) and in some cases of vitamin E deficiency associated with other malabsorption syndromes (Elias et al. 1981; Burck et al. 1981; Tomasi 1979; Guggenheim et al. 1982). In a number of cases, however, oral vitamin E supplements were ineffective even when a water-miscible preparation was administered, and parenteral administration was necessary to raise the serum vitamin E levels to normal (Elias et al. 1981; Guggenheim et al. 1982).

Necrotizing Myopathy

Myopathy was a very minor pathologic feature of the human cases described above. In most patients histologic examination of muscle showed only neurogenic atrophy, although mild CPK elevations were present in some cases. In contrast, myopathy is the most common abnormality in animals with vitamin E deficiency, and it has been observed in every species studied including chickens, ducks, rats, and monkeys. This muscle disorder is so easily induced by commercial animal feeds that "nutritional muscular dystrophy" is a common problem in domestic animals. In some species there is a frank necrotizing myopathy heralded by a steep rise in serum enzyme activities (Machlin et al. 1978) and rapidly reversed by vitamin E, which fosters brisk muscle regeneration. In other species active muscle necrosis is less obvious, but the muscle fiber profile is gradually transformed into a type 2 predominance (Parry and Montpetit 1978), probably as a result of continual proteolytic degradation of type 1 muscle fibers (Dayton et al. 1979). It is not clear why similar muscle changes have not been observed in patients with vitamin E deficiency, or to what extent a primary myopathy is responsible for the muscle weakness found in such patients. Muscle weakness and creatinuria are frequently present in children with cystic fibrosis, though the weakness has not been described in detail. Most such patients are vitamin E deficient; administration of tocopherol reduces the creatinuria but seems to have no significant effect on muscle strength (Levin et al. 1961).

Pathophysiology. The biochemical mechanism of muscle degeneration in vitamin E deficiency has been studied in considerable detail. Like selenium, vitamin E is thought to act as an antioxidant, protecting unsaturated membrane lipids and possibly some proteins from oxidative degradation. Polymerization of peroxidized fatty acids with polysaccharides is thought to account for the accumulation of the brown lipochrome pigment (ceroid) that is deposited in many tissues and causes the distinctive "brown-bowel" syndrome in patients with vitamin E deficiency (Braunstein 1961). Vitamin E may act at an early stage in this process by preventing the formation of hydroperoxides from unsaturated fatty acids, while selenium is a cofactor for glutathione peroxidase, which destroys hydrogen peroxide and fatty acid hydroperoxides when they have formed (Rotruck et al. 1973). Thus, vitamin E and selenium appear to have complementary actions, and deficiency of one substance increases the dietary requirement for the other (Van Vleet 1980).

The dietary requirement for vitamin E is increased with a diet high in polyunsaturated fatty acids. Administration of the sulfur-containing amino acid cystine, a precursor of glutathione, also helps to prevent nutritional muscular dystrophy in some species, but muscle levels of reduced glutathione are *higher* than normal in vitamin E-deficient animals. However, the ratio of disulfide to sulfhydryls in muscle proteins is markedly increased in vitamin E-deficient chicks, and Shih and coworkers (1977) suggested that sulfhydryl compounds such as cysteine (the reduced form of cystine) may prevent oxidative degradation of muscle proteins by reversing the oxidation of protein sulfhydryl groups to protein sulfonates; this would prevent the irreversible oxidation of sulfonates to disulfides. Studies carried out with erythrocytes have shown that oxidized proteins are rapidly degraded by a soluble, ATP-dependent proteolytic system (Goldberg and Boches 1982).

Administration of the antioxidant ethoxyquin protects vitamin E-deficient rats from the development of necrotizing myopathy (Gabriel et al. 1980). Biochemical and structural abnormalities of mitochondria are a prominent feature of the myopathy in vitamin E-deficient rabbits, an observation that may partly explain the special vulnerability of type 1 muscle fibers (Heffron et al. 1978). So far, the biochemical effects of vitamin E deficiency on muscle have not been studied in human patients with muscle weakness.

Occurrence of Vitamin E Deficiency

The only known cause of vitamin E deficiency in man is malabsorption. Absorption of vitamin E from the proximal small intestine begins with the hydrolysis of vitamin E esters by pancreatic enzymes, a reaction that requires bile salts as cofactors. Bile salts are also important for intraluminal solubilization of nonpolar lipids such as vitamin E, through the formation of micelles that are absorbed via the intestinal lymphatics. The extremely low serum levels of vitamin E in abetalipoproteinemia suggest that chylomicron synthesis in the intestinal mucosa is also essential for the absorption of tocopherol.

Muller and associates (1974) examined absorption of vitamin E in groups of children with five disorders causing malabsorption. Children with abetalipoproteinemia were totally deficient in vitamin E, but serum vitamin E levels rose when massive oral doses were given in either a fat-soluble or a water-miscible form, reflecting, perhaps, absorption via the portal vein rather than the lymphatic system. Vitamin E deficiency was nearly as severe in children with obstructive jaundice, but serum levels could not be raised by massive oral vitamin E therapy, emphasizing the essential role of bile salts in vitamin E absorption. Cystic fibrosis was associated with moderate vitamin E deficiency, which was more easily corrected by administration of a water-miscible form of vitamin E than of the fat-soluble preparation. Malabsorption of lipid-soluble vitamins in cystic fibrosis and other forms of pancreatic insufficiency appears to result both from reduced secretion of the pancreatic enzyme that hydrolizes vitamin E esters, and from inadequate micellar solubilization owing to reduced availability of bile acids, which are insufficiently reabsorbed in the distal ileum. Oral administration of pancreatic enzymes corrects these abnormalities (Scott et al. 1977). Children with intestinal lymphangiectasia have a moderate degree of vitamin E deficiency that is easily corrected by small oral supplements of fat-soluble vitamin E. The mildest degree of vitamin E deficiency is found in children with celiac disease; in these patients the vitamin deficiency responds to a gluten-free diet without vitamin supplementation.

Vitamin D Deficiency

The relation of vitamin D deficiency to proximal muscular weakness is discussed in Chapter 3.

Essential Fatty Acid Deficiency

Essential fatty acid (EFA) deficiency can occur in infants and growing children as a result of dietary inadequacy or malabsorption of fats, but it is rare in adults because the plentiful stores of arachidonic and linoleic acids are readily mobilized from body lipids during starvation. However, total parenteral alimentation with lipid-free solutions has been found to produce biochemical evidence of EFA deficiency after only 1 week, and within 4 weeks some patients developed typical symptoms such as hair loss, a dry, scaly dermatitis, and delayed wound healing (McCarthy et al. 1981; Goodgame et al. 1978). It appears that high plasma carbohydrate and insulin levels suppress lipolysis, so that the body stores of EFA become unavailable.

Recently Stewart and Hensley (1981) described four patients who developed generalized muscle pain, tenderness, and swelling, with abrupt elevations of serum CPK activity to very high levels (1500 to 2200 units per liter), after 2 to 3 weeks of lipid-free total parenteral nutrition. The clinical muscle status was not described; EMG was said to confirm an acute myopathy, but muscle biopsy was not performed. Serum electrolytes and minerals were normal, and all the patients had received standard amounts of vitamins and trace elements, including vitamin E and selenium. High ratios of 5,8,11-eicosatrienoic acid to arachidonic acid in plasma confirmed the presence of EFA deficiency in all of the cases. The symptoms and laboratory abnormalities subsided rapidly on stopping parenteral alimentation; administration of intravenous linoleate (Intralipid) was equally effective, even when total parenteral nutrition was continued.

Acute, necrotizing myopathy has not previously been recognized as a complication of EFA deficiency, and none of the patients had the usual skin and hair changes of that disorder, so the cause of this new muscle syndrome is uncertain. It is clear, however, that it can be prevented by periodic intravenous administration of EFA during total parenteral nutrition.

MINERAL AND ELECTROLYTE DEFICIENCIES

Potassium, Magnesium, and Phosphorus Deficiencies

These minerals are discussed in Chapter 2.

Trace Metals Deficiency

Chromium

Chromium deficiency appeared to be the cause of a peripheral neuropathy that developed in a patient who had been treated by total parenteral nutrition for a period of 3 years (Jeejeebhoy et al. 1977). The patient complained of paresthesias and ataxia of the legs. EMG showed reduced recruitment of motor unit potentials in a foot muscle, and motor nerve conduction was slow in the peroneal and posterior tibial nerves; no other details were given. Weight loss, a marked increase in the number of calories needed to sustain weight, and mild diabetes mellitus were additional features. The respiratory quotient was low, suggesting predominant use of lipid fuel despite a high carbohydrate content of the parenteral formula. Further investigation disclosed a negative chromium balance with low blood and hair levels of chromium, and the disorder resolved with chromium supplementation.

The function of chromium is not well understood; chromium deficiency causes glucose intolerance, but insulin levels are normal. In this patient the increased caloric intake needed to maintain constant weight, despite insulin therapy, and the low respiratory quotient, imply a block of cellular metabolism of carbohydrate fuels.

Selenium

Selenium deficiency is rare in human beings but is a frequent cause of disease in grazing animals, giving rise to disorders such as "white muscle disease," necrotizing myopathy, myoglobinuria, liver necrosis, and cardiomyopathy (Van Vleet 1980). The principal cause of selenium deficiency in domestic animals is a low selenium content of foliage plants grown on acidic, poorly aerated soils, but high intake of copper, silver, tellurium, or zinc may antagonize the action of selenium, increasing the dietary requirement. As mentioned above, vitamin E and selenium have complementary actions; deficiency of either substance may produce similar manifestations, combined deficiency occurs in domestic animals, and to some extent either substance may be used to treat this deficiency (Van Vleet 1980).

Congestive cardiomyopathy is endemic in a selenium-deficient zone of China and has been attributed to selenium deficiency. Recently a fatal cardiomyopathy occurred in an occidental patient after 2 years of total parenteral nutrition without selenium supplements (Johnson et al. 1981). Total parenteral nutrition for more than 3 weeks produced asymptomatic selenium deficiency in patients living in a low-selenium area of New Zealand (van Rij et al. 1979), and one patient developed pain and tenderness of the thigh muscles, responding to selenium replacement (no clinical or laboratory details were given). An American patient developed muscle pain and tenderness, with markedly elevated CPK levels in the serum, after 2 years of total parenteral nutrition. Selenium deficiency was discovered, and the muscle disorder responded to selenium replacement (Kien and Ganther 1983).

Because of the low selenium levels of soil in many parts of New Zealand, plasma and electrolyte selenium levels are substantially lower in New Zealanders than in the inhabitants of most other countries. The activity of the selenium-dependent enzyme erythrocyte glutathione peroxidase is correspondingly reduced. In one rural area of New Zealand, where selenium deficiency occurs commonly in livestock, nearly half of the inhabitants complain of myalgia and muscle tenderness, but a placebo-controlled trial of selenium supplements showed no effect on these symptoms (Thomson and Robinson 1980).

Iron Deficiency

Excessive fatigue and reduced physical stamina are the classical symptoms of iron-deficiency anemia. Although these symptoms are plausibly attributable to the anemia itself, recent animal studies have shown that the capacity for sustained running is reduced even when the anemia is corrected (Finch et al. 1976; Davies et al. 1982). The muscle content of iron-containing oxidative enzymes and the maximum oxidative capacity are about half of normal (McLane et al. 1981). Muscle fatigue (measured as a decline of contractile force) and lactic acid release were nearly twice normal during indirect stimulation of muscles of the perfused rat hind limb. The abnormalities were most marked in fast-twitch red muscle fibers, which are rich in both oxidative and glycolytic enzymes.

The consequences of a reduced aerobic capacity of muscle in the anemic animal or patient are not known. Severe anemia alone increases lactic acidemia during exercise, by reducing the rate of delivery of oxygen to the working muscle; lactic acidosis, in turn, induces hyperpnea, tachycardia, hyperkinetic circulation, and early fatigue. Reduction of the oxidative capacity of muscle also causes lactic acidosis, but by reducing muscle oxygen consumption it would *lower* peripheral oxygen utilization, permitting more of the circulating oxygen to be utilized by the brain and other organs. Thus, the reduced exercise capacity of iron-deficient muscle may simply be appropriate for the reduced oxygen-carrying capacity of the blood.

COMPLICATIONS OF PARENTERAL ALIMENTATION

Metabolic derangements that occur during parenteral alimentation are often signaled by neuromuscular symptoms. The incidence of these com-

TABLE 26. Neuromuscular Complications of Parenteral Alimentation

Syndrome	Metabolic Disorder
Acute or subacute necrotic myopathy	Hypophosphatemia Potassium deficiency Essential fatty acid deficiency Selenium deficiency (?)
Acute reversible paralysis	Hypokalemia Hyperkalemia Hypophosphatemia
Tetany	Hypocalcemia Hypomagnesemia
Polyneuropathy	Chromium deficiency

plications has diminished considerably in the past decade as a result of experience gained from early catastrophes, and the requirements for electrolytes, minerals, vitamins and other nutrients have been well defined. It is still important, however, to monitor serum chemistries carefully during the institution of hyperalimentation in sick or malnourished patients. The specific neuromuscular disorders that may be encountered during parenteral fluid or alimentary therapy are listed in Table 26. A detailed discussion of each disorder will be found in other parts of this book.

INTESTINAL MALABSORPTION

The neuromuscular complications encountered in patients with intestinal malabsorption are listed in Table 27. Some of these complications have well-defined causes, such as myopathy owing to vitamin D deficiency, neuropathy and myeloneuropathy owing to vitamin B_{12} deficiency, tetany owing to hypocalcemia or magnesium deficiency, and acute flaccid paralysis owing to potassium depletion. Other complications are suspected to result from prolonged deficiency of vitamin E (neuromyopathy, sensory myeloneuropathy, and external ophthalmoplegia), though evidence for this is still incomplete. There remain a number of cases of myopathy, peripheral neuropathy, and myeloneuropathy, the nutritional basis of which is not understood; in some cases the neuromuscular symptoms improve when the malabsorption is controlled, but others resist all attempts at treatment. Some patients have few or no gastrointestinal symptoms, the presenting symptoms being neuromuscular. Malabsorption is thus an important, little-known cause of neuropathy and myopathy of obscure origin.

Tropical Sprue and Celiac Disease

Tropical sprue is a diffuse disorder of the small-intestinal mucosa that is endemic to Southern India, Sri Lanka, Southeast Asia, and the Caribbean Islands. The cause is unknown but is thought to be infectious, because it may occur in epidemic form and often responds to treatment with antibiotics. Celiac disease (gluten-sensitive enteropathy) has many clinical and pathologic similarities to tropical sprue, and neuromuscular complications appear to have a similar incidence in the two disorders (Table 28). Both disorders can cause neuromuscular symptoms without obvious gastrointestinal symptoms.

TABLE 27. Neuromuscular Complications of Intestinal Malabsorption

Neuromuscular Syndrome	Sprue, Celiac Disease	Bacterial Overgrowth	Gastric Resection	Diffuse Ileal Disease	Chronic Pancreatitis	Cystic Fibrosis	Chronic Cholestatic Liver Disease
Myopathy due to vitamin D deficiency	+		+				
Myopathy due to other causes	+		+		+	+	+
Sensorimotor polyneuropathy	+	+	+		+	+	+
Myelopathy due to vitamin B-12 deficiency	+	+	+	+			
Myelopathy, cause unknown	+	+	+		+	+	+
Acute hypokalemic paralysis	+		+	+			
Tetany	+			+			
External ophthalmoplegia		+				+	+

TABLE 28. Neuromuscular Complications of Tropical Sprue and Celiac Disease

	Incidence (%)	
	Tropical Sprue*	Celiac Disease†
Myopathy	33%	12%
Polyneuropathy	0	5%
Myeloneuropathy due to:		
vitamin B-12 deficiency	4%	2%
cause unknown	0	5%
Acute hypokalemic paralysis	0	5%
Tetany	4%	12%
Restless legs syndrome	0	5%

*Iyer et al, 1973.
†Banerji and Hurwitz, 1971A.

The most common neuromuscular syndrome encountered in these disorders is a myopathy characterized by proximal muscle weakness and atrophy, with myopathic changes on EMG. This type of myopathy was present in one third of 24 unselected patients with tropical sprue in South India (Iyer et al. 1973) and in 12 percent of 42 partly selected adults with celiac disease in Northern Ireland (Banerji and Hurwitz 1971a). Serum enzymes are usually normal, and muscle biopsy shows scattered atrophy of single muscle fibers. In the few cases in which histochemical studies have been reported, type 2 atrophy has been found. Hall (1968) interpreted these histologic abnormalities as evidence of a neuropathy, a view that has been repeated uncritically by later authors, but the clinical and laboratory features of his two cases were typical of a metabolic myopathy such as that associated with osteomalacia. Banerji and Hurwitz (1971a) found biochemical and radiologic evidence of osteomalacia in all five of their celiac patients with myopathy, and all of them complained of bone pain. Thus, it is likely that vitamin-D deficiency is the major cause of myopathy in celiac disease.

Peripheral neuropathy is uncommon, and when present is usually associated with spinal cord signs referable to the posterior and lateral columns, giving a picture similar to that of vitamin B_{12} deficiency. In a few instances laboratory evidence of vitamin B_{12} deficiency was obtained and the neurologic symptoms responded to treatment with this vitamin (Iyer et al. 1973; Banerji and Hurwitz 1971a; Jeejeebhoy et al. 1967). But Cooke and Smith (1966) saw no response to vitamin B_{12} in a series of 16 patients with myeloneuropathy complicating adult celiac disease, and the findings at autopsy were not compatible with subacute combined degeneration.

Nerve conduction studies have given conflicting results. Nerve conduction was abnormal in a third of the patients with tropical sprue (Iyer et al. 1973), but only 7 percent of adults with celiac disease had reduced nerve conduction velocities (Morris et al. 1970; Banerji and Hurwitz 1971a). However, Binder and colleagues (1967) reported a patient with celiac disease who had a severe sensorimotor neuropathy with normal nerve conduction velocities, though the sensory nerve responses were diminished in amplitude. Unfortunately, none of the electrophysiologic studies has been reported in adequate detail, and nerve biopsies have not been studied by modern neuropathologic techniques.

Gastric Resection

The incidence of neurologic disorders following partial gastrectomy is surprisingly high. The exact incidence is unknown because a prospective study has not been carried out, but the careful retrospective study of 106 patients by Banerji and Hurwitz (1971b) probably gives a good approximation (Table 29). The interval from the gastric operation to the onset of neurologic symptoms ranged from 1 to 25 years, averaging 12 years in the 16 patients with neurologic signs. Of the six cases of myopathy, three were associated with steatorrhea and osteomalacia, one was due to potassium deficiency, and two were of uncertain cause. The osteomalacic myopathy was clinically identical to the myopathy of vitamin D deficiency, and all three patients responded to treatment with vitamin D. Five patients had a sensorimotor polyneuropathy with moderate slowing of motor nerve conduction velocity; in three of the five there was deficiency or malabsorption of vitamin B_{12}, and treatment with vitamin B_{12} was followed by improvement. Only two of these patients had steatorrhea.

Behse and Buchthal (1977) reported detailed electrophysiologic and pathologic studies in six patients who developed neuropathy between 1 and 15 years after a subtotal gastrectomy. All the patients had suffered severe weight loss and had evidence of malabsorption, but blood levels of vitamin B_{12} and Schilling tests were normal. The neurologic examination revealed a distal pattern of sensory loss, muscle weakness, and amyotrophy, without signs of spinal cord involvement. The spinal fluid protein was normal or slightly increased. Motor and sensory nerve conduction were slowed to a moderate or marked degree in proximal and distal nerve segments, and the amplitude of sensory nerve responses was markedly reduced. Microscopic examination of sural nerve biopsy specimens revealed segmental demyelination, remyelination, and regeneration. EMG showed signs of denervation and reinnervation in all muscles.

The nutritional factors responsible for this demyelinating neuropathy are completely unknown. None of the vitamin deficiencies is known to cause a demyelinating neuropathy. There are several reasons that malabsorption occurs rather frequently in patients who have undergone gastric resection (Greenberger and Isselbacher 1977). The usual Billroth II operation bypasses the duodenum, reducing the secretion of duodenal hormones that stimulate pancreatic secretion. The altered anatomic relationships may hamper the mixing of food with bile salts and pancreatic enzymes in the jejunum. If there is stasis in the afferent loop, bacterial overgrowth can lead to deconjugation of bile salts, which are then absorbed prematurely. All of these factors may result in steatorrhea and malabsorption of lipids and fat-soluble vitamins. Calcium deficiency results both from vitamin D deficiency

TABLE 29. Nervous System Disorders in 106 Patients Who Had a Previous Gastrectomy (Banerji and Hurwitz, 1971B)

	Number of Patients
Myopathy	6
Polyneuropathy	5
Myelopathy	5
Acute hypokalemic paralysis	1
Motor neuron disease	1
Restless legs syndrome	12

and from the formation of insoluble calcium soaps in the lumen of the bowel. Accelerated passage of food through the small bowel likewise interferes with digestion and absorption. As in sprue, unidentified components of malnutrition may contribute to the genesis of neuromuscular disorders.

Malabsorption of vitamin B_{12} is not uncommon, primarily as a result of reduced production of intrinsic factor by the gastric remnant, which in many cases undergoes atrophic gastritis. Partial gastrectomy was responsible for half of the reported cases of myelopathy caused by nonaddisonian vitamin B_{12} deficiency reviewed by Pallis and Lewis (1974). The complication is rare, however, since none of the 106 postgastrectomy patients examined by Bannerji and Hurwitz (1971b) had subacute combined degeneration of the cord; 5 patients had a myelopathy unresponsive to vitamin B_{12}, and 3 patients had a peripheral neuropathy that the authors attributed to vitamin B_{12} deficiency on rather slender evidence.

Some authors have claimed, without autopsy documentation, that amyotrophic lateral sclerosis or a syndrome resembling it is sometimes a consequence of subtotal gastrectomy (Ask-Upmark 1950; Kniffen and Quick 1969). It is unlikely, however, that the association of these two conditions is other than coincidental. Reports of pancreatic dysfunction in amyotrophic lateral sclerosis (Quick and Greer 1967) can probably be explained as a secondary result of malnutrition (Pallis and Lewis 1974).

Pancreatic Insufficiency

Chronic pancreatitis and cystic fibrosis are the main causes of chronic pancreatic insufficiency. Most cases of chronic pancreatitis are associated with alcoholism, and any neuromuscular complications that occur are usually attributed to alcoholism rather than to malabsorption; at any rate there are only two reports of neuromuscular disease attributed to chronic pancreatitis. One patient, whose intake of alcohol was not mentioned, had generalized weakness, a sensory polyneuropathy, severe steatorrhea, and diabetes mellitus; the vitamin E level was not measured, but bowel biopsy did not reveal ceroid pigment. Muscle biopsy was normal, and nerve conduction testing was said to show a sensory neuropathy (Binder et al. 1967). The second patient was a known alcoholic who developed painful proximal muscle weakness and wasting; vibration and position sense were reduced in the distal extremities, but reflexes and superficial pain sensation were intact. Diabetes mellitus and vitamin E deficiency were also present, and the bowel was stained brown by ceroid pigment. Serum enzymes were normal, EMG showed myopathic changes, motor nerve conduction velocities were moderately reduced, and muscle biopsy showed a combination of myopathic and neurogenic abnormalities (Bauman et al. 1968).

In these two cases it is difficult to know to what extent malabsorption was responsible for the neuromuscular abnormalities. However, alcoholic myopathy is usually associated with elevated serum enzyme levels, nerve conduction velocity is usually normal or only slightly reduced in alcoholic neuropathy, and diabetes had been present for a relatively short time. The role of vitamin E deficiency is also unclear. Deposits of ceroid pigment in various organs were found at autopsy in 61 percent of patients with chronic pancreatitis (Braunstein 1961), but the distinctive neuropathologic abnormalities associated with vitamin E deficiency have not been described in patients with chronic pancreatitis.

Cystic fibrosis is one of the leading causes of malabsorption in the United States. Children with cystic fibrosis tend to have poor muscular development and creatinuria, but their neuromuscular status has not been described in any detail. Vitamin E deficiency is usually present, but administration of vitamin E, while reducing creatinuria (Nitowsky 1956) and correcting the sensitivity of erythrocytes to peroxide hemolysis (Farrell et al. 1977), does not seem to improve muscle power (Levin et al. 1961). At autopsy, degeneration of skeletal muscle fibers has been noted in some patients, but no clinical details were reported (Weinberg et al. 1958). After many years of malabsorption, a few patients have developed sensory neuropathy, areflexia, signs of dorsal and lateral column involvement, ataxia, and external ophthalmoplegia, a syndrome that has been linked to vitamin E deficiency. A 19-year-old man with previously undiagnosed cystic fibrosis presented this constellation of neurologic abnormalities, together with rickets and a proximal myopathy. The bone and muscle symptoms resolved after treatment with vitamin D, but the other neurologic signs did not improve (Scott et al. 1977). In that case the myopathy was presumably caused by vitamin D deficiency. In summary, myopathy and motor neuropathy appear to be infrequent in cystic fibrosis, even in patients with neurologic signs suggestive of vitamin E deficiency.

Chronic Cholestatic Liver Disease

Some children with infantile obstructive cholangiopathy eventually develop a slowly progressive sensory ataxia that may be related to vitamin E deficiency. These cases were described earlier in this chapter. Some of the children also exhibit distal limb weakness and paralysis of extraocular muscles.

Jejunal Diverticulosis and Other Bacterial Overgrowth Syndromes

Neurologic disorders occur frequently in patients with jejunal diverticulosis, but neuromuscular disorders are uncommon. In a survey by Cooke and colleagues (1963), 12 of 33 patients had neurologic symptoms; 5 had vitamin B_{12} deficiency myelopathy, another 5 had sensory ataxia and impaired reflexes that did not respond to vitamin B_{12}, and 2 had subjective sensory symptoms. The main factor responsible for malabsorption is bacterial proliferation in the diverticula; this causes vitamin B_{12} deficiency and steatorrhea, the former because of bacterial consumption of the vitamin, the latter because of bacterial deconjugation of bile salts. Antibiotic therapy may improve both abnormalities, and may relieve neurologic symptoms that do not respond to treatment with vitamin B_{12}. Other intestinal disorders associated with bacterial overgrowth, such as fistula, stricture, and blind loop, have been reported to cause vitamin B_{12} deficiency myeloneuropathy (Pallis and Lewis 1974).

Binder and associates (1967) reported a patient with jejunal diverticulosis who developed severe, diffuse muscle weakness and wasting, areflexia, loss of vibration and position sense, and external ophthalmoplegia. Electrodiagnostic tests revealed a peripheral neuropathy. Ceroid lipopigment deposits were found in the intestinal mucosa, and peroxide-induced hemolysis was increased, but the neurologic signs did not respond to parenteral administration of vitamin E, vitamin B_{12}, and other water-soluble vitamins, and the steatorrhea was not controlled by antibiotics. Aside from this case, severe neuromuscular disease has not been reported in the bacterial overgrowth syndromes.

Regional Enteritis and Ileal Resection

Regional enteritis may cause malabsorption in several ways. The inflammatory changes may reduce the area of the absorptive surface of the bowel. Strictures and fistulas may cause bacteria overgrowth, resulting in deconjugation of bile salts, and bile salt deficiency is augmented by impaired reabsorption of bile salts in the distal ileum. The predilection of the disease for the distal ileum may impair vitamin B_{12} absorption, but there are no well-documented reports of subacute combined degeneration in patients who had not undergone resection of the distal ileum (Pallis and Lewis 1974).

Malnutrition, cachexia, steatorrhea, and deficiencies of potassium, calcium, and magnesium are well-recognized complications of severe regional enteritis. Tetany and hypokalemic myopathies occur in this setting, but for some reason the other neuromuscular disorders associated with sprue and the postgastrectomy syndrome have not been reported in patients with regional enteritis.

Diagnosis of Malabsorption

Since myopathy and peripheral neuropathy may develop in patients with subclinical malabsorption, a careful search for evidence of malabsorption (Greenberger and Isselbacher 1977; Oslen 1979) should be included in the standard workup for neuromuscular disease of unknown cause.

The first step is to determine whether there is steatorrhea, since significant malabsorption is unlikely to be present without increased fecal excretion of fat. The most reliable screening test is a quantitative fat determination on a 3-day stool collection, obtained while the patient ingests a normal diet containing 60 to 100 g of fat per day. If fat excretion is increased (more than 6 g per day or more than 30 percent of the dry weight of the stool), the second step is to determine whether steatorrhea is due to maldigestion or to a mucosal abnormality. The most useful initial studies are (1) microscopic examination of the stool for undigested fibers; (2) plain x-ray of the abdomen for pancreatic calcifications, which are present in most cases of chronic pancreatitis; (3) barium meal x-ray examination, which can reveal abnormal barium patterns associated with malabsorption, anatomic abnormalities such as diverticulosis and blind loop, and disease processes like regional enteritis; and (4) D-xylose absorption test and Schilling test, which measure, respectively, absorption of simple sugars from the proximal small bowel and absorption of vitamin B_{12} from the distal ileum. Usually at least one of these absorption tests is abnormal in patients with diffuse mucosal diseases such as sprue and in patients with bacterial overgrowth syndromes. (Xylose and vitamin B_{12} are assimilated by the bacteria.)

In patients with neuromuscular complications, special interest centers on identifying deficiencies of vitamin D, vitamin E, and vitamin B_{12}. Measurements of serum levels of vitamin D and E can be performed in some clinical laboratories, but measurement of vitamin D metabolites and erythrocyte fragility tests for vitamin E deficiency are research procedures. However, vitamin D deficiency is usually accompanied by biochemical and radiologic signs of osteomalacia, while in long-standing vitamin E deficiency lipopigment deposits in smooth muscle fibers may be found in a biopsy of the intestine. Vitamin B_{12} deficiency is readily identified by measurement of the serum vitamin B_{12} level and the Schilling test. Low absorption of cyanocobalamin is usually corrected by intrinsic factor in patients with malabsorption caused by partial gastrectomy, while treatment with antibiotics or pancreatic enzymes may improve cyanocobalamin absorption in patients with bacterial overgrowth or pancreatic insufficiency, respectively.

ALCOHOLISM

Many of the devastating neurologic complications of alcoholism have been attributed to malnutrition, but with the single exception of Wernicke's disease, which is universally acknowledged to be due to thiamine deficiency, no specific nutritional disturbance has been incriminated, and the relative importances of ethanol toxicity and nutritional deficiency continue to be argued. Since the cause of the neuromuscular complications of alcoholism is still unknown, and since alcoholism is frequently associated with malnutrition, it is instructive to compare the clinical features of the alcoholic disorders with the better-defined complications of nutritional deficiency.

Polyneuropathy

Occurrence

Except for the alcohol withdrawal syndromes, alcoholic neuropathy is probably the commonest neurologic complication of alcoholism. The precise incidence is unknown, but peripheral neuropathy was identified in 9 percent of alcoholics at the Boston City Hospital (Victor 1975), in 30 percent of alcoholics at the Harlem Hospital in New York (Thornhill et al. 1973), and in 14 percent of alcoholics in an Edinburgh Hospital (Boyd et al. 1981). In some series men and women are affected nearly equally (Victor and Adams 1953; Behse and Buchthal 1977), even though three fourths of alcoholics are men, a finding that suggests that women may be more susceptible to this complication.

In nearly every case there is a long history of heavy alcohol consumption amounting to about 100 ml of ethanol per day for at least 3 years. Beer, wine, and whiskey appear to be equally potent in causing neuropathy. The patients who develop neuropathy have been characterized as chronic, steady drinkers rather than spree drinkers. In Western countries, the large majority of patients are between 40 and 60 years of age (Behse and Buchthal 1977; Bischoff 1971; Walsh and McLeod 1970); one rarely sees alcoholic neuropathy in persons under the age of 30.

Clinical Features

The authoritative articles by Victor and Adams (1953) and Victor (1975) record an unrivaled experience with hundreds of cases of alcoholic neuropathy. Bischoff (1971) and Behse and Buchthal (1977) have added statistical details without materially changing the established clinical descriptions.

In many cases, neuropathy is discovered incidentally in patients with other alcoholic complications such as Wernicke's disease or cirrhosis of the liver. Among the 86 patients with Wernicke's disease studied by Victor and Adams (1953) there were 48 (56 percent) with polyneuropathy. The onset and progression of the neuropathy are usually gradual; however, an acute onset over a few days or weeks is sometimes encountered. The presenting complaints are mainly weakness, paresthesias, and pain in the feet and legs

TABLE 30. Incidence of Neuromuscular Symptoms and Signs in 145 Cases of Alcoholic Polyneuropathy (Bischoff, 1971)

Symptoms		Signs	
Muscle weakness	46%	Diminished reflexes	97%
Spontaneous pain	45%	Sensory loss:	
Paresthesia	37%	vibration	90%
Muscle cramps	30%	touch	60%
Numbness	30%	deep sensation	48%
Ataxia of gait	29%	pain	36%
Burning pain	12%	temperature	26%
		Muscle weakness	55%
		Proximal muscle weakness	22%
		Foot drop	24%
		Tenderness of leg muscles	28%
		Autonomic disturbances	4%
		Cranial nerve palsies	3%

(Table 30), though in Bischoff's series 29 percent of the patients complained of unsteadiness of gait. Paresthesias without pain and subjective coldness of the feet are frequently mentioned. The pain is usually an aching muscular discomfort in the legs and feet; lancinating pains and burning pain in the soles of the feet are infrequent symptoms. About half of the patients have a mild neuropathy with no muscle weakness except in the intrinsic foot muscles; in these patients appreciation of pin prick, touch and vibration is diminished in the feet and sometimes in the hands, the ankle jerks are sluggish or absent, and the lower leg muscles are tender to pressure. In severe cases, the sensory deficits are more extensive, and muscle weakness is present in a distal distribution, greater in the legs than in the arms; the proximal leg muscles and neck flexors may also be weak. Victor (1975) and Bischoff (1971) both observed that deep and superficial sensation were usually involved to approximately the same degree.

Severe trophic changes of the feet have been encountered in South African Blacks with alcoholic polyneuropathy (Perdikis and Bremner 1969, Isaacson 1977, Miller and Hunt 1978), and the same picture is found in alcoholic derelicts in New York (Fig. 41) (Thornhill et al. 1973) and in France (Bureau and Bearriere 1958). The feet and lower legs show severe alterations consisting of chronic edema, hyperpigmentation of the skin, perforating ulcers of the feet (especially overlying the metatarsal heads), and deformities of the toes including clawing, dislocation, and bony resorption. The skin is moist, warm and shiny, and the peripheral pulses are strong; in fact, oscillometry often shows increased arterial pulsation. Secondary infection is often present, sometimes necessitating amputation. Radiography shows phalangeal and metatarsal shortening and tapering, and subluxation of the interphalangeal and metatarsal phalangeal joints, while arteriography shows numerous beaded, tortuous digital vessels resembling a tumor blush, with early venous filling due to arteriovenus shunting. Under light microscopy, the walls of small arteries and arterioles appear markedly thickened by smooth muscle hyperplasia. The neurologic findings have not been described in much detail, but loss of pain and temperature sensation in the feet is a frequent finding, and most of the trophic changes, like those of leprosy, are probably due to degeneration of the small-diameter pain, temperature, and sympathetic nerves, combined with chronic trauma, cold injury, and secondary infection.

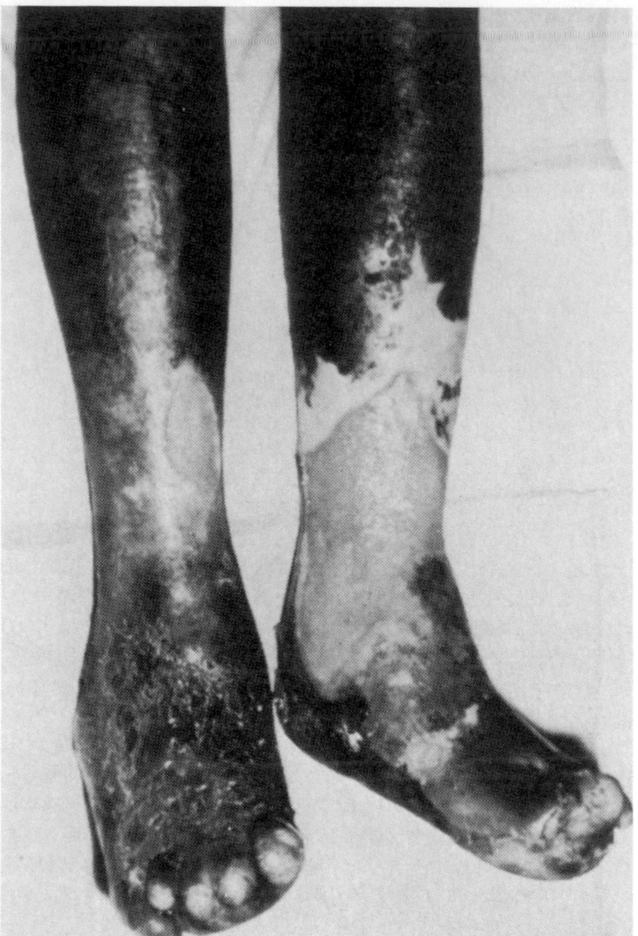

FIGURE 41. Ulceromutilating arthropathy in a patient with alcoholic neuropathy. The feet show chronic edema, increased pigmentation, ulceration, resorption of digits, clawing, and hallux vulgus deformities. (From Thornhill et al., 1973, with permission.)

Laboratory Studies

Motor nerve conduction is normal or mildly slowed, but the amplitude of the muscle responses is frequently reduced. EMG shows evidence of denervation and reinnervation, especially in the distal muscles of the lower extremities. These findings suggest that axonal degeneration is the underlying pathologic change. Sensory nerve amplitudes are severely reduced, and sensory conduction velocities range from normal to moderately slow, reflecting a loss of large-diameter nerve fibers (Walsh and McLeod 1970, Behse and Buchthal 1977). F-wave latencies in the lower extremities, reflecting proximal motor nerve conduction, are likely to be normal when conduction velocity below the knee is slow, indicating that the distal segments of the peripheral nerves are most severely affected (Ahmed 1980). The CSF protein is usually normal but may be slightly increased.

Although some older pathologic studies reported segmental demyelination, recent investigations show that the primary neuropathologic change is axonal degeneration of both myelinated and unmyelinated fibers, and that regeneration is relatively sparse compared with that seen in some other types of neuropathy (Walsh and McLeod 1970; Tredici and Minazzi 1975; Behse and Buchthal 1977).

Course and Treatment

If the patient abstains from alcohol and follows a nutritious diet supplemented with thiamine and other B vitamins, the neuropathy will certainly not get worse, but the degree of recovery will depend on the severity and acuteness of the neuropathy; mild or recent nerve damage carries a better prognosis than severe or chronic disease. In mild cases, improvement may begin within a few weeks; in severe cases there may be no change for several months, slow improvement may continue for two or three years, and neuropathic deficits may be severe and permanent. Since many patients continue to drink, the actual prognosis for alcoholic neuropathy is rather poor. There is no reliable information as to whether vitamin supplements or good nutrition can prevent the neuropathy from deteriorating in a patient who continues to drink.

Pathogenesis

Victor (1975) has strongly argued that alcoholic neuropathy is caused by nutritional deficiency, and specifically by lack of thiamine. His view is that there is no important difference between alcoholic neuropathy and beriberi. Nutritional deficiency is certainly very common in alcoholism. In a recent dietary survey of alcoholic patients, Boyd and associates (1981) found caloric deficiency in 66 percent, protein deficiency in 9 percent, and inadequate intake of thiamine, riboflavin, and niacin in 80 percent, 48 percent and 51 percent, respectively. Thiamine intake was inadequate in 12 of 13 patients with Wernicke's disease and in 9 of 10 patients with polyneuropathy. These dietary defects are compounded by malabsorption of thiamine and other nutrients, demonstrable in at least 50 percent of alcoholics (Hoyumpa 1980; Green and Tall 1979).

However, there are several difficulties with the thiamine hypothesis. In the first place, the cardiovascular features of beriberi are rarely observed, even in the subacute form of alcoholic neuropathy. Alcoholic cardiomyopathy (which many investigators attribute to a toxic effect of alcohol) occurs independently of neuropathy and, unlike beriberi, is a low-output disorder unresponsive to thiamine. Moreover, in beriberi superficial sensory loss is more prominent than deep sensory loss (Yabuki et al. 1976, Denny-Brown 1958), while the reverse is usually found in alcoholic polyneuropathy (Bischoff 1971).

Another difficulty is that malnutrition and thiamine deficiency are so common that many alcoholics without neuropathy or Wernicke's disease show biochemical evidence of thiamine deficiency. Langhor and associates (1981) found biochemical evidence of thiamine, riboflavin, or pyridoxine deficiency in 88 percent of alcoholics with cerebellar or brain stem signs (most of whom also had neuropathy) but in only 29 percent of alcoholics with simple polyneuropathy. Among alcoholics with neurologic disorders, 81 percent of those with B-vitamin deficiency had cerebellar or brain stem signs and 88 percent had neuropathy; of the alcoholics without B-vitamin deficiency, 19 percent had cerebellar or brain stem signs and 77 percent had neuropathy. Similarly, Meyer and associates (1981) found no correlation between the severity of alcoholic polyneuropathy and the biochemical indices of thiamine deficiency. In contrast, biochemical evidence of thiamine deficiency was present in 88 percent of patients with Wernicke's disease, and Wernicke's disease was present in 30 percent of alcoholic patients with thiamine deficiency but in only 2 percent of alcoholics without thiamine deficiency (Wood et al. 1977). These findings suggest that B-vitamin deficiency has much less to do with the pathogenesis of alcoholic neuropathy than with that of Wernicke's disease. However, the methods available for assessing thiamine deficiency give inconsistent and confusing results (Wood et al. 1977), and the pathophysiology of thiamine deficiency is still poorly understood.

Even less is known about the role of nutritional factors other than thiamine. Pyridoxine deficiency and vitamin B_{12} deficiency have been convincingly excluded (Langohr et al. 1981, Behse and Buchthal 1977), and no other single nutritional deficiency is known to cause polyneuropathy. This does not exclude a nutritional cause, for neuropathies and myelopathies of obscure origin also occur in patients with malabsorption, presumably as a result of some unidentified nutritional disturbance (though the neuropathy in those cases is usually of the demyelinative type).

As for a direct toxic effect of alcohol, animal experiments have yielded only meager results. Bosch and associates (1979) detected mild, distal axonal degeneration in tail nerves of rats fed 11 to 12 grams of ethanol per kilogram body weight daily for 16 to 18 weeks, the equivalent of more than 3 quarts of whiskey a day for an averaged-sized man. More equivocal changes were reported in the posterior tibial nerves of rats consuming 6 to 9 grams of ethanol per day (Juntunen et al. 1978), even in the presence of thiamine deficiency (Juntunen et al. 1979). Clinical weakness did not develop in any of these experiments. Of course, rats may be inappropriate animals for these experiments, and the duration of alcohol feeding may not have been long enough. Baboons fed on ethanol (4.5 to 8.3 grams per kilogram per day) for 9 months to 4 years develop alcoholic hepatitis and cirrhosis, but some animals show only fatty changes in the liver after 3 to 4 years of this regimen (Rubin and Lieber 1974). Postmortem examination of three baboons who died after 4 years showed no lesions outside the liver, but the peripheral nerves were not specifically commented on. Like Laennec's cirrhosis, alcoholic neuropathy is most common between the ages of 40 and 60, usually appears after many years of steady consumption of large amounts of alcohol, and may be acutely exacerbated by bouts of very heavy drinking. These similarities suggest that alcohol or its metabolites may play a direct role in the pathogenesis of both diseases, perhaps in combination with poorly understood nutritional factors.

Alcoholic Myopathies

In the 1950s, Hed and his Swedish colleagues drew attention to an acute necrotizing myopathy occurring during a protracted alcoholic debauch. Since then several varieties of muscular disorder have been linked to alcoholism, and there are indications that different pathogenic mechanisms may be responsible for these syndromes.

Serum Enzyme Elevations Following an Alcoholic Bout

Nygren (1966) and Perkoff and associates (1967) found elevated serum CPK levels without muscle symptoms in 60 to 75 percent of chronic alcoholics who were admitted to hospital during a period of heavy drinking. Lafair and Myerson(1968) made the interesting observation that the CPK level was often normal on admission, began to rise 24 to 48 hours later, and reached a peak 3 to 5 days after admission, returning to normal within 2 weeks. In order to examine the effect of diet on this phenomenon, Dimberg and associates (1967) administered 500 ml of 40 percent ethanol daily for 5 days to 12 chronic alcoholic men who had recently recovered from an alcoholic debauch. Six patients were given a normal diet, and six other patients were given a 1300 calorie, low-carbohydrate diet. CPK level remained normal in all subjects during alcoholic administration but afterwards rose transiently in two of the six subjects who were taking a low carbohydrate diet, remaining normal in the six subjects on a normal diet.

The significance of this delayed rise of serum CPK is still uncertain, but Knochel and his colleagues (1977) have suggested that acute phosphorus deficiency may be responsible. Muscle phosphorus content is markedly reduced in chronic alcoholics following a period of heavy drinking, and after admission to the hospital such patients are often given high-calorie feedings that are low in phosphorus. As discussed in Chapter 2, this diet may promote rapid uptake of extracellular phosphorus by muscle; the resulting hypophosphatemia may block glycolysis and prevent the regeneration of ATP. Knochel (1977) observed that serum phosphorus levels usually fell to very low values just before the serum CPK levels rose in alcoholic patients admitted to the hospital. The only role for alcohol in this hypothesis is its nutritional effect on phosphorus metabolism, which can be duplicated by starvation combined with phosphorus depletion. This hypothesis is plausible, but it has not been tested in a prospective study of alcoholic patients.

Acute Necrotizing Myopathy and Myoglobinuria

Hed and associates (1962) described 11 alcoholic patients with an acute syndrome of focal or generalized muscle pain, tenderness, swelling and weakness, beginning abruptly during a drinking bout *before* admission to the hospital. Several of the patients had had repeated attacks of a similar type, and half of the patients developed myoglobinuria. Other investigators have reported similar cases (Perkoff et al. 1967; Lafair and Myerson 1968; Walsh and Conomy 1977).

The onset of muscle symptoms is usually sudden, occurring 1 or 2 days before admission to the hospital. Convulsions, delirium tremens, and other types of motor hyperactivity may predispose patients to this complication. In many cases the affected muscles are swollen, extremely tender and indurated, and the overlying skin may be edematous with a dusky, mottled color. When the calf muscles are affected the condition is frequently mistaken for acute thrombophlebitis, but the muscle damage may be concentrated in other locations such as thighs, buttocks, arms, or back. Low-output cardiac failure and disturbances of cardiac rhythm and conduction are sometimes associated, and there may be severe dysphagia due to weakness of the pharyngeal muscles (Seneviratne 1975; Weber et al. 1981).

The serum CPK level is elevated to a moderate or marked degree, depending on the extent of the muscle damage. In severe cases there is myoglobinuria that may cause acute renal failure and hyperkalemia. EMG of affected muscles shows myopathic abnormalities as well as spontaneous fibrillations. Muscle biopsy reveals massive necrosis of muscle fibers in severe cases and scattered necrosis of muscle fibers in milder cases; in time the necrotic fibers are invaded by phagocytes and there is a proliferation of regenerating fibers, eventually leading to restitution of normal muscle structure except for residual fibrosis and increased fat in some cases.

Following admission to the hospital or withdrawal from alcohol, the muscle pain and swelling subside gradually, and muscle power recovers over a period of 3 weeks to 3 months. In a few cases, especially after repeated episodes, the patient is left with permanent muscle weakness. Cardiac function usually returns to normal but the conduction defects tend to be permanent (Seneviratne 1975).

In most cases of this sort there is no laboratory clue to suggest a metabolic origin of the rhabdomyolysis. However, there have been several case reports of acute hypokalemic paralysis occurring during an alcoholic debauch (Martin et al. 1971; Rubenstein and Wainapel 1977). Those patients developed progressive limb weakness over several days, and at the time of admission they had severe quadriparesis sparing the bulbar and respiratory musculature. Although CPK levels were moderately or markedly elevated there was no myoglobinuria, and none of the patients had muscle pain, tenderness or swelling. This feature seems to distinguish alcoholic hypokalemic myopathy from the painful, necrotizing myopathy described above. In the hypokalemic cases, intravenous infusion of large amounts of potassium leads to improvement of strength within 24 to 48 hours and full recovery within 7 days, suggesting that reversible loss of muscle function, rather than necrosis, is responsible for most of the weakness. EMG shows myopathic abnormalities together with profuse spontaneous fibrillation, both of which resolve rapidly during potassium replacement. Muscle biopsy shows vacuolation and scattered necrosis of muscle fibers, as found in other types of hypokalemic myopathy.

The pathogenesis of acute, painful alcoholic myopathy remains unknown. Knochel (1977), as mentioned above, suggested that most cases of acute alcoholic myopathy were due to phosphate depletion aggravated by overzealous refeeding. However, in nearly all of the reported cases the myopathy came on abruptly *before* admission to the hospital, while the patient was still drinking heavily. Indeed, a recent study by Knochel's group (Anderson et al. 1980) showed that the serum CPK activities of 10 alcoholics with rhabdomyolysis were already markedly elevated on the day of admission; in some cases the CPK levels rose further after admission, while in other cases they fell steeply. Others have shown that administration of alcohol to patients who have recently recovered from acute alcoholic myopathy causes myalgia and CPK elevations within 24 hours; serum phosphorus levels were not mentioned (Curran and Wetmore 1972; Myerson and Lafair 1970; Spector et al 1979), but it is unlikely that hypophosphatemia was involved.

Thus, the weight of clinical evidence is against Knochel's hypothesis and favors a direct toxic effect of alcohol. Until recently, experiments with animals (Munsat et al. 1973; Teräväinen et al. 1978) and normal human volunteers (Song and Rubin 1972) had produced only mild histologic muscle damage and CPK elevation through prolonged feeding of alcohol, but Haller and Drachman (1980) produced more impressive muscle necrosis in rats who were fasted for three days after three weeks of continuous exposure to alcohol vapor. Before fasting the serum CPK levels remained normal or rose slightly, but during fasting the serum CPK levels rose sharply in 60 percent of the rats, and myoglobinuria was detected in half of those animals. On histologic study the skeletal muscles showed various degrees of muscle fiber necrosis. Serum phosphorus and potassium levels were normal before the onset of muscle necrosis, but muscle phosphorus and adenine nucleotide levels were not reported.

This experimental model, which seems to reproduce the clinical pattern of acute alcoholic myopathy, suggests that both nutritional factors and a direct effect of alcohol may be involved in that disorder. The "toxic" effect of alcohol has still not been defined, despite indications of ultrastructural and biochemical alterations in mitochondria and microsomes of cardiac and skeletal muscle (Rubin et al. 1976), but the deleterious effect of fasting suggests that alterations of energy metabolism may be the key to the abrupt onset of cellular necrosis.

Chronic Proximal Weakness

Some chronic alcoholics develop proximal muscle weakness and atrophy over a period of several weeks or months, with little or no muscle pain. The lower extremities are affected more than the upper extremities, the tendon reflexes are preserved, and signs of peripheral neuropathy are usually mild or absent. The patients are usually middle-aged, have been drinking heavily for a number of years, and often have other alcoholic complications such as fatty liver, cirrhosis, Wernicke's disease, or cerebellar ataxia. When patients with these findings abstain from alcohol and receive a good diet with vitamin supplements, the muscle weakness generally begins to improve in a week or two and continues to improve for several months, though muscle power may never return completely to normal (Ekbom et al. 1964; Rossouw et al. 1976; Perkoff et al. 1967).

Serum CPK activity is normal in some cases but may be elevated, especially after a recent bout of heavy drinking. EMG usually shows myopathic abnormalities in the proximal muscles; neurogenic abnormalities or normal findings occur in a minority of cases. Muscle biopsies show mild abnormalities, including small numbers of degenerating muscle fibers, atrophy of scattered single fibers, muscle fiber regeneration, a mild increase of internal nuclei, occasional fiber splitting, and an increase in the amount of endomysial fat (Klinkerfuss et al. 1967; Ekbom et al. 1964). With histochemical stains the main finding is a selective atrophy of type 2 muscle fibers (Rossouw et al. 1976; Hanid et al. 1981).

Ekbom et al. (1964) made the unexpected observation that myopathic EMG abnormalities were also present in asymptomatic alcoholics without clinical muscle abnormalities. Faris and associates (1967) also reported myopathic EMG abnormalities in the proximal muscles of 18 out of 24 chronic alcoholics without muscle weakness. Muscle biopsies in those cases often showed minor abnormalities similar to those encountered in patients with chronic alcoholic myopathy; in particular there was atrophy of scattered muscle fibers and of small groups of muscle fibers (Faris and Reyes 1971) with selective atrophy of type 2 muscle fibers (Hanid et al. 1981).

Some authors have interpreted this atrophic reaction as evidence that chronic proximal weakness in alcoholics has a purely neurogenic cause, but the arguments are no more persuasive here than in discussions of corticosteroid myopathy and other metabolic disorders characterized by proximal weakness, a myopathic EMG, and type 2 muscle fiber atrophy. It is equally possible (and more plausible) that chronic alcoholic indulgence has a selective effect on the metabolism of type 2 muscle fibers, but this has not been studied experimentally, and the relative importance of malnutrition and of alcohol itself in producing this change is likewise unknown.

NONNUTRITIONAL COMPLICATIONS OF GASTROINTESTINAL AND HEPATIC DISEASE

Celiac Disease

Henriksson and associates (1982) uncovered five undiagnosed cases of gluten-sensitive enteropathy among 119 patients with polymyositis. Two of the five patients had no important gastrointestinal symptoms, and none had laboratory evidence of osteomalacia. The clinical and laboratory features of the neuromuscular illness were typical of polymyositis, and several of the patients responded to treatment with steroids or azathioprine; only two of the patients improved with a gluten-free diet, but in the other three cases the diet was started many years after the onset of muscular weakness.

The authors speculated that the inflammatory myopathy might be a consequence of gluten ingestion, but did not suggest how this might come about. There is at best incomplete evidence for an immune pathogenesis of the intestinal changes in celiac disease, and extraintestinal inflammatory manifestations are highly unusual. Nevertheless, it is reasonable to add celiac disease to the list of systemic illnesses that should be searched for, by history if not by jejunal biopsy, in patients with idiopathic polymyositis.

Crohn's Disease and Ulcerative Colitis

Extraintestinal complications are very frequent in inflammatory bowel disease, but no neuromuscular complications were mentioned in a recent survey of 700 patients with these disorders, except for a single case of orbital myositis (Greenstein et al. 1976). Another case of bilateral orbital myositis was recently reported in a 14-year-old girl with Crohn's disease (Young et al. 1981). There was a good clinical response to steroid therapy, but the eye disease relapsed during tapering and did not resolve until the patient underwent resection of the terminal ileum.

Polymyositis is rarely associated with inflammatory bowel disease, and random muscle biopsies from patients without neuromuscular symptoms show no abnormality (Tydd and Dyer 1974). There are two reports of painful muscle nodules in patients with Crohn's disease. In one case the nodules arose in the gastrocnemius and quadriceps muscles, and biopsy of a nodule showed necrotizing vasculitis involving small arteries, with deposits of complement but not of immunoglobulin. The adjacent muscle showed atrophic changes without inflammatory or necrotic features, and the nodular lesions resolved with steroid therapy (Gilliam et al. 1981). In the second case, biopsy of a gastrocnemius nodule showed discrete granulomas with Langhans giant cells, and the adjacent muscles showed muscle fiber necrosis and regeneration, interstitial infiltration by lymphocytes, and increased endomysial connective tissue. Initially the serum CPK was normal, but subsequently the patient developed generalized proximal weakness, and the muscle symptoms responded to high-dose steroid therapy (Menard et al. 1976). This case can be classified as an example of focal nodular myositis (see Chapter 5), but the granulomatous histopathology suggests an etiologic link with the underlying bowel disease.

Infectious Hepatitis

Myopathy

There have been several reports of severe polymyositis appearing simultaneously with infectious hepatitis (Mihas et al. 1978; Schwartz 1978; Pittsley et al. 1978). Hepatitis B surface antigen was present in the serum in three of the patients. Muscle weakness, pain and tenderness developed over 2 to 8 weeks without overt jaundice, although two patients had enlargement of the liver. Two patients had arthralgia, one had generalized lymphadenopathy, and one had a skin eruption that resembled dermatomyositis. Two patients died; the third recovered coincident with steroid therapy. In one case (Mihas et al. 1978) deposits of immunoglobulin and complement were detected in the cytoplasm and nucleus of muscle fibers, but tests for the presence of hepatitis B surface antigen in muscle were not performed.

Recently, Damjanov and associates (1980) reported a patient on chronic hemodialysis who developed polymyositis two years after he was discovered to have chronic hepatitis B antigenemia. Immunofluorescence microscopy showed deposits of IgG, C3, and hepatitis B surface antigen on the basement membrane of scattered muscle fibers and in the walls of small muscle arteries and arterioles, though vasculitis was not present. Thus, it is possible that deposition of immune complexes in muscle is responsible for the occurrence of polymyositis in patients with hepatitis B antigenemia. Nevertheless, a pathogenic role for immune complexes has never been directly demonstrated in polymyositis. Hepatitis B antigenemia is not a frequent finding in polymyositis; a search for the antigen in muscle and serum was negative in 29 patients with polymyositis who did not have clinical or laboratory evidence of liver disease (Whitaker et al. 1973).

Myalgia is a very common symptom in infectious hepatitis, but muscle weakness is rarely present and the cause of the myalgia, as in other viral infections, is unknown. Patten and associates (1977) described a patient who had severe myalgia with a febrile illness that proved to be mild hepatitis B. Because of the presence of severe muscle tenderness the patient's muscle power could not be assessed accurately, but serum CPK activity was normal. Muscle biopsy, however, showed many lipid droplets, which were present in all of the muscle fibers but were more numerous in type 1 fibers. There was no inflammation or muscle necrosis. With steroid therapy the myalgia resolved very rapidly, and a repeat muscle biopsy no longer showed lipid accumulation. The relation of the lipid storage to the patient's myalgia is unknown.

Neuropathy

Twenty-six cases of Guillain-Barré syndrome have been recorded in association with viral hepatitis (Berger et al. 1981), but some of these may have been caused by cytomegalovirus or Epstein-Barr virus, since most of the reports were published before specific serologic tests were available. Three of the patients had proven Type B hepatitis. The average age was 27 years, considerably younger than the median age (46 to 52 years) reported in unselected series of patients with Guillain-Barré syndrome. In 62 percent of the cases polyneuritis began in the convalescent period; in the remainder the neuropathy preceded or accompanied the onset of jaundice. The clinical course was similar to that of other cases of Guillain-Barré syndrome. In a recently-studied case (Berger et al. 1981), in vitro tests showed that peripheral blood mononuclear cells and T-cell lymphocytes were sensitized to peripheral nerve myelin basic protein, as is true in cases of Guillain-Barré syndrome unassociated with infectious hepatitis.

Chari and associates (1977) found evidence of mild, predominantly sensory nerve conduction abnormalities in 75 percent of 12 patients with active hepatitis of unspecified type, who were compared with healthy controls from the same socioeconomic group. Symptoms of hepatitis had been present for 4 to 60 days (average 25 days). Two of the patients had minor clinical signs of a sensorimotor neuropathy in the lower extremities; in the remaining patients the neuropathy was subclinical. The mean value of motor nerve conduction velocity was reduced in the peroneal nerves, but the conduction velocity was below the normal range in only one patient. Median nerve sensory responses were absent in three patients, and the latency was prolonged in two others. Examination of teased sural nerve fibers showed segmental demyelination in 9 of the 12 cases, and the mean internodal distances were strikingly reduced, probably indicating remyelination. This mild demyelinative polyneuropathy may have no connection with Guillain-Barré syndrome, which occurs very rarely in infectious hepatitis and is primarily a motor disorder.

Primary Biliary Cirrhosis

Primary biliary cirrhosis is a progressive and ultimately fatal form of chronic liver disease of unknown cause, occurring mainly in middle-aged women. In nearly all cases, the presence of antimitochondrial antibodies in the serum suggests that autoimmune mechanisms may be important, and the disease is often associated with other autoimmune manifestations such as keratoconjunctivitis sicca, renal tubular acidosis, scleroderma, and arthropathy (Clarke et al. 1978).

A few reports have documented the rare association of primary biliary cirrhosis with various neuromuscular disorders. Polymyositis has been reported in three patients in association with features of scleroderma (Benoist et al. 1977; Epstein et al. 1981). One patient had proximal muscle wasting and weakness in all four extremities, while another had the clinical picture of focal nodular myositis, with painful swellings of the thighs. Myasthenia gravis developed following penicillamine therapy in a patient with asymptomatic primary biliary cirrhosis who also had Hashimoto's thyroiditis. The serum titer of antibodies to acetylcholine receptor was high, and the thymus gland showed lymphoid hyperplasia (Rajaraman et al. 1980). Another patient with asymptomatic biliary cirrhosis had the syndrome of progressive external ophthalmoplegia accompanied by limb-girdle muscular weakness and dysphagia. A muscle biopsy sample showed "ragged-red" staining alterations due to the presence of mitochondrial aggregates in type 1 muscle fibers (Remacle et al. 1980).

Patients with advanced biliary cirrhosis often develop cutaneous xanthomata, which may encroach on cutaneous nerves, causing focal sensory neuropathies (Asbury 1975). One patient developed a generalized sensory polyneuropathy that preceded the diagnosis of biliary cirrhosis (Charron 1980). Examination of a specimen of sural nerve revealed axonal degeneration predominantly affecting large-diameter nerve fibers. Motor neuropathy has not been reported in this disorder. In the late stages of biliary cirrhosis, steatorrhea may lead to malabsorption of vitamin D, osteomalacia, and bone pain; muscular wasting and weakness may develop, presumably as a result of vitamin D deficiency.

REFERENCES

AGAMANOLIS, DP, CHESTER, EM, VICTOR, M, ET AL: *Neuropathology of experimental vitamin B_{12} deficiency in monkeys.* Neurology 26:905–914, 1976.

AGAMANOLIS, DP, VICTOR, M, HARRIS, JW, ET AL: *An ultrastructural study of subacute combined degeneration of the spinal cord in vitamin B_{12}-deficient rhesus monkeys.* J Neuropathol Exp Neurol 37:273–299, 1978.

AHMED, I: *F-wave conduction velocity in alcoholic polyneuropathy.* South Med J 73:273–299, 1980.

AMESS, JAL, REES, GM, BURMAN, JF, ET AL: *Megaloblastic haemopoiesis in patients receiving nitrous oxide.* Lancet ii:339–342, 1978.

ANDERSON, R, COHEN, M, HALLER, R, ET AL.: *Skeletal muscle phosphorus and magnesium deficiency in alcoholic myopathy.* Mineral Electrolyte Metab 4:106–112, 1980.

ASBURY, AK: *Hepatic neuropathy.* In DYCK, PJ, THOMAS, PK, and Lambert, EH (EDS): *Peripheral Neuropathy.* WB Saunders, Philadelphia, 1975, pp 993–998.

ASK-UPMARK, E: *Amyotrophic lateral sclerosis observed in five persons after gastric resection.* Gastroenterology 15:257–259, 1950.

BANERJI, NK, AND HURWITZ, LJ: *Neurological manifestations in adult steatorrhoea (probable gluten enteropathy).* J Neurol Sci 14:125–141, 1971(A).

BANERJI, NK, AND HURWITZ, LJ: Nervous system manifestations after gastric surgery. Acta Neurol Scand 47:485–513, 1971(B).

BAUMAN, MB, DI MASE, JD, OSKI, F, ET AL: *Brown bowel and skeletal myopathy associated with vitamin E depletion in pancreatic insufficiency.* Gastroenterology 54:93–100, 1968.

BAYOUMI, RA AND ROSALKI, SB: *Evaluation of methods of coenzyme activation of erythrocyte enzymes for detection of deficiency of vitamins B_1, B_2, and B_6.* Clin Chem 22:327–335, 1976.

BEHSE, F, AND BUCHTHAL, F: *Alcoholic neuropathy: Clinical, electrophysiological and biopsy findings.* Ann Neurol 2:95–110, 1977.

BENOIST, M, HENIN, D, KAHN, M-F, ET AL: *Cirrhose biliaire primitive associée à une polyarthrite rheumatoïde et à une polymyosite aiguë.* Nouv Presse Med 6:2427–2429, 1977.

BERGER, JR, AYYAR, R, AND SHEREMATA, WA: *Guillain-Barré syndrome complicating acute hepatitis B. A case with detailed electrophysiological and immunological studies.* Arch Neurol 38:366–368, 1981.

BINDER, HJ, SOLITAIRE, GB, AND SPIRO, HM: *Neuromuscular disease in patients with steatorrhea.* Gut 8:605–611, 1967.

BISCHOFF, A: *Die alkoholische Polyneuropathie: Klinische, ultrastrukturelle und pathogenetische Aspekte.* Dtsch Med Wochenschr 96:317–322, 1971.

BOSCH, EP, PELHAM, RW, RASOOL, CG, ET AL: *Animal models of alcoholic neuropathy: Morphological, electrophysiological and biochemical findings.* Muscle Nerve 2:133–144, 1979.

BOYD, DHA, MACLAREN, DS, AND STODDARD, ME: *The nutritional status of patients with an alcohol problem.* Acta Vitaminol Enzymol 3:75–82, 1981.

BRAUNSTEIN, H: *Tocopherol deficiency in adults with chronic pancreatitis.* Gastroenterology 40:224–231, 1961.

BRENNAN, MF: *Uncomplicated starvation versus cancer cachexia.* Cancer Res 37:2359–2364, 1977.

BUCHTHAL, F: *Electrophysiological abnormalities in metabolic myopathies and neuropathies.* Acta Neurol Scand 46 (Suppl 43):129–176, 1970.

BUNDSCHER, HD, SUCHENWIRTH, R, AND D'AVIS, W: *Histochemical changes in disuse atrophy of human skeletal muscle. Proceedings of the Second International Congress on Muscle Diseases, Perth, 1971.* Part 1. Excerpta Medica, Amsterdam, 1973, pp 108–112.

BURCK, U, GOEBEL, HH, KUHLENDAHL, HD, ET AL: *Neuromyopathy and vitamin E deficiency in man.* Neuropediatrics 12:267–278, 1981.

BUREAU, Y, AND BARRIERE, H: *Ulcerating and mutilating trophic lesions of the lower limbs.* Brit J Derm 70:372–377, 1958.

BUTLER, WM, TAYLOR, HG, AND DIEHL, LF: *Lhermitte's sign in cobalamin (vitamin B_{12}) deficiency.* JAMA 245:1059, 1981.

CHARI, VR, KATIYAR, BC, AND RASTOGI, BL: *Neuropathy in hepatic disorder. A clinical, electrophysiological and histopathological appraisal.* J Neurol Sci 31:93–111, 1977.

CHARRON, L, PEYRONNARD, J-M, AND MARCHAND, L: *Sensory neuropathy associated with primary biliary cirrhosis. Histologic and morphometric studies.* Arch Neurol 37:84–87, 1980.

CLARK, CM, AND GOODLAD, GAJ: *Depletion of proteins of phasic and tonic muscles in tumour-bearing rats.* Europ J Cancer 7:3–9, 1971.

CLARK, CM, AND GOODLAD, GAJ: *Muscle protein biosynthesis in the tumour-bearing rat. A defect in a post-initiating stage of translation.* Biochim Biophys Acta 378:230–240, 1975.

CLARKE, AK, GALBRAITH, RM, HAMILTON, EBD, ET AL: *Rheumatic disorders in primary biliary cirrhosis.* Ann Rheum Dis 37:42–47, 1978.

COOKE, WT, AND SMITH, WT: *Neurological disorders associated with adult celiac disease.* Brain 89:683–722, 1966.

COOKE, WT, COX, EV, FONE, DJ, ET AL: *The clinical and metabolic significance of jejunal diverticulosis.* Gut 4:115–131, 1963.

COSTA, G: *Cachexia, the metabolic component of neoplastic diseases.* Cancer Res 37:2327–2335, 1977.

COX-KLAZINGA, M AND ENDTZ, LJ: *Peripheral nerve involvement in pernicious anaemia.* J Neurol Sci 45:367–371, 1980.

CURRAN, JR AND WETMORE, SJ: *Alcoholic myopathy.* Dis Nerv Syst 33:19–22, 1972.

DAMJANOV, ID, MOSER, RL, KATZ, SM, ET AL: *Immune complex myositis associated with viral hepatitis.* Hum Pathol 11:478–481, 1980.

DASTUR, DK, MANGHANI, DK, OSUNTOKUN, BO, ET AL: *Neuromuscular and related changes in malnutrition. A review.* J Neurol Sci 55:207–230, 1982.

DAVIES, KJA, MAGUIRE, JJ, BROOKS, GA, ET AL: *Muscle mitochondrial bioenergetics, oxygen supply, and work capacity during dietary iron deficiency and repletion.* Am J Physiol 242:E418–E427, 1982.

DAYTON, WR, SCHALLMEYER, JV, CHAN, AC, ET AL: *Elevated levels of a calcium-activated muscle protease in rapidly atrophying muscles from vitamin E-deficient rabbits.* Biochim Biophys Acta 584:216–230, 1979.

DEACON, R, LUMB, M, PERRY, J, ET AL: *Selective inactivation of vitamin B_{12} in rats by nitrous oxide.* Lancet ii:1023–1024, 1978.

DENNY-BROWN, D: *Neurological conditions resulting from prolonged and severe dietary restriction. (Case reports in prisoners-of-war, and general review).* Medicine 26:41–113, 1947.

DENNY-BROWN, D: *The neurological aspects of thiamine deficiency.* Fed Proc 17 (Suppl 2):35–43, 1958.

DIMBERG, R, HED, R, KALLNER, G, ET AL: *Liver-muscle enzyme activities in the serum of alcoholics on a diet poor in carbohydrates.* Acta Med Scand 181:227–232, 1967.

DINN, JJ, MCCANN, S, WILSON, P, ET AL: *Animal model for subacute combined degeneration.* Lancet ii:1154, 1978.

DINN, JJ, WEIR, DG, MCCANN, S, ET AL: *Methyl group deficiency in nerve tissue: A hypothesis to explain the lesion of subacute combined degeneration.* Ir J Med Sci 149:1–4, 1980.

DIREKZE, M: *Progressive external ophthalmoplegia: Some clinical associations.* Acta Neurol Scand 49:195–204, 1973.

EKBOM, K, HED, R, KIRSTEIN, R, ET AL: *Muscular affections in chronic alcoholism.* Arch Neurol 10:449–458, 1964.

ELIAS, SE, MULLER, DPR, AND SCOTT, J: *Association of spinocerebellar disorders with cystic fibrosis or chronic childhood cholestasis and very low serum vitamin E.* Lancet ii:1319–1321, 1981.

ELLIS, JM, AZUMA, J, WATANABE, T, ET AL: *Survey and new data on treatment with pyridoxine of patients having a clinical syndrome including the carpal tunnel and other defects.* Res Commun Chem Pathol Pharmacol 17:165–177, 1977.

ELLIS, JM, KISHI, T, AZUMA, J, ET AL: *Vitamin B_6 deficiency in patients with a clinical syndrome including the carpal tunnel defect. Biochemical and clinical response to therapy with pyridoxine.* Res Commun Chem Pathol Pharmacol 13:743–757, 1976.

ENGLAND, JM, AND LINNEL, JC: *Problems with the serum vitamin B_{12} assay.* Lancet ii:1072–1074, 1980.

ENGSNER, G AND WOLDEMARIAM, T: *Motor nerve conduction velocity in marasmus and in kwashiorkor.* Neuropädiatrie 5:34–48, 1974.

EPSTEIN, O, BURROUGHS, AK, AND SHERLOCK, S: *Polymyositis and acute onset systemic sclerosis in a patient with primary biliary cirrhosis: A clinical syndrome similar to the mixed connective tissue disease.* J Roy Soc Med 74:456–458, 1981.

FARIS, AA AND REYES, MG: *Reappraisal of alcoholic myopathy.* J Neurol Neurosurg Pychiatry 34:86–92, 1971.

Faris, AA, Reyes, MG, and Abrams, BM: *Subclinical alcoholic myopathy: Electromyographic and biopsy study.* Trans Am Neurol Assoc 92:102–106, 1967.

Farrell, PM, Bieri, JG, Fratantoni, JF, et al: *The occurrence and effects of human vitamin E deficiency. A study in patients with cystic fibrosis.* J Clin Invest 60:233–241, 1977.

Feit, H, Glasberg, M, Ireton, C, et al: *Peripheral neuropathy and starvation after gastric partitioning for morbid obesity.* Ann Intern Med 96:453–455, 1982.

Finch, CA, Miller, LR, Imadar, AR, et al: *Iron deficiency in the rat. Physiological and biochemical studies of muscle dysfunction.* J Clin Invest 58:447–453, 1976.

Finch, CA, Gollnick, PD, Hlastala, MP, et al: *Lactic acidosis as a result of iron deficiency.* J Clin Invest 64:129–137, 1979.

Folkers, K, Ellis, J, Watanabe, T, et al: *Biochemical evidence for a deficiency of vitamin B_6 in the carpal tunnel syndrome based on a crossover clinical study.* Proc Nat Acad Sci 75:3410–3412, 1978.

Gabriel, E, Machlin, EJ, Filipski, R, et al: *Influence of age on the vitamin E requirement for resolution of necrotizing myopathy.* J Nutr 110:1372–1379, 1980.

Gandy, G, Jacobson, W, Sidman, R: *Inhibition of transmethylation reaction in the central nervous system—An experimental model for subacute combined degeneration of the cord.* J Physiol 233:1–3, 1973.

Gardiner, PF, Montanaro, G, Simpson, DR, et al: *Effects of glucocorticoid treatment and food restriction on rat hindlimb muscles.* Am J Physiol 238:E124–E130, 1980.

Gautier-Smith, PC: *Lhermitte's sign in subacute combined degeneration of the cord.* J Neurol Neurosurg Psychiatry 36:861–863, 1973.

Geller, A, Gilles, F, Schwachman, H: *Degeneration of fasciculus gracilis in cystic fibrosis.* Neurology 27:185–187, 1977.

Gilliam, JH, III, Challa, VR, Agudelo, CA, et al: *Vasculitis involving muscle associated with Crohn's colitis.* Gastroenterology 81:787–790, 1981.

Goldberg, AL and Boches, FS: *Oxidized proteins in erythrocytes are rapidly degraded by the adenosine triphosphate-dependent proteolytic system.* Science 215:1107–1109, 1982.

Gomez, MR, Engel, AG, and Dyck, PJ: *Progressive ataxia, retinal degeneration, neuromyopathy, and mental subnormality in a patient with true hypoparathyroidism, dwarfism, malabsorption, and cholelithiasis.* Neurology 22:849–855, 1972.

Goodgame, JT, Lowry, SF, Brennan, MF: *Essential fatty acid deficiency in total parenteral nutrition: Time course of development and suggestions for therapy.* Surgery 84:271–277, 1978.

Goodlad, GAJ and Clark, CM: *Activity of gastrocnemius and soleus polyribosomes in rats bearing the Walker 256 carcinoma.* Eur J Cancer 8:647–651, 1972.

Green, PHR and Tall, AR: *Drugs, alcohol and malabsorption.* Am J Med 67:1066–1076, 1979.

Greenberger, NJ and Isselbacher, KJ: *Disorders of absorption.* In Thorn, GA, Adams, RD, Braunwald, E, et al (eds): *Harrison's Principles of Internal Medicine,* Ed 8, McGraw-Hill, New York, 1977, pp 1518–1537.

Greenstein, AJ, Janowitz, HD, and Sachar, DB: *The extra-intestinal complications of Crohn's disease and ulcerative colitis: A study of 700 patients.* Medicine 55:401–412, 1976.

Guggenheim, MA, Ringel, SP, Silverman, A, et al: *Progressive neuromuscular disease in children with chronic cholestasis and vitamin E deficiency: Diagnosis and treatment with alpha-tocopherol.* J Pediat 100:51–58, 1982.

Haggmark, T and Eriksson, E: *Cylinder or mobile cask brace after knee ligament surgery: A clinical analysis and morphologic and enzymatic studies of changes in the quadriceps muscle.* Am J Sports Med 7:48–56, 1979.

Hall, CA: *Vitamin B_{12} deficiency and early rise in mean corpuscular volume.* JAMA 245:1144–1146, 1981.

Hall, WH: *Proximal muscle atrophy in adult celiac disease.* Am J Dig Dis 13:697–704, 1968.

Haller, RG and Drachman, DB: *Alcoholic rhabdomyolysis: An experimental model in the rat.* Science 208:412–415, 1980.

Hanid, A, Slavin, G, Mair, W, et al: *Fibre type changes in striated muscle of alcoholics.* J Clin Pathol 34:991–995, 1981.

Harriman, DGF: *Muscle cachexia. Some aspects of its pathology and clinical features. Proceedings of the Fifth International Congress of Neuropathology, Zurich, 1965.* Excerpta Medica International Congress Series 100:677–683, 1966.

Hed, R, Lundmark, C, Fahlgren, H, et al: *Acute muscular syndrome in chronic alcoholism.* Acta Med Scand 171:585–599, 1962.

HEFFRON, JJA, CHAN, AC, GRONERT, GA, ET AL: *Decreased phosphorylative capacity and respiratory rate of rabbit skeletal muscle mitochondria in vitamin E dystrophy.* Int J Biochem 9:539–543, 1978.

HENRIKSSON, KG, HALLERT, C, NORRBY, K, ET AL: *Polymyositis and adult coeliac disease.* Acta Neurol Scandinav 65:301–319, 1982.

HERBERT, PN, GOTTO, AM, AND FREDERICKSEN, DS: *Familial lipoprotein deficiency (abetalipoproteinemia, hypobetalipoproteinemia, and Tangier disease).* In STANBURY, JB, WYNGAARDEN, JB, AND FREDERICKSEN, DS (EDS): *The Metabolic Basis of Inherited Disease,* ed. 4, McGraw-Hill, New York, 1978 pp 544–588.

HNIK, P, HOLAS, M, AND PAYNE, R: *Reflex muscle atrophy induced by chronic peripheral nociceptive stimulation.* J Physiol (Paris) 73:241–250, 1977.

HOYUMPA, AM, JR: *Mechanisms of thiamin deficiency in chronic alcoholism.* Am J Clin Nutr 33:2750–2761, 1980.

ISAACSON, C: *Idiopathic neurotrophic feet in Blacks. A pathological study.* S Afr Med J 52:845–848, 1977.

IYER, GV, TAORI, GM, KAPADIA, CR, ET AL: *Neurological manifestations in tropical sprue: A clinical and electrodiagnostic study.* Neurology 23:959–966, 1973.

JEEJEEBHOY, KN, CHU, RC, MARLISS, ER, ET AL: *Chromium deficiency, glucose intolerance, and neuropathy reversed by chromium supplementation, in a patient receiving long-term total parenteral nutrition.* Am J Clin Nutr 30:531–538, 1977.

JEEJEEBHOY, KN, WADIA, NH, AND DESAI, HG: *Role of vitamin B_{12} deficiency in tropical "nutritional" neuromyelopathy.* J Neurol Neurosurg Psychiatry 30:7–12, 1967.

JOHNSON, RA, BAKER, SS, FALLON, JT, ET AL: *An occidental case of cardiomyopathy and selenium deficiency.* N Engl J Med 304:1210–1212, 1981.

JUNTUNEN, J, TERÄVÄINEN, H, ERIKSON, K, ET AL: *Experimental alcoholic neuropathy in the rat: Histological and electrophysiological study on the myoneural junctions and peripheral nerves.* Acta Neuropath (Berl) 41:131–137, 1978.

JUNTUNEN, J, TERÄVÄINEN, H, ERIKSON, K, ET AL: *Peripheral neuropathy and myopathy. An experimental study of rats on alcohol and variable dietary thiamine.* Virchows Arch A (Path Anat Histol) 383:241–252, 1979.

KARK, RAP, BROWN, J, EDGERTON, R, ET AL: *Experimental thiamine deficiency. Neuropathic and mitochondrial changes induced in rat muscle.* Arch Neurol 32:818–825, 1975.

KIEN, CL AND GANTHER, HE: *Manifestations of chronic selenium deficiency in total parenteral nutrition.* Am J Clin Nutr 37:319–328, 1983.

KLINKERFUSS, G, BLEISCH, V, DIOSO, MM, ET AL: *A spectrum of myopathy associated with alcoholism. II. Light and electron microscopic observations.* Ann Intern Med 67:493–510, 1967.

KNIFFEN, JC AND QUICK, DT: *Neuromuscular disorder following gastric resection.* Arch Intern Med 124:336–340, 1969.

KNOCHEL, JP: *The pathophysiology and clinical characteristics of severe hypophosphatemia.* Arch Intern Med 137:203–220, 1977.

KOSIK, KS, MULLINS, TF, BRADLEY, WG, ET AL: *Coma and axonal degeneration in vitamin B_{12} deficiency.* Arch Neurol 37:590–592, 1980.

KRUMHOLZ, A, WEISS, HD, GOLDSTEIN, PJ, ET AL: *Evoked responses in vitamin B_{12} deficiency.* Ann Neurol 9:407–409, 1981.

LAFAIR, JS AND MYERSON, RM: *Alcoholic myopathy, with special reference to the significance of creatine phosphokinase.* Arch Intern Med 122:417–422, 1968.

LANGOHR, HD, PETRUCH, F, AND SCHROTH, G: *Vitamin B_1, B_2 and B_6 deficiency in neurological disorders.* J Neurol 225:95–108, 1981.

LAYZER, RB: *Myeloneuropathy after prolonged exposure to nitrous oxide.* Lancet ii:1227–1230, 1978.

LAYZER, RB, FISHMAN, RA, AND SCHAFER, JA: *Neuropathy following abuse of nitrous oxide.* Neurology 28:504–506, 1978.

LE QUESNE, PM: *Neuropathy due to drugs.* In DYCK, PJ, THOMAS, PK, AND LAMBERT, EH (EDS): *Peripheral Neuropathy.* WB SAUNDERS, Philadelphia, 1975, pp 1263–1280.

LEVIN, S, GORDON, MH, AND NITOWSKY, HM: *Studies of tocopherol deficiency in infants and children. VI. Evaluation of muscle strength and effect of tocopherol administration in children with cystic fibrosis.* Pediatrics 27:578–588, 1961.

LI, JB, AND GOLDBERG, AL: *Effects of food deprivation on protein synthesis and degradation in rat skeletal muscles.* Am J Physiol 231:441–448, 1976.

LINDBOE, CF AND PLATOU, CS: *Disuse atrophy of human skeletal muscle. An enzyme histochemical study.* Acta Neuropathol 56:241–244, 1982.

LINDBOE, CF AND TORVIK, A: *The effects of ageing, cachexia and neoplasms on striated muscle. Quantitative histological and histochemical observations on an autopsy material.* Acta Neuropathol 57:85–92, 1982.

LINDBOE, CF, ASKEVOLD, F, AND SLETTEBØ, M: *Changes in skeletal muscles of young women with anorexia nervosa. An enzyme histochemical study.* Acta Neuropathol 56:299–302, 1982.

LUNDHOLM, K, BYLUND, A-C, HOLM, J, ET AL: *Skeletal muscle metabolism in patients with malignant tumor.* Eur J Cancer 12:465–473, 1976.

MACHLIN, LJ, GABRIEL, E, SPIEGEL, HE, ET AL: *Plasma activity of pyruvate kinase and glutamic oxalacetic transaminase as indices of myopathy in the vitamin E deficient rat.* J Nutr 108:1963–1968, 1978.

MARTIN, JB, CRAIG, JW, ECKEL, RE, ET AL: *Hypokalemic myopathy in chronic alcoholism.* Neurology 21:1160–1168, 1971.

MCCARTHY, MC, COTTAM, GL, AND TURNER, WW, JR: *Essential fatty acid deficiency in critically ill surgical patients.* Am J Surg 142:747–751, 1981.

MCLANE, JA, FELL, RD, MCKAY, RH, ET AL: *Physiological and biochemical effects of iron deficiency on rat skeletal muscle.* Am J Physiol 241:C47–C54, 1981.

MENARD, DB, HADDAD, H, BLAIN, JG, ET AL: *Granulomatous myositis and myopathy associated with Crohn's colitis.* N Eng J Med 295:818–819, 1976.

MENDELL, JR: *Experimental myopathies.* In VINKEN, PJ AND BRUYN, GW (EDS): *Handbook of Clinical Neurology, vol 40.* North-Holland Publishing, Amsterdam, 1979, pp 133–182.

MESULAM, M-M, VAN HOESEN, GW, AND BUTTERS, N: *Clinical manifestations of chronic thiamine deficiency in the rhesus monkey.* Neurology 27:239–245, 1979.

MEYER, JG, NEUDORFER, B, RETHEL, R, ET AL: *Uber die Beziehung zwischen alkoholischer Polyneuropathie und Vitamin B_1, B_{12} und Folsaure.* Nervenarzt 52:329–332, 1981.

MIHAS, AA, KIRBY, JD, AND KENT, SR: *Hepatitis B antigen and polymyositis.* JAMA 239:221–222, 1978.

MILLER, RG, DAVIS, CJF, AND ILLINGWORTH, DR: *The neuropathy of abetalipoproteinemia.* Neurology 30:1286–1291, 1980.

MILLER, RM AND HUNT, JA: *The radiological features of alcoholic ulcero-osteolytic neuropathy in Blacks.* S Afr Med J 54:159–161, 1978.

MONTGOMERY, RD: *Muscle morphology in infantile protein malnutrition.* J Clin Pathol 15:511–521, 1962.

MORRIS, JS, ADJUKIEWICZ, AB, AND READ, AE: *Neurological disorders and adult coeliac disease.* Gut 11:549–554, 1970.

MULLER, DPR, HARRIES, JT, AND LLOYD, JK: *The relative importance of the factors involved in the absorption of vitamin E in childhood.* Gut 15:966–971, 1974.

MUNSAT, T, NEUSTEIN, H, HIGGINS, J, ET AL: *Experimental acute alcoholic myopathy.* Neurology 23:407, 1973.

MYERSON, RM, AND LAFAIR, JS: *Alcoholic muscle disease.* Med Clin North Am 54:723–730, 1970.

NELSON, JS, FITCH, CD, FISCHER, VW, ET AL: *Progressive neuropathologic lesions in vitamin E-deficient rhesus monkeys.* J Neuropath Exp Neurol 40:166–186, 1981.

NITOWSKY, HM, GORDON, HH, AND TILDON, JT: *Studies of tocopherol deficiency in infants and children. IV. The effect of alpha-tocopherol on creatinuria in patients with cystic fibrosis of the pancreas and biliary atresia.* Bull Johns Hopkins Hosp 98:361–371, 1956.

NYGREN, A: *Serum creatine phosphokinase activity in chronic alcoholism, in connection with acute alcohol intoxication.* Acta Med Scand 179:623–630, 1966.

OCHOA, J: *Isoniazid neuropathy in man: Quantitative electron microscopy study.* Brain 93:831–850, 1970.

OLSEN, WA: *A pathophysiologic approach to diagnosis of malabsorption.* Am J Med 67:1007–1013, 1979.

OSUNTOKUN, BO: *Motor nerve conduction in kwashiorkor (protein-calorie deficiency) before and after treatment.* Afr J Med Sci 2:109–119, 1971.

PALLIS, CA AND LEWIS, PD: *The Neurology of Gastrointestinal Disease.* WB Saunders, Philadelphia, 1974.

PANT, SH, ASBURY, AK, AND RICHARDSON, EP: *The myelopathy of pernicious anemia—A neuropathological reappraisal.* Acta Neurol Scand 44:Suppl, 35, 1968.

PARRY, DJ, AND MONTPETIT, VJA: *Histochemical changes in fast and slow muscles of nutritionally dystrophic rabbits.* J Neuropathol Exp Neurol 37:231–243, 1978.

PATTEN, BM, SHABOT, JM, ALPERIN, J, ET AL: *Hepatitis-associated lipid storage myopathy.* Ann Intern Med 87:417–421, 1977.

Pawlik, F, Bischoff, A, and Bitsch, I: *Peripheral nerve changes in thiamine deficiency and starvation. An electron microscopic study.* Acta Neuropath 39:211–218, 1977.

Perdikis, P, and Bremner, C: *Idiopathic neurotrophic feet in Bantu patients.* S Afr J Surg 7:171–178, 1969.

Perkoff, GT, Dioso, MM, Blisch, V, et al: *A spectrum of myopathy associated with alcoholism. I. Clinical and laboratory features.* Ann Intern Med 67:481–492, 1967.

Pittsley, RA, Shearn, MA, Kaufman, L: *Acute hepatitis B simulating dermatomyositis.* JAMA 239:959, 1978.

Platt, BS: *Clinical features of endemic beriberi.* Fed Proc 17 (Suppl 2):8–18, 1958.

Potera, C, Rose, DP, and Brown, RR: *Vitamin B_6 deficiency in cancer patients.* Am J Clin Nutr 30:1677–1679, 1977.

Prineas, JW: *Peripheral nerve changes in thiamine deficient rats.* Arch Neurol 23:541–548, 1970.

Quick, D and Greer, M: *Pancreatic dysfunction in patients with amyotrophic lateral sclerosis.* Neurology 17:112–116, 1967.

Rajaraman, S, Deodhar, SD, Carey, WD, et al: *Hashimoto's thyroiditis, primary biliary cirrhosis, and myasthenia gravis.* Am J Clin Pathol 74:831–834, 1980.

Raju, NV: *Effect of exercise during rehabilitation on swimming performance, metabolism and function of muscle in rats.* Br J Nutr 38:157–165, 1977.

Remacle, J-P, Pellisier, J-F, Chamlian, A, et al: *Progressive ophthalmoplegia associated with asymptomatic primary biliary cirrhosis. Histologic, histochemical, cytochemical, and ultrastructural studies of muscle and liver biopsy specimens.* Hum Pathol 11:540–548, 1980.

Reynolds, EH, Rothfeld, P, and Pincus, JH: *Neurological disease associated with folate deficiency.* Br Med 2:398–400, 1973.

Richards, JR: *Current concepts in the metabolic responses to injury, infection and starvation.* Proc Nutr Soc 39:113–123, 1980.

Rosenblum, JL, Keating, JP, Prensky, AL, et al: *A progressive neurologic syndrome in children with chronic liver disease.* N Engl J Med 304:503–508, 1981.

Rossouw, JE, Keeton, RG, and Hewlett, RH: *Chronic proximal muscular weakness in alcoholics.* S Afr Med J 50:2095–2098, 1976.

Rotruck, JT, Pope, AL, Ganther, HE, et al: *Selenium: Biochemical role as a component of glutathione peroxidase.* Science 179:588–590, 1973.

Rubenstein, AE and Wainapel, SF: *Acute hypokalemic myopathy in alcoholism.* Arch Neurol 34:553–555, 1977.

Rubin, E and Lieber, CS: *Fatty liver, alcoholic hepatitis and cirrhosis produced by alcohol in primates.* N Engl J Med 290:128–135, 1974.

Rubin, E, Katz, A, Lieber, CS, et al: *Muscle damage produced by chronic alcohol consumption.* Am J Pathol 83:499–516, 1976.

Sachdev, KK, Taori, GM, and Pereira, SM: *Neuromuscular status in protein-calorie malnutrition. Clinical, nerve conduction, and electromyographic studies.* Neurology 21:801–805, 1971.

Sargeant, AJ, Davies, CTM, Edwards, RHT, et al: *Functional and structural changes after disuse of human muscle.* Clin Sci Molec Med 52:337–342, 1977.

Satyanarayana, K, Naidu, AN, and Rao, BSN: *Nutritional deprivation in childhood and the body size, activity, and physical work capacity of young boys.* Am J Clin Nutr 32:1769–1775, 1979.

Satyanarayana, K, Naidu, AN, and Rao, BSN: *Studies on the effect of nutritional deprivation during childhood on body composition of adolescent boys: creatinine excretion.* Am J Clin Nutr 34:161–165, 1981.

Schwartz, IS: *Acute hepatitis with myositis.* JAMA 240:1953–1954, 1978.

Scobie, IN, Durward, WF, and MacCuish, SC: *Proximal myopathy after prolonged total therapeutic starvation.* Br Med J 1:1212–1213, 1980.

Scott, J, Elias, E, Moult, PJA, et al: *Pancreatic rickets in adult cystic fibrosis with myopathy and proximal renal tubular dysfunction.* Am J Med 63:488–492, 1977.

Scott, JM, Wilson, P, Dinn, JJ, et al: *Pathogenesis of subacute combined degeneration: A result of methyl group deficiency.* Lancet ii:334–337, 1981.

Seneviratne, BIB: *Acute cardiomyopathy with rhabdomyolysis in chronic alcoholism.* Br Med J 4:378–380, 1975.

Shih, JCH, Jonas, RH, and Scott, ML: *Oxidative deterioration of the muscle proteins during nutritional muscular dystrophy in chicks.* J Nutr 107:1786–1791,1977.

Shorvon, SD, Carney, MWP, Chanarin, I, et al: *The neuropsychiatry of megaloblastic anaemia.* Br Med J 281:1036–1038, 1980.

SINGH, N, KUMAR, A, AND GHAI, OP: *Conduction velocity of motor nerves in children suffering from protein-calorie malnutrition and marasmus.* Electromyogr Clin Neurophysiol 16:381–392, 1976.

SMALL, DH AND CARNEGIE, PR: *Myelopathy associated with vitamin B-12 deficiency. New approaches to an old problem.* Trends Neuro Sci 4:x-xi, 1981.

SONG, SK AND RUBIN, E: *Ethanol produces muscle damage in human volunteers.* Science 175:327–328, 1972.

SPECTOR, R, CHOUDHURY, A, CONCILLA, P, ET AL: *Acoholic myopathy. Diagnosis by alcoholic challenge.* JAMA 242:1648–1649, 1979.

STEWART, PM AND HENSLEY, WJ: *Acute polymyopathy during total parenteral nutrition.* Br Med J 283:1578, 1981

STRAIN, AJ: *Cancer cachexia in man: A Review.* Invest Cell Pathol 2:181–193, 1979.

STRAIN, AJ, EASTY, GC AND NEVILLE, AM: *A new experimental model of human cachexia.* Invest Cell Pathol 2:87–96, 1979.

SUNG, JH, PARK, SH, MASTRI, AR, ET AL: *Axonal dystrophy in the gracile nucleus in congenital biliary atresia and cystic fibrosis (mucoviscidosis): Beneficial effect of vitamin E therapy.* J Neuropathol Exp Neurol 39:584–597, 1980.

TAKAHASHI, K, AND NAKAMURA, H: *Axonal degeneration in beri-beri neuropathy.* Arch Neurol 33:836–841, 1976.

TEEHAN, BP, SMITH, LJ, SIGLER, MH, ET AL: *Plasma pyridoxal-5′-phosphate levels and clinical correlations in chronic hemodialysis patients.* Am J Clin Nutr 31:1932–1936, 1978.

TELERMAN-TOPPET, N, COËRS, C, AND DESENEUX, JJ: *Ophthalmoplégie externe progressive associée à une polyneuropathie sensitivo-motrice chez un patient atteint de maladie coeliaque.* Rev Neurol 121:57–70, 1969.

TERÄVÄINEN, H, JUNTUNEN, J, ERIKSON, K, ET AL: *Myopathy associated with chronic alcohol drinking. Histological and electrophysiological study.* Virchows Arch A (Path Anat Histol) 378:45–53, 1978.

THOMSON, CD AND ROBINSON, MF: *Selenium in human health and disease with emphasis on those aspects peculiar to New Zealand.* Am J Clin Nutr 33:303–323, 1980.

THORNHILL, HL, RICHTER, RW, AND SHELTON, ML: *Neuropathic arthropathy (Charcot forefeet) in alcoholics.* Orthoped Clin North Am 4:7–20, 1973.

TOMASI, LG: *Reversibility of human myopathy caused by vitamin E deficiency.* Neurology 29:1182–1186, 1979.

TOMLINSON, BE, WALTON, JN, AND REBEIZ, JJ: *The effect of aging and of cachexia upon skeletal muscle. A histopathological study.* J Neurol Sci 9:321–346, 1969.

TORRES, I, SMITH, WT, AND OXNARD, CE: *Peripheral neuropathy associated with vitamin B_{12} deficiency in captive monkeys.* J Pathol 105:125–146, 1971.

TREDICI, G AND MINAZZI, M: *Alcoholic neuropathy: An electronmicroscopic study.* J Neurol Sci 25:333–346, 1975.

TYDD, TF AND DYER, NH: *Muscle biopsy in Crohn's disease.* Lancet ii:1574–1575, 1974.

VAN RIJ, AM, THOMSON, CD, MCKENZIE, JM, ET AL: Selenium deficiency in total parenteral nutrition. Am J Clin Nutr 32:2076–2085, 1979.

VAN VLEET, JF: *Current knowledge of selenium-vitamin E deficiency in domestic animals.* J Amer Vet Med Assoc 176:321–325, 1980.

VICTOR, M AND ADAMS, RD: *The effect of alcohol on the nervous system.* Proc Assoc Res Nerv Ment Dis 32:526–573, 1953.

VICTOR, M: *Polyneuropathy due to nutritional deficiency and alcoholism.* In DYCK, PJ, THOMAS, PK, AND LAMBERT, EH (EDS): *Peripheral Neuropathy.* WB Saunders, Philadelphia, 1975, pp 1030–1066.

WALSH, JC AND CONOMY, AB: *The effect of ethyl alcohol on striated muscle: Some clinical and pathological observations.* Aust NZ J Med 7:485–490, 1977.

WALSH, JC AND MCLEOD, JG: *Alcoholic neuropathy: An electrophysiological and histological study.* J Neurol Sci 10:457–469, 1970.

WEBER, LD, NASHEL, DJ, AND MELLOW, MH: *Pharyngeal dysphagia in alcoholic myopathy.* Ann Intern Med 95:189–191, 1981.

WEINBERG, T, GORDON, HH, OPPENHEIMER, EH, ET AL: *Myopathy in association with tocopherol deficiency in cases of congenital biliary atresia and cystic fibrosis of the pancreas.* Am J Pathol 34:565–566, 1958.

WHITAKER, JN, HOLLAND, PV, ALTER, HJ, ET AL: *Idiopathic inflammatory myopathy. Failure to detect hepatitis B antigen in serum and muscle.* Arch Neurol 28:410–411, 1973.

Wood, B, Breen, KJ, and Penington, DG: *Thiamine status in alcoholism.* Aust NZ J Med 7:475–484, 1977.

Yabuki, S, Nakaya, K, Sugimura, T, et al: *Juvenile polyneuropathy due to vitamin B_1 deficiency—Clinical observations and pathogenetic analysis of 24 cases.* Folia Psychiat Neurol 30:517–529, 1976.

Young, RSK, Hodes, BL, Cruse, RP, et al: *Orbital pseudotumor and Crohn disease.* J Pediatrics 99:250–252, 1981.

Chapter 10

COMPLICATIONS OF MEDICAL AND SURGICAL TREATMENT

RADIATION NEUROPATHY AND NEURONOPATHY

Until recently the peripheral nervous system was thought to be quite resistant to radiation injury. With the old kilovoltage machines, the permissible dose of internal radiation was limited by the skin tolerance, so doses over 4,000 rads were rarely given. In the past 20 years, however, the advent of megavoltage radiation has permitted doses in the range of 5,000 to 7,000 rads to be delivered to the brachial and lumbosacral plexuses and to nerves of the head and neck, and cases of delayed radiation neuropathy have become more numerous. The incidence, latency, and severity of these neuropathies depend on the total dose of radiation, the size of the fractional doses, and the length of time over which radiation is administered (Svensson et al. 1975). Additional sensitizing factors, such as high-oxygen atmosphere or the simultaneous administration of neurotoxic agents such as vincristine (Cassady et al. 1980), can increase the risks of radiation injury.

Brachial Plexus Neuropathies

Incidence

Brachial plexopathy appears to be the most common type of radiation neuropathy, and this complication is especially frequent in patients given prophylactic or therapeutic radiation for carcinoma of the breast. The incidence is difficult to determine; radiation protocols vary widely, the complication may not appear until many years later, and it is often unclear whether neuropathies are due to nerve injuries during mastectomy (Partanen and Nikkanen 1978), to invasion of the plexus by cancer, to lymphedema of the arm, or to radiation neuropathy. Thus, Stoll and Andrews (1966) reported a 73 percent incidence of brachial plexopathy in a large series of breast cancer patients treated with 6,300 rads (peak dose) of megavoltage radiation. In most of the patients, symptoms appeared 10 to 22 months after completion of the radiation. Edema of the arm appeared to play some role in causing the nerve symptoms, which were sometimes alleviated by diuretic or steroid therapy, by reducing edema with a pressure bandage, or by decompressive surgery at the carpal tunnel or thoracic outlet. However, the authors did not comment on the possibility that some plexus lesions were due to recurrent cancer or to surgical trauma.

Ganel and associates (1979) attempted to assess the role of lymphedema by studying 90 women who underwent radical mastectomy, usually followed by 3,500 to 4,000 rads of kilovoltage radiation. Radiation neuropathy would not be expected from this dose, but 20 to 30 percent of the patients subsequently developed symptoms and signs of carpal tunnel syndrome or other nerve dysfunction. Nerve conduction tests (including F-wave measurements) showed median nerve conduction delay across the wrist or slowing of proximal conduction, which were attributed to carpal tunnel syndrome or thoracic outlet compression, respectively. These abnormalities were nearly twice as common in patients with lymphedema, and the carpal tunnel symptoms were relieved by decompressive surgery. The authors concluded that lymphedema was largely responsible for these nerve complaints.

In another series, only 3 percent of 490 breast cancer patients developed plexopathy after receiving 6,000 rads (plexus dose) of cobalt therapy over 40 days (Basso-Ricci et al. 1980). When the radiation treatment was modified to exclude the axilla, reducing the plexus dose to 4,900 rads, no cases of brachial plexopathy occurred in the next 200 patients.

Based on the rather scanty data available, Svensson et al. (1975) estimated that a reasonably low risk of radiation injury to the brachial plexus would result from a Cumulative Radiation Effect (CRE) of less than 1,900.* For example, 5,000 rads given over 5 weeks in fractions of 200 rads yields a CRE of 1,572; when the same dose is given in 4 weeks, the CRE is 1,702, and in both circumstances the risk of plexus injury is very small. Six thousand rads given in 240-rad fractions over 5 weeks gives a CRE of 1,886, with a risk of 3 to 5 percent, and the same dose given in 300-rad fractions over 4 weeks yields a CRE of 2,043, which carries approximately a 15 percent risk of injury to the plexus.

Latency

The interval between the end of radiation therapy and the onset of radiation plexopathy ranged from 5 months to 20 years in one series of cases (Thomas and Colby 1972) and from 3 months to 26 years in another series (Kori et al. 1981); in both series the mean interval was about 6 years. Surprisingly, the latent interval was similar in patients with plexopathy caused by recurrent cancer, averaging 6 years in the first series (nearly all cases of breast cancer) and 3.5 years in the second series (only 35 percent breast cancer cases); the largest latent interval was 16 years.

PATHOPHYSIOLOGY. Most authors think that radiation damage is caused by extraneural fibrosis, which envelopes and constricts the nerve trunks. This process, abetted by endoneurial and perineurial fibrosis, leads to obliteration of blood vessels,

---

$$\text{*CRE} = \frac{\text{total absorbed dose to plexus in rads}}{(\text{number of treatments})^{0.24} \times (\text{total number of days})^{0.11}}$$

disintegration of myelin sheaths and axons, and Wallerian degeneration of the distal nerve fibers (Sunderland 1978). The same process is responsible for obliteration of the lymph channels, producing the lymphedema that frequently accompanies the neuropathy and may add to the damage by increasing intraneural pressure and reducing neural blood flow.

However, animal experiments have shown that the peripheral nerves are damaged directly by radiation doses of 5,000 rads or more; axons and myelin begin to degenerate about 2 months after radiation (Sunderland 1978). Delayed radiation damage to the cauda equina of rats begins as late as 7 months after a single dose of 3,500 rads. This type of radiation damage is not due to fibrosis; the actual mechanism is unknown, although damage to the microvasculature has been postulated (Bradley et al. 1977). Furthermore, severe fibrosis and lymphedema are not invariable accompaniments of radiation plexopathy. Thus, it is unclear whether delayed radiation neuropathy should be attributed to the mechanical effects of extraneural fibrotic proliferation, or whether fibrosis is merely an additional result of radiation, the nerve damage being caused by direct effects on intraneural structures. Both factors may operate; direct effects may be responsible for the small proportion of cases of brachial plexopathy that appear 3 to 6 months after treatment, and fibrosis for the later complications.

Clinical Features

Numbness, paresthesia, and dysesthesia in the hand or arm are the most frequent presenting symptoms; pain is absent initially in 80 percent of cases, and later on pain is not usually severe. Muscle weakness usually appears somewhat later but may accompany or even precede the earliest sensory symptoms. Spontaneous finger twitching, jerking, and cramps occur in some patients. Lymphedema is found in 75 percent of the cases. Kori et al. (1981) found primarily upper trunk (C-5, C-6) involvement in 75 percent of their cases, the remainder showing diffuse involvement of the entire plexus, but Thomas and Colby (1972) found diffuse involvement in 75 percent of their cases, with distal predominance more often than proximal. These differences could reflect the inclusion of different types of cancer patients in the two series; radiation of the axilla may have different effects from radiation of the supraclavicular area.

Typically, the plexus damage grows steadily worse over the course of months and years. Thomas and Colby (1972) noted that deterioration could continue for as long as 30 years, but in 4 of their 14 cases a plateau was reached after 4 to 9 years. Aside from measures designed to reduce lymphedema, and surgical decompression of the carpal tunnel in a few instances, no treatment has been found to arrest the relentless progression.

Diagnosis

The main diagnostic problem is to distinguish this complication from neoplastic involvement of the plexus or nerve roots. Other causes of pain, weakness, or sensory disturbance in the arm can be identified without much difficulty: nerve injuries caused by radical mastectomy, nerve entrapment in the carpal tunnel or other parts of the arm, and degenerative disk disease or arthritis.

Both metastatic and radiation-induced plexopathy often appear many years after the original treatment and progress gradually for several years; the main difference is the fact that severe pain is an early and frequent feature of cancerous lesions, while pain is absent in many patients with radiation plexopathy, and when present it appears late and is not severe (Thomas

TABLE 31. Differences Between Metastatic and Radiation-Induced Brachial Plexopathies*

	Percentage of Patients with Clinical Finding	
	Metastatic	Radiation
Pain at presentation	80	18
Lymphedema	14	73
Horner syndrome	54	14
Upper trunk (C-5, C-6)	4	77
Lower trunk (C-8, T-1)	72	0
Whole plexus	24	23

*Data are from Kori et al. (1981).

and Colby 1972). Lymphedema is more frequent in radiation neuropathy, while a Horner syndrome is more common in cancerous lesions (Kori et al. 1981). Kori and associates (1981) found that cancerous lesions usually involved the lower trunk, while radiation damage favored the upper trunk and never presented with isolated lower-trunk involvement (Table 31). Another factor to be considered is whether the CRE was high enough (over 1,800) to give an appreciable risk of radiation damage.

Electromyography may provide valuable diagnostic aid. In about half of patients with radiation neuropathy, EMG shows continuous, repetitive bursts of motor unit potentials (myokymia) (Fig. 42). These are clinically inapparent in half of the cases; the remaining patients have visible muscle twitching or even myoclonic jerks (Stohr 1982). Nerve block studies show that the spontaneous activity originates in the proximal nerves, presumably at the site of radiation damage (Stohr 1982). This type of spontaneous motor nerve activity does not occur in metastatic cancer (Albers et al. 1981).

When metastases are present elsewhere, it is very likely that the plexus symptoms are also metastatic in origin. However, in the series of Kori et al. (1981), plexus involvement was the only sign of recurrent tumor in 15 percent of the metastatic cases. There may be no signs of local recurrence either, and the nerve symptoms may progress for as long as 4 years before the cancer surfaces. Surgical exploration of the plexus is almost the only way to confirm a strong suspicion of recurrent cancer; this can be done safely, although the result is negative in 20 percent of the cases. Breast cancer is especially likely to grow slowly, infiltrating the plexus where it is hard to find amidst the scar tissue. In such patients, the clinical diagnosis may be sufficient justification for performing a neurosurgical procedure to relieve the pain.

Lumbosacral Radiculopathy and Plexopathy

There are only a few reports of lumbosacral plexopathy due to radiation damage. The two best documented cases, described by Ashenhurst and associates (1977), were in patients who received 5,900 to 6,760 rads to the pelvic tissues; signs of plexus damage appeared 6 months and 4 years later, respectively, and the patients survived for 9 years with progressive neuropathy and with no evidence of recurrent cancer. Sensory loss, muscle weakness and atrophy, fasciculations, and loss of reflexes were present in both lower extremities in a pattern indicating asymmetric and patchy involvement of the entire plexus. The spinal fluid was entirely normal.

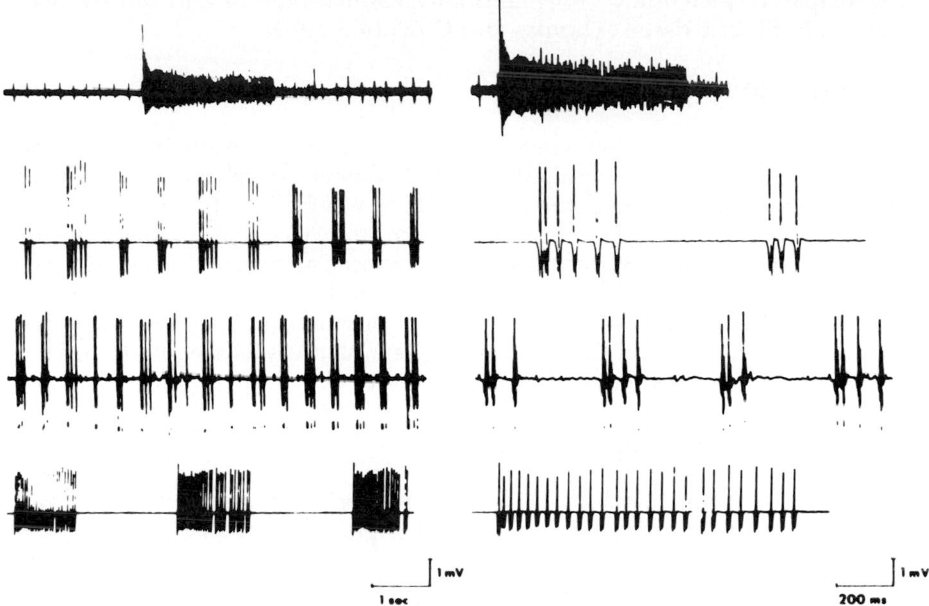

FIGURE 42. Myokymic EMG discharges from four patients with radiation plexopathy. Each discharge is shown at a slow sweep speed on the left and at a fast sweep speed on the right. (From Albers et al., 1981, with permission.)

Pathophysiology. The cause of the plexopathy is presumed to be fibrosis, just as in the brachial plexus cases. One patient developed bowel obstruction due to radiation fibrosis 8 months after completion of radiation therapy, 3 years before the plexus symptoms began. There is experimental evidence, however, that the lumbosacral nerve roots are more sensitive to direct radiation damage than either the lumbosacral spinal cord or the thoracic nerve roots (van der Kogel and Barendsen 1974; Bradley et al. 1977). A single dose of 2,000 rads, delivered to either the lumbar cord or the cauda equina of rats, produced paraplegia after an interval of 3 to 7 months; there was severe degeneration of the lumbosacral spinal roots, the posterior roots being much more severely affected than the anterior roots. Larger total doses of radiation were necessary when the radiation was divided into fractions (van der Kogel and Barendsen 1974). However, when the total x-ray dose was a little below the level producing overt paralysis, nerve root degeneration was most striking in the *ventral* roots, beginning 8 to 9 months after radiation. The root damage was characterized initially by demyelination, and this was followed by marked proliferation and hyperplasia of Schwann cells in 25 percent of the animals (van der Kogel 1977). The motor neurons in the spinal cord were unaffected, though there was mild damage in the white matter. In contrast, cervical or thoracic irradiation severely damaged the white matter of the spinal cord, paraplegia appearing 4 to 5 months later, but the nerve roots were spared.

Similar experiments have not been performed with other animal species, and it is not known whether the human cauda equina is also susceptible to radiation damage. A picture of selective lower motor neuron degeneration has been reported in patients following irradiation of the lumbosacral spinal cord, but it is not known whether the anterior horn cells or the lumbosacral nerve roots were damaged in those cases (see below).

The main diagnostic difficulty is to distinguish recurrent tumor from radiation plexopathy. This is an especially challenging problem when a pelvic cancer recurs many years after primary treatment, infiltrating the retroperitoneal tissues and exciting an exuberant fibroplastic response. When such patients present with neurologic symptoms, a pelvic mass is not usually palpable (McKinney 1973), and surgical exploration and biopsy may yield only fibrous tissue (Thomas and Chisholm 1973).

Femoral Neuropathy

Laurent (1975) reported four cases of delayed femoral neuropathy following radiation directed at the inguinal region. In each case there was a palpable mass of dense scar tissue in the groin, which was believed to be compressing the femoral nerve. The presenting symptom was pain in the anterior thigh and medial leg, appearing 12 to 16 months after radiation treatment; this was followed, in several months, by weakness and atrophy of the quadriceps muscle, diminished sensation in the femoral and saphenous nerve distributions, and loss of the knee jerk reflex. Neurolysis seemed to relieve the pain but did not change the motor deficits.

Cranial Neuropathies

The lower cranial nerves may be injured by megavoltage radiation therapy of cancers of the head and neck. The hypoglossal nerve is the one most frequently affected; damage to this nerve developed in 19 of 25 patients with cranial neuropathies appearing 1 to 14 years after radiation, the mean latency being 5 years. The radiation doses ranged from 6,250 rads over 41 days to 10,000 rads over 43 days. The 10th nerve was injured in 9 cases, the 11th nerve in 5 cases, and multiple nerves in 6 cases (Berger and Bataini 1977). Several patients were followed for up to 6 years after the onset of neurological symptoms, but there was no autopsy proof that the neuropathy was not due to recurrent cancer (Cheng and Schulz 1975).

Delayed Lumbosacral Motor Neuron Degeneration

In the cervical and thoracic spinal cord, delayed radiation myelopathy is mainly a disorder of the white matter, though when necrosis is extensive it may extend into the gray matter of the anterior horns. However, a clinical picture resembling a selective motor neuronopathy has been encountered in a small number of patients following lumbosacral spinal cord irradiation. Maier and associates (1969) summarized the findings in 15 cases of this sort, 9 of which had been reported previously in greater detail. All of the patients had been treated for testicular tumor, and the radiation field included the lumbar and lower thoracic spinal cord. More recently, Sadowsky and associates (1976) reported another example of selective lumbosacral neuronopathy in an adolescent girl who was given whole neuroaxis radiation for a medulloblastoma of the vermis. In all of the cases there was a gradual progression of painless, asymmetrical, patchy denervation in the lower extremity muscles, beginning between 4 months and 13 years after treatment. In some cases, progression continued to the point of paraplegia, while in others the process stabilized after several years. Muscular weakness, atrophy, and fasciculations were present without any sensory symptoms or signs, and sphincter function was surprisingly unaffected. Electrodiagnostic tests showed abnormalities compatible with anterior horn cell degeneration. The spinal fluid protein concentration was often increased to as much as 200 mg/dl, but the cell count was normal.

Pathophysiology. As yet no pathologic examination has been performed in a case of this sort, but the high spinal fluid protein values could indicate that the ventral nerve roots, rather than the anterior horn cells, are the primary site of the damage.

Rat experiments suggest that the cauda equina is more vulnerable to radiation damage than the motor neurons (van der Kogel and Barendsen 1974; Bradley et al. 1977). There is no clue as to why the lumbosacral motor neurons or ventral roots are particularly vulnerable to ionizing radiation. Fifteen cases of motor neuronopathy were found in a review of 343 patients given similar radiation treatment for testicular cancer, an incidence of 4 percent (Maier et al. 1969); this is comparable to the incidence of white matter damage in patients receiving cervical and thoracic radiation. Progressive motor neuron degeneration has also been reported following electrical injury of the spinal cord, but in that syndrome the brunt of the damage falls on the region of the cord through which the electric current passed, whether cervical or lumbosacral (Panse 1970).

NERVE INJECTION INJURIES

Nerve Injuries During Venous and Arterial Punctures

Serious injuries from this cause are quite uncommon (Britt and Gordon 1964; Gastaut et al. 1982; Berry and Wallis 1977). The median nerve is subject to injury in the medial aspect of the antecubital space; in this location the nerve lies medial to the brachial artery and to the median basilic vein, where it is easily pierced during attempts at introducing a needle into the vein or artery (Figs. 43 and 44). In the center of the cubital fossa, directly underneath the median cubital vein, lies the lateral cutaneous nerve of the forearm, which is occasionally injured during venipuncture or during a cutdown. Lateral to this, the radial nerve and its deep motor branch, the posterior interosseous nerve, are vulnerable to a needle probing for the median cephalic vein. The ulnar nerve, on the medial aspect of the forearm, is less frequently punctured than the more superficial medial cutaneous nerve of the forearm. Subclavian vein catheterization carries a slight risk of injury to the brachial plexus or the oculosympathetic, recurrent laryngeal, and phrenic nerves. The brachial plexus can be injured during axillary arteri-

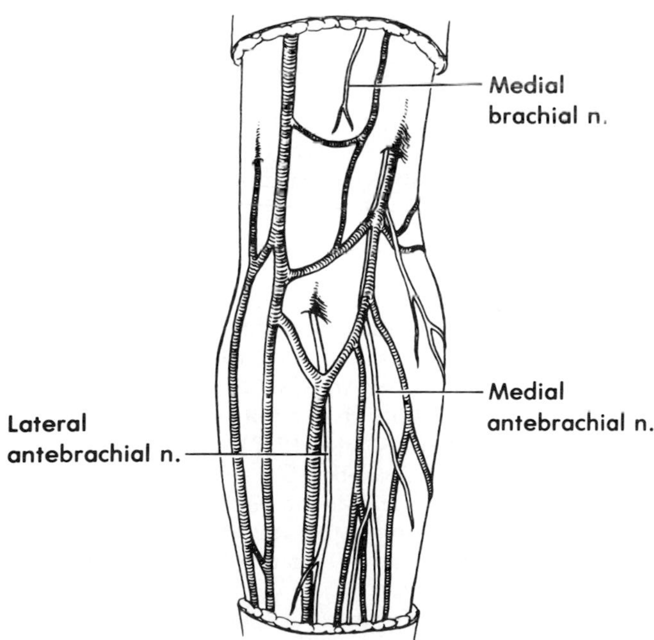

FIGURE 43. Relation of superficial veins of antecubital region to cutaneous nerves.

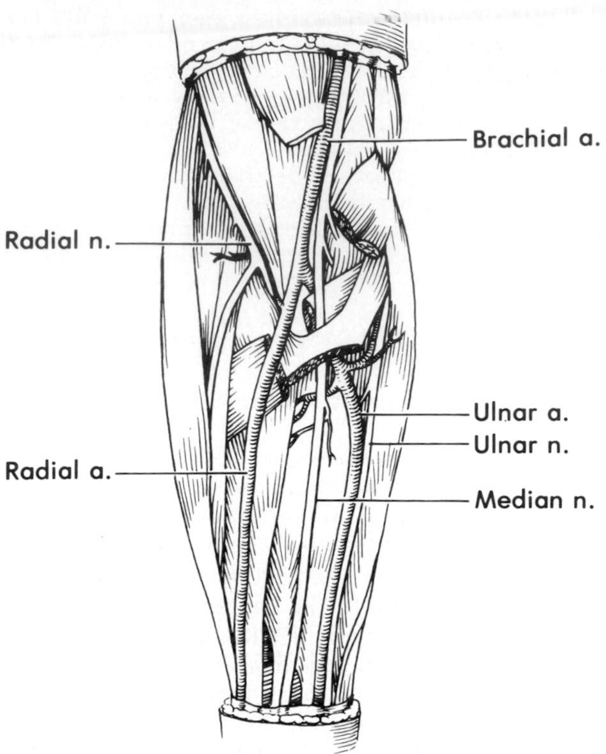

FIGURE 44. Relation of antecubital arteries to median, ulnar, and radial nerves.

ography, as a result of compression by a hematoma or a pseudoaneurysm. Prompt surgical decompression is indicated in such cases (O'Keefe 1980).

Selander and associates (1977), in animal experiments, showed that a long-beveled needle can pierce a nerve fascicle and transect nerve fibers, especially if the bevel is oriented transversely to the nerve; this would be the case in venipuncture, where the needle is usually held with the bevel facing up. Also, the needle may slice through the perineurium, allowing herniation of nerve fibers, which may cause focal demyelination; or the needle may cause endoneurial hemorrhage. The nerve may also be compressed by a large hematoma or by extravasated fluid.

Nerve Block Procedures

In performing a nerve block for regional anesthesia, the operator probes with the needle until paresthesias are elicited by contact with the nerve trunk, and then injects the local anesthetic around the nerve. Nerves can be injured if they are penetrated, if anesthetic solution is injected into the nerve, or if a hematoma forms around or within a nerve, but serious injury is uncommon. Selander and associates (1977) suggest that the risk of injury can be minimized by using a short-beveled fine needle, by probing gently so that the needle stops advancing at the point when paresthesias are produced (touching but not piercing the nerve), and by withdrawing the needle a bit if paresthesias occur at the start of injection, to avoid intraneural injection.

Follow-up studies of supraclavicular brachial plexus blocks, which are especially subject to complications, indicate that 5 to 7 percent of patients have persistent sensory complaints (pain or paresthesia) for up to a year after the procedure, but motor deficits of the upper limb hardly ever occur (Woolley and Vandam 1959). Phrenic, recurrent laryngeal, and oculosympathetic nerve paralysis are rare complications. Similar accidents may occur in the course of a stellate ganglion block. The lumbar nerve roots may be injured during paraspinal lumbar sympathetic block. A painful, unilateral neuropathy of the sacral plexus has been observed following paracervical block in obstetric patients. The manifestations, which appear 12 hours to 10 days after delivery, include severe pain in the buttock and posterior lower extremity, hypesthesia, and reduced reflexes, but the motor findings have not been commented on. A transient fever and the presence of a palpable mass overlying the sacroiliac joint suggest that a retroperitoneal hematoma is the cause of this complication (Gaylord and Pearson 1982).

Intramuscular Injections

Nearly all of these injuries involve the sciatic or gluteal nerves in the buttock or the radial nerve inferior to the deltoid muscle. Infants, small children and agitated adult patients are the most frequent victims of misplaced injections, and the risk of injury is much greater when a patient receives a large number of injections. When the nerve is injected directly, the damage is often serious because of the deleterious effects of the drug or its vehicle on nerve structures. The long list of substances that are harmful to nerves includes penicillin and many other antibiotics, propylene glycol (a commonly used vehicle), meperidine, barbiturates, phenothiazines, and paraldehyde (Sunderland 1978; Gentili et al. 1980). Damage occurs mainly with intrafascicular injections; injection of a drug outside of the nerve produces at most delayed symptoms of nerve irritation without motor or sensory deficits, and extrafascicular injection (within the epineurial connective tissue) tends to produce little or no damage (Gentili et al. 1980; Hudson et al. 1980) (Fig. 45). In a few cases, however, the drug is inadvertently injected into an

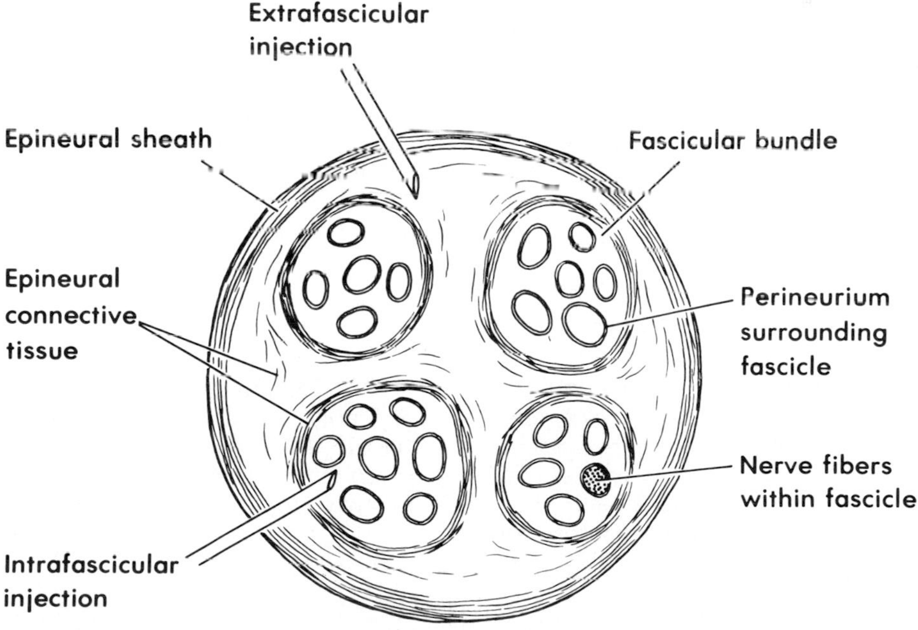

FIGURE 45. Diagram of a nerve trunk in cross section, showing how intrafascicular and extrafascicular injection injuries occur.

artery, causing ischemic necrosis of the skin and muscle and gravely damaging the regional nerves.

Intrafascicular injection produces immediate, severe pain radiating into the deep and superficial sensory territories of the injected nerve fascicles. A neurologic deficit is usually noticed immediately or within a few minutes; motor fibers are more vulnerable, and the motor deficit is generally more severe than the sensory deficit. In the case of the sciatic nerve, the peroneal division is usually more severely injured because of its lateral position, overlapping the tibial division slightly. In about half of the cases the pain persists and becomes a major clinical problem; in sciatic injuries, the pain is aggravated by sitting on the injected buttock and also by stretching of the nerve when the patient bends over or when the leg is advanced during walking.

The amount of recovery will depend on the nature of the original injury (Sunderland 1978). In a small proportion of cases the lesion consists of demyelination with transient conduction block; the axons are preserved, subsequent fibrosis is not extensive, and complete recovery usually occurs within 6 weeks. Unfortunately, in the large majority of cases there is some degree of axonal breakdown, and the subsequent incursion of intraneural and extraneural fibrosis may impede the attempts of regenerating nerve fibers to cross the zone of damage. Recovery through regeneration is still possible, though it may take 2 years or longer in the case of sciatic lesions of the buttock, and recovery is usually incomplete.

Because the outcome of untreated injection injuries is so often poor, surgical methods of assisting repair have been developed (Hudson et al. 1980), but the results are difficult to evaluate. Sunderland (1978) advocates waiting for 6 weeks to give time for conduction block to resolve. If recovery is inadequate, the nerve is then explored and the damage assessed with the aid of an operating microscope and an apparatus for stimulating and recording directly from nerve fascicles (Hudson et al. 1980). Nerve fascicles that are completely destroyed and will therefore not recover spontaneously are excised and repaired, using a nerve graft if necessary. Less severe or doubtful injuries can be treated by internal and external neurolysis, in the hope that this will improve the chance for successful regeneration by removing constricting scar tissue. If recovery is still poor after waiting 12 months (in the case of the sciatic nerve), the nerve can be re-explored and the injured fascicles excised and repaired. Unfortunately, the results of nerve excision and repair in high sciatic lesions are poor in any case, and since a controlled trial has not been performed there is no evidence that surgical treatment, whether by neurolysis or by repair, improves the outcome.

DRUG-INDUCED DISORDERS

Disorders of Muscle

In a recent review, Lane and Mastaglia (1978) classified the drug-induced myopathies into several categories based on modes of clinical presentation. I have modified their classification slightly to match the diagnostic approach to muscle weakness outlined in Chapter 1 (Table 32). Although the number of drugs causing myopathy is fairly large, only a few drugs in each category are in common use.

Muscle Injury by Injections

Inserting an EMG needle produces a linear tract of muscle fiber necrosis; over the next week, this excites an inflammatory reaction, phagocytosis, and

TABLE 32. Drug-Induced Myopathies

Clinical Syndrome	Drugs
Injection myopathy	Antibiotics (in infants); pentazocine; meperidine
Acute hypokalemic paralysis	Drugs causing potassium depletion; thyroid hormones
Acute necrotic myopathy	Drugs causing potassium depletion; drug-induced coma; dopamine-blocking neuroleptics; aminocaproic acid
Subacute and chronic myopathies	
Atrophic type	Corticosteroids; anticonvulsants; rifampin; colchicine
Necrotic type	Drugs causing potassium depletion; clofibrate; beta-adrenergic blockers; emetine; penicillamine
Degenerative type	Chloroquine

regenerative changes (Engel 1967). Serum CPK activity rises slightly, the peak of activity occurring 6 hours afterward and returning to normal by 48 hours (Chrissian et al. 1976). The average increase of CPK activity amounts to only 50 percent in normal individuals, and even in patients with muscle disease the increase is not usually large enough to cause diagnostic confusion (Cherington et al. 1968; Maeyens and Pitner 1968). Frequency analysis of the EMG signal showed high-frequency displacement (similar to that found in myopathies and in reinnervating nerve lesions) in 21 percent of muscles re-examined during the first week after EMG needling (Sandstedt 1981). Because of the possibility of producing misleading pathologic alterations, it is important to avoid EMG examination near the site of a planned muscle biopsy.

Needles used for injection of drugs are likely to be more traumatic than slender EMG needles. Small hemorrhages from injured blood vessels probably add to the damage in many instances, and large hematomas can form in patients with bleeding diatheses. Nevertheless, the major cause of muscle injury following intramuscular injections is the injected material itself, either the drug or its vehicle. Animal and human studies have shown moderate or marked elevations of serum CPK activity following intramuscular injection of a wide variety of drugs, including chlorpromazine, diazepam, local anesthetics, digoxin, phenobarbital, penicillin, and meperidine (Batsakis et al. 1968; Meltzer et al. 1970; Klein et al. 1973; Gloor et al. 1977; Yagiela et al. 1981; Steiness et al. 1978). The enzyme activity reaches a maximum between 2 and 24 hours after the injection. The CPK activity remains elevated up to 84 hours after a single injection of 50 mg of chlorpromazine (Meltzer et al. 1970). Multiple injections and large volumes of drug increase the likelihood of tissue damage. Histologic studies show large areas of muscle necrosis at the injection site (Benoit and Belt 1972; Steiness et al. 1978; Gloor et al. 1977; Rasmussen and Svendsen 1976; Yagiela et al. 1981). Drug vehicles such as glycerol formal and propylene glycol produce similar degrees of muscle necrosis (Rasmussen and Svendsen 1976).

Benoit and associates (1980) demonstrated that muscle necrosis produced by injection of local anesthetic agents was prevented by verapamil, a drug that inhibits the translocation of calcium across biologic membranes. They suggested that many drugs produce muscle necrosis by increasing the sarcoplasmic free calcium concentration, a mechanism similar to that postulated for ischemic necrosis. Some drugs, such as phenytoin (Serrano et al. 1973; Wilensky and Lowden 1973), are poorly absorbed from muscle tissue and remain there in large collections, probably because they precipitate as crystals at tissue pH, causing hemorrhage and necrosis. Paraldehyde is readily absorbed from muscle but can cause muscle necrosis, sterile abscesses, and injury to adjacent nerves. Even so, long-lasting harm rarely results from a few injections of injurious drugs.

The situation is different, however, when repeated intramuscular injections are given into the same muscle; sometimes an exuberant fibrotic reaction ensues, eventually producing a fibrous contracture of the muscle. This unfortunate complication has been observed in two clinical settings: repeated injections of antibiotics into the quadriceps muscles of infants (Norman et al. 1970; Bergeson et al. 1982) and self-injection of pentazocine or meperidine by narcotic-dependent persons (Aberfeld et al. 1968; Steiner et al. 1973; Levin and Engel 1975; De Lateur and Halliday 1978).

In infants, quadriceps contractures are usually detected when they cause limitation of knee flexion and hip adduction; at this time the muscles may be palpably indurated. As few as 10 antibiotic injections can cause such contractures. Some cases respond to muscle stretching therapy, while others require surgical lysis of the fibrous bands.

The syndrome of narcotic-induced muscle fibrosis is even more dramatic. Typically the patient has given himself several injections a day, for a period of months or years, in the accessible deltoid, triceps, quadriceps, and gluteal muscles. The muscles become indurated and contracted, although strength is normal. In places, the overlying skin is fibrotic and bound down to the muscle, and there may be ulceration and abscesses. The taut deltoid muscles, shortened by fibrous contractures, prevent the arms from reaching the sides and pull the scapulae away from the back, producing a bizarre appearance that has been dubbed "arm levitation" (Fig. 46) (Levin and Engel 1975). The quadriceps contractures produce a ludicrous, stiff-legged gait and cause the knees to extend rigidly when the patient sits down, while gluteal contractures limit hip flexion so that sitting becomes difficult or impossible. Entrapment neuropathies of the radial, femoral, or sciatic nerves may develop, adding distal paralytic complications that increase the diagnostic confusion.

Serum enzyme levels, surprisingly enough, are usually normal. EMG shows a variety of findings depending upon the portions of muscle sampled by the electrode: some areas are normal; some show myopathic motor unit potentials accompanied by increased insertional activity, pseudomyotonic bursts, or fibrillations; and others, which have the gritty resistance of scar tissue, are electrically silent. Muscle biopsy specimens likewise show fields of normal muscle adjacent to fields of degenerating muscle fibers undergoing phagocytosis, with chronic inflammation, muscle fiber regeneration, and abundant perimysial and endomysial fibrosis. Similar pathologic changes were produced experimentally by injecting pentazocine into rat leg muscles for 5 to 6 weeks. Fibrotic changes were not seen in control animals injected with saline (Oh 1977).

Surgical release of the muscle contractures has been reported to help in restoring muscle function, and external neurolysis may relieve the nerve entrapments.

Acute Reversible Paralysis

Acute hypokalemic paralysis occurs in some patients with chronic potassium depletion resulting from treatment with thiazide diuretics, ammonium chloride, laxatives, mineralocorticoids, licorice, glycyrrhizic acid, or

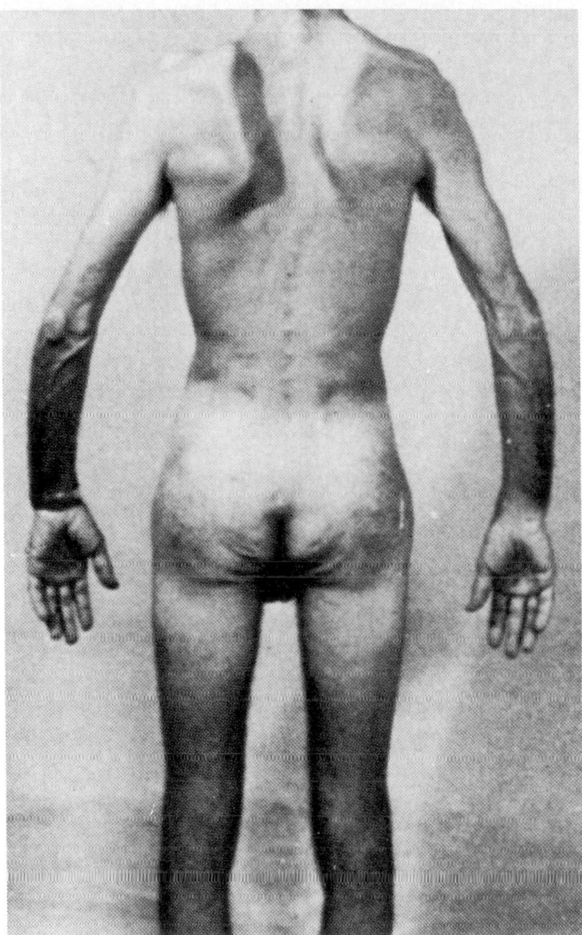

FIGURE 46. A patient with fibrosclerotic myopathy due to repeated intramuscular injections of pentazocine. Contractures of the deltoid muscles prevent the arms from reaching the sides; the weight of the arms exerts traction on the scapulae, causing scapular winging. (From Steiner et al., 1973, with permission.)

amphotericin B. In addition, surreptitious ingestion of large amounts of thyroid hormone may induce thyrotoxic periodic paralysis. Transient hyperkalemic paralysis is a rare complication of drug treatment; the few examples have been patients with chronic renal insufficiency who were treated with either triamterene or spironolactone. These syndromes are discussed in Chapters 2 and 3.

Acute Necrotic Myopathy

The distinctive features of this syndrome are myalgia, generalized muscle weakness, and high serum enzymes or outright myoglobinuria. One cause of this syndrome is *coma induced by an overdose of sedative drugs,* such as barbiturates or narcotics. Here the drug effect is mainly indirect, causing muscle compression and ischemia through prolonged immobility, insensitivity to pain, hypotension, and hypoxia (Chapter 8). The drugs most frequently responsible for myoglobinuria are probably those causing *potassium depletion;* this topic is discussed in Chapter 2.

The *neuroleptic malignant syndrome* is a state of hyperthermia, muscular rigidity, altered consciousness and autonomic instability, caused by the major tranquilizers including phenothiazines, butyrophenones and thioxanthenes. It appears to be an idiosyncratic reaction to ordinary therapeutic doses of these drugs, but it may be more likely to occur when a tranquilizer is administered together with a tricyclic antidepressant, an anticholinergic drug, or lithium. Marked elevation of the serum CPK activity is a regular feature (Smego and Durack 1982), presumably as a result of the intense, sustained muscle contraction. The syndrome resembles the anesthetic complication malignant hyperthermia, and in both conditions intravenous administration of dantrolene has been reported to be useful in controlling the hyperthermia and muscle damage, which may otherwise have fatal consequences (Goekoops and Carbaat 1982); however, it is likely that the intense muscle rigidity originates in the central nervous system, while anesthesia-induced malignant hyperthermia is a disorder of the muscle contractile mechanism.

About a dozen cases of myoglobinuria have been reported in patients taking epsilon-aminocaproic acid (EACA), an antifibrinolytic substance used in the management of hyperfibrinolytic states and of ruptured cerebral aneurysms. In the latter condition, the drug is employed to reduce the likelihood of rebleeding while awaiting a favorable time for performing aneurysm surgery. In almost all of the cases where myoglobinuria occurred, the drug was administered for 4 to 8 weeks in doses ranging from 12 to 36 grams per day. The patients developed rapidly progressive, generalized pain and weakness of the muscles, sometimes to the point of respiratory insufficiency. Serum CPK levels were markedly elevated, and EMG showed myopathic abnormalities with fibrillations. Muscle biopsy specimens give no clue to the pathogenesis, merely showing extensive muscle fiber necrosis without inflammation or any convincing abnormalities of the microvasculature. Following withdrawal of the drug there is brisk muscle fiber regeneration, bringing complete recovery of muscle function within 3 months (Brodkin 1980; Britt et al 1980; Kennard et al. 1980).

The incidence of this complication is uncertain; MacKay and associates (1978) encountered two cases in one year among six patients with subarachnoid hemorrhage who were treated with EACA. It does not appear to be an idiosyncratic reaction, because there was no recurrence of symptoms in five patients who were given the drug a second time (Brodkin 1980). Intravascular coagulation would be a plausible explanation for the muscle damage, but careful histologic studies have not shown this (Britt et al. 1980), and animal experiments have not yet revealed a direct toxic effect on muscle (Kennard et al. 1980). It appears, however, that serious muscle damage can almost always be avoided if the drug is not given for more than 3 weeks. It would be prudent to follow serum CPK levels closely during therapy.

Subacute and Chronic Myopathies

At least three clinical syndromes of slowly progressive, proximal muscle weakness can be distinguished: atrophic, necrotic, and degenerative myopathies.

Atrophic Myopathies. These disorders, exemplified by steroid myopathy and osteomalacic myopathy, usually manifest proximal muscular weakness and atrophy without muscle pain or tenderness, though bone pain may be present. Serum CPK levels are normal, EMG may be normal or may show myopathic changes without fibrillations, and muscle biopsy often shows type 2 muscle fiber atrophy without muscle fiber necrosis or other distinctive features. These disorders are described in Chapter 3. A similar myopathy has been reported in a patient treated with the antituberculous drug rifampin (Jenkins and Emerson 1981). Four years of daily colchicine therapy apparently led to progressive weakness and atrophy of the lower extremity muscles in another reported patient (Kontos 1962). EMG showed myopathic abnormalities and motor nerve conduction velocity was slightly reduced, while serum enzyme levels and muscle histology were normal. Recovery occurred after the drug was withdrawn. Atrophic hindlimb weakness has also been reported in cats given colchicine for several weeks (Ferguson 1952).

Necrotic Myopathies. These myopathies are distinguished by elevated CPK levels, usually in association with a histologic appearance of scattered muscle fiber necrosis and with EMG findings of fibrillations and other irritable features, in addition to the usual myopathic changes. Myalgia is a prominent symptom in some of the myopathies in this category. The most common cause is chronic potassium deficiency; this myopathy is discussed in Chapter 2.

The cholesterol-lowering drug clofibrate (also used in the treatment of diabetes insipidus) sometimes causes myalgia and CPK elevation, which may progess to overt muscle weakness. Myoglobinuria has been reported only once (Smals et al. 1977). The clinical and laboratory abnormalities may begin after a few days of treatment but usually develop over a period of several weeks or months, and they resolve quickly when the drug is withdrawn. In the original report (Langer and Levy 1968), CPK elevations developed in 9 percent of 60 treated patients, though only 2 of the 5 patients had muscle symptoms. In a much larger series, Smith and associates (1970) found that after 6 months of clofibrate therapy, CPK elevations were no more frequent than in untreated controls, and none of the patients developed myalgia. Nevertheless, a number of well-documented cases of clofibrate myopathy have been reported, especially in patients with renal insufficiency (Pierides et al. 1975), nephrotic syndrome (Bridgman et al. 1972), or diabetes insipidus (Matsukura et al. 1980). In patients with overt muscle weakness, EMG was either normal or showed myopathic abnormalities without fibrillations, and light microscopic and electron microscopic examination of muscle tissue showed nonspecific degeneration of muscle fibers (Abourizk et al. 1979).

PATHOPHYSIOLOGY. The unusual susceptibility of patients with renal disease to clofibrate-induced muscle damage may be related to the fact that the active molecule, de-esterified clofibrate, is strongly bound to serum albumin. In normal individuals, only 3 to 4 percent of the de-esterified clofibrate in the serum is unbound, while in uremic or nephrotic patients the unbound fraction may be 20 to 30 percent of the total (Bridgman et al. 1972; Pierides et al. 1975). Other drugs that bind to serum albumin could displace clofibrate, raising the free fraction of the drug. For these reasons, it is desirable to reduce the dosage of clofibrate in patients with low serum albumin levels, and to measure both total and free serum drug levels during long-term therapy.

The mechanism of clofibrate myopathy is unknown. Clofibrate produces a myopathy in rats (Teräväinen et al. 1977), and in rat muscle it reduces palmitate oxidation and the activity of carnitine palmityltransferase (Paul and Adibi 1979), inhibits the oxidation of branched-chain amino acids (Pardridge et al. 1980), and reduces the intracellular pool of Krebs-cycle intermediates (Pardridge et al. 1981). It is possible that these effects on muscle oxidative metabolism are responsible for the occasional occurrence of muscle damage in human patients, but clofibrate, like other aromatic monocarboxylic acids, also induces myotonia by blocking chloride channels in the outer membrane (Peter and Campion 1977); this could be another factor in the development of muscle damage.

There are rare reports of a myopathy with marked CPK elevations occurring during treatment with adrenergic-receptor blocking agents. Labetalol, an antihypertensive agent that blocks both alpha- and beta-adrenergic receptors, may cause transient myalgia, and in one case this was accompanied by a moderate rise in serum enzymes; although weakness was not detected clinically, the EMG showed myopathic abnormalities with increased insertional activity and fibrillations. Electron microscopy of a muscle sample showed numerous subsarcolemmal vacuoles, though light microscopy did not reveal muscle necrosis or other abnormalities. The symptoms and serum enzyme elevations subsided rapidly when the drug was withdrawn, and reappeared in a few days when treatment was resumed (Teicher et al. 1981). Another report described severe, painless proximal weakness, with markedly elevated CPK levels, in a patient treated for 6 months with sotalol; the symptoms subsided rapidly on withdrawl of the drug, but returned when propranolol was given. The EMG was myopathic with fibrillation potentials, but a muscle sample showed no abnormality (Forfar et al. 1979). The rarity of these toxic reactions suggests that a few individuals may be particularly susceptible to beta blockers, but the mechanism is unknown, and the patients had no neuromuscular symptoms when not taking the drug. Muscle weakness due to neuromuscular blockade has also been reported with adrenergic blocking agents; this complication is discussed later in this chapter.

In rodents, vincristine produces a necrotizing myopathy, but in man vincristine therapy mainly causes a distal, sensorimotor polyneuropathy. Many patients, however, experience proximal myalgia in the first few weeks of therapy, when distal paresthesias and subjective numbness first appear. Serum CPK (Allen 1978) and EMG of proximal muscles (Bradley et al. 1970) are usually normal, though biopsy of a proximal muscle may show scattered necrosis and regeneration of muscle fibers (Bradley et al. 1970). The myalgia often disappears spontaneously in a few months despite continuing treatment. After prolonged treatment, autopsy studies show patchy, segmental necrosis of muscle fibers in both proximal and distal muscles (Bradley et al. 1970). Serum CPK levels have been normal and EMG findings have been purely neurogenic in the few patients who have developed severe, generalized muscle weakness during vincristine therapy (Wheeler and Votaw 1974; Mueller and Flaherty 1978).

Because of its toxicity, emetine has been largely replaced as an amebacide by metronidazole, but it is still used occasionally in cases of amebiasis that do not respond to the latter drug. Emetine causes a necrotizing myopathy and myocardopathy in man and animals. Toxic symptoms are uncommon when the drug is given in a daily dose of 1.0 mg per kg for 10 days, but daily doses of 1.25 mg per kg or more may produce muscle weakness within 2 weeks. Cardiac and skeletal muscle damage may begin or continue to grow worse after the drug has been stopped (Fewings et al. 1971; Yang and Dubick 1980). The myopathy is characterized by diffuse muscle weakness, pain and tenderness, more pronounced in the proximal portions of the limbs and in the bulbar, neck, trunk, and respiratory muscles. Serum CPK levels are moderately elevated, and muscle pathology is notable for extensive muscle fiber necrosis. Experiments in rats have shown that the skeletal muscle weakness is entirely due to a direct toxic effect on muscle, without significant impairment of peripheral nerves or neuromuscular transmission. Type 1 and type 2 muscle fibers were involved to an equal degree in one study (Bradley et al. 1976), while in another study, Type 1 fibers were more affected (Duane and Engel 1970). Complete recovery of muscle function may be expected if the patient survives the myocardial injury. Though emetine has several toxic effects on cellular metabolism, the mechanism of emetine myopathy is still uncertain. The drug inhibits protein synthesis, but it appears that this action may not account for its cardiotoxicity (Yang and Dubick 1980).

A few cases of inflammatory myopathy have occurred during treatment of rheumatoid arthritis with penicillamine, a drug notorious for inducing hypersensitivity reactions. (Myasthenia gravis is a more frequent complication, as described below.) Both polymyositis (Morgan et al. 1981) and a dermatomyositis-like picture (Fernandes et al. 1977) have been reported, though in the latter case the facial rash could have been due to drug-induced lupus erythematosus. Withdrawal of the drug and treatment with prednisone were effective in eliminating the myositis over a period of several months.

Degenerative Myopathies. This term seems appropriate for the muscular disorder caused by prolonged treatment with chloroquine and other 4-aminoquinoline drugs (Whisnant et al. 1963; Hughes et al. 1971; Godeau et al. 1976; Mastaglia et al. 1977). Muscular weakness and atrophy, unaccompanied by pain or tenderness, develop insidiously, usually beginning in the lower extremities and eventually spreading to the upper extremities, trunk, anterior neck muscles, and sometimes the face and upper eyelids. The weakness may progress fairly rapidly over a period of several weeks or may develop slowly over many months. The weakness is diffuse, though usually the proximal muscles are more severely affected. The muscle stretch reflexes are usually depressed, even in relatively strong muscles, but no other symptoms or signs of neuropathy are present. Following withdrawal of the drug, muscle strength begins to improve within a few weeks, and normal strength usually returns within 6 months.

Many of the patients have taken ordinary doses (250 to 300 mg per day); most have been treated continuously for a year or more, but weakness can develop after as little as one month of treatment (Whisnant et al. 1963). In some cases there is a simultaneous loss of pigment from the hair and eyebrows (Godeau et al. 1976), or there is slit-lamp evidence of corneal edema (Whisnant et al. 1963), but the well-known chloroquine retinopathy rarely occurs in patients with neuropathy. Electrocardiographic conduction defects and cardiomyopathy are sometimes present (Godeau et al. 1976; Hughes et al. 1971). The serum enzyme levels are normal or slightly elevated. EMG abnormalities, most striking in proximal muscles, include myopathic motor unit potentials, an early recruitment pattern, increased irritability, fibrillations, and pseudomyotonic discharges. Myotonic discharges have occasionally been noted (Mastaglia et al. 1977), and one patient actually developed clinical myotonia (Blomberg 1965). Examination of muscle biopsies by light microscopy usually shows striking vacuolation of muscle fibers, and electron microscopy shows an accumulation of autophagic vacuoles (lysosomes) laden with membranous debris (Hughes et al. 1971). The vacuoles appear to arise by proliferation of transverse and longitudinal tubular membranes; this change is more striking in type 1 muscle fibers in animal experiments (MacDonald and Engel 1970), but in human cases both fiber types are affected. Mitochondrial vacuolation has also been observed. There may be similar vacuolar changes in endothelial cells and Schwann cells (Godeau et al. 1976). Chloroquine also causes vacuolar changes in cultured macrophages and sensory ganglia, and animal experiments show widespread lamellar inclusions in many cell types of the central and peripheral nervous systems.

It has been speculated that this accumulation of membranous inclusions may result either from stabilization of lysosomal membranes, from inhibition of lysosomal enzymes, or from binding of the drug to membranes so as to prevent their degradation. The last mechanism would link chloroquine toxicity to the lipid storage syndromes induced by other amphophilic drugs (Lüllmann et al. 1975).

Disorders of Neuromuscular Transmission

There are two mechanisms by which drugs give rise to myasthenic weakness. The first mechanism is induction of autoimmune myasthenia gravis, a condition closely resembling the spontaneous disorder. The second mechanism involves a pharmacological action of the drug on neuromuscular transmission; this may become evident either as an exacerbation of weakness in a myasthenic patient, or as weakness arising de novo in apparently normal patients. (Another manifestation, prolonged postoperative apnea, is discussed later in this chapter). Argov and Mastaglia (1979A) have recently reviewed the drug-induced disorders of neuromuscular transmission.

Drug-Induced Autoimmune Myasthenia Gravis

Penicillamine is now the most important cause of drug-induced myasthenia gravis. Most of the cases have occurred in patients with rheumatoid arthritis or other collagen diseases (Seitz et al. 1976; Vincent et al. 1978; Russell and Lindstrom 1978; Torres et al. 1980), but two cases have been reported in patients with Wilson's disease (Czlonskowska 1975, Masters et al. 1977). Almost all of the affected persons have been women, and the full range of myasthenic severity has been seen—from a purely ocular syndrome to generalized, fulminating weakness. Elevated serum titers of antibodies to acetylcholine receptor were found in almost all of the cases, and the clinical features of the myasthenic disorder were indistinguishable from the naturally-occurring disease. In most cases, after cessation of penicillamine therapy, the neuromuscular disorder gradually resolved over a period of several months; during this time, the antireceptor antibody titers fell slowly, suggesting resolution of an autoimmune process (Vincent et al. 1978; Fawcett et al. 1982).

The incidence of this complication is fairly low. Masters and associates (1977) found only one case among 56 patients with rheumatoid arthritis treated with penicillamine, though 20 percent of the patients had antistriational (antimuscle) antibodies. Argov and associates (1980) found neither clinical nor electrophysiologic evidence of myasthenia gravis in 25 rheumatoid patients receiving penicillamine for 2 to 5 years, and the serum titers of antibodies to acetylcholine receptor were all normal. Martin and associates (1980) did not observe myasthenic weakness in 57 rheumatoid patients on penicillamine for 2 to 55 months, though two patients had mildly elevated antireceptor antibody titers. They suggested that the presence of the HLA-B8 genotype (found in 60 to 80 percent of young females with myasthenia gravis) may predispose to development of this autoimmune complication during penicillamine therapy, but this genetic trait is not present in all cases (Torres et al. 1980). The antireceptor antibodies in penicillamine-induced myasthenia gravis are mainly directed against human acetylcholine receptor, while in spontaneous myasthenia gravis antireceptor antibodies have a broad range of cross-reactivity, though the pattern is different in each patient (Garlepp et al. 1981).

Hydantoin drugs have also caused a few cases of myasthenia gravis. Single examples have been reported with phenytoin (Brumlik and Jacobs 1974) and mephenytoin (Regli and Guggenheim 1965), and two cases were caused by trimethadione (Peterson 1966; Booker et al. 1970). In the trimethadione cases, antinuclear antibodies were present initially and disappeared after the drug was withdrawn. Antibodies to acetylcholine receptor have not been measured in hydantoin-induced myasthenia gravis, but antistriational antibodies were present in one case (Peterson 1966).

Pathophysiology. Both penicillamine and hydantoin drugs tend to induce antinuclear antibodies and the LE-cell phenomenon, and both drugs have been incriminated in the development of autoimmune disorders including systemic lupus erythematosus and immune-complex nephritis. (So far myasthenia gravis has not developed in patients treated with other drugs capable of inducing autoimmunity, such as hydralazine and procainamide.) The great variety of these autoimmune consequences suggests that the drugs induce a general disposition toward autoimmunity (Schoen and Trentham 1981). This phenomenon resembles the genetic disposition to autoimmune diseases that is linked to the HLA-B8 genotype. Unlike the natural diseases, however, drug-induced lupus and myasthenia gravis usually go away when the drug is withdrawn. If the mechanism of drug-induced myasthenia gravis were clarified, it might help to explain how autoimmune diseases start, why they persist, and how they can be controlled.

Neuromuscular Blocking Drugs

A number of commonly used drugs have a mild neuromuscular blocking action that occasionally results in clinical weakness (Argov and Mastaglia 1979A) (Table 33). This complication is rare except in the case of the peptide and aminoglycoside antibiotics, and even in patients with myasthenia gravis the danger of using these drugs has been somewhat exaggerated. Still, it is important to be aware of the risks, to use the drugs cautiously in patients with renal insufficiency or with known disorders of neuromuscular transmission, and to recognize such paralytic symptoms promptly if they do occur.

Antibiotics. Reviewing the English medical literature up to 1971, Wright and McQuillen (1971) found 138 cases of postoperative apnea that could be

TABLE 33. Drugs Reported to Cause Weakness Because of Neuromuscular Blocking Properties

Therapeutic Class	Drug
Antibiotics	Aminoglycosides, polypeptides, tetracyclines
Adrenergic blockers	Bretylium, beta blockers, trimethaphan
Membrane stabilizers	Quinine, quinidine, procainamide
Psychotropic drugs	Chlorpromazine, lithium
Anti-inflammatory drugs	Corticosteroids, chloroquine
Lipotropic drugs	D, L-carnitine

attributed to antibiotic treatment. The antibiotics included aminoglycosides (streptomycin, neomycin, kanamycin, gentamycin, lincomycin, and clindamycin), polypeptide antibiotics (polymyxin and colistin), and tetracyclines (oxytetracycline, rolitetracycline). Many of the cases occurred when a large dose of antibiotic was instilled into the peritoneal cavity near the end of an abdominal operation, respiratory failure occurring 10 to 30 minutes afterward. In other cases the drugs were placed in the pleural cavity, beneath skin flaps, in the extradural space, in the bowel lumen, or in the esophagus. When antibiotics were administered by the intramuscular route, paralysis developed up to 24 hours after the last dose. Apnea is often the presenting event, but patients who are observed closely also show flaccid paralysis of the limbs and trunk, ptosis, ophthalmoplegia, and bulbar weakness. Internal ophthalmoplegia (dilated, unreactive pupils) is a distinctive feature which indicates that muscarinic synapses are also blocked, as may occur in cases of botulism.

In most patients there are contributing factors such as renal insufficiency (causing the drug to accumulate in the body), inadvertent drug overdosage, hypocalcemia, myasthenia gravis, botulism (Santos et al. 1981), or residual effects of anesthetic neuromuscular blocking drugs. In patients with renal insufficiency, muscle weakness may last for several days, but recovery is eventually complete in all cases (McQuillen et al. 1968; Pittinger et al. 1970; Lindesmith et al. 1968).

The nature of the neuromuscular blockade produced by the aminoglycoside antibiotics is complex, and contradictory effects have been reported in different studies. There is evidence for both a presynaptic blocking effect, resembling that produced by magnesium and antagonized by calcium, and a postsynaptic competitive block antagonized by anticholinesterase drugs (Elmqvist and Josefsson 1962; Dretchen et al. 1973; Lee et al. 1976; Rubbo et al. 1977). Polymyxin and colistin produce a noncompetitive, depolarizing, postsynaptic block that is not reversed by neostigmine; anticholinesterase drugs may in fact increase the block (Lindesmith et al. 1968). Rolitetracyline has a postsynaptic blocking effect similar to that of d-tubocurarine (Wright and Collier 1976).

These differences determine the type of treatment that should be given, though in all cases ventilatory support and protection of the airway are the mainstays of treatment. In cases of aminoglycoside intoxication, intravenous calcium gluconate and intramuscular anticholinesterase drugs may be used together, but for paralysis due to the polypeptide antibiotics the best course is to rely on general supportive measures until the paralysis resolves.

Adrenergic Blocking Drugs. The antihypertensive drugs bretylium and guanethidine prevent the release of norepinephrine from sympathetic nerve endings. The former drug is no longer used in the treatment of hypertension but is still used as an anti-arrhythmia agent. Both drugs are notable for side effects of asthenia and subjective weakness, symptoms that can only partly be accounted for by orthostatic hypotension, but overt weakness has rarely occurred. One patient developed an acute myasthenic syndrome during treatment with bretylium, but subsequently tolerated guanethidine without difficulty (Campbell and Montuschi 1960). Studies in rat diaphragm and frog sartorius preparations show that bretylium has a hemicholinium-like, presynaptic blocking effect on the release of acetylcholine, while guanethidine reduces the electrical and mechanical responses of muscle to direct stimulation (Chang et al. 1967). Bretylium markedly potentiates the neuromuscular block produced by d-tubocurarine (Welch and Waud 1982).

Various beta-receptor antagonists, including propranolol, have been responsible for a few case reports of acute myasthenic weakness or of prolonged curarization following surgery (Rozen and Whan 1972; Herishanu and Rosenberg 1975; Hughes and Zacharias 1976). In animal experiments, propranolol enhances the blocking effect of curare and causes neuromuscular block in the presence of neostigmine. These pharmacologic actions are poorly understood; they have been attributed to a combination of quinine-like depression of muscle excitability and presynaptic and postsynaptic blocking effects (Lillehei and Roed 1971). Although one might be apprehensive about administering propranolol to patients with myasthenia gravis, I have done this without observing any untoward effects, and others have made similar observations (Kornfeld et al. 1976).

A much more common side effect of the beta blockers is excessive fatigue and inability to walk quickly up hills or upstairs (Editorial 1980). This symptom does not seem to relate to muscle weakness, but it may be a consequence of altered physiologic responses to exercise. Beta blockers reduce the maximum work capacity of normal persons, and they reduce oxygen consumption at all work loads, probably by inhibiting the consumption of lipid substrates. More importantly, perhaps, the drugs increase "perceived exertion" at any given work load (Pearson et al. 1979). The biochemical basis for these effects is still being investigated; it is not known, for example, whether the excessive fatigue is related to an increased rate of lactic acid production (Twentyman et al. 1981) or to a reduced rate of ATP generation during exercise. Some beta blockers seem to be more troublesome than others in this respect, and switching to another agent may eliminate this side effect.

Trimethaphan, a quaternary ammonium ganglionic blocking agent, has produced acute respiratory paralysis and flaccid paralysis of the extremities when administered intravenously in large doses (Dale and Schroeder 1976). Trimethaphan has also been responsible for prolonged postoperative apnea in patients given succinylcholine during surgery. Experimental studies have demonstrated that the drug has a curariform neuromuscular blocking action, which is not unexpected given its structural resemblance to other quaternary compounds with nicotinic blocking activity.

Membrane Stabilizers. Quinine, quinidine, and procainamide have long been known to have deleterious effects in patients with myasthenia gravis (Kornfeld et al. 1976; Drachman and Skom 1965; Stoffer and Chandler 1980). These drugs have similar actions, both as anti-arrhythmia agents and at the neuromuscular junction. They interfere with neuromuscular transmission in a complex fashion, producing a block that is not effectively reversed, and may even be intensified, by anticholinesterase drugs. These actions include depression of excitability of presynaptic nerve terminals and of the electrically-excitable muscle membrane, reduction of acetylcholine release from nerve terminals, and antagonism of the effect of acetylcholine on the postsynaptic membrane. The last effect appears to be unimportant at clinically-encountered drug levels (Miller et al. 1968). Chloroquine, another antimalarial drug with membrane stabilizing properties, has similar neuromuscular blocking properties and has been reported to produce acute muscle weakness in cats with doses as low as those used in clinical practice (Vartanian and Chinyanga 1972). Chloroquine has caused postoperative respiratory depression (Jui-Ten 1971), and may have been responsible for a transient episode of autoimmune myasthenia gravis in a patient with rheumatoid arthritis (Schumm et al. 1981).

Phenytoin slightly depresses neuromuscular transmission by both presynaptic and postsynaptic mechanisms (Yaari et al. 1977), but the drug appears to be comparatively safe even in myasthenic patients. In fact, a patient whose myasthenia was exacerbated by procainamide in a dose of 1500 mg daily showed no deleterious effect from phenytoin (Kornfeld et al. 1976).

Psychotropic Drugs. The mild neuromuscular blocking effects of these agents rarely have any clinical importance. Chlorpromazine, in a daily dose of 500 to 600 mg, exacerbated myasthenic weakness in one patient; the resulting neuromuscular block was only partly reversed by neostigmine (McQuillen et al. 1963). No similar cases have been reported subsequently. In vitro studies of chlorpromazine showed multiple effects on the frog neuromuscular junction: inhibition of transmitter release at nerve terminals, probably due to reduction of inward calcium flux during nerve action potentials, and reduced amplitude of miniature end-plate potentials, suggesting a curariform action (Argov and Yaari 1979).

Lithium carbonate has been reported to prolong the neuromuscular block produced by pancuronium (Borden et al. 1974) and succinycholine (Hill et al. 1976) in single cases. Two other patients developed cranial and limb weakness resembling myasthenia gravis during oral lithium therapy (Neil et al. 1976; Granacher 1977). The symptoms subsided when the drug was withdrawn and reappeared when treatment was resumed. In dogs, a blood lithium level of 1.6 mEq per liter prolonged both competitive and depolarizing neuromuscular block induced by pancuronium and succinylcholine, respectively (Reimherr et al. 1977), but lithium had little neuromuscular blocking activity in guinea pigs (Waud et al. 1982). A subjective feeling of weakness or heaviness of the limbs is a common complaint during the first week of lithium therapy, but weakness is rarely mentioned by patients on long-term therapy (Schou et al. 1970).

Corticosteroid Hormones. Initial treatment with prednisone and other corticosteroids often intensifies muscle weakness in patients with myasthenia gravis. This dose-related effect, which has not been encountered in any other disease, occurs in 40 to 50 percent of myasthenic patients starting prednisone therapy at a dose of about 60 mg daily. The deterioration begins 1 to 21 days after the start of treatment, and usually lasts for a week (Mann et al. 1976). The exacerbation of weakness can be sudden and severe; it is especially likely to occur when large, single steroid doses are given daily or on alternate days, and is much less noticeable when treatment is begun at a low dose that is increased gradually (Seybold and Drachman 1974). The peak of weakness tends to occur a few hours after the dose, suggesting a direct pharmacologic effect of the drug on neuromuscular function. For that reason, dividing the daily dose into 2 or 3 fractions helps to avoid serious deterioration of muscle strength. My own practice is to start with a low dose, such as 5 mg twice a day, and to increase the dose every few days, up to a final dose of 20 to 25 mg twice a day, pausing along the way if the patient gets weaker. Presumably the anti-inflammatory action of the steroid medication eventually improves neuromuscular transmission to such a degree that the deleterious effects of the drug no longer have any clinical impact.

Pathophysiology. Animal studies have shown a confusing variety of corticosteroid effects on neuromuscular transmission. In one study, prednisone antagonized the weakness produced by hemicholinium (which depletes presynaptic stores of acetylcholine) and curare (which blocks the postsynaptic response to acetylcholine) (Arts and Oosterhuis 1975). In another study, prednisolone and dexamethasone antagonized the action of hemicholinium but not of curare (Leeuwin and Wolters 1977). Others have shown that prednisolone in high concentration (0.2 to 1.0 mM) reduces the amplitude of miniature endplate potentials and endplate potentials (Wilson et al. 1974; Kim et al. 1979), but this effect is unlikely to be clinically relevant. In patients with myasthenia gravis, Miller and associates (1981) showed that a single dose of methylprednisolone increased the myasthenic decrement in response to repetitive nerve stimulation, and reduced the mechanical tension of a single muscle twitch without reducing the amplitude of the accompanying compound muscle action potential. These effects reached a maximum 1 to 3 hours after an oral dose of the drug, a time course similar to that observed clinically. These clinical tests of neuromuscular transmission confirm the existence of a mild neuromuscular blocking action of corticosteroids, but they also suggest that impaired contractility may contribute to the transient weakness. Why this should be is still unclear; contractility has not been studied in experimental autoimmune myasthenia gravis.

D-Carnitine. Carnitine deficiency has been documented in some chronic hemodialysis patients, and it was thought that replacement of carnitine might not only correct their abnormalities of lipid metabolism but might prevent the development of myopathy. Instead, a myasthenic syndrome developed in three patients after 2 to 3 weeks of treatment with D,L-carnitine, which was given intravenously in a dose of 2 grams after each hemodialysis session. There was severe weakness of jaw and limb muscles, which improved transiently with hemodialysis and responded to edrophonium. Repetitive nerve stimulation showed a typical myasthenic decrement during the weakness. The authors speculated that accumulation of acylcarnitine esters, chemically similar to acetylcholine, produced a competitive postsynaptic block (De Grandis et al. 1980). Since L-carnitine did not produce this effect, D-carnitine was presumably responsible (Bazzato et al. 1981).

Peripheral Neuropathies

The number of drugs capable of causing peripheral neuropathy is exceedingly large; the reader will find a useful compendium of most of these agents in several recent reviews (Argov and Mastaglia 1979B; D'Arcy and Griffin 1979 and 1981). For our purposes, we can omit mention of agents that cause a sensory neuropathy without muscle weakness, as well as those that cause neuropathy only in the context of an allergic reaction. Drug-induced serum sickness may be accompanied by mononeuritis, plexitis, or polyneuritis, and drug-induced vasculitis can give rise to mononeuritis multiplex. In contrast, the drugs listed in Table 34 cause motor or sensorimotor polyneuropathies by some sort of toxic mechanism, though for the most part these mechanisms are poorly understood. All of these agents are in common use and have been responsible for numerous reported cases of neuropathy.

Pathophysiology

With one exception, the principal pathologic mechanism of the drug-induced neuropathies is axonal degeneration, either in the form of a dying-back process (e.g., vincristine) or in a patchy, diffuse distribution throughout the nerves and roots (e.g., isoniazid). Perhexilene neuropathy alone is

Table 34. Drug-Induced Motor Polyneuropathies

Drug (Refs)	Duration of Treatment Drug	Mode of Onset	Anatomic Pattern*	Pain	Autonomic Manifestations	Other Manifestations	Slowing of MNCV†	CSF	Nerve Pathology‡	Recovery
Amiodarone (Dudognon et al. 1979, Fischer et al. 1977, Larre et al. 1981, Meier et al. 1979, Lemaire et al. 1982)	6 months to 3 years	Gradual	DSM	Frequent	Constipation	Tremor, gait ataxia, nervousness, corneal deposits, photodermatitis, hypothyroidism	0, + (++)	Protein slightly or moderately increased	AD (SD) of myelinated and unmyelinated fibers; lipid body inclusions	Slow, sometimes incomplete
Dapsone (Gutman et al. 1976)	6 weeks to 5 years	Gradual	Purely motor; distal, occasionally proximal, or in hands only	0	0	0	0, +	?	?	Slow, complete
Disulfiram (Mokri et al. 1981, Nukada and Pollock 1981, Ansbacher et al. 1982)	10 days to 5 years	Subacute or gradual	DSM	Infrequent	0	0	0, +	Normal	Dying-back neurofilamentous AD, mainly of large fibers	Slow, incomplete
Ethambutol (Tugwell and James 1972, Takeuchi et al. 1980A,B, Matsuoka et al. 1981)	4–9 months	Gradual	DSM (predominantly sensory)	Infrequent	0	Optic neuropathy, myelopathy	0, +	?	AD	Slow, sometimes incomplete
Gold (Katrak et al. 1981, Endtz 1958, Mitsumoto et al. 1982)	One injection to 6 months	Acute, subacute or gradual	Distal, proximal, or diffuse; sensorimotor or purely motor	Frequent	0	Myokymia, anxiety, insomnia, confusion, psychosis	0, +, ++	In 50%, protein and IgG increased, pleocytosis	AD, SD of large and small fibers	Slow, sometimes incomplete

Isoniazid (LeQuesne 1975, Ochoa 1970)	2 weeks to 39 months	Gradual	DSM	Frequent	0	0	0, +, ++	?	AD, myelinated and unmyelinated fibers	Slow, complete
Methaqualone (Marks and Sloggem 1976)	2–4 days	Acute	DSM	0	0	0	?	?	?	Rapid, complete
Nitrofurantoin (LeQuesne 1975, Toole and Parrish 1973)	3 days to 6 months	Acute or subacute	DSM (rarely, purely motor)	Frequent	0	0	0, +	Normal, or protein slightly increased		Rapid and complete or slow and incomplete
Perhexilene (Nick et al. 1978, Fardeau et al. 1979, Said 1978)	3–29 months	Gradual	DSM (may be proximal in lower extremities)	Frequent	Pupillary paralysis, orthostatic hypotension, sphincter malfunction	Facial weakness, sensory ataxia, numbness of face and trunk, tremor, cerebellar signs, papilledema, mental impairment, liver damage	++, +++	Increased protein, up to 590 mg/dl	SD, (AD). Larger fibers predominantly affected. Lipid body inclusions.	Slow, sometimes incomplete
Podophyllum (Chamberlain et al. 1972, Filley et al. 1982)	Within hours or in 1–2 weeks after contact	Acute	Diffuse, motor and sensory, with respiratory and cranial nerve signs	0	0	Confusion, coma, vomiting, pancytopenia, liver damage	?	Normal	?	Slow, complete
Vincristine (Casey et al. 1973, Bradley et al. 1970, Allen 1978, Goldstein et al. 1981)	Loss of reflexes after 4–19 mg; sensory and motor loss after 9–32 mg	Gradual or subacute	DSM (weakness of extensors of wrist and fingers first, then becomes diffuse)	Early myalgia (transient)	Ileus, constipation, orthostatic hypotension, bladder dysfunction, impotence, pupillary paralysis	Ptosis, paralysis of cranial nerves 6, 7, 10, hypersecretion of ADH, alopecia, cardiomyopathy	0, +	Normal	AD, dying-back type	Rapid and complete or slow and incomplete. Reflex loss often permanent.

*DSM: distal, sensorimotor.
†+, ++, +++: mild, moderate, or marked slowing.
‡AD: axonal degeneration; SD: segmental demyelination.

clearly established as predominantly demyelinative in type; however, a minor degree of segmental demyelination and remyelination is found in some of the other neuropathies, and axonal degeneration also occurs in perhexilene cases. Thus, motor nerve conduction velocities are normal or mildly slow except in perhexilene neuropathy, where velocities are markedly reduced, and electromyography reveals the usual changes of acute and chronic denervation whenever there is substantial muscular weakness.

Clinical Patterns

Usually, sensory symptoms of distal paresthesias and numbness precede the motor involvement, and sensory impairment always assumes a stocking-glove distribution. However, dapsone nearly always produces a pure motor polyneuropathy. Muscle weakness and atrophy usually have a distal, symmetrical distribution, but proximal weakness sometimes predominates (e.g., some cases of dapsone and perhexilene neuropathy), and weakness is sometimes more striking in the hands than in the feet (dapsone, vincristine). Autonomic neuropathy is a prominent toxic feature of amiodarone, perhexilene, and vincristine, and some drugs cause striking CNS symptoms (amiodarone, ethambutol, gold, perhexilene, podophyllum).

Relation of Drug Dose to Incidence of Neuropathy

Several temporal patterns can be discerned. Perhexilene and amiodarone induce phospholipid storage in Schwann cells and other tissues, and the drugs are excreted slowly; as a result, the incidence of neuropathy increases with the dosage and the duration of treatment. Latent neuropathy was detected by electrophysiologic testing in 65 percent of patients taking perhexilene, although none had clinical signs (Sebille 1978). These neuropathies usually appear gradually after several months of treatment. In contrast, with gold and nitrofurantoin the incidence of neuropathy bears little relation to the dose of the drug or the duration of treatment; neuropathy may appear after a single dose or after several months of treatment. These neuropathies tend to worsen rapidly once they begin, and may even begin or continue to progress after the drug has been stopped. A third group of drugs (vincristine, dapsone, disulfiram) show marked variation in individual susceptibility as well as a dose-related or cumulative effect. Podophyllum poisoning usually results from a single topical application or oral ingestion; neuropathy may develop within a few hours or may appear several days later.

Drug metabolism. Patients who acetylate isoniazid slowly have a much higher incidence of neuropathy than those who inactivate the drug rapidly. Among patients taking perhexilene, those with neuropathy have been found to oxidize other drugs more slowly than those who do not have neuropathy, but whether this is a genetic trait or a toxic effect of perhexilene on liver function is unclear (Shah et al. 1982).

Drug excretion is a major determinant of nitrofurantoin neuropathy, which occurs in about 4 percent of azotemic patients treated with the drug but is rare in patients with normal renal function. Azotemic patients have much higher blood levels of nitrofurantoin and its metabolites, but uremic neuropathy could also have something to do with this increased susceptibility.

Pre-existing neuropathy may make some persons more vulnerable to toxic neuropathies, especially vincristine neuropathy, but this relationship is hard to prove. Prudence suggests that all of these drugs should be used cautiously in patients with neuromuscular disorders.

Concomitant treatment sometimes contributes to the development of neuropathy. Vincristine toxicity is increased by drugs that impair liver function (e.g., asparaginase) and possibly by other cytotoxic drugs not known to be either neurotoxic or hepatotoxic. Simultaneous treatment with two neurotoxic drugs should probably be avoided (e.g., procarbazine, a mildly neurotoxic agent, with vincristine).

Nutritional and other medical factors may be important. Infants and poorly-nourished patients are unusually susceptible to vincristine toxicity (Allen 1978). Patients with lymphoma are four times more likely to develop vincristine neuropathy than patients with leukemia or carcinoma (Watkins and Griffin 1978). The dietary intake of pyridoxine markedly affects the incidence of neuropathy due to drugs that interfere with pyridoxine metabolism, such as isoniazid, hydralazine (Raskin and Fishman 1965), and penicillamine (Pool et al. 1981). Cellular stores of glutathione may be an important factor in nitrofurantoin toxicity; nitrofurantoin metabolites deplete glutathione in lymphocytes, and are more toxic to lymphocytes deficient in the enzyme glutathione synthetase (Spielberg et al. 1981).

Factors Affecting Recovery

Since recovery from neuropathy due to axonal degeneration requires nerve regeneration, improvement is slow whenever there is severe weakness, and permanent deficits may remain. In the lipid-storage neuropathies (perhexilene and amiodarone), recovery involves a slow elimination of the drug, which is bound to lipid inclusions, a process that takes many months. In other neuropathies there is pathologic evidence that a considerable amount of nerve regeneration occurs simultaneously with axonal degeneration (gold, isoniazid). With vincristine and some other drugs, the neurologic deficits may resolve while drug treatment continues at a reduced dose.

COMPLICATIONS OF ANESTHESIA AND SURGERY

Ischemic Muscle Injury During Surgery

Myoglobinuria has been reported following spinal operations in two patients who were placed in the knee-chest or "tuck" position (Keim et al. 1970). In this position, the patient lies prone with knees and hips tightly flexed; presumably this angulation obstructs circulation in the lower extremities. This clinical picture is analogous to the occurrence of myoglobinuria in patients rendered comatose by drugs or carbon monoxide. The knee-chest position has been used many times without apparent ill effects, though no attempt has been made to look for subclinical muscle damage in the postoperative period. Clearly the knee-chest position is somewhat risky; if it is used, padding should be placed to prevent compression of the major limb arteries.

CPK Elevations Due to Operative Trauma

Any surgical procedure in which muscles are cut or injured tends to elevate the serum CPK activity. In dog experiments, thoracotomy caused a 19-fold elevation of CPK, the peak values occurring 12 to 14 hours after the operation (Klein et al. 1973). Human patients exhibit 3-fold to 5-fold elevations

24 hours following renal transplantation or abdominal surgery (Miller et al 1972)

Muscular Effects of Succinylcholine

Succinylcholine is routinely administered to facilitate tracheal intubation during the induction of anesthesia. The usual dose of 1 mg per kg causes transient fasciculations, which are occasionally vigorous enough to produce gross movement of the limbs (Ryan et al. 1971; Charak and Dhar 1981). Some patients experience postoperative *muscle soreness,* which is said to result from the intense, transitory muscle contractions. However, a recent study showed that myalgia after abdominal surgery was no more frequent with succinylcholine than with pancuronium, a non-depolarizing blocker that does not cause muscle twitching (Brodsky and Ehrenwerth 1980).

A slight *rise of serum potassium* concentration tends to occur in normal persons, reaching a peak 2 to 5 minutes after the injection of succinylcholine; the increase amounts to 0.5 mEq per liter or less and rarely exceeds 1.0 mEq per liter (Evers et al. 1969). Ordinarily, this transient potassium rise has no clinical effect, but in hyperkalemic patients there is a risk of inducing cardiac arrhythymias. Moreover, a much larger rise of serum potassium can occur when succinylcholine is administered to patients with extensive burns (Schaner et al. 1969), massive muscle injuries (Birch et al. 1969), recent radiation therapy involving muscle (Cairoli et al. 1982), tetanus (Roth and Wüthrich 1969), or muscle paralysis caused by central nervous system or motor unit disorders (Tobey et al. 1972; Cooperman 1970; Smith 1971). In such patients, the serum potassium level sometimes increases by several mEq per liter, producing cardiac arrhythmia or arrest. Patients with chronic renal failure do not show any greater rise of serum potassium than normal subjects (Miller et al. 1972; Koide and Waud 1972), though pre-existing hyperkalemia puts these patients at an increased risk (Roth and Wüthrich 1969). In normal subjects, the hyperkalemic response and the fasciculations are both reduced or abolished by prior administration of a small dose of a non-depolarizing neuromuscular blocking drug (Famewo 1981A, B), but the result is less predictable in highly susceptible patients (Smith 1971), and it is safer not to use succincylcholine in such cases.

Pathophysiology. The mechanism of hyperkalemia following succinylcholine has been extensively studied. It is clear that the potassium comes from skeletal muscle, presumably as a result of the normal efflux of potassium that occurs during muscle activity. When muscle is denervated, sensitivity to acetylcholine spreads from the endplate region to the entire muscle membrane; exposure to succinylcholine causes prolonged depolarization and contracture, and potassium efflux increases 20-fold. A similar increase of acetylcholine sensitivity occurs in muscle segments severed from their connection with the endplate region, and in disuse atrophy (Gronert et al. 1973). These changes develop 10 to 14 days after denervation or spinal cord section and persist for about 3 months.

Succinylcholine also causes an *increase of serum CPK activity,* beginning a few hours after administration and continuing for 24 hours or longer. The magnitude of the rise, ordinarily quite small, can be correlated with the observed intensity of the fasciculations (Charak and Dahr 1981), and is much increased with halothane anesthesia or when succinylcholine is administered repeatedly, though not when the drug is infused continuously (Tammisto and Airaksinen 1966). Pretreatment with a small dose of either d-tubocurarine or succinylcholine reduces this effect, as does preliminary administration of thiopental (Tammisto et al. 1967, Charak and Dhar 1981). Subclinical myoglobinuria and myoglobinemia have been noted following the administration of single or multiple doses of succinylcholine during halothane anesthesia (Airaksinen and Tammisto 1966; Ryan et al. 1971); children are especially susceptible to this effect. The clinical importance of this phenomenon is less than at first appears, since frank rhabdomyolysis is a rare consequence (Jensen et al. 1968) and may indicate an underlying metabolic myopathy (Bennike and Jarnum 1964).

Pathophysiology. The mechanism by which succinylcholine causes CPK and myoglobin to escape from muscle is somewhat unclear. It is unlikely to be a simple permeability change, for the effect is delayed and persists long after the drug has been eliminated. The simplest explanation is that vigorous contraction or contracture injures some muscle fibers, either mechanically or by exhausting their energy stores, as may occur in seizures, tetanus, or catatonic rigidity. The main objection to this explanation is that patients who are susceptible to succinylcholine-induced hyperkalemia, and whose muscle fibers respond to succinylcholine with a prolonged contracture, do not seem to be unusually prone to develop myoglobinuria. However, serum CPK responses to succinylcholine have not been reported in those patients.

Malignant Hyperthermia

This grave anesthetic complication is actually a primary muscle disorder, in which exposure to succinylcholine and other anesthetic agents provokes a massive acceleration of muscle energy metabolism resulting in fever, metabolic acidosis, and rhabdomyolysis (Gronert 1980; Denborough 1980). Outside of anesthesia, most susceptible persons appear normal and have no neuromuscular complaints, though several cases have been linked to the congenital myopathy known as central core disease (Eng et al. 1978) and to other, ill-defined musculoskeletal abnormalities. There is a strong familial clustering of cases, which sometimes suggest an autosomal dominant pattern of inheritance, but multifactorial inheritance fits the genetic data better, and many susceptible individuals give a negative family history. Thus, the appearance of muscular rigidity and hyperthermia during anesthesia is often unanticipated, and this catastrophic emergency carries a 60 to 70 percent mortality rate.

The most potent *triggering agents* are the depolarizing neuromuscular blocking drugs (succinylcholine and decamethonium) and the volatile anesthetics other than nitrous oxide. Phenothiazines, ketamine, and amide-type local anesthetic drugs may act as weak triggering agents.

Clinical Features

An attack begins with intense muscular rigidity in 75 percent of patients; whether the non-rigid cases have a different pathogenesis is still uncertain. The rigidity represents a muscle contracture, with no EMG activity but intense hydrolysis of ATP, at several hundred times the resting rate of ATP consumption. In response to this expenditure of energy, aerobic and anaerobic energy metabolism rise dramatically, generating heat, carbon dioxide, and lactic acid. The rising body temperature and metabolic acidosis soon produce a high-output cardiovascular state, and metabolic exhaustion eventually leads to disintegration of muscle fibers with release of potassium, CPK, and myoglobin. Myoglobinuria and shock may bring on oliguric renal failure, and hyperkalemia causes cardiac arrest. Patients who survive have diffuse weakness, tenderness and swelling of the muscles and extremely high serum CPK levels, but the muscular system recovers completely within a few weeks.

Treatment

Treatment (Gronert 1980) consists of stopping anesthesia immediately and giving intravenous dantrolene in a dose of 1 to 2 mg per kg, repeated if necessary every 5 to 10 minutes to a total dose of 10 mg per kg. Dantrolene inhibits the intracellular release of calcium from sarcoplasmic reticulum, and it has been effective in controlling malignant hyperthermia in pigs and in several human cases (Kolb et al. 1982). Additional measures include artificial cooling, increased ventilation, intravenous administration of bicarbonate, and fluid loading. Temperature, blood gases and pH, venous pressure, and urine output are closely monitored for 24 hours, and dantrolene is given orally in a dose of 2 mg per kg q.i.d. for 1 to 3 days afterward.

Prevention

Much work has gone into devising reliable methods for *identifying susceptible individuals*, especially among relatives of persons who have had an episode of malignant hyperthermia. About 70 percent of survivors of such an episode show persistent elevation of the serum CPK activity; thus, a person with a positive family history and several abnormal CPK tests should be considered susceptible. For persons at risk but with consistently normal CPK levels, several diagnostic tests have been devised. The one most widely used involves exposing a freshly-biopsied muscle sample to various concentrations of halothane, caffeine, or succinylcholine, while measuring the tension and contracture thresholds. These tests are difficult to perform but are fairly sensitive and reliable when carried out in an experienced research laboratory. Unfortunately, there are only a few such laboratories in the world; fresh tissue is required; and children must be exposed to the risk of anesthesia in order to obtain a muscle sample. Other tests are either less specific or have not yet been fully validated.

The current recommendations for administering anesthesia to a patient known or suspected to be susceptible to malignant hyperthermia are as follows (Gronert 1980, 1981): (1) During the 24 hour period before surgery, dantrolene is given orally in 3 or 4 divided doses, to a total of 4 mg per kg. (2) Preanesthetic sedation should be generous, in the form of barbiturates or opiates, omitting atropine. (3) For general anesthesia, the safe agents are nitrous oxide, barbiturates, opiates, althesin, droperidol, and pancuronium. (4) For regional anesthesia, the ester-type agents (procaine, chloroprocaine, piperocaine, tetracaine) are safer than amide agents (lidocaine, mepivacaine). (5) Body temperature and blood gases should be monitored closely. With these precautions, episodes of malignant hyperthermia occur rarely and can usually be aborted quickly.

PATHOPHYSIOLOGY. The existence of a similar syndrome in several breeds of swine has facilitated laboratory investigation, but it must be remembered that the human syndrome is not a uniform disease, and the porcine disease differs from the human in that episodes of malignant hyperthermia are triggered by exercise or excitement as well as by drugs.

It is generally believed that the key abnormality in malignant hyperthermia is an excessive release of calcium from intracellular binding sites in the sarcoplasmic reticulum and possibly in mitochondria. However, this defect has never been demonstrated directly. What has been shown is that muscle from affected humans and pigs develops contracture more readily than normal upon exposure to halothane, succinylcholine, caffeine, or potassium chloride. As shown in Figure 47, contracture could result from an abnormality of the myofibrillar proteins; from excessive release of calcium from the sarcoplasmic reticulum (SR); from inadequate reuptake of calcium by SR; or from excessive depolarization of the plasma membrane or transverse tubular system in response to normal stimulation. An abnormality of the contractile proteins can be excluded by the fact that the contracture is prevented by dantrolene and by deuterium oxide, substances that block transmission of the signal from the transverse tubular system to the sarcoplasmic reticulum without affecting the contractility of the myofibrils (Okumura et al. 1980). The other possible mechanisms cannot be sorted out using the available data. There are reports that fragmented preparations of SR and of plasma membranes respond abnormally to caffeine and other triggering agents in vitro, but the results obtained in different laboratories are not consistent. Taken together, however, the data suggest that there may be abnormalities at several sites in the excitation-contraction coupling system, perhaps reflecting a more general membrane abnormality (Gronert 1980; Okumura et al. 1980). This supposition gains some support from reports of increased erythrocyte fragility and abnormal mitochondrial function in malignant hyperthermic swine (Cheah and Cheah 1979). Temperature perturbation studies of SR suggest that the porcine defect may involve altered physicochemical properties of the membrane lipids (Nelson and Bee 1979).

Postoperative Apnea

During recovery from anesthesia, a few patients exhibit signs of persistent neuromuscular blockade in the form of ocular and bulbar weakness, difficulty handling secretions, and inadequate ventilation. The explanation for this occurrence must be sought in an examination of the drugs administered before and during surgery and of the previous medical condition of the patient.

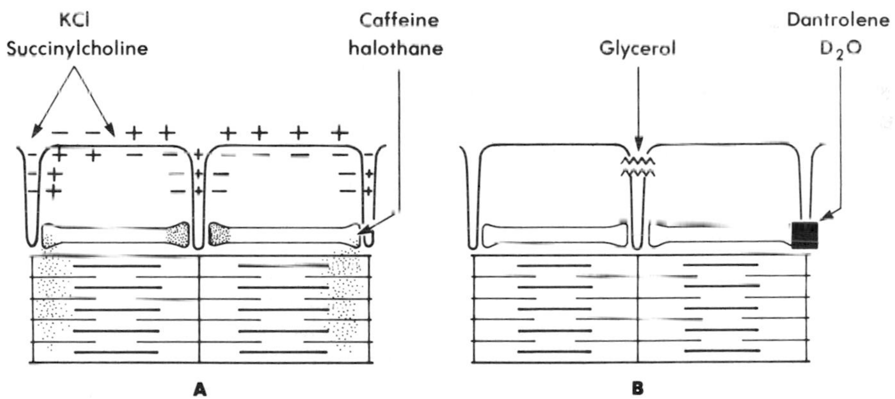

FIGURE 47. Mechanism of contracture in malignant hyperthermia. *A:* The site of action of chemical agents inducing contracture. High-concentration KCl depolarizes the sarcolemma and T-tubules, triggering the release of calcium *(small dots)* from the sarcoplasmic reticulum (SR). Caffeine and halothane directly trigger release of calcium from the SR. *B:* Contractures induced by KCl or succinylcholine are prevented by treatment with glycerol, which disrupts the T-tubules; caffeine and halothane still produce contracture, however. Succinylcholine thus appears to act on the sarcolemma and T-tubules, like KCl. Dantrolene and deuterium oxide, both of which block transmission of signals from the T-tubules to the SR, inhibit the induction of contracture by KCl, succinylcholine, caffeine and halothane. These observations suggest that, in malignant hyperthermia, the T-tubules and SR are abnormally sensitive to chemical agents that trigger release of calcium. (Based on Okumura et al., 1980.)

Prolonged Action of Succinylcholine

This depolarizing muscle relaxant is rapidly hydrolyzed and inactivated by plasma cholinesterase. The action of succinylcholine may be prolonged if the plasma cholinesterase activity is less than 50 percent of the normal mean activity; when the enzyme activity is very low the neuromuscular block may last for 2 to 3 hours. In infants up to 6 months of age, plasma cholinesterase activity is about 50 percent of the adult value. In adults, low plasma cholinesterase activity may be due to (a) the presence of a genetic enzyme variant; (b) a physiologic decrease in activity during pregnancy (declining about 25 percent between the 10th week and the early postpartum period); (c) reduced synthesis of the enzyme due to liver disease, inanition, or other disease states; (d) removal of the enzyme during plasmapheresis (Wood and Hall 1978; Evans et al. 1980); (e) partial inactivation of cholinesterase by drugs such as pancuronium, neostigmine, pyridostigmine, lithium, monoamine oxidase inhibitors, and oral contraceptives (Whittaker 1980). The action of succinylcholine may also be prolonged by drugs acting directly on neuromuscular transmission, such as anticholinesterase drugs, ketamine, procaine, and oxytocin (Argov and Mastaglia 1979A).

Side Effects of Non-Anesthetic Drugs

A wide variety of drugs have undesired neuromuscular blocking properties and may cause postoperative apnea by themselves or in conjunction with the neuromuscular blockers administered during anesthesia. These drugs were discussed earlier in this chapter.

Latent or Unrecognized Disorders of Neuromuscular Transmission

Patients with myasthenia gravis or Lambert-Eaton syndrome are extremely sensitive to the paralyzing effects of d-tubocurarine; weakness is induced by less than one-tenth of the dose necessary to cause weakness in normal individuals. In these patients, the duration of action of neuromuscular blocking agents is unduly prolonged, since even small amounts of residual drug may cause clinical weakness. Ordinarily, this effect is only encountered when long-acting nondepolarizing agents are used, such as d-tubocurarine or pancuronium.

Anesthetic Error

Excessive doses of long-acting neuromuscular blocking agents account for some cases of postoperative apnea occurring in normal individuals. In one survey of "succinylcholine-sensitive" patients, 28 percent had normal plasma cholinesterase activity, and in more than half of these cases the apnea could be attributed to errors in anesthetic technique (Viby-Mogensen and Hanel 1978).

The safest way to manage postoperative apnea is to re-intubate the trachea and support respiration until the effect of the medication wears off. In patients with genetic variants of plasma cholinesterase, prolonged succinylcholine block has desensitizing as well as depolarizing features, and pharmacologic reversal may require the successive administration of a purified cholinesterase preparation and neostigmine (Viby-Mogensen 1981). Paralysis caused by antibiotics and other non-anesthetic drugs responds unpredictably to pharmacotherapy and may be made worse by neostigmine.

Furthermore, there is usually not enough time to analyze the precise cause of the apnea.

Peripheral Nerve Injuries During Anesthesia and Surgery

Neuropathies Due to Body Position

During surgical procedures, the major nerves of the extremities are subject to traction or compression when patients are placed in unusual positions or are left in one position for long periods, unable to heed the sensory warnings that would cause a sleeping person to shift position. Despite improvements in positioning techniques, neuropathies continue to occur, but their incidence is uncertain because no prospective study has been done. Retrospective chart reviews, which undoubtedly underestimate the incidence of mild neuropathies, have given estimates varying from 0.14 percent (Parks 1973) to 6 percent (Morin et al. 1982). Pre-existing nerve disease, such as diabetes mellitus and uremic neuropathy, makes peripheral nerves more susceptible to injury by compression and traction. The duration of surgery is another important factor; Parks (1973) reported that most of the cases occurred after operations lasting at least 6 hours.

Brachial plexus palsy is by far the most common major nerve injury, accounting for 39 percent of the episodes in one series (Parks 1973). The major factors appear to be stretching of the plexus by abduction, dorsal extension, and external rotation of the arm, posterior displacement of the shoulder, and rotation of the head to the opposite side (Britt and Gordon 1964). Compression of the plexus between the clavicle and first rib may also occur. In the supine position, plexus injury can occur when the arm is placed on an armboard; in the lateral decubitus position, the plexus may be injured when the arm is suspended from an ether screen or is allowed to hang across the chest.

The upper roots of the plexus are most frequently injured, but in some cases the entire plexus or only the lower roots are involved. There is usually pain in the shoulder and tenderness in the supraclavicular area, but sensory deficits are slight or absent. A Horner syndrome may accompany lower trunk palsies, indicating that the injury involves the proximal nerve roots. In a follow-up study, recovery occurred within 9 days in 32 percent of patients and within 6 months in another 56 percent while 12 percent of patients had residual deficits after 1 year (Parks 1973).

Radial neuropathies are nearly always due to compression in the spiral groove of the humerus; this injury can be prevented by proper positioning, but it accounted for 15 percent of postoperative neuropathies in a recent series (Parks 1973).

The *ulnar nerve* is harder to protect from injury. When the elbow is extended and the forearm pronated, the nerve may be compressed against the posterior aspect of the medial epicondyle of the humerus, while flexion of the elbow may cause a traction injury, perhaps aggravated by entrapment in the cubital tunnel (Miller and Camp 1979). In most reports the radial and ulnar neuropathies recovered rapidly (within 6 weeks), but Miller and Camp (1979) reported a selected series of eight patients with severe postoperative ulnar neuropathy persisting for 6 to 96 months. A good elbow pad may help to prevent this complication (Murphy and Devers 1974).

Median nerve injuries rarely occur except as a result of intravenous injections in the antecubital fossa.

The *peroneal nerve* accounts for 21 percent of operative injuries (Parks 1973). Compression against the head of the fibula, the usual mechanism, can occur in the lateral decubitus position or when the outer aspect of the upper leg rests against a metal brace or a leg strap. The nerve can also be stretched by flexion of the hip and knee in the lithotomy position (Britt and Gordon 1964). Recovery is incomplete after one year in 15 percent of cases (Parks 1973). The *sciatic nerve* is occasionally injured by compression of the buttock, especially in an emaciated patient or when the opposite buttock is elevated during surgery (Britt and Gordon 1964). Unilateral or bilateral *femoral neuropathy* occurs rarely following surgery or childbirth in the lithotomy position; compression of the femoral nerve against the inguinal ligament or excessive stretching of the nerve by abduction and external rotation of the thighs, are the postulated mechanisms (Montag and Mead 1981).

Tourniquet Paralysis

The tourniquet is widely used to obtain a bloodless field in extremity surgery. A few decades ago, when an Esmarch bandage or rubber tubing was used for this purpose, postoperative paralysis was a common occurrence, but since the introduction of the pneumatic tourniquet, which permits accurate control of the applied pressure, only a few cases of tourniquet paralysis have been reported. In the upper extremity, a cuff pressure of 250 to 300 torr applied for up to 2 hours is almost always safe (see Chapter 8); higher pressures may injure nerves by direct compression by the edges of the tourniquet. The calibration of the tourniquet is not always accurate, however, and a few patients may be unusually susceptible to nerve compression palsies.

Electrophysiologic studies of two patients who developed nearly complete motor and sensory paralysis of the arm distal to a tourniquet showed a combination of conduction block and Wallerian degeneration. Recovery of function, associated with resolution of the conduction block, did not begin until more than 2 months after the injury, and was still incomplete after 4 to 6 months (Rudge 1974; Bolton and MacFarlane 1978). Experiments with human subjects show that, following release of a pneumatic tourniquet that has compressed the arm at a pressure of 300 torr for 30 to 60 minutes, nerve function recovers within 1 hour in most cases and within 24 hours in all cases (Yates et al. 1981).

While tourniquet paralysis is rare in the upper extremity, Weingarten and associates (1979) found EMG abnormalities suggesting denervation in leg muscles distal to the tourniquet site in 72 percent of 25 patients studied 3 weeks after knee surgery. The quadriceps muscle was involved in nearly all of these cases, and in some patients the muscles supplied by the tibial, peroneal, or obturator nerves were also affected. The average tourniquet time was 41 minutes in the patients without EMG abnormalities and 55 minutes in the affected patients. The EMG abnormalities resolved within 5 months. These observations are surprising, since denervation changes in muscle imply Wallerian degeneration, which would not be expected to occur in the absence of severe conduction block. Unfortunately, the authors did not describe the neurologic findings, and nerve conduction tests were not done. It does seem, however, that there is a need for more clinical and electrophysiologic studies of extremity function following the use of a pneumatic tourniquet.

Complications of Spinal Anesthesia

Damage to the spinal cord or lumbosacral nerve roots is a rare complication of spinal anesthesia. The incidence of transient paralysis of the legs following either intradural or extradural block is about 0.1 percent, and permanent paralysis occurs in about 0.02 percent of cases (Kane 1981).

Single nerve roots are sometimes injured directly by the needle; in such cases, focal pain and sensory or motor symptoms are noted immediately after the procedure and usually clear completely within a few weeks.

Epidural or subdural hemorrhage is a serious complication occurring almost exclusively in patients with a bleeding tendency; symptoms of cauda equina or spinal cord compression develop hours or days after the procedure and increase rapidly (see Chapter 8).

Some patients manifest paraplegia, lumbosacral sensory loss, and urinary and fecal incontinence immediately after spinal anesthesia; this is usually a toxic effect of the local anesthetic, or some other constituent of the solution, upon the cauda equina. This type of toxic injury is primarily encountered with intrathecal anesthesia; when it occurs with epidural block there has usually been an inadvertent penetration of the dura. The neurologic symptoms may resolve within a few weeks, but permanent deficits may remain. Acute cauda equina compression due to lumbar spinal stenosis has occasionally been precipitated by spinal anesthesia (Kane 1981).

Ischemic necrosis of the lumbar spinal cord, primarily a complication of epidural block, also presents with immediate paraplegia and sensory loss, but can usually be distinguished from the cauda equina syndrome by the presence of a lower thoracic sensory level, dissociated sensory loss, and Babinski sign. The cause of this syndrome is uncertain, but prolonged hypotension, the effects of the epinephrine in the anesthetic solution, and preexisting atherosclerosis may be contributing factors (Kane 1981).

A delayed syndrome of slowly progressive weakness and sensory loss in the legs following spinal anesthesia may be due to spinal adhesive arachnoiditis. The neurologic deficits, which derive from constrictive, ischemic damage to both nerve roots and spinal cord, usually begin a few weeks or months after the procedure, and they ascend gradually over the course of weeks, months, or years until they become arrested or lead to a fatal outcome. This complication is now extremely rare; when it was more common, several decades ago, it was attributed to contamination of syringes by detergents or to the presence of toxic preservatives in the anesthetic solutions.

Adhesive arachnoiditis also occurs following myelography with iodinated contrast media, especially oil-soluble materials such as iophendylate (Pantopaque). Other factors, such as the presence of blood in the spinal fluid, surgical procedures, and repeated myelography, are thought to increase the risk of developing arachnoiditis. Some water-soluble contrast media also cause arachnoiditis, but so far metrizamide seems to be very safe in this respect (Shaw et al. 1978). Some cases of adhesive arachnoiditis are caused by injections of drugs or, as in the case of Depo-Medrol, of the vehicle in which the drug is dissolved (Bernat et al. 1976). Syphilis, tuberculosis, and other infections used to be the main cause of adhesive arachnoiditis; such cases are now rare in developed countries, but in tropical regions such as India, Southeast Asia, and Africa, idiopathic arachnoiditis, presumably infectious in origin, is still an important cause of spinal cord and cauda equina syndromes (Jenik et al. 1981).

Neuropathy Due to Surgical Trauma

Operative injury of motor nerves is an uncommon complication that has not received much attention in the surgical literature. The following are some of the neuropathies that have been recognized, listed according to body region.

Neck surgery is notoriously hazardous to nerves, and in the performance of major cancer surgery some nerves are nearly always sacrificed (Conley 1979). The facial nerve is vulnerable during operations on or near the parotid gland. The vagus nerve may be resected during radical neck operations; its recurrent laryngeal branch may be injured during thyroid surgery. The latter injury is less serious, because vocal cord paralysis can be ameliorated by an injection of Teflon, while proximal vagus injury disturbs the swallowing mechanism. The accessory nerve is particularly vulnerable because of its superficial location as it crosses diagonally through the posterior triangle of the neck; it is all too frequently divided during biopsy of an adjacent lymph node. Accessory nerve paralysis causes uncomfortable sagging of the shoulder and inability to raise the arm laterally above the horizontal. The nerve can be repaired if the injury is recognized promptly. Hypoglossal nerve resection is usually a deliberate result of radical cancer surgery.

The motor nerve complications of *radical mastectomy* have never been adequately analyzed. The thoracodorsal nerve (latissimus dorsi muscle), long thoracic nerve (serratus anterior muscle) and axillary nerve (deltoid muscle) are the ones most often damaged, in descending order of frequency. Latissimus weakness occurred in 5 percent of patients in one series and in 23 percent in another series (Partanen and Nikkanen 1978). While uncomplicated radical mastectomy causes little functional impairment, the addition of a motor neuropathy can seriously impair shoulder girdle movements.

Median sternotomy seems to be attended by brachial plexus neuropathy more often than other operations. In a recent prospective study of patients undergoing coronary bypass surgery, 5 percent of the patients developed brachial plexus neuropathy (Lederman et al. 1982), and in another study the incidence was about 2.6 percent (Morin et al. 1982). The plexus involvement was usually unilateral and was almost always confined to the lower trunk or medial cord. Nearly all of the patients recovered completely within 3 months. Presumably, wide retraction of the divided halves of the anterior chest wall compresses the plexus in the thoracic outlet. Fracture of the first rib may be another important factor; in some cases the fractured rib actually penetrates the brachial plexus (Vander Salm et al. 1980, 1982). The incidence of brachial plexus injury can be reduced by placing the retractor at the lower end of the sternum and opening it as little as possible.

During *pelvic surgery* through an abdominal incision, the femoral nerve is subject to injury by pressure exerted by retractor blades. In 1966, Rosenblum and associates found 36 examples of this complication in the literature and contributed 10 additional cases. The injury was bilateral in 22 percent of the cases. A prospective study at a university hospital in Denmark revealed an 11.6 percent incidence of femoral neuropathy following abdominal hysterectomy. Muscle weakness was present in half of the cases. The symptoms resolved within 2 months in nearly all of the cases, and the remaining patients had non-disabling residual sensory loss without motor deficit (Kvist-Poulsen and Borel 1982). Self-retaining retractors are more hazardous, and thin women are said to be more vulnerable. The mechanism appears to involve indirect compression of the nerve through compression of the adjacent psoas muscle by the tip of the retractor blade. This would explain why neuropathy of the genitofemoral nerve is sometimes associated, for this sensory nerve lies superficial to the psoas muscle throughout its length. Painful sensory neuropathies of the ilioinguinal and iliohypogastric nerves are not uncommon after lower abdominal surgery (Stulz and

Pfeiffer 1982). Major cancer surgery in the pelvis sometimes injures the sciatic or obturator nerve.

Hip joint surgery may injure the sciatic nerve and less often the obturator nerve, femoral nerve, or lumbar plexus. Insertion of a hip joint prosthesis is especially hazardous, producing ipsilateral EMG abnormalities in 70 percent of cases, though clinically important nerve damage occurs in only 0.7 percent (Weber et al. 1976). Traction is the principal mechanism of nerve damage; however, the sciatic nerve has also been damaged directly by the polymerization of methyl methacrylate, and delayed sciatic injury has occurred from a projecting spur of methyl methacrylate (Edwards et al. 1981). Peroneal nerve palsy occurred in 0.9 percent of 2,626 patients who underwent *total knee arthroplasty;* only 20 percent of the patients recovered full motor function during a follow-up period of 6 months to 7 years, and none of the sensory deficits resolved completely (Rose et al. 1982).

Placement of an arteriovenous shunt in the upper extremity can cause a variety of neuropathic symptoms. These are discussed in Chapter 7.

Neuromuscular Consequences of Induced Hypothermia

Peripheral Neuropathy

When surgical hypothermia was introduced in the 1950s, the anesthetized patient was immersed in a bath of ice water, so skin and muscle had to be cooled to 0 to 5°C to bring the core temperature down to 26 to 30°C. Delayed peripheral neuropathy was a frequent complication of that procedure (Stephens and Appleby 1955). At the present time, the principal use of profound hypothermia is during cardiac surgery, where it is achieved by cooling the blood during extracorporeal circulation. As a result, none of the body tissues are cooled below 20°C, and peripheral neuropathy does not occur. Schaumburg and associates (1967) showed that cat sciatic nerves were not damaged by cooling unless the temperature went below 20°C.

The clinical picture of peripheral neuropathy following external cooling in ice water was described by Stephens and Appleby (1955). More than 30 minutes of immersion was required to produce symptoms; mild neuropathy occurred in 46 percent of patients following immersion for 30 to 60 minutes, and more severe neuropathy occurred in 83 percent of patients who had been cooled for more than 60 minutes. There was no disturbance of skin color, sweating, or peripheral pulses. In mild cases, distal limb paresthesias, accompanied by slight distal blunting of touch and pain sensation, began 2 to 5 days after surgery and resolved completely within 2 weeks. In more severe cases, distal paresthesia began on the first postoperative day and became progressively worse over a period of several days, as distal sensory and motor deficits developed. Severe neuropathies resolved slowly, often leaving permanent muscle weakness and wasting. Neuropathy did not appear in a limb that had not been immersed, a fact that confirmed the importance of external cooling in the genesis of the nerve damage. The clinical picture is similar to that observed in soldiers whose lower limbs were injured by prolonged exposure to ice-cold water (trench foot or immersion foot). In those cases, however, hyperemia and soft tissue edema occurred soon after rewarming, and there was severe burning pain, features not seen following surgical hypothermia.

PATHOPHYSIOLOGY. Recent experimental studies in rats (Nukada et al. 1981) showed that cooling the sciatic nerve to 3°C for 2 hours resulted in a delayed loss of motor and sensory function, beginning 24 hours after rewarming and progressing for 3 to 7 days. Clinical recovery began in 2 weeks, and by 4 weeks only slight weakness remained. Histologic examination showed axonal swelling and endoneurial edema 24 hours after cooling, with increased permeability of the endoneurial blood vessels. The endoneurial edema progressed during the next week, accompanied by degeneration of myelinated nerve fibers. After 2 weeks, there was extensive regeneration of nerve fibers, accounting for the clinical recovery. It is unclear whether the nerve damage was caused by endoneurial edema or was related to unidentified metabolic disturbances.

Serum CPK Elevation

Accidental hypothermia may be associated with a moderate increase of serum CPK activity (Maclean et al. 1974). Similar serum enzyme elevations, without myoglobinuria, were produced in dogs cooled externally for 6 hours with ice bags; the serum CPK activity rose during rewarming, reaching a peak 9 to 16 hours later (Carlson et al. 1978). The pathologic basis of these changes was not investigated, but the fact that the CPK elevation occurred during rewarming is reminiscent of the CPK elevations occurring when the circulation of a limb is restored after circulatory arrest (see Chapter 8). Serum enzyme levels have not been measured following surgical hypothermia.

Postoperative Inflammatory Neuropathies

Acute idiopathic polyneuritis (Guillain-Barré syndrome) and acute brachial neuritis sometimes occur in the postoperative period. This subject was discussed in Chapter 5.

Neuropathy from Chronic Exposure to Nitrous Oxide

A sensorimotor polyneuropathy or myeloneuropathy has resulted from chronic abuse of nitrous oxide, and this complication has also occurred in a few dentists who were heavily exposed to nitrous oxide in their professional activities. This subject is discussed in Chapter 9. The results of a recent inquiry by questionnaire (Brodsky et al. 1981) suggest that sensorimotor complaints are much higher (1.5 percent) in dentists and dental assistants exposed to nitrous oxide than in the unexposed, but some of the positive responders could have been abusing the agent. There does not seem to be any neurologic risk to patients, although hemopoiesis may suffer from even 12 hours of continuous exposure to nitrous oxide (O'Sullivan et al. 1981), and shorter periods of exposure cause megaloblastic bone marrow changes in critically ill patients (Amos et al. 1982). The nervous system appears to be much more resistant to nitrous oxide toxicity than the bone marrow; a patient with porphyric polyneuropathy developed megaloblastosis of the bone marrow after repeated administration of nitrous oxide for 15 to 20 minutes, 2 to 3 times daily, but the neuropathy continued to improve slowly (Nunn et al. 1982). Nevertheless, the practice of administering nitrous oxide repeatedly to facilitate physiotherapy, or to assist in the care of burned patients, should be considered potentially hazardous to the nervous system.

REFERENCES

Aberfeld, DC, Bienenstock, H, Shapiro, MS, et al: *Diffuse myopathy related to meperidine addiction in a mother and daughter.* Arch Neurol 19:384–388, 1968.

ABOURIZK, N, KHALIL, BA, BAHUTH, N, ET AL: *Clofibrate-induced muscular syndrome. Report of a case with clinical, electromyographic and pathologic observations.* J Neurol Sci 42:1–9, 1979.

AIRAKSINEN, MM AND TAMMISTO, T: *Myoglobinuria after intermittent administration of succinylcholine during halothane anesthesia.* Clin Pharmcol Ther 7:583–587, 1966.

ALBERS, JW, ALLEN, AA, II, BASTRON, JA, ET AL: *Limb myokymia.* Muscle Nerve 4:494–504, 1981.

ALLEN, JC: *The effects of cancer therapy on the nervous system.* J Pediat 93:903–909, 1978.

AMOS, RJ, HINDS, CJ, AMESS, JAL, ET AL: *Incidence and pathogenesis of acute megaloblastic bone-marrow change in patients receiving intensive care.* Lancet ii:835–839, 1982.

ANSBACHER, LE, BOSCH, EP, CANCILLA, PA: *Disulfiram neuropathy: A neurofilamentous distal axonopathy.* Neurology 32:424–428, 1982.

ARGOV, Z AND MASTAGLIA, FL: *Disorders of neuromuscular transmission caused by drugs.* N Engl J Med 301:409–413, 1979A.

ARGOV, Z AND MASTAGLIA, FL: *Drug-induced peripheral neuropathies.* Br Med J 1:663–666, 1979B.

ARGOV, Z AND YAARI, Y: *The action of chlorpromazine at an isolated cholinergic synapse.* Brain Res 164:227–236, 1979.

ARGOV, Z, NICHOLSON, L, FAWCETT, PRW, ET AL: *Neuromuscular transmission and acetylcholine receptor antibodies in rheumatoid arthritis patients on D-penicillamine.* Lancet i:203, 1980.

ARTS, WF AND OOSTERHUIS, HJ: *Effect of prednisolone on neuromuscular blocking in mice in vitro.* Neurology 25:1088–1090, 1975.

ASHENHURST EM, QUARTEY, GRC, AND STARREVELD, A: *Lumbosacral radiculopathy induced by radiation.* Can J Neurol Sci 4:259–263, 1977.

BASSO-RICCI, S, DELLA COSTA, C, VIGANOTTI, G, ET AL: *Report on 42 cases of postirradiation lesions of the brachial plexus and their treatment.* Tumori 66:117–122, 1980.

BATSAKIS, JG, PRESTON, JA, BRIERE, RO, ET AL: *Iatrogenic aberrations of serum enzyme activity.* Clin Biochem 2:125–133, 1968.

BAZZATO, G, COLI, U, LANDINI, S, ET AL: *Myasthenia-like syndrome after D,L- but not L-carnitine.* Lancet i:1209, 1981.

BENNIKE, K-A AND JARNUM, S: *Myoglobinuria with acute renal failure possibly induced by suxamethonium. A case report.* Br J Anaesth 36:730–736, 1964.

BENOIT, PW AND BELT, WD: *Some effects of local anesthetic agents on skeletal muscle.* Exp Neurol 34:264–278, 1972.

BENOIT, PW, YAGIDA, JA, AND FORT, NF: *Pharmacologic correlation between local anesthetic-induced myotoxicity and disturbance of intracellular calcium distribution.* Toxicol Appl Pharmacol 52:187–198, 1980.

BERGER, PS AND BATAINI, JP: *Radiation-induced cranial nerve palsy.* Cancer 40:152–155, 1977.

BERGESON, PS, SINGER, SA, AND KAPLAN, AM: *Intramuscular injections in children.* Pediatrics 70:944–948, 1982.

BERNAT, JL, SADOWSKY, CH, VINCENT, FM, ET AL: *Sclerosing spinal pachymeningitis. A complication of intrathecal administration of Depo-Medrol for multiple sclerosis.* J Neurol Neurosurg Psychiatry 39:1124–1128, 1976.

BERRY, PR, AND WALLIS, WE: *Venepuncture nerve injuries.* Lancet i:1236–1237, 1977.

BIRCH, AA, JR, MITCHELL, GD, PLAYFORD, GA, ET AL: *Changes in serum potassium response to succinylcholine following trauma.* JAMA 210:490–493, 1969.

BLOMBERG, LH: *Dystrophia myotonica probably caused by chloroquine.* Acta Neurol Scand 41(Suppl 13, Part II):647–651, 1965.

BOLTON,CF AND MACFARLANE, RM: *Human pneumatic tourniquet paralysis.* Neurology 28:787–793, 1978.

BOOKER, HE, CHUN, RWM, SANGUINO M: *Myasthenia gravis syndrome associated with trimethadione.* JAMA 212:2262–2263, 1970.

BORDEN, H, CLARK, MT, AND KATZ, H: *The use of pancuronium bromide in patients receiving lithium carbonate.* Can Anaesth Soc J 21:79–82, 1974.

BRADLEY, WG, LASSMAN, LP, PEARCE, GW, ET AL: *The neuromyopathy of vincristine in man. Clinical, electrophysiological and pathological studies.* J Neurol Sci 10:107–131, 1970.

BRADLEY, WG, FEWINGS, JD, HARRIS, JB, ET AL: *Emetine myopathy in the rat.* Br J Pharmacol 57:29–41, 1976.

BRADLEY, WG, FEWINGS, JD, CUMMING, WJK, ET AL: *Delayed myeloradiculopathy produced by spinal x-irradiation in the rat.* J Neurol Sci 31:63–82, 1977.

BRIDGMAN, JF, ROSEN, SM, AND THORP, JM: *Complications during clofibrate treatment of nephrotic-syndrome hyperlipoproteinaemia.* Lancet ii:506–509, 1972.

Britt, BA and Gordon, RA: *Peripheral nerve injuries asociated with anaesthesia.* Can Anaesth Soc J 11:514–536, 1964.

Britt, CW, Jr, Light, RR, Peters, BH, et al: *Rhabdomyolysis during treatment with epsilon-aminocaproic acid.* Arch Neurol 37:187–188, 1980.

Brodkin, HM: *Myoglobinuria following epsilon-aminocaproic acid (EACA) therapy.* J Neurosurg 53:690–692, 1980.

Brodsky, JB and Ehrenwerth, J: *Postoperative muscle pains and suxamethonium.* Br J Anaesth 52:215–217, 1980.

Brodsky, JB, Cohen, EN, Brown, BW, Jr, et al: *Exposure to nitrous oxide and neurologic disease among dental professionals.* Anesth Analg 60:297–301, 1981.

Brumlik, J and Jacobs, RS: *Myasthenia gravis assocated with diphenylhydantoin therapy for epilepsy.* Can J Neurol Sci 1:127–129, 1974.

Cairoli, VJ, Ivankovich, AD, Vucicevic, D, et al: *Succinylcholine-induced hyperkalemia in the rat following radiation injury to muscle.* Anesth Analg 61:83–86, 1982.

Campbell, EDR and Montuschi, E: *Muscle weakness caused by bretylium tosylate.* Lancet ii:789, 1960.

Carlson CJ, Emilson, B, and Rapaport, E: *Creating phosphokinase MB isoenzyme in hypothermia: Case reports and experimental studies.* Am Heart J 95:352–368, 1978.

Casey, EB, Jellife, AM, Le Quesne, PM, et al: *Vincristine neuropathy. Clinical and electrophysiological observations.* Brain 96:69–86, 1973.

Cassady, JR, Tonnesen, GL, Wolfe, LC, et al: *Augmentation of vincristine neurotoxicity by irradiation of peripheral nerves.* Cancer Treat Rep 64:963–965, 1980.

Chamberlain, MJ, Reynolds AL, and Yeoman, WB: *Toxic effects of podophyllum application in pregnancy.* Br Med J 3:391–392, 1972.

Chang, CC, Chen, TF, and Cheng, HC: *On the mechanism of neuromuscular blocking action of bretylium and guanethidine.* J Pharmacol Exp Ther 158:89–98, 1967.

Charak, DS and Dhar, CL: *Suxamethonium-induced changes in serum creatine phosphokinase.* Br J Anaesth 53:955–957, 1981.

Cheah, KS and Cheah, AM: *Mitochondrial calcium, erythrocyte fragility and porcine malignant hyperthermia.* FEBS Lett 107:265–268, 1979.

Cheng, VST and Schulz, MD: *Unilateral hypoglossal nerve atrophy as a late complication of radiation therapy of head and neck carcinoma. A report of four cases and a review of the literature on peripheral and cranial nerve damages after radiation therapy.* Cancer 35:1537–1544, 1975.

Cherington, M, Lewin, E, and McCrimmon, A: *Serum creatine phosphokinase changes following needle electromyographic studies.* Neurology 18:271–272, 1968.

Chrissian, SA, Stolov, WC, and Hongladarom, T: *Needle electromyography: Its effect on serum creatine phosphokinase activity.* Arch Phys Med Rehabil 57:114–119, 1976.

Conley, JJ: *Complications of Head and Neck Surgery.* WB Saunders, Philadelphia, 1979, pp 137–141.

Cooperman, LH: *Succinylcholine-induced hyperkalemia in neuromuscular disease.* JAMA 213:1867–1871, 1970.

Czlonskowska, A: *Myasthenia syndrome during penicillamine treatment.* Br Med J 2:726–727, 1975.

Dale, RC and Schroeder, ET: *Respiratory paralysis during treatment of hypertension with trimethaphan camsylate.* Arch Intern Med 136:816–818, 1976.

D'Arcy, PF and Griffin, JP: *Iatrogenic Diseases,* ed 2. Oxford University Press, Oxford, 1979.

D'Arcy, PF and Griffin, JP: *Iatrogenic Diseases,* ed 2. Update 1981. Oxford University Press, Oxford, 1981.

De Grandis, D, Mezzina, C, Fiaschi, A, et al: *Myasthenia due to carnitine treatment.* J Neurol Sci 46:365–371, 1980.

De Lateur, BJ and Halliday, WR: *Pentazocine fibrous myopathy: Report of two cases and literature review.* Arch Phys Med Rehabil 59:394–397, 1978.

Denborough, MA: *The pathopharmacology of malignant hyperpyrexia.* Pharmacol Ther 9:357–365, 1980.

Drachman, DA and Skom JH: *Procainamide—a hazard in myasthenia gravis.* Arch Neurol 13:316–320, 1965.

Dretchen, KL, Sokoll, MD, Gergis, SD, et al: *Relative effects of streptomycin on motor nerve terminal and endplate.* Eur J Pharmacol 22:10–16, 1973.

Duane, DD and Engel, AG: *Emetine myopathy.* Neurology 20:733–739, 1970.

Dudognon, P, Hauw, JJ, de Baecque, C, et al: *Neuropathie au chlorohydrate d'amiodarone. Etude clinique et histopathologique d'une nouvelle lipidose médicamenteuse.* Rev Neurol (Paris) 135:527–540, 1979.

EDITORIAL: *Fatigue as an unwanted effect of drugs.* Lancet i:1285–1286, 1980.

EDWARDS, MS, BARBARO, NM, ASHER, SW, et al: *Delayed sciatic palsy after total hip replacement: Case report.* Neurosurgery 9:61–63, 1981.

EISER, AR, NEFF, MS, AND SLIFKIN, RF: *Acute myoglobinuric renal failure. A consequence of the neuroleptic malignant syndrome.* Arch Intern Med 142:601–603, 1982.

ELMQVIST, D AND JOSEFSSON, JO: *The nature of the neuromuscular block produced by neomycin.* Acta Physiol Scand 54:105–110, 1962.

ENDTZ, LJ: *Complications nerveuses du traitment aurique. Aperçu des symptomes neurologiques et psychiatriques. Résultats du traitement par le B.A.L.* Rev Neurol (Paris) 99:395–410, 1958.

ENG, GD, EPSTEIN, BS, ENGEL, WK, ET AL: *Malignant hyperthermia and central core disease in a child with congenital dislocating hips.* Arch Neurol 35:189–197, 1978.

ENGEL, WK: *Focal myopathic changes produced by electromyographic and hypodermic needles. "Needle myopathy."* Arch Neurol 16:509–511, 1967.

EVANS, RT, MACDONALD, R, AND ROBINSON, A: *Suxamethonium apnoea associated with plasmapheresis.* Anaesthesia 35:198–201, 1980.

EVERS, W, RACZ, GB, DOBKIN, AB: *A study of plasma potassium and electrocardiographic changes after a single dose of succinylcholine.* Can Anesth Soc J 16:273–281, 1969.

FAMEWO, CE: *Effect of fazadinium (Fazadon) on muscle fasciculations induced by succinylcholine.* Can Anaesth Soc J 28:459–462, 1981A.

FAMEWO, CE: *The influence of fazadinium on the potassium efflux produced by succinylcholine.* Can Anesth Soc J 28:463–466, 1981B.

FARDEAU, M, TOMÉ, FMS, AND SIMON, P: *Muscle and nerve changes induced by perhexilene maleate in man and mice.* Muscle Nerve 2:24–36, 1979.

FAWCETT, PRW, MCLACHLAN, SM, NICHOLSON, SM, ET AL: *D-penicillamine-associated myasthenia gravis: Immunological and electrophysiological studies.* Muscle Nerve 5:328–334, 1982.

FERGUSON, FC, JR: *Colchicine. I. General pharmacology.* J Pharmacol Exp Ther 106:261–270, 1952.

FERNANDES, L, SWINSON, DR, HAMILTON, EBD: *Dermatomyositis complicating penicillamine treatment.* Ann Rheumat Dis 36:94–95, 1977.

FEWINGS, JD, BURNS, RJ, AND KAKULAS, BA: *A case of acute emetine myopathy.* In KAKULAS, BA (ED): *Clinical Studies in Myology.* Excerpta Medica, Amsterdam, 1971, pp 594–598.

FILLEY, CM, GRAFF-RADFORD, NR, LACY, JR, ET AL: *Neurologic manifestations of podophyllin toxicity.* Neurology 32:308–311, 1982.

FISCHER, C, BADY, B, TRILLET, M, ET AL: *Deux cas de neuropathie périphérique à l'amiodarone.* Nouv Presse Med 6:3645–3646, 1977.

FORFAR, JC, BROWN, GJ, CULL, RE: *Proximal myopathy during beta-blockade.* Br Med J 2:1331–1332, 1979.

GANEL, A, ENGEL, J, SELA, M, ET AL: *Nerve entrapments associated with postmastectomy lymphedema.* Cancer 44:2254–2259, 1979.

GARLEPP, M, KAY, P, DAWKINS, RL, ET AL: *Cross-reactivity of anti-acetylcholine receptor autoantibodies.* Muscle Nerve 4:282–288, 1981.

GASTAUT, JL, GASTAUT, JA, POUGET, J, ET AL: *Les blessures des nerfs périphériques par ponction veineuse.* Nouv Presse Med 11:513–515, 1982.

GAYLORD, TG AND PEARSON, JW: *Neuropathy following paracervical block in the obstetric patient.* Obstet Gynecol 60:521–524, 1982.

GENTILI, F, HUDSON, AR, AND HUNTER, D: *Clinical and experimental aspects of injection injuries of peripheral nerves.* Can J Neurol Sci 7:143–151, 1980.

GLOOR, HO, VORBURGER, C, AND SCHÄDELIN, J: *Intramuskuläre injecktionen und serumkreatinphosphokinase-aktivität.* Schweiz Med Wschr 107:948–952, 1977.

GODEAU, P, HERREMAN, G, HIMMICH, H, ET AL: *Neuromyopathie due à la chloroquine au cours du lupus érythémateux. Deux nouvelles observations, soulignant la nécessité de l'étude ultrastructurelle de la biopsie musculaire.* Ann Med Interne 127:544–551, 1976.

GOEKOOP, JG AND CARBAAT, PAT: *Treatment of neuroleptic malignant syndrome with dantrolene.* Lancet ii:49–50, 1982.

GOLDSTEIN, BD, LOWNDES, HE, AND CHO, E: *Neurotoxicology of vincristine in the cat. Electrophysiological studies.* Arch Toxicol 48:253–264, 1981.

GRANACHER, RP, JR: *Neuromuscular problems associated with lithium.* Am J Psychiatry 134:702, 1977.

GRONERT, GA: *Malignant hyperthermia.* Anesthesiology 53:395–423, 1980.

GRONERT, GA: *Puzzles in malignant hyperthermia.* Anesthesiology 54:1–2, 1981.

GRONERT, GA, LAMBERT, EH, AND THEYE, RA: *The response of denervated skeletal muscle to succinylcholine.* Anesthesiology 39:13–22, 1973.

GUTMANN, L, MARTIN, JD, AND WELTON, W: *Dapsone motor neuropathy—an axonal disease.* Neurology 26:514–516, 1976.

HERISHANU, Y, ROSENBERG, P: *β-Blockers and myasthenia gravis.* Ann Intern Med 83:834–835, 1975.

HILL, G, WONG, KC, HODGES, MR: *Potentiation of succinylcholine neuromuscular blockade by lithium carbonate.* Anesthesiology 44:439–442, 1976.

HUDSON, AR, KLINE, D, GENTILI, F: *Peripheral nerve injection injury.* In OMER, GE, JR AND SPINNER, M (EDS): *Management of Peripheral Nerve Problems.* WB Saunders, Philadelphia, 1980, pp 639–653.

HUGHES, JT, ESIRI, M, OXBURY, JM, ET AL: *Chloroquine myopathy.* Quart J Med 40:85–93, 1971.

HUGHES, RO AND ZACHARIAS, FJ: *Myasthenic syndrome during treatment with practolol.* Br Med J 1:460–461, 1976.

JENIK, F, TEKLE-HAIMANOT, R, AND HAMORY, BH: *Non-traumatic adhesive arachnoiditis as a cause of spinal cord syndromes. Investigation on 507 patients.* Paraplegia 19:140–154, 1981.

JENKINS, P AND EMERSON, PA: *Myopathy induced by rifampicin.* Br Med J 283:105–106, 1981.

JENSEN, K, BENNIKE, KA, HANEL, HK, ET AL: *Myoglobinuria following anesthesia including suxamethonium.* Br J Anaesth 40:329–334, 1968.

JUI-TEN, T: *Clinical and experimental studies on the mechanism of neuromuscular blockade by chloroquine diorotate.* Jpn J Anesth 20:491–503, 1971.

KANE, RE: *Neurologic deficits following epidural and spinal anesthesia.* Anesth Analg 60:150–161, 1981.

KATRAK, SM, POLLOCK, M, O'BRIEN, CP, ET AL: *Clinical and morphological features of gold neuropathy.* Brain 103:671–693, 1980.

KEIM, HA AND WEINSTEIN, JD: *Acute renal failure—A complication of spine fusion in the tuck position.* J Bone Joint Surg 52A:1248–1250, 1970.

KENNARD, C, SWASH, M, AND HENSON, RA: *Myopathy due to epsilon-aminocaproic acid.* Muscle Nerve 3:202–206, 1980.

KIM, YI, GOLDNER, MM, AND SANDERS, DB: *Short-term effects of prednisolone on neuromuscular transmission in normal rats and those with experimental autoimmune myasthenia gravis.* J Neurol Sci 41:223–234, 1979.

KLEIN, MS, SHELL, WE, AND SOBEL, BE: *Serum creatine phosphokinase (CPK) isoenzymes after intramuscular injections, surgery, and myocardial infarction. Experimental and clinical studies.* Cardiovasc Res 7:412–418, 1973.

KOIDE, M AND WAUD, BE: *Serum potassium concentrations after succinylcholine in patients with renal failure.* Anesthesiology 36:142–145, 1972.

KOLB, ME, HORNE, ML, AND MARTZ, R: *Dantrolene in human malignant hyperthermia.* Anesthesiology 56:254–262, 1982.

KONTOS, HA: *Myopathy associated with chronic colchicine toxicity.* N Eng J Med 266:38–39, 1962.

KORI, SH, FOLEY, KM, AND POSNER, JB: *Brachial plexus lesions in patients with cancer: 100 cases.* Neurology 31:45–50, 1981.

KORNFELD, P, HOROWITZ, SH, GENKINS, G, ET AL: *Myasthenia gravis unmasked by antiarrhythmic agents.* Mt Sinai J Med NY 43:10–14, 1976.

KVIST-POULSEN, H AND BOREL, J: *Iatrogenic femoral neuropathy subsequent to abdominal hysterectomy: Incidence and prevention.* Obstet Gynecol 60:516–520, 1982.

LANE, RJM AND MASTAGLIA, FL: *Drug-induced myopathies in man.* Lancet ii:562–566, 1978.

LANGER, T AND LEVY, RI: *Acute muscular syndrome associated with administration of clofibrate.* N Engl J Med 279:856–858, 1968.

LARRE, P, COQUET, M, MAUPETIT, J: *Neuropathie à l'amiodarone.* Nouv Presse Med 10:2750, 1981.

LAURENT, LE: *Femoral nerve compression syndrome with paresis of the quadriceps muscle caused by radiotherapy of malignant tumors. A report of four cases.* Acta Orthop Scand 46:804–808, 1975.

LEDERMAN, RJ, BREUER, AC, HANSON, MR, ET AL: *Peripheral nervous system complications of coronary artery bypass graft surgery.* Ann Neurol 12:297–301, 1982.

LEE, C, CHEN, D, BARNES, A, ET AL: *Neuromuscular block by neomycin in the cat.* Can Anaesth Soc J 23:527–533, 1976.

Leeuwin, RS and Wolters, ECMJ: *Effect of corticosteroids on sciatic nerve-tibialis anterior muscle of rats treated with hemicholinium-3. An experimental approach to a possible mechanism of action of corticosteroids in myasthenia gravis.* Neurology 27:171–177, 1977.

Lemaire, JF, Autret, A, Biziere, K, et al: *Amiodaron neuropathy: Further arguments for human drug-induced neurolipidosis.* Eur Neurol 21:65–68, 1982.

Le Quesne, PM: *Neuropathy due to drugs.* In Dyck, PJ, Thomas, PK, and Lambert, EH (eds): *Peripheral Neuropathy.* WB Saunders, Philadelphia, 1975, pp 1263–1280.

Levin, B and Engel, WK: *Iatrogenic muscle fibrosis. Arm levitation as an initial sign.* JAMA 234:621–624, 1975.

Lillehei, G and Røed, A: *Antitetanic effect of propranolol on mammalian motor-nerve and skeletal muscle and combined action of propranolol and neostigmine on the neuromuscular transmission.* Arch Int Pharmacol Ther 194:129–140, 1971.

Lindesmith, LA, Baines, RD, Jr, Bigelow, DB, et al: *Reversible respiratory paralysis associated with polymyxin therapy.* Ann Intern Med 68:318–327, 1968.

Lüllmann, H, Lüllmann-Rauch, R, and Wasermann, O: *Drug-induced phospholipidosis.* CRC Crit Rev Toxicol 41:185–218, 1975.

MacDonald, RD and Engel, AG: *Experimental chloroquine myopathy.* J Neuropath Exp Neurol 29:479–499, 1970.

MacKay, AR, U, HS, and Weinstein, PR: *Myopathy associated with epsilon-aminocaproic acid (EACA) therapy.* J Neurosurg 49:597–601, 1978.

Maclean, D, Murison, J, Griffiths, PD: *Serum enzyme activities in accidental hypothermia and hypothermic myxoedema.* Clin Chim Acta 52:197–200, 1974.

Maeyens, E, Jr and Pitner, SE: *Effects of electromyography on CPK and aldolase levels.* Arch Neurol 19:538–539, 1968.

Maier, JG, Perry, RH, Saylor, W, et al: *Radiation myelitis of the dorsolumbar spinal cord.* Radiology 93:153–160, 1969.

Mann, JD, Johns, TR, and Campa, JF: *Long-term administration of corticosteroids in myasthenia gravis.* Neurology 26:729–740, 1976.

Marks, P and Sloggem, J: Peripheral neuropathy caused by methaqualone. Am J Med Sci 272:323–326, 1976.

Martin, VM, Vincent, A, and Clarke, C: *Anti-acetylcholine receptor antibodies in penicillamine treated patients without myasthenia gravis.* Lancet ii:705, 1980.

Mastaglia, FL, Papadimitriou, JM, Dawkins, RL, et al: *Vacuolar myopathy associated with chloroquine, lupus erythematosus and thymoma.* J Neurol Sci 34:315–328, 1977.

Masters, CL, Dawkins, RL, Zilko, PJ, et al : *Penicillamine-associated myasthenia gravis, antiacetylcholine receptor and antistriational antibodies.* Am J Med 63:689–694, 1977.

Matsukura, S, Matsumoto, J, Chihara, K, et al: *Clofibrate-induced myopathy in patients with diabetes insipidus.* Endocrinol Japon 27:401–403, 1980.

Matsuoka, Y, Takayanagi, T, and Sobue, I: *Experimental ethambutol neuropathy in rats. Morphometric and teased-fibre studies.* J Neurol Sci 51:89–99, 1981.

McKinney, AS: *Neurologic findings in retroperitoneal mass lesions.* South Med J 66:862–864, 1973.

McQuillen, MP, Gross, M, and Johns, RJ: *Chlorpromazine-induced weakness in myasthenia gravis.* Arch Neurol 8:286–290, 1963.

McQuillen, MP, Cantor, HE, and O'Rourke, JR: *Myasthenic syndrome associated with antibiotics.* Arch Neurol 18:402–415, 1968.

Meier, C, Kauer, B, Müller, U, et al: *Neuromyopathy during chronic amiodarone treatment. A case report.* J Neurol 220:231–239, 1979.

Meltzer, HY, Mrozak, S, and Boyer, M: *Effect of intramuscular injections on serum creatine phosphokinase activity.* Am J Med Sci 259:42–48, 1970.

Miller, RD, Way, WL, and Katzung, BG: *Neuromuscular effects of quinidine.* Proc Soc Exp Biol Med 129:215–218, 1968.

Miller, RD, Way, WL, Hamilton, WK, et al: *Succinylcholine-induced hyperkalemia in patients with renal failure?* Anesthesiology 36:138–141, 1972.

Miller, RG and Camp, PE: *Postoperative ulnar neuropathy.* JAMA 242:1636–1639, 1979.

Miller, RG, Maxfield, M, Mirika, A, et al: *Acute inhibition of neuromuscular function by corticosteroids in myasthenia gravis.* Neurology 31:97, 1981.

Mitsumoto, H, Wilbourn, AJ, and Subramony, SH: *Generalized myokymia and gold therapy.* Arch Neurol 39:449–450, 1982.

Mokri, B, Ohnishi, A, Dyck, PJ: *Disulfiram neuropathy. Neurology* 31:730–735, 1981.

MONTAG, TW AND MEAD, PB: *Postpartum femoral neuropathy.* J Reprod Med 26:563–566, 1981.

MORGAN, GJ, JR, MCGUIRE, JL, AND OCHOA, J: *Penicillamine-induced myositis in rheumatoid arthritis.* Muscle Nerve 4:137–140, 1981.

MORIN, JE, LONG, R, ELLEKER, MG, ET AL: *Upper extremity neuropathies following median sternotomy.* Ann Thorac Surg 34:181–184, 1982.

MUELLER, JM AND FLAHERTY, MJ: *Vincristine-induced quadriparesis.* South Med J 71:1310–1311, 1978.

MURPHY, JP AND DEVERS, JC: *Prevention of postsurgical ulnar neuropathy.* JAMA 227:1123–1124, 1974.

NEIL, JF, HIMMELBOCH, JM AND LICATA, SM: *Emergence of myasthenia gravis during treatment with lithium carbonate.* Arch Gen Psychiatry 33:1090–1092, 1976.

NELSON, TE AND BEE, DE: *Temperature perturbation studies of sarcoplasmic reticulum from malignant hyperthermia pig muscle.* J Clin Invest 64:895–901, 1979.

NICK, J, DUDOGNON, P, ESCOUROLLE, R, ET AL: *Manifestations neurologiques en rapport avec le traitement par le maleate de perhexilene.* Rev Neurol 134:103–114, 1978.

NORMAN, MG, TEMPLE, AR, MURPHY, JV: *Infantile quadriceps-femoris contracture resulting from intramuscular injections.* N Engl J Med 282:964–966, 1970.

NUKADA, H AND POLLOCK, M: *Disulfiram neuropathy. A morphometric study of sural nerve.* J Neurol Sci 51:51–67, 1981.

NUKADA, H, POLLOCK, M, AND ALLPRESS, S: *Experimental cold injury to peripheral nerve.* Brain 104:779–811, 1981.

NUNN, JF, GORCHEIN, A, SHARER, NM, ET AL: *Megaloblastic haemopoiesis after multiple short-term exposure to nitrous oxide.* Lancet i:1379–1381, 1982.

OCHOA, J: *Isoniazid neuropathy in man: Quantitative electron microscopic study.* Brain 93:831–850, 1970.

OH, SJ: *Experimental pentazocine-induced fibrous myopathy.* Alabama J Med Sci 14:64–67, 1977.

O'KEEFE, DM: *Brachial plexus injury following axillary arteriography. Case report and review of the literature.* J Neurosurg 53:853–857, 1980.

OKUMURA, F, CROCKER, BD, AND DENBOROUGH, MA: *Site of the muscle cell abnormality in swine susceptible to malignant hyperpyrexia.* Br J Anaesth 52:377–383, 1980.

O'SULLIVAN, H, JENNINGS, F, WARD, K, ET AL: *Human bone marrow biochemical function and megaloblastic hematopoiesis after nitrous oxide anesthesia.* Anesthesiology 55:645–649, 1981.

PANSE, F: *Electrical lesions of the nervous system.* In VINKEN, PJ AND BRUYN, GW (EDS): *Handbook of Clinical Neurology, vol. 7.* North-Holland Publishing, Amsterdam, 1970, pp 344–387.

PARDRIDGE, WM, CASANELLO-ERTL, D, AND DUDUGGIAN-VARTAVARIAN, L: *Branched chain amino acid oxidation in cultured rat skeletal muscle cells. Selective inhibition by clofibric acid.* J Clin Invest 66:88–93, 1980.

PARDRIDGE, WM, DUDUGGIAN-VARTAVARIAN, L, AND CASANELLO-ERTL, D, ET AL: *Effects of clofibric acid on amino acid metabolism in cultured rat skeletal muscle.* Am J Physiol 240:E203–E208, 1981.

PARKS, BJ: *Postoperative peripheral neuropathies.* Surgery 74:348–357, 1973.

PARTANEN, VSJ AND NIKKANEN, TAV: *Electromyography in the estimation of nerve lesions after surgical and radiation therapy for breast cancer.* Strahlentherapie 154:489–494, 1978.

PAUL, HS AND ADIBI, SA: *Paradoxical effects of clofibrate on liver and muscle metabolism in rats. Induction of myotonia and alteration of fatty acid and glucose oxidation.* J Clin Invest 64:405–412, 1979.

PEARSON, SB, BANKS, DC, AND PATRICK, JM: *The effect of β-adrenoceptor blockade on factors affecting exercise tolerance in normal man.* Br J Clin Pharmacol 8:143–148, 1979.

PETER, JB AND CAMPION, DS: *Animal models of myotonia.* In ROWLAND, LP (ED): *Pathogenesis of Human Muscular Dystrophies.* Excerpta Medica, Amsterdam-Oxford, 1977, pp 739–746.

PETERSON, HD: *Association of trimethadione therapy and myasthenia gravis.* N Engl J Med 274:506–507, 1966.

PHILLIPS, OC, EBNER, H, NELSON, AT, ET AL: *Neurologic complications following spinal anesthesia with lidocaine: A prospective review of 10,440 cases.* Anesthesiology 30:285–289, 1969.

PIERIDES, AM, ALVAREZ-UDE, F, KERR, DNS, ET AL: *Clofibrate-induced muscle damage in patients with chronic renal failure.* Lancet ii:1279–1282, 1975.

PITTINGER, CB, ERYASA, Y, AND ADAMSON, R: *Antibiotic-induced paralysis.* Anesth Analg 49:487–501, 1970.

POOL, KD, FEIT, H, AND KIRKPATRICK, J: *Penicillamine-induced neuropathy in rheumatoid arthritis.* Ann Intern Med 95:457–458, 1981.

RASKIN, NH AND FISHMAN, RA: *Pyridoxine-deficiency neuropathy due to hydralazine.* N Engl J Med 273:1182–1185, 1965.

RASMUSSEN, F AND SVENDSEN, O: *Tissue damage and concentration at the injection site after intramuscular injection of chemotherapeutics and vehicles in pigs.* Res Vet Sci 20:55–60, 1976.

REGLI, F AND GUGGENHEIM, P: *Myasthenisches Syndrom als seltene Komplikation unter Hydantoinbehandlung.* Nervenarzt 36:315–318, 1965.

REIMHERR, FW, HODGES, MR, HILL, GE, ET AL: *Prolongation of muscle relaxant effects by lithium carbonate.* Am J Psychiatry 134:205–206, 1977.

ROSE, HA, HOOD, RW, OTIS, JC, ET AL: *Peroneal-nerve palsy following total knee arthroplasty. A review of the Hospital for Special Surgery experience.* J Bone Joint Surg 64-A:347–351, 1982.

ROTH, F AND WÜTHRICH, H: *The clinical importance of hyperkalaemia following suxamethonium administration.* Br J Anaesth 41:311–316, 1969.

ROZEN, MS AND WHAN, FM: *Prolonged curarization associated with propranolol.* Med J Aust 1:467–468, 1972.

ROSENBLUM, J, SCHWARZ, GA, AND BENDLER, E: *Femoral neuropathy—A neurological complication of hysterectomy.* JAMA 195:409–414, 1966.

RUBBO, JT, GERGIS, SD, AND SOKOLL, MD: *Comparative neuromuscular effects of lincomycin and clindamycin.* Anesth Analg 56:329–332, 1977.

RUDGE, P: *Tourniquet paralysis with prolonged conduction block. An electro-physiological study.* J Bone Joint Surg 56B:716–720, 1974.

RUSSELL, AS AND LINDSTROM, JM: *Penicillamine-induced myasthenia gravis associated with antibodies to acetylcholine receptor.* Neurology 28:847–849, 1978.

RYAN, JF, KAGEN, LJ, AND HYMAN, AL: *Myoglobinemia after a single dose of succinylcholine.* N Engl J Med 285:824–827, 1971.

SADOWSKY, CH, SACHS, E, JR, AND OCHOA, J: *Postradiation motor neuron syndrome.* Arch Neurol 33:786–787, 1976.

SAID, G: *Perhexilene neuropathy: A clinico-pathological study.* Ann Neurol 3:259–266, 1978.

SANDSTEDT, PER: *Effects of a previous electromyographic examination studied by frequency analysis, muscle biopsy and creatine kinase.* Acta Neurol Scand 64:303–309, 1981.

SANTOS, JI, SWENSEN, P, GLASGOW, LA: *Potentiation of clostridium botulinum toxin by aminoglycoside antibiotics: Clinical and laboratory observations.* Pediatrics 68:50–54, 1981.

SCHANER, PJ, BROWN, RL, KIRKSEY, TD, ET AL: *Succinylcholine-induced hyperkalemia in burned patients.* Anesth Analg 48:764–770, 1969.

SCHAUMBURG, H, BYCK, R, HERMAN, R, ET AL: *Peripheral nerve damage by cold.* Arch Neurol 16:103–109, 1967.

SCHOEN, RT AND TRENTHAM, DE: *Drug-induced lupus: An adjuvant disease?* Am J Med 71:5–8, 1981.

SCHOU, M, BAASTRUP, PC, AND GROF, P: *Pharmacological and clinical problems of lithium prophylaxis.* Br J Psychiatry 116:615–619, 1970.

SCHUMM, F, WIETHÖLTER, H, FATEH-MOGHADAM, A: *Myasthenie-Syndrom unter Chloroquin Therapie.* Dtsch Med Wochenschr 106:1745–1747, 1981.

SEBILLE, A: *Prevalence of latent perhexilene neuropathy.* Br Med J 1:1321–1322, 1978.

SEITZ, D, HOPF, HC, JANZEN, RWC, ET AL: *Penicillamin-induzierte Myasthenie bei chronischer Polyarthritis.* Dtsch Med Wochenschr 101:1153–1158, 1976.

SELANDER, D, DHUNER, K-G, AND LUNDBORG, G: *Peripheral nerve injury due to injection needles used for regional anesthesia.* Acta Anaesth Scand 21:182–188, 1977.

SERRANO, EE, ROYE, DB, HAMMER, RH, ET AL: *Plasma diphenylhydantoin values after oral and intramuscular administration of diphenylhydantoin.* Neurology 23:311–317, 1973.

SEYBOLD, ME AND DRACHMAN, DB: *Gradually increasing doses of prednisone in myasthenia gravis: Reducing the hazards of treatment.* N Engl J Med 290:81–84, 1974.

SHAH, RR, OATES, NS, IDLE, JR, ET AL: *Impaired oxidation of debrisoquine in patients with perhexilene neuropathy.* Br Med J 284:295–299, 1982.

SHAW, MDM, RUSSELL, JA, AND GROSSART, KW: *The changing pattern of spinal arachnoiditis.* J Neurol Neurosurg Psychiat 41:97–107, 1978.

SMALS, AGH, BEEX, LVAM AND KLOPPENBORG, PWC: *Clofibrate-induced muscle damage with myoglobinuria and cardiomyopathy.* New Engl J Med 296:942, 1977.

SMEGO, RA, JR AND DURACK, DT: *The neuroleptic malignant syndrome.* Arch Intern Med 142:1183–1185, 1982.

SMITH, AF, MACFIE, WG, AND OLIVER, MF: *Clofibrate, serum enzymes, and muscle pain.* Br Med J 2:26–88, 1970.

SMITH, RB: *Hyperkalaemia following succinylcholine administration in neurological disorders: A review.* Can Anaesth Soc J 18:199–201, 1971.

SPIELBERG, SP, GORDON, GB, AND LOMBARDI, L: *Nitrofurantoin cytotoxicity. In vitro assessment of risk based on glutathione metabolism.* J Clin Invest 67:37–41, 1981.

STEINER, JC, WINKLEMAN, AC, DE JESUS, PV, JR: *Pentazocine-induced myopathy.* Arch Neurol 28:408–409, 1973.

STEINESS, E, RASMUSSEN, F, SVENDSEN, O, ET AL: *A comparative study of serum creatine phosphokinase (CPK) activity in rabbits, pigs and humans after intramuscular injection of local damaging drugs.* Acta Pharmacol Toxicol (Copenhagen) 42:357–364, 1978.

STEPHENS, J AND APPLEBY, S: *Polyneuropathy following induced hypothermia.* Trans Am Neurol Assoc 80:102–104, 1955.

STOFFER, SS AND CHANDLER, JH: *Quinidine-induced exacerbation of myasthenia gravis in patient with Graves' disease.* Arch Intern Med 140:283–284, 1980.

STÖHR, M: *Special types of spontaneous electrical activity in radiogenic nerve injuries.* Muscle Nerve 5:S78–S83, 1982.

STOLL, BA AND ANDREWS, JT: *Radiation-induced peripheral neuropathy.* Br Med J 1:834–837, 1966.

STULZ, P AND PFEIFFER, KM: *Peripheral nerve injuries resulting from common surgical procedures in the lower portion of the abdomen.* Arch Surg 117:324–327, 1982.

SUNDERLAND, S: *Nerves and Nerve Injuries,* ed 2. Churchill Livingstone, Edinburgh-London-New York, 1978, pp 173–181.

SVENSSON, H, WESTLING, P, AND LARSSON, L-G: *Radiation-induced lesions of the brachial plexus correlated to the dose-time-fraction schedule.* Acta Radiol (Ther) 14:228–238, 1975.

TAKEUCHI, H, TAKAHASHI, M, KONG, J, ET AL: *Ethambutol neuropathy: Clinical and electromyographic studies.* Folia Psychiat Neurol Jap 34:45–55, 1980A.

TAKEUCHI, H, TAKAHASHI, H, TARUI, S, ET AL: *Peripheral nerve conduction function in patients treated with antituberculotic agents, with special reference to ethambutol and isoniazid.* Folia Psychiat Neurol Jap 34:57–64, 1980B.

TAMMISTO, T AND AIRAKSINEN, M: *Increase of creatine kinase activity in serum as sign of muscular injury caused by intermittently administered suxamethonium during halothane anesthesia.* Br J Anaesth 8:510–514, 1966.

TAMMISTO, T, LEIKKONEN, P, AND AIRAKSINEN, M: *The inhibitory effect of d-tubocurarine on the increase of serum-creatine-kinase activity produced by intermittent suxamethonium administration during halothane anaesthesia.* Acta Anaesth Scand 11:333–340, 1967.

TEICHER, A, ROSENTHAL, T, KISSIN, E, ET AL: *Labetalol-induced toxic myopathy.* Br Med J 282:1824–1825, 1981.

TERÄVÄINEN, H, LARSEN, A, AND HILLBOM, M: *Clofibrate-induced myopathy in the rat.* Acta Neuropathol 39:135–138, 1977.

THOMAS, JE AND COLBY, MY, JR: *Radiation-induced or metastatic brachial plexopathy? A diagnostic dilemma.* JAMA 222:1392–1395, 1972.

THOMAS, MH AND CHISHOLM, GD: *Retroperitoneal fibrosis associated with malignant disease.* Br J Cancer 28:453–458, 1973.

TOBEY, RE, JACOBSEN, PM, KAHLE, CT, ET AL: *The serum potassium response to muscle relaxants in neural injury.* Anesthesiology 37:332–337, 1972.

TOOLE, JF AND PARRISH, ML: *Nitrofurantoin polyneuropathy.* Neurology 23:554–559, 1973.

TORRES, CF, GRIGGS, RC, BAUM, J, ET AL: *Penicillamine-induced myasthenia gravis in progressive systemic sclerosis.* Arthritis Rheum 23:505–508, 1980.

TUGWELL, P AND JAMES, SL: *Peripheral neuropathy with ethambutol.* Postgrad Med J 48:667–670, 1972.

TWENTYMAN, OP, DISLEY, A, GRIBBIN, HR, ET AL: *Effect of β-adrenergic blockade on respiratory and metabolic responses to exercise.* J Appl Physiol: Respirat Environ Exercise Physiol 51:788–793, 1981.

VAN DER KOGEL, AJ: *Radiation-induced nerve root degeneration and hypertrophic neuropathy in the lumbosacral spinal cord of rats: The relation with changes in aging rats.* Acta Neuropathol 39:139–145, 1977.

VAN DER KOGEL, AJ AND BARENDSEN, GW: *Late effects of spinal cord irradiation with 300 kV X-rays and 15 MeV neutrons.* Br J Radiol 47:393–398, 1974.

VANDER SALM, TJ, CEREDA, J-M, AND CUTLER, BS: *Brachial plexus injury following median sternotomy.* J Thorac Cardiovasc Surg 80:447–452, 1980.

VANDER SALM, TJ, CUTLER, BJ, AND OKIKE, ON: *Brachial plexus injury following median sternotomy. Part II.* J Thorac Cardiovasc Surg 83:914–917, 1982.

Vartanian, GA and Chinyanga, HM: *The mechanism of acute neuromuscular weakness induced by chloroquine.* Can J Physiol Pharmacol 50:1099–1103, 1972.

Viby-Mogensen, J: *Succinylcholine neuromuscular blockade in subjects homozygous for atypical plasma cholinesterase.* Anesthesiology 55:429–434, 1981.

Viby-Mogensen, J and Hanel, HK: *Prolonged apnoea after suxamethonium: An analysis of the first 225 cases reported to the Danish Cholinesterase Research Unit.* Acta Anaesth Scand 22:371–380, 1978.

Vincent, A, Newsom-Davis, J, and Martin, V: *Anti-acetylcholine receptor antibodies in D-penicillamine-associated myasthenia gravis.* Lancet i:1254, 1978.

Watkins, SM and Griffin, JP: *High incidence of vincristine-induced neuropathy in lymphomas.* Br Med J 1:610–612, 1978.

Waud, BE, Farrell, L, and Waud, DR: *Lithium and neuromuscular transmission.* Anesth Analg 61:399–402, 1982.

Weber, ER, Daube, JR, and Conventry, MB: *Peripheral neuropathies, associated with total hip arthroplasty.* J Bone Joint Surg 58A:66–69, 1976.

Weingarten, SI, Louis, DL, and Waylonis, GW: *Electromyographic changes in postmeniscectomy patients. Role of the pneumatic tourniquet.* JAMA 241:1248–1250, 1979.

Welch, GW and Waud, BE: *Effect of bretyllium on neuromuscular transmission.* Anesth Analg 61:443–444, 1982.

Wheeler, RH and Votaw, M: *Vincristine and quadriparesis.* Ann Intern Med 81:709–710, 1974.

Whisnant, JP, Espinosa, RE, Kierland, RR, et al: *Chloroquine neuromyopathy.* Mayo Clin Proc 38:501–513, 1963.

Whittaker, M: *Plasma cholinesterase variants and the anaesthetist.* Anaesthesia 35:174–197, 1980.

Wilensky, AJ and Lowden, JA: *Inadequate serum levels after intramuscular administration of diphenylhydantoin.* Neurology 23:318–324, 1973.

Wilson, RW, Ward, MD, and Johns, TR: *Corticosteroids—A direct effect at the neuromuscular junction.* Neurology 24:1091–1095, 1974.

Wood, GJ and Hall, GM: *Plasmapheresis and plasma cholinesterase.* Br J Anaesth 50:945–949, 1978.

Woolley, EJ and Vandam, LD: *Neurological sequelae of brachial plexus nerve block.* Ann Surg 149:53–60, 1959.

Wright, EA and McQuillen, MP: *Antibiotic-induced neuromuscular blockade.* Ann NY Acad Sci 183:358–368, 1971.

Wright, JM and Collier, B: *The site of the neuromuscular block produced by polymyxin B and rolitetracycline.* Can J Physiol Pharmacol 54:926–936, 1976.

Yaari, Y, Pincus, JH, and Argov, Z: *Depression of synaptic transmission by diphenylhydantoin.* Ann Neurol 1:334–338, 1977.

Yagiela, JA, Benoit, PW, Buoncristiani, RD, et al: *Comparison of myotoxic effects of lidocaine with epinephrine in rats and humans.* Anesth Analg 60:471–480, 1981.

Yang, WCT and Dubick, M: *Mechanism of emetine cardiotoxicity.* Pharmacol Ther 10:15–26, 1980.

Yates, SK, Hurst, LN, and Brown, WF: *The pathogenesis of pneumatic tourniquet paralysis in man.* J Neurol Neurosurg Psychiat 44:759–767, 1981.

INDEX

An *italic* number indicates a figure. A "t" indicates a table.